RN Pharmacology for Nursing
REVIEW MODULE EDITION 7.0

Contributors

Norma Jean E. Henry, MSN/Ed, RN

Mendy McMichael, DNP, MSN

Janean Johnson, MSN, RN, CNE

Agnes DiStasi, DNP, RN, CNE

Brenda S. Ball, MEd, BSN, RN

Carrie B. Elkins, DHSc, MSN

Mary Jane Janowski, RN, MA

Kellie L. Wilford, MSN, RN

Marsha S. Barlow, MSN, RN

Peggy Leehy, MSN, RN

Terri Lemon, DNP, MSN, RN

Consultants

Susan Adcock, RN, MS

Tracey Bousquet, BSN, RN

Lakeisha Wheless, MSN, RN

Virginia Tufano, EdD, MSN, RN

Megan Jester, MS, RN

Lisa Kongable, MA, PMH–CNS, ARNP, CNE

Melanie Schrader, MSN, RN

Betty Daniel, MSN Nursing Education, RN

Jenni L. Hoffman, DNP, FNP–C, CLNC

Jessica Johnson, MSN, RN

Director of content review: Kristen Lawler

Director of development: Derek Prater

Project management: Janet Hines, Nicole Burke

Coordination of content review: Norma Jean E. Henry, Mendy McMichael

Copy editing: Kelly Von Lunen, Derek Prater

Layout: Spring Lenox, Randi Hardy

Illustrations: Randi Hardy

Online media: Morgan Smith, Ron Hanson, Nicole Lobdell, Brant Stacy

Cover design: Jason Buck

Interior book design: Spring Lenox

IMPORTANT NOTICE TO THE READER

User's Guide

Welcome to the Assessment Technologies Institute® RN Pharmacology for Nursing Review Module Edition 7.0. The mission of ATI's Content Mastery Series® Review Modules is to provide user-friendly compendiums of nursing knowledge that will:

- Help you locate important information quickly.
- Assist in your learning efforts.
- Provide exercises for applying your nursing knowledge.
- Facilitate your entry into the nursing profession as a newly licensed nurse.

This newest edition of the Review Modules has been redesigned to optimize your learning experience. We've fit more content into less space and have done so in a way that will make it even easier for you to find and understand the information you need.

ORGANIZATION

This Review Module is organized into units covering pharmacological principles (Unit 1) and medications affecting the body systems and physiological processes (Units 2 to 12). Chapters within these units conform to one of two organizing principles for presenting the content.

- Nursing concepts
- Medications

Nursing concepts chapters begin with an overview describing the central concept and its relevance to nursing. Subordinate themes are covered in outline form to demonstrate relationships and present the information in a clear, succinct manner.

Medications chapters include an overview describing a disorder or group of disorders. Medications used to treat these disorders are grouped according to classification. A specific medication can be selected as a prototype or example of the characteristics of medications in this classification. These sections include information about how the medication works and its therapeutic uses. Next, you will find information about complications, contraindications/precautions, and interactions, as well as nursing interventions and client education to help prevent and/or manage these issues. Finally, the chapter includes information on nursing administration of the medication and evaluation of the medication's effectiveness.

ACTIVE LEARNING SCENARIOS AND APPLICATION EXERCISES

Each chapter includes opportunities for you to test your knowledge and to practice applying that knowledge. Active Learning Scenario exercises pose a nursing scenario and then direct you to use an ATI Active Learning Template (included at the back of this book) to record the important knowledge a nurse should apply to the scenario. An example is then provided to which you can compare your completed Active Learning Template. The Application Exercises include NCLEX-style questions, such as multiple-choice and multiple-select items, providing you with opportunities to practice answering the kinds of questions you might expect to see on ATI assessments or the NCLEX. After the Application Exercises, an answer key is provided, along with rationales.

NCLEX® CONNECTIONS

To prepare for the NCLEX-RN, it is important to understand how the content in this Review Module is connected to the NCLEX-RN test plan. You can find information on the detailed test plan at the National Council of State Boards of Nursing's website, www.ncsbn.org. When reviewing content in this Review Module, regularly ask yourself, "How does this content fit into the test plan, and what types of questions related to this content should I expect?"

To help you in this process, we've included NCLEX Connections at the beginning of each unit and with each question in the Application Exercises Answer Keys. The NCLEX Connections at the beginning of each unit point out areas of the detailed test plan that relate to the content within that unit. The NCLEX Connections attached to the Application Exercises Answer Keys demonstrate how each exercise fits within the detailed content outline. These NCLEX Connections will help you understand how the detailed content outline is organized, starting with major client needs categories and subcategories and followed by related content areas and tasks. The major client needs categories are:

- Safe and Effective Care Environment
  - Management of Care
  - Safety and Infection Control
- Health Promotion and Maintenance
- Psychosocial Integrity
- Physiological Integrity
  - Basic Care and Comfort
  - Pharmacological and Parenteral Therapies
  - Reduction of Risk Potential
  - Physiological Adaptation

An NCLEX Connection might, for example, alert you that content within a unit is related to:

- Pharmacological and Parenteral Therapies
  - Adverse Effects/Contraindications/Side Effects/Interactions
    - Identify a contraindication to the administration of a medication to the client.

QSEN COMPETENCIES

As you use the Review Modules, you will note the integration of the Quality and Safety Education for Nurses (QSEN) competencies throughout the chapters. These competencies are integral components of the curriculum of many nursing programs in the United States and prepare you to provide safe, high-quality care as a newly licensed nurse. Icons appear to draw your attention to the six QSEN competencies.

Safety: The minimization of risk factors that could cause injury or harm while promoting quality care and maintaining a secure environment for clients, self, and others.

Patient-Centered Care: The provision of caring and compassionate, culturally sensitive care that addresses clients' physiological, psychological, sociological, spiritual, and cultural needs, preferences, and values.

Evidence-Based Practice: The use of current knowledge from research and other credible sources, on which to base clinical judgment and client care.

Informatics: The use of information technology as a communication and information-gathering tool that supports clinical decision-making and scientifically based nursing practice.

Quality Improvement: Care related and organizational processes that involve the development and implementation of a plan to improve health care services and better meet clients' needs.

Teamwork and Collaboration: The delivery of client care in partnership with multidisciplinary members of the health care team to achieve continuity of care and positive client outcomes.

ICONS

Icons are used throughout the Review Module to draw your attention to particular areas. Keep an eye out for these icons.

(N) This icon is used for NCLEX Connections.

(G) This icon indicates gerontological considerations, or knowledge specific to the care of older adult clients.

Qs This icon is used for content related to safety and is a QSEN competency. When you see this icon, take note of safety concerns or steps that nurses can take to ensure client safety and a safe environment.

Qpcc This icon is a QSEN competency that indicates the importance of a holistic approach to providing care.

Qebp This icon, a QSEN competency, points out the integration of research into clinical practice.

Qi This icon is a QSEN competency and highlights the use of information technology to support nursing practice.

Qqi This icon is used to focus on the QSEN competency of integrating planning processes to meet clients' needs.

Qtc This icon highlights the QSEN competency of care delivery using an interprofessional approach.

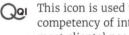 This icon appears at the top-right of pages and indicates availability of an online media supplement, such as a graphic, animation, or video. If you have an electronic copy of the Review Module, this icon will appear alongside clickable links to media supplements. If you have a hard copy version of the Review Module, visit www.atitesting.com for details on how to access these features.

FEEDBACK

ATI welcomes feedback regarding this Review Module. Please provide comments to comments@atitesting.com.

Table of Contents

When reviewing the following chapters, keep in mind the relevant topics and tasks of the NCLEX outline, in particular:

Client Needs: Safety and Infection Control

ACCIDENT/ERROR/INJURY PREVENTION
Assess client for allergies intervene as needed.

Verify appropriateness and/or accuracy of a treatment order.

**REPORTING OF INCIDENT/EVENT/
IRREGULAR OCCURRENCE/VARIANCE**
Identify need/situation where reporting of incident/event/ irregular occurrence/variance is appropriate.

Acknowledge and document practice error.

Client Needs: Pharmacological and Parenteral Therapies

**ADVERSE EFFECTS/CONTRAINDICATIONS/
SIDE EFFECTS/INTERACTIONS**
Identify a contraindication to the administration of a medication to the client.

Identify symptoms/evidence of an allergic reaction.

DOSAGE CALCULATION: Perform calculations needed for medication administration.

MEDICATION ADMINISTRATION
Prepare and administer medications, using rights of medication administration.

Review pertinent data prior to medication administration.

PARENTERAL/INTRAVENOUS THERAPIES: Apply knowledge and concepts of mathematics/nursing procedures/psychomotor skills when caring for a client receiving intravenous and parenteral therapy.

UNIT 1   PHARMACOLOGICAL PRINCIPLES

CHAPTER 1 # Pharmacokinetics and Routes of Administration

Pharmacokinetics refers to how medications travel through the body. They undergo a variety of biochemical processes that result in absorption, distribution, metabolism, and excretion.

PHASES OF PHARMACOKINETICS

ABSORPTION

Absorption is the transmission of medications from the location of administration (gastrointestinal [GI] tract, muscle, skin, mucous membranes, or subcutaneous tissue) to the bloodstream. The most common routes of administration are enteral (through the GI tract) and parenteral (by injection). Each of these routes has a unique pattern of absorption.
- The rate of medication absorption determines how soon the medication will take effect.
- The amount of medication the body absorbs determines the intensity of its effects.
- The route of administration affects the rate and amount of absorption.

Oral

BARRIERS TO ABSORPTION: Medications must pass through the layer of epithelial cells that line the GI tract.

ABSORPTION PATTERN: Varies greatly due to
- Stability and solubility of the medication
- GI pH and emptying time
- Presence of food in the stomach or intestines
- Other concurrent medications
- Forms of medications (enteric-coated pills, liquids)

Sublingual, buccal

BARRIERS TO ABSORPTION: Swallowing before dissolution allows gastric pH to inactivate the medication.

ABSORPTION PATTERN: Quick absorption systemically through highly vascular mucous membranes

Other mucous membranes (rectal, vaginal)

BARRIERS TO ABSORPTION: Presence of stool in the rectum or infectious material in the vagina limits tissue contact.

ABSORPTION PATTERN: Easy absorption with both local and systemic effects

Inhalation via mouth, nose

BARRIERS TO ABSORPTION: Inspiratory effort

ABSORPTION PATTERN: Rapid absorption through alveolar capillary networks

Intradermal, topical

BARRIERS TO ABSORPTION: Close proximity of epidermal cells

ABSORPTION PATTERN
- Slow, gradual absorption
- Effects primarily local, but systemic as well, especially with lipid-soluble medications passing through subcutaneous fatty tissue

Subcutaneous, intramuscular

BARRIERS TO ABSORPTION: Capillary walls have large spaces between cells. Therefore, there is no significant barrier.

ABSORPTION PATTERN
- Solubility of the medication in water: Highly soluble medications have rapid absorption (10 to 30 min); poorly soluble medications have slow absorption.
- Blood perfusion at the site of injection: Sites with high blood perfusion have rapid absorption; sites with low blood perfusion have slow absorption.

Intravenous

BARRIERS TO ABSORPTION: No barriers

ABSORPTION PATTERN
- **Immediate:** enters directly into the blood
- **Complete:** reaches the blood in its entirety

DISTRIBUTION

Distribution is the transportation of medications to sites of action by bodily fluids. Factors influencing distribution include the following.

Circulation: Conditions that inhibit blood flow or perfusion, such as peripheral vascular or cardiac disease, can delay medication distribution.

Permeability of the cell membrane: The medication must be able to pass through tissues and membranes to reach its target area. Medications that are lipid-soluble or have a transport system can cross the blood-brain barrier and the placenta.

Plasma protein binding: Medications compete for protein binding sites within the bloodstream, primarily albumin. The ability of a medication to bind to a protein can affect how much of the medication will leave and travel to target tissues. Two medications can compete for the same binding sites, resulting in toxicity.

METABOLISM

Metabolism (biotransformation) changes medications into less active or inactive forms by the action of enzymes. This occurs primarily in the liver, but it also takes place in the kidneys, lungs, intestines, and blood.

FACTORS INFLUENCING THE RATE OF MEDICATION METABOLISM

- **Age:** Infants have a limited medication-metabolizing capacity. The aging process also can influence medication metabolism, but varies with the individual. In general, hepatic medication metabolism tends to decline with age. Older adults require smaller doses of medications due to the possibility of accumulation in the body. ©
- **Increase in some medication-metabolizing enzymes:** This can metabolize a particular medication sooner, requiring an increase in dosage of that medication to maintain a therapeutic level. It can also cause an increase in the metabolism of other concurrent-use medications.
- **First-pass effect:** The liver inactivates some medications on their first pass through the liver, and thus they require a nonenteral route (sublingual, IV) because of their high first-pass effect.
- **Similar metabolic pathways:** When the same pathway metabolizes two medications, it can alter the metabolism of one or both of them. In this way, the rate of metabolism can decrease for one or both of the medications, leading to medication accumulation.
- **Nutritional status:** Clients who are malnourished can be deficient in the factors that are necessary to produce specific medication-metabolizing enzymes, thus impairing medication metabolism.

OUTCOMES OF METABOLISM

- Increased renal excretion of medication
- Inactivation of medications
- Increased therapeutic effect
- Activation of pro-medications (also called pro-drugs) into active forms
- Decreased toxicity when active forms of medications become inactive forms
- Increased toxicity when inactive forms of medications become active forms

EXCRETION

Excretion is the elimination of medications from the body, primarily through the kidneys. Elimination also takes place through the liver, lungs, intestines, and exocrine glands (such as in breast milk). Kidney dysfunction can lead to an increase in the duration and intensity of a medication's response, so it is important to monitor BUN and creatinine levels.

MEDICATION RESPONSES

Medication dosing attempts to regulate medication responses to maintain plasma levels between the minimum effective concentration (MEC) and the toxic concentration. A plasma medication level is in the therapeutic range when it is effective and not toxic. Nurses use therapeutic levels of many medications to monitor clients' responses.

THERAPEUTIC INDEX

Medications with a high therapeutic index (TI) have a wide safety margin. Therefore, there is no need for routine serum medication-level monitoring. Medications with a low TI require close monitoring of serum medication levels. Nurses should consider the route of administration when monitoring for peak levels (highest plasma level when elimination = absorption). For example, an oral medication can peak from 1 to 3 hr after administration. If the route is IV, the peak time might occur within 10 min. (Refer to a drug reference or a pharmacist for specific medication peak times.) For trough levels, obtain a blood sample immediately before the next medication dose, regardless of the route of administration. A plateau is a medication's concentration in plasma during a series of doses.

HALF-LIFE

Half-life ($t^{1/2}$) refers to the time for the medication in the body to drop by 50%. Liver and kidney function affect half-life. It usually takes four half-lives to achieve a steady state of serum concentration (medication intake = medication metabolism and excretion).

SHORT HALF-LIFE

- Medications leave the body quickly (4 to 8 hr).
- Short-dosing interval or MEC drops between doses.

LONG HALF-LIFE

- Medications leave the body more slowly: over more than 24 hr: with a greater risk for medication accumulation and toxicity.
- Can give medications at longer intervals without loss of therapeutic effects.
- Medications take a longer time to reach a steady state.

PHARMACODYNAMICS

Pharmacodynamics describes the interactions between medications and target cells, body systems, and organs to produce effects. These interactions result in functional changes that are the mechanism of action of the medication. Medications interact with cells in one of two ways or in both ways.

Agonists are medications that bind to or mimic the receptor activity that endogenous compounds regulate. For example, morphine is an agonist because it activates the receptors that produce analgesia, sedation, constipation, and other effects. (Receptors are the medication's target sites on or within the cells.)

Antagonists are medications that can block the usual receptor activity that endogenous compounds regulate or the receptor activity of other medications. For example, losartan, an angiotensin II receptor blocker, is an antagonist. It works by blocking angiotensin II receptors on blood vessels, which prevents vasoconstriction.

Partial agonists act as agonists and antagonists, with limited affinity to receptor sites. For example, nalbuphine acts as an antagonist at mu receptors and an agonist at kappa receptors, causing analgesia with minimal respiratory depression at low doses.

ROUTES OF ADMINISTRATION

ORAL OR ENTERAL

Tablets, capsules, liquids, suspensions, elixirs, lozenges

Most common route

NURSING ACTIONS

- Contraindications for oral medication administration include vomiting, decreased GI motility, absence of a gag reflex, difficulty swallowing, and a decreased level of consciousness.
- Have clients sit upright at a 90° angle to facilitate swallowing.
- Administer irritating medications, such as analgesics, with small amounts of food.
- Do not mix with large amounts of food or beverages in case clients cannot consume the entire quantity.
- Avoid administration with interacting foods or beverages, such as grapefruit juice.
- In general, administer oral medications on an empty stomach (30 min to 1 hr before meals, 2 hr after meals).
- Follow the manufacturer's directions for crushing, cutting, and diluting medications. Break or cut scored tablets only. (See the Institute for Safe Medication Practices website, www.ismp.org).
- Make sure clients swallow enteric-coated or time-release medications whole.
- Use a liquid form of the medication to facilitate swallowing whenever possible.

ADVANTAGES

- Safe
- Inexpensive
- Easy and convenient

DISADVANTAGES

- Oral medications have highly variable absorption.
- Inactivation can occur in the GI tract or by first-pass effect.
- Clients must be cooperative and conscious.
- Contraindications include nausea and vomiting.

SUBLINGUAL AND BUCCAL

Sublingual: under the tongue

Buccal: between the cheek and the gum

Directly enters the bloodstream and bypasses the liver

NURSING ACTIONS

- Instruct clients to keep the medication in place until complete absorption occurs.
- Clients should not eat or drink while the tablet is in place or until it has completely dissolved.

LIQUIDS, SUSPENSIONS, AND ELIXIRS

NURSING ACTIONS

- Follow directions for dilution and shaking.
- When administering the medication, pour it into a cup on flat surface. Make sure the base of the meniscus (lowest fluid line) is at the level of the dose.

TRANSDERMAL

Medication in a skin patch for absorption through the skin, producing systemic effects

NURSING ACTIONS

Instruct clients to:
- Apply patches to ensure proper dosing.
- Wash the skin with soap and water, and dry it thoroughly before applying a new patch.
- Place the patch on a hairless area, and rotate sites daily to prevent skin irritation.

TOPICAL

- Painless
- Limited adverse effects

NURSING ACTIONS

- Apply with a glove, tongue blade, or cotton-tipped applicator.
- Do not apply with a bare hand.

INSTILLATION (DROPS, OINTMENTS, SPRAYS)

Generally used for eyes, ears, and nose

NURSING ACTIONS

Eyes
- Have clients sit upright or lie supine, tilt their head slightly, and look up at the ceiling.
- Rest your dominant hand on the clients' forehead, hold the dropper above the conjunctival sac about 1 to 2 cm, drop the medication into the center of the sac, avoid placing it directly on the cornea, and have them close the eye gently. If they blink during instillation, repeat the procedure.
- Apply gentle pressure with your finger and a clean facial tissue on the nasolacrimal duct for 30 to 60 seconds to prevent systemic absorption of the medication.
- If instilling more than one medication in the same eye, wait at least 5 min between them.
- For eye ointment, apply a thin ribbon to the edge of the lower eyelid from the inner to the outer canthus.

Ears
- Have clients sit upright or lie on their side.
- Straighten the ear canal by pulling the auricle upward and outward for adults or down and back for children. Hold the dropper 1 cm above the ear canal, instill the medication, and then gently apply pressure with your finger to the tragus of the ear unless it is too painful.
- Do not press a cotton ball deep into the ear canal. If necessary, gently place it into the outermost part of the ear canal.
- Have clients remain in the side-lying position if possible for 2 to 3 min after instilling ear drops.

Nose
- Use medical aseptic technique when administering medications into the nose.
- Have clients lie supine with their head positioned to allow the medication to enter the appropriate nasal passage.
- Use your dominant hand to instill the drops, supporting the head with your nondominant hand.
- Instruct clients to breathe through the mouth, stay in a supine position, and not blow their nose for 5 min after drop instillation.

INHALATION

Administered through metered dose inhalers (MDI) or dry-powder inhalers (DPI)

NURSING ACTIONS

MDI

Instruct clients to:
- Remove the cap from the inhaler's mouthpiece.
- Shake the inhaler vigorously five or six times.
- Hold the inhaler with the mouthpiece at the bottom.
- Hold the inhaler with your thumb near the mouthpiece and your index and middle fingers at the top.
- Hold the inhaler about 2 to 4 cm (1 to 2 in) away from the front of your mouth or close your mouth around the mouthpiece of the inhaler with the opening pointing toward the back of your throat.
- Take a deep breath and then exhale.
- Tilt your head back slightly, press the inhaler, and, at the same time, begin a slow, deep inhalation breath. Continue to breathe in slowly and deeply for 3 to 5 seconds to facilitate delivery to the air passages.
- Hold your breath for 10 seconds to allow the medication to deposit in your airways.
- Take the inhaler out of your mouth and slowly exhale through pursed lips.
- Resume normal breathing.
- A spacer keeps the medication in the device longer, thereby increasing the amount of medication the device delivers to the lungs and decreasing the amount of medication in the oropharynx.
- For clients who use a spacer:
  ○ Remove the covers from the mouthpieces of the inhaler and of the spacer.
  ○ Insert the MDI into the end of the spacer.
  ○ Shake the inhaler five or six times.
  ○ Exhale completely, and then close your mouth around the spacer's mouthpiece. Continue as with an MDI.

DPI

Instruct clients to:
- Do not shake the device.
- Take the cover off the mouthpiece.
- Follow the manufacturer's directions for preparing the medication, such as turning the wheel of the inhaler or loading a medication pellet.
- Exhale completely.
- Place the mouthpiece between your lips and take a deep inhalation breath through your mouth.
- Hold your breath for 5 to 10 seconds.
- Take the inhaler out of your mouth and slowly exhale through pursed lips.
- Resume normal breathing.
- Clients who need more than one puff should wait the length of time the provider specifies before self-administering the second puff.
- Instruct clients to rinse their mouth out with water or brush their teeth if using a corticosteroid inhaler to reduce the risk of fungal infections of the mouth.
- Instruct clients to remove the canister and rinse the inhaler, cap, and spacer once a day with warm running water and dry them completely before using the inhaler again.

NASOGASTRIC AND GASTROSTOMY TUBES

NURSING ACTIONS
- Verify proper tube placement.
- Use a syringe and allow the medication to flow in by gravity or push it in with the plunger of the syringe.
- To prevent clogging, flush the tubing before and after each medication with 15 to 30 mL of warm sterile water.
- Flush with another 15 to 30 mL of warm sterile water after instilling all the medications.
- **General guidelines**
  ○ Use liquid forms of medications; if not available, consider crushing medications if appropriate guidelines allow.
  ○ Do not administer sublingual medications through the NG tube (may give sublingual medications under the tongue).
  ○ Do not crush specifically prepared oral medications (extended/time-release, fluid-filled, enteric-coated).
  ○ Administer each medication separately.
  ○ Do not mix medications with enteral feedings.
  ○ Completely dissolve crushed tablets and capsule contents in 15 to 30 mL of sterile water prior to administration.

SUPPOSITORIES

NURSING ACTIONS
- Follow the manufacturer's directions for storage.
- Wear gloves for the procedure.
- Remove the wrapper, and lubricate the suppository if necessary.
- **Rectal suppositories (thin, bullet-shaped medication)**
  ○ Position clients in the left lateral position or Sims' position.
  ○ Insert the suppository just beyond the internal sphincter.
  ○ Instruct clients to remain flat or in the left lateral position for at least 5 min after insertion to retain the suppository. Absorption times vary with the medication.
- **Vaginal suppositories**
  ○ Position clients supine with their knees bent and their feet flat on the bed and close to their hips (modified lithotomy or dorsal recumbent position).
  ○ Use the applicator, if available.
  ○ Insert the suppository along the posterior wall of the vagina 7.5 to 10 cm (3 to 4 in).
  ○ Instruct clients to remain supine for at least 5 min after insertion to retain the suppository.
  ○ If using an applicator, wash it with soap and water. (If it is disposable, discard it.)

PARENTERAL

NURSING ACTIONS

- The vastus lateralis is best for infants 1 year and younger.
- The ventrogluteal site is preferable for IM injections and for injecting volumes exceeding 2 mL.
- The deltoid site has a smaller muscle mass and can only accommodate up to 1 mL of fluid.
- Use a needle size and length appropriate for the type of injection and the client's size. Syringe size should approximate the volume of medication.
- Use a tuberculin syringe for solution volumes smaller than 0.5 mL.
- Rotate injection sites to enhance medication absorption, and document each site.
- Do not use injection sites that are edematous, inflamed, or have moles, birthmarks, or scars.
- For IV administration, immediately monitor clients for therapeutic and adverse effects.
- Discard all sharps (broken ampule bottles, needles) in leak- and puncture-proof containers.

INTRADERMAL

NURSING ACTIONS

- Use for tuberculin testing or checking for medication or allergy sensitivities.
- Use small amounts of solution (0.01 to 0.1 mL) in a tuberculin syringe with a fine-gauge needle (26- to 27-gauge) in lightly pigmented, thin-skinned, hairless sites (the inner surface of the mid-forearm or scapular area of the back) at a 10° to 15° angle.
- Insert the needle with the bevel up. A small bleb should appear.
- Do not massage the site after injection.

SUBCUTANEOUS AND INTRAMUSCULAR

NURSING ACTIONS

Subcutaneous

- Use for small doses of nonirritating, water-soluble medications, such as insulin and heparin.
- Use a 3/8- to 5/8-inch, 25- to 27-gauge needle or a 28- to 31-gauge insulin syringe. Inject no more than 1.5 mL of solution.
- Select sites that have an adequate fat-pad size (abdomen, upper hips, lateral upper arms, thighs).
- For average-size clients, pinch up the skin and inject at a 45° to 90° angle. For clients who are obese, use a 90° angle.

Intramuscular

- Use for irritating medications, solutions in oils, and aqueous suspensions.
- The most common sites are ventrogluteal, dorsogluteal, deltoid, and vastus lateralis (pediatric).
- Use a needle size 18- to 27-gauge (usually 22- to 25-gauge), 1- to 1.5-inch long, and inject at a 90° angle. Solution volume is usually 1 to 3 mL. Divide larger volumes into two syringes and use two different sites.

ADVANTAGES

- Use for poorly soluble medications.
- Use for administering medications that have slow absorption for an extended period of time (depot preparations).

DISADVANTAGES

- IM injections are more costly.
- IM injections are inconvenient.
- There can be pain with the risk for local tissue damage and nerve damage.
- There is a risk for infection at the injection site.

Z-TRACK

NURSING ACTIONS

- Use this technique for all IM injections because it is less painful and it prevents medication from leaking back into subcutaneous tissue.
- Use for medications that cause visible or permanent skin stains, such as iron preparations.

INTRAVENOUS

NURSING ACTIONS

- Use for administering medications, fluid, and blood products.
- Vascular access devices can be for short-term use (catheters) or long-term use (infusion ports). Use 16-gauge devices for clients who have trauma, 18-gauge during surgery and for blood administration, and 22- to 24-gauge for children, older adults, and clients who have medical issues or are stable postoperatively.
- Peripheral veins in the arm or hand are preferable. Ask clients which site they prefer. For newborns, use veins in the head, lower legs, and feet. After administration, immediately monitor for therapeutic and adverse effects.

ADVANTAGES

- Onset is rapid, and absorption into the blood is immediate, which provides an immediate response.
- This route allows control over the precise amount of medication to administer.
- It allows for administration of large volumes of fluid.
- It dilutes irritating medications in free-flowing IV fluid.

DISADVANTAGES

- IV injections are even more costly.
- IV injections are inconvenient.
- Absorption of the medication into the blood is immediate. This is potentially dangerous if giving the wrong dosage or the wrong medication.
- There is an increased risk for infection or embolism with IV injections.
- Poor circulation can inhibit the medication's distribution.

EPIDURAL

NURSING ACTIONS

- Use for IV opioid analgesia (morphine or fentanyl).
- The clinician advances the catheter through the needle into the epidural space at the level of the fourth or fifth vertebra.
- Use an infusion pump to administer medication.

Application Exercises

1. A provider prescribes phenobarbital for a client who has a seizure disorder. The medication has a long half-life of 4 days. How many times per day should the nurse expect to administer this medication?

    A. One
    B. Two
    C. Three
    D. Four

2. A staff educator is reviewing medication dosages and factors that influence medication metabolism with a group of nurses at an in-service presentation. Which of the following factors should the educator include as a reason to administer lower medication dosages? (Select all that apply.)

    A. Increased renal excretion
    B. Increased medication-metabolizing enzymes
    C. Liver failure
    D. Peripheral vascular disease
    E. Concurrent use of medication the same pathway metabolizes

3. A nurse is preparing to administer eye drops to a client. Which of the following actions should the nurse take? (Select all that apply.)

    A. Have the client lie on her side.
    B. Ask the client to look up at the ceiling.
    C. Tell the client to blink when the drops enter her eye.
    D. Drop the medication into the center of the client's conjunctival sac.
    E. Instruct the client to close her eye gently after instillation.

4. A nurse is completing discharge teaching for a client who has a new prescription for transdermal patches. Which of the following statements should the nurse identify as an indication that the client understands the instructions?

    A. "I will clean the site with an alcohol swab before I apply the patch."
    B. "I will rotate the application sites weekly."
    C. "I will apply the patch to an area of skin with no hair."
    D. "I will place the new patch on the site of the old patch."

5. A nurse reviewing a client's medical record notes a new prescription for verifying the trough level of the client's medication. Which of the following actions should the nurse take?

    A. Obtain a blood specimen immediately prior to administering the next dose of medication.
    B. Verify that the client has been taking the medication for 24 hr before obtaining a blood specimen.
    C. Ask the client to provide a urine specimen after the next dose of medication.
    D. Administer the medication, and obtain a blood specimen 30 min later.

PRACTICE Active Learning Scenario

A nurse is showing a client how to use a metered-dose inhaler (MDI) with a spacer. What should the nurse include in the instructions? Use the ATI Active Learning Template: Therapeutic Procedure to complete this item.

INDICATIONS: Identify the medication absorption pattern and a barrier to absorption.

CLIENT EDUCATION: Describe the steps to follow when using an MDI with a spacer.

Application Exercises Key

1. A. **CORRECT:** Medications with long half-lives remain at their therapeutic levels between doses for long periods of time. The nurse should expect to administer this medication once a day.

   B. Medications with long half-lives remain at their therapeutic levels between doses for long periods of time. A medication the nurse administers twice a day would have a shorter half-life. An example is vancomycin.

   C. Medications with long half-lives remain at their therapeutic levels between doses for long periods of time. A medication the nurse administers three times a day would have a shorter half-life. An example is zidovudine.

   D. Medications with long half-lives remain at their therapeutic levels between doses for long periods of time. A medication the nurse administers four times a day would have a shorter half-life. An example is ibuprofen.

   Ⓝ *NCLEX® Connection: Pharmacological and Parenteral Therapies, Medication Administration*

2. A. Increased renal excretion decreases the concentration of the medication, requiring an increased dosage.

   B. Increased medication-metabolizing enzymes decrease the concentration of the medication, requiring an increased dosage.

   C. **CORRECT:** Liver failure decreases metabolism and thus increases the concentration of a medication. This requires decreasing the dosage.

   D. Peripheral vascular disease impairs distribution, requiring an increased dosage.

   E. **CORRECT:** When the same pathway metabolizes two medications, they compete for metabolism, thereby increasing the concentration of one or both medications. This requires decreasing the dosage of one or both medications.

   Ⓝ *NCLEX® Connection: Pharmacological and Parenteral Therapies, Adverse Effects/Contraindications/Side Effects/Interactions*

3. A. The client should be sitting or in a supine position to facilitate the instillation of eye drops.

   B. **CORRECT:** The client should look upward to keep the drops from falling onto her cornea.

   C. Ideally, the client should not blink so that she doesn't eject the eye drops. If she does blink, the nurse should repeat the instillation.

   D. **CORRECT:** The nurse should drop the medication into the center of the conjunctival sac to promote distribution.

   E. **CORRECT:** The client should close her eye gently to promote distribution of the medication.

   Ⓝ *NCLEX® Connection: Pharmacological and Parenteral Therapies, Medication Administration*

4. A. The client should wash his skin with soap and water and dry it thoroughly before applying a transdermal patch.

   B. The client should rotate application sites daily to prevent skin irritation.

   C. **CORRECT:** The client should apply the patch to a hairless area of skin to promote absorption of the medication.

   D. The client should rotate application sites daily to prevent skin irritation.

   Ⓝ *NCLEX® Connection: Pharmacological and Parenteral Therapies, Medication Administration*

5. A. **CORRECT:** To verify trough levels of a medication, the nurse should obtain a blood specimen immediately before administering the next dose of medication.

   B. The length of time the client has been taking the medication does not affect trough levels.

   C. Trough levels are from serum, not urine.

   D. Trough levels reflect the least concentration of the medication in the client's blood. It will be higher after administration of the medication.

   Ⓝ *NCLEX® Connection: Pharmacological and Parenteral Therapies, Parenteral/Intravenous Therapies*

PRACTICE Answer

Using the ATI Active Learning Template: Therapeutic Procedure

INDICATIONS

- Medication Absorption Pattern: rapid absorption through the alveolar capillary network. A spacer keeps the medication in the device longer, thereby increasing the amount of medication the device delivers to the lungs and decreasing the amount of medication in the oropharynx.
- Barrier to Absorption: Inadequate respiratory effort

CLIENT EDUCATION

- Remove the covers from the mouthpieces of the inhaler and of the spacer.
- Insert the MDI into the end of the spacer.
- Shake the inhaler five or six times.
- Exhale completely, and then close your mouth around the spacer's mouthpiece.
- Take a deep breath and then exhale.
- Tilt your head back slightly, press the inhaler, and, at the same time, begin a slow, deep inhalation breath. Continue to breathe in slowly and deeply for 3 to 5 seconds to facilitate delivery to the air passages.
- Hold your breath for 10 seconds to allow the medication to deposit in your airways.
- Take the mouthpiece out of your mouth and slowly exhale through pursed lips.
- Resume normal breathing.

Ⓝ *NCLEX® Connection: Pharmacological and Parenteral Therapies, Medication Administration*

UNIT 1   PHARMACOLOGICAL PRINCIPLES

CHAPTER 2

Safe Medication Administration and Error Reduction

The providers who may legally write prescriptions in the United States include physicians, advanced practice nurses, dentists, and physician assistants. These providers are responsible for obtaining clients' medical history, performing a physical examination, diagnosing, prescribing medications, monitoring response to therapy, and modifying prescriptions as necessary.

Nurses are responsible for having knowledge of federal, state (nurse practice act), and local laws, and facilities' policies that govern the prescribing, dispensing and administration of medications; preparing, administering, and evaluating response to medications; developing and maintaining an up-to-date knowledge base of medications they administer, including uses, mechanisms of action, routes of administration, safe dosage range, adverse and side effects, precautions, contraindications, and interactions; maintaining acceptable practice and skills competencies; determining the accuracy of medication prescriptions; reporting all medication errors; safeguarding and storing medications; following legal mandates when administering controlled substances; calculating medication doses accurately; and understanding the responsibilities of other members of the health care team regarding medications. Qs

2.1 Knowledge required prior to medication administration

Medication category/class
Medications have a pharmacological action, therapeutic use, body system target, chemical makeup, and classification for use during pregnancy.

For example, lisinopril is an ACE inhibitor (pharmacological action) and an antihypertensive (therapeutic use).

Mechanism of action
This is how medications produce their therapeutic effect.

For example, glipizide is an oral hypoglycemic agent that lowers blood glucose levels primarily by stimulating pancreatic islet cells to release insulin.

Therapeutic effect
This is the expected effect (physiological response) for which the nurse administers a medication to a specific client. One medication can have more than one therapeutic effect.

For example, one client receives acetaminophen to lower fever, whereas another client receives it to relieve pain.

Side effects
These are expected and predictable effects that result at therapeutic dosages.

For example, morphine for pain relief usually results in constipation.

Adverse effects
These are undesirable, inadvertent, unexpected and potentially dangerous responses to a medication. Some are immediate, whereas others take weeks or months to develop.

For example, the antibiotic gentamicin can cause hearing loss.

Toxic effects
Medications can have specific risks and manifestations of toxicity. They develop after taking a medication for a lengthy period of time or when toxic amounts build up due to faulty metabolism or excretion.

For example, nurses monitor clients taking digoxin for dysrhythmias, a manifestation of cardiotoxicity. Hypokalemia places these clients at greater risk for digoxin toxicity.

Medication interactions
Medications can interact with each other, resulting in beneficial or harmful effects.

For example, giving the beta-blocker atenolol concurrently with the calcium channel blocker nifedipine helps prevent reflex tachycardia.

An example of an undesirable interaction is giving omeprazole, a proton pump inhibitor, concurrently with phenytoin, an anticonvulsant. This can increase the serum level of phenytoin.

Obtain a complete medication history, and be knowledgeable of clinically significant interactions.

Be aware that medications can also interact beneficially or harmfully with food and with herbal and dietary supplements.

Precautions/Contraindications
These are conditions (diseases, age, pregnancy, lactation) that make it risky or completely unsafe for clients to take specific medications.

For example, tetracyclines can stain developing teeth. Therefore, children younger than 8 years should not take these medications. Another example is that myasthenia gravis is a contraindication for fentanyl, an opioid analgesic.

Some medications require caution with some conditions.

For example, the kidneys excrete vancomycin without changing it. Therefore, renal impairment requires caution when administering this medication.

Preparation, dosage, administration
It is important to know any specific considerations for preparation, safe dosages, dosage calculations, and how to administer the medication.

For example, morphine is available in many formulations. Oral doses of morphine are generally higher than parenteral doses due to extensive first-pass effect. Clients who have chronic, severe pain, such as with cancer, generally take oral doses of morphine.

Nursing implications
Know how to monitor therapeutic effects and side effects, prevent and treat adverse effects, provide comfort, and instruct clients about the safe use of medications.

MEDICATION CATEGORY AND CLASSIFICATION

NOMENCLATURE

Chemical name is the name of the medication that reflects its chemical composition and molecular structure (isobutylphenylpropanoic acid).

Generic name is the official or nonproprietary name the United States Adopted Names Council gives a medication. Each medication has only one generic name (ibuprofen).

Trade name is the brand or proprietary name the company that manufactures the medication gives it. One medication can have multiple trade names (Advil, Motrin).

CONSIDERATIONS

Nurses administer prescription medications under the supervision of providers. Some medications can be habit-forming, or have potential harmful effects and require more stringent supervision. Qs

Uncontrolled substances require monitoring by a provider, but do not generally pose risks of abuse and addiction. Antibiotics are an example of uncontrolled prescription medications.

Controlled substances have a potential for abuse and dependence and have a "schedule" classification. Heroin is in Schedule I and has no medical use in the United States. Medications in Schedules II through V have legitimate applications. Each subsequent level has a decreasing risk of abuse and dependence. For example, morphine is a Schedule II medication that has a greater risk for abuse and dependence than phenobarbital, which is a Schedule IV medication.

- New drugs in development undergo the rigorous testing procedures of the U.S. Food and Drug Administration (FDA) to determine both effectiveness and safety before approval. However, new drugs can have unidentified or unreported adverse effects; nurses observing these can report them online at www.fda.gov/medwatch.
- The FDA's Pregnancy Risk Categories (A, B, C, D, X) classify medications according to their potential harm during pregnancy, with Category A being the safest and Category X the most dangerous. Teratogenesis from unsafe medications is most likely to occur during the first trimester. Before administering any medication to a woman who is pregnant or could be pregnant, determine whether it is safe for use during pregnancy.

MEDICATION PRESCRIPTIONS

Each facility has written policies for medication prescriptions, including which providers may write, receive, and transcribe medication prescriptions. Qtc

Types of medication prescriptions

Routine or standard prescriptions
- A routine or standard prescription identifies medications nurses give on a regular schedule with or without a termination date or a specific number of doses. Without a termination date, the prescription remains in effect until the provider discontinues it or discharges the client.
- Providers must re-prescribe some medications, such as opioids and antibiotics, within a specific amount of time or they will automatically discontinue.

Single or one-time prescriptions: A single or one-time prescription is for administration once at a specific time or as soon as possible. These prescriptions are common for preoperative or preprocedural medications. For example, a one-time prescription instructs the nurse to administer lorazepam 2 mg IM at 0700.

Stat prescriptions: A stat prescription is only for administration once and immediately, typically in emergencies when a client's condition changes suddenly. For example, a stat prescription instructs the nurse to administer digoxin 0.125 mg IV bolus stat.

PRN prescriptions: A PRN (*pro re nata*) prescription specifies at what dosage, what frequency, and under what conditions a nurse may administer the medication. The nurse uses clinical judgment to determine the client's need for the medication. For example, a PRN prescription instructs the nurse to administer morphine 2 mg IV bolus every 1 hr PRN for chest pain. When administering PRN medications, the nurse documents the findings that demonstrate the client's need for the medication and the time of administration.

Standing prescriptions: Providers write standing prescriptions for specific circumstances or for specific units. For example, a critical care unit has standing prescriptions for treating clients who have asystole. Another example is a heparin protocol.

Components of a medication prescription

- Client's full name
- Date and time of the prescription
- Name of the medication (generic or brand)
- Strength and dosage of the medication
- Route of administration
- Time and frequency of administration: exact times or number of times per day (according to the facility's policy or the specific qualities of the medication)
- Quantity to dispense and the number of refills
- Signature of the prescribing provider

Communicating medication prescriptions

Origin of medication prescriptions: Providers or nurses who take verbal or telephone prescriptions from a provider write medication prescriptions on the client's medical record. When the nurse writes a medication prescription on the client's medical record, the facility's policy specifies how much time the provider has to sign the prescription. Nurses transcribe medication prescriptions onto the medication administration record (MAR).

Taking a telephone prescription

- If possible, have a second nurse listen on an extension or on a speaker in a private area (to ensure confidentiality).
- Make sure that the prescription is complete and correct by reading back to the provider the client's name, the name of the medication, the dosage, the time of administration, the frequency, and the route.
- To ensure correct spelling, use aids such as "b as in boy." State numbers separately, such as "one, five" for 15.
- Remind the provider to verify the prescription and sign it within the amount of time the facility's policy specifies.
- Enter the prescription in the client's health record.

Medication reconciliation

The Joint Commission requires policies and procedures for medication reconciliation. Nurses compile a list of each client's current medications, including all medications with their dosages and frequency. They compare the list with new medication prescriptions and reconcile it with the provider to resolve any discrepancies. This process should take place at admission, when transferring clients between units or facilities, and at discharge.

PREASSESSMENT FOR MEDICATION THERAPY

Nurses obtain the following information before initiating medication therapy, and update it as necessary.

Health history

- Age
- Health problems and current reason for seeking care
- All medications currently taken (prescription and nonprescription): name, dose, route, and frequency of each
- Any adverse or side effects possibly from medication therapy, as well as therapeutic effects
- Use of herbal or natural products for medicinal purposes
- Use of caffeine, tobacco, alcohol, and street drugs
- Clients' understanding of the purpose of the medications along with the client's beliefs, feelings, and concerns Qpcc
- All medication and food allergies

Physical examination

A systematic physical examination provides a baseline for evaluating the therapeutic effects of medication therapy and for detecting possible side and adverse effects.

RIGHTS OF SAFE MEDICATION ADMINISTRATION

Right client

Verify clients' identification before each medication administration. The Joint Commission requires two client identifiers.

- Acceptable identifiers include the client's name, an assigned identification number, telephone number, birth date, or another person-specific identifier, such as a photo identification card.
- Check identification bands for name and identification number.
- Check for allergies by asking clients, looking for an allergy bracelet or medal, and reviewing the MAR.
- Use bar-code scanners to identify clients. Ql

Right medication

Correctly interpret medication prescriptions, verifying completeness and clarity.

- Read medication labels and compare them with the MAR three times: before removing the container, when removing the amount of medication from the container, and in the presence of the client before administering the medication.
- Leave unit-dose medication in its package until administration.
- When using automated medication dispensing systems, perform the same checks and adapt them as necessary. Ql

Right dose

- Use a unit-dose system to decrease errors. If not available, calculate the correct medication dose.
- Check a drug reference to ensure the dose is within the usual range.
- When performing medication calculations or conversions, have another qualified nurse check the calculated dose.
- Prepare medication dosages using standard measurement devices, such as graduated cups or syringes. Some medication dosages require a second verifier or witness, such as some cytotoxic medications. Automated medication dispensing systems use a machine to control the dispensing of medications.

Right time

Administer medication on time to maintain a consistent therapeutic blood level.

- It is generally acceptable to administer the medication 30 min before or after the scheduled time. Refer to the drug reference or the facility's policy for exceptions.
- Give priority to time-critical medications that must act at specific times (preoperatively).

Right route

The most common routes of administration are oral, topical, subcutaneous, IM, and IV. Additional routes include sublingual, buccal, intradermal, transdermal, epidural, inhalation, nasal, ophthalmic, otic, rectal, vaginal, intraosseous, and via enteral tubes.

- Select the correct preparation for the route the provider prescribed (otic versus ophthalmic topical ointment or drops).
- Always use different syringes for enteral and parenteral medication administration.
- Know how to administer medication safely and correctly.

Right documentation

- Immediately record the medication, dose, route, time, and any pertinent information, including the client's response to the medication. Document the medication after administration, not before.
- For some medications, in particular those to alleviate pain, evaluate the client's response and document it later, perhaps after 30 min.

Right client education

- Inform clients about the medication: its purpose, what to expect, how to take it, and what to report.
- To individualize the teaching, determine what the clients already know about the medication, need to know about the medication, and want to know about the medication.

Right to refuse

- Respect clients' right to refuse any medication.
- Explain the consequences, inform the provider, and document the refusal.

Right assessment

Collect any essential data before and after administering any medication. For example, measure apical heart rate before giving digoxin.

Right evaluation

Follow up with clients to verify therapeutic effects as well as side and adverse effects.

MEDICATION ERROR PREVENTION

COMMON MEDICATION ERRORS

- Wrong medication or IV fluid
- Incorrect dose or IV rate
- Wrong client, route, or time
- Administration of an allergy-inducing medication
- Omission of a dose or administration of extra doses
- Incorrect discontinuation of a medication or IV fluid
- Inaccurate prescribing
- Inadvertently giving a medication that has a similar name

USING THE NURSING PROCESS TO PREVENT MEDICATION ERRORS Qs

Assessment

- Be knowledgeable about the medications administered. Use appropriate resources.
  - Providers, including nurses, physicians, and pharmacists
  - Poison control centers
  - Sales representatives from drug companies
  - Nursing pharmacology textbooks and drug handbooks
  - *Physicians' Desk Reference*
  - Professional journals
  - Professional websites
- Obtain information about medical diagnoses and conditions that affect medication administration, such as the ability to swallow, allergies, and heart, liver, and kidney disorders.
  - Identify allergies.
  - Obtain necessary preadministration data (heart rate, blood pressure, serum levels) to assess the appropriateness of the medication and to obtain baseline data for evaluating the effectiveness of medications.
  - Omit or delay doses as necessary due to clients' status.
- Determine whether the medication prescription is complete, including the name of the client, date and time, name of medication, dosage, route of administration, times of administration or frequency, and signature of the prescribing provider.
- Interpret the medication prescription accurately. The Institute for Safe Medication Practices (ISMP) is a nonprofit organization working to educate health care providers and consumers about safe medication practices. The ISMP and the FDA identify the most common medical abbreviations that result in misinterpretation, mistakes, and injury. For a complete list, go to www.ismp.org.
  - **Error-Prone Abbreviation List:** abbreviations that have caused a high number of medication errors
  - **Confused Medication Name List:** sound-alike and look-alike medication names
  - **High-Alert Medication List:** medications that, if a nurse administers them in error, have a high risk for resulting in significant harm to clients. Strategies to prevent errors include limiting access; using auxiliary labels and automated alerts; standardizing the prescription, preparation, and administration; and using automated or independent double checks.
- Question the provider if the prescription is unclear or seems inappropriate for the client. Refuse to administer a medication if it seems unsafe, and notify the charge nurse or supervisor.
- Providers usually make dosage changes gradually. Question them about abrupt and excessive changes.

Planning

- Identify client outcomes for medication administration.
- Set priorities (which medications to give first or before specific treatments or procedures).

Implementation

- Avoid distractions during medication preparation (poor lighting, ringing phones). Interruptions can increase the risk of error.
- Prepare medications for one client at a time.
- Check the labels for the medication's name and concentration. Read labels carefully. Measure doses accurately, and double-check dosages of high-alert medications, such as insulin and heparin, with a colleague. Check the medication's expiration date.
- Doses are usually one to two tablets or one single-dose vial. Question multiple tablets or vials for a single dose.
- Follow the rights of medication administration consistently and carefully. Take the MAR to the bedside.
- Do not administer medications that someone else prepared.
- Encourage clients to become part of the safety net, teaching them about medications and the importance of proper identification before medication administration. Omit or delay a dose when clients question the size of a dose or the appearance of a medication.
- Follow correct procedures for all routes of administration.
- Communicate clearly both verbally and in writing.
- Use verbal prescriptions only for emergencies, and follow the facility's protocol for telephone prescriptions. Nursing students *may not* accept verbal or telephone orders.
- Follow all laws and regulations for preparing and administering controlled substances. Keep them in a secure area. Have another nurse witness the discarding of controlled substances.
- Do not leave medications at the bedside. Some facilities' policies allow exceptions, such as for topical medications.
- Follow the principles of client and family education for medications.

Evaluation

- Evaluate clients' responses to medications, and document and report them.
- Use knowledge of the therapeutic effect and common side and adverse effects of medications to compare expected outcomes with actual findings.
- Identify side and adverse effects, and document and report them.
- Report all errors, and implement corrective measures immediately.
  - Complete an incident report within the time frame the facility specifies, usually 24 hr. This report should include Qoɪ
    - Client's identification
    - Name and dose of the medication
    - Time and place of the incident
    - Accurate and objective account of the event
    - Who you notified
    - What actions you took
    - Your signature (or that of the person who completed the report)
  - Do not reference or include this report in the client's medical record.
  - Medication errors relate to systems, procedures, product design, or practice patterns. Report all errors to help the facility's risk managers determine how errors occur and what changes to make to avoid similar errors in the future.

Application Exercises

1. A nurse is preparing a client's medications. Which of the following actions should the nurse take in following legal practice guidelines? (Select all that apply.)
   - A. Maintain skill competency.
   - B. Determine the dosage.
   - C. Monitor for adverse effects.
   - D. Safeguard medications.
   - E. Identify the client's diagnosis.

2. A nurse reviewing a client's health record notes a new prescription for lisinopril 10 mg PO once every day. The nurse should identify this as which of the following types of prescription?
   - A. Single
   - B. Stat
   - C. Routine
   - D. Standing

3. A nurse is reviewing a new prescription for ondansetron 4 mg PO PRN for nausea and vomiting for a client who has hyperemesis gravidarum. The nurse should clarify which of the following parts of the prescription with the provider?
   - A. Name
   - B. Dosage
   - C. Route
   - D. Frequency

4. A nurse is admitting a client and completing a preassessment before administering medications. Which of the following data should the nurse include in the preassessment? (Select all that apply.)
   - A. Use of herbal teas
   - B. Daily fluid intake
   - C. Current health status
   - D. Previous surgical history
   - E. Food allergies

5. A nurse orienting a newly licensed nurse is reviewing the procedure for taking a telephone prescription. Which of the following statements should the nurse identify as an indication that the newly licensed nurse understands the process?
   - A. "A second nurse enters the prescription into the client's medical record."
   - B. "Another nurse should listen to the phone call."
   - C. "The provider can clarify the prescription when he signs the health record."
   - D. "I should omit the 'read back' if this is a one-time prescription."

Application Exercises Key

1. A. **CORRECT:** Maintaining skill competency and using appropriate administration techniques are legal responsibilities of the nurse.

    B. Determining the medication's dosage is the provider's responsibility.

    C. **CORRECT:** A nurse is legally responsible for monitoring for side and adverse effects of medications.

    D. **CORRECT:** Safeguarding of medications, such as controlled substances, is a legal responsibility of the nurse.

    E. A nurse should know about a client's diagnosis, but identifying a diagnosis is the provider's responsibility.

    Ⓝ *NCLEX® Connection: Safety and Infection Control, Accident/Error/Injury Prevention*

2. A. A single or one-time prescription is for administration once at a specific time or as soon as possible.

    B. A stat prescription is only for administration once and immediately.

    C. **CORRECT:** A routine or standard prescription identifies medications to give on a regular schedule with or without a termination date or a specific number of doses. The nurse will administer this medication every day until the provider discontinues it.

    D. Providers write standing prescriptions for specific circumstances or for specific units.

    Ⓝ *NCLEX® Connection: Pharmacological and Parenteral Therapies, Medication Administration*

3. A. This prescription includes the medication's generic name, ondansetron.

    B. This prescription includes the medication's dosage of 4 mg.

    C. This prescription includes the medication's route, which is oral (PO).

    D. **CORRECT:** This prescription does not include the time or frequency of medication administration. The nurse must clarify this with the prescribing provider.

    Ⓝ *NCLEX® Connection: Safety and Infection Control, Accident/Error/Injury Prevention*

4. A. **CORRECT:** The nurse should inquire about the client's use of herbal products, which often contain caffeine, prior to medication administration because caffeine can affect medication biotransformation.

    B. Daily fluid intake is important for ensuring adequate hydration, but it is not part of the preassessment the nurse completes prior to medication administration.

    C. **CORRECT:** The nurse should review the client's current health status because new prescriptions can cause alterations in current health status.

    D. Surgical history is important for determining any risks or alterations in the client's health status, but it is not part of the preassessment the nurse completes prior to medication administration.

    E. **CORRECT:** The nurse should inquire about food allergies during the preassessment to identify any potential reactions or interactions.

    Ⓝ *NCLEX® Connection: Safety and Infection Control, Accident/Error/Injury Prevention*

5. A. The nurse who accepts the telephone prescription should enter it into the client's medical record to prevent errors in translation.

    B. **CORRECT:** A second nurse should listen to a telephone prescription to prevent errors in communication.

    C. The nurse should verify that the prescription is complete and accurate at the time she takes it by reading it back to the prescribing provider.

    D. A telephone prescription includes reading back all types of medication prescriptions.

    Ⓝ *NCLEX® Connection: Pharmacological and Parenteral Therapies, Adverse Effects/Contraindications/Side Effects/Interactions*

PRACTICE Active Learning Scenario

A staff educator is reviewing the prevention of medication errors with a group of newly licensed nurses. What should the educator include about using the nursing process to prevent medication errors? Use the ATI Active Learning Template: Basic Concept to complete this item.

NURSING INTERVENTIONS: Using the nursing process to prevent medication errors, list the following.

- Three assessment actions
- One planning action
- Four implementation actions
- Three evaluation actions

PRACTICE Answer

Using the ATI Active Learning Template: Basic Concept

NURSING INTERVENTIONS

Assessment
- Be knowledgeable about the medication to administer. Use appropriate resources.
- Obtain information about medical diagnoses and conditions that affect medication administration.
- Determine whether the medication prescription is complete.
- Interpret the medication prescription accurately.
- Question the provider if the prescription is unclear or seems inappropriate for the client.
- Question the provider about abrupt and excessive changes in dosage.

Planning
- Identify clients' outcomes for medication administration.
- Set priorities (which medications to give first or before specific treatments or procedures).

Implementation
- Avoid distractions and interruptions during medication preparation.
- Prepare medications for one client at a time.
- Check the labels for the medication's name and concentration.
- Question multiple tablets or vials for a single dose.
- Follow the rights of medication administration consistently and carefully.
- Do not administer medications that someone else prepared.
- Encourage clients to become part of the safety net.
- Follow correct procedures for all routes of administration.
- Communicate clearly both verbally and in writing.
- Use verbal prescriptions only for emergencies, and follow the facility's protocol for telephone prescriptions.
- Follow all laws and regulations for preparing and administering controlled substances.
- Do not leave medications at the bedside.
- Follow the principles of client and family education for medications.

Evaluation
- Evaluate clients' responses to medications, and document and report them.
- Use knowledge of the therapeutic effect and common side and adverse effects of medications to compare expected outcomes with actual findings.
- Identify side and adverse effects, and document and report them.
- Report all errors, and implement corrective measures immediately.

Ⓝ *NCLEX® Connection: Safety and Infection Control, Reporting of Incident/Event/Irregular Occurrence Variance*

UNIT 1   PHARMACOLOGICAL PRINCIPLES

CHAPTER 3 *Dosage Calculation*

Basic medication dose conversion and calculation skills are essential for providing safe nursing care.

Nurses are responsible for administering the correct amount of medication by calculating the precise amount of medication to give. Nurses can use three different methods for dosage calculation: ratio and proportion, formula (desired over have), and dimensional analysis.

TYPES OF CALCULATIONS

- Solid oral medication
- Liquid oral medication
- Injectable medication
- Correct doses by weight
- IV infusion rates

STANDARD CONVERSION FACTORS

- 1 mg = 1,000 mcg
- 1 g = 1,000 mg
- 1 kg = 1,000 g
- 1 oz = 30 mL
- 1 L = 1,000 mL
- 1 tsp = 5 mL
- 1 tbsp = 15 mL
- 1 tbsp = 3 tsp
- 1 kg = 2.2 lb
- 1 gr = 60 mg

GENERAL ROUNDING GUIDELINES

ROUNDING UP: If the number to the right is equal to or greater than 5, round up by adding 1 to the number on the left.

ROUNDING DOWN: If the number to the right is less than 5, round down by dropping the number, leaving the number to the left as is.

For dosages less than 1.0: Round to the nearest hundredth.
- For example (rounding up): 0.746 mL = 0.75 mL. The calculated dose is 0.746 mL. Look at the number in the thousandths place (6). Six is greater than 5. To round to hundredths, add 1 to the 4 in the hundredths place and drop the 6. The rounded dose is 0.75 mL.
- Or (rounding down): 0.743 mL = 0.74 mL. The calculated dose is 0.743 mL. Look at the number in the thousandths place (3). Three is less than 5. To round to the hundredth, drop the 3 and leave the 4 as is. The rounded dose is 0.74 mL.

For dosages greater than 1.0: Round to the nearest tenth.
- For example (rounding up): 1.38 = 1.4. The calculated dose is 1.38 mg. Look at the number in the hundredths place (8). Eight is greater than 5. To round to the tenth, add 1 to the 3 in the tenth place and drop the 8. The rounded dose is 1.4 mg.
- Or (rounding down): 1.34 mL = 1.3 mL. The calculated dose is 1.34 mL. Look at the number in the hundredths place (4). Four is less than 5. To round to the tenth, drop the 4 and leave the 3 as is. The rounded dose is 1.3 mL.

Solid dosage

Example: A nurse is preparing to administer phenytoin 0.2 g PO every 8 hr. The amount available is phenytoin 100 mg/capsule. How many capsules should the nurse administer per dose? (Round the answer to the nearest whole number. Use a leading zero if it applies. Do not use a trailing zero.)

USING RATIO AND PROPORTION

STEP 1: What is the unit of measurement the nurse should calculate?

capsules

STEP 2: What is the dose the nurse should administer? Dose to administer = Desired

0.2 g

STEP 3: What is the dose available? Dose available = Have

100 mg

STEP 4: Should the nurse convert the units of measurement? Yes (g ≠ mg)

1 g = 1,000 mg (1 × 1,000)

0.2 g = 200 mg (0.2 × 1,000)

STEP 5: What is the quantity of the dose available? = Quantity

1 capsule

STEP 6: Set up the equation and solve for X.

$$\frac{Have}{Quantity} = \frac{Desired}{X}$$

$$\frac{100\ mg}{1\ cap} = \frac{200\ mg}{X\ cap}$$

$$X = 2$$

STEP 7: Round, if necessary.

STEP 8: Reassess to determine whether the amount to administer makes sense. If there are 100 mg/capsule and the prescription reads 0.2 g (200 mg), it makes sense to administer 2 capsules. The nurse should administer phenytoin 2 capsules PO.

USING DESIRED OVER HAVE

STEP 1: What is the unit of measurement the nurse should calculate?

capsules

STEP 2: What is the dose the nurse should administer? Dose to administer = Desired

0.2 g

STEP 3: What is the dose available? Dose available = Have

100 mg

STEP 4: Should the nurse convert the units of measurement? Yes (g ≠ mg)

1 g = 1,000 mg (1 × 1,000)

0.2 g = 200 mg (0.2 × 1,000)

STEP 5: What is the quantity of the dose available? = Quantity

1 capsule

STEP 6: Set up the equation and solve for X.

$$\frac{Desired \times Quantity}{Have} = X$$

$$\frac{200 \text{ mg} \times 1 \text{ cap}}{100 \text{ mg}} = X \text{ cap}$$

$$X = 2$$

STEP 7: Round, if necessary.

STEP 8: Reassess to determine whether the amount to administer makes sense. If there are 100 mg/capsule and the prescription reads 0.2 g (200 mg), it makes sense to administer 2 capsules. The nurse should administer phenytoin 2 capsules PO.

USING DIMENSIONAL ANALYSIS

STEP 1: What is the unit of measurement the nurse should calculate?

capsules

STEP 2: What is the quantity of the dose available? = Quantity

1 capsule

STEP 3: What is the dose available? Dose available = Have

100 mg

STEP 4: What is the dose the nurse should administer? Dose to administer = Desired

0.2 g

STEP 5: Should the nurse convert the units of measurement? Yes (g ≠ mg)

1,000 mg = 1 g

0.2 g = 200 mg (0.2 × 100)

STEP 6: Set up the equation and solve for X.

$$X = \frac{Quantity}{Have} \times \frac{Conversion\ (Have)}{Conversion\ (Desired)} \times Desired$$

$$X \text{ cap} = \frac{1 \text{ cap}}{100 \text{ mg}} \times \frac{1,000 \text{ mg}}{1 \text{ g}} \times 0.2 \text{ g}$$

$$X = 2$$

STEP 7: Round, if necessary.

STEP 8: Reassess to determine whether the amount to administer makes sense. If there are 100 mg/capsule and the prescription reads 0.2 g (200 mg), it makes sense to administer 2 capsules. The nurse should administer phenytoin 2 capsules PO.

Liquid dosage

Example: A nurse is preparing to administer amoxicillin 0.25 g PO every 8 hr. The amount available is amoxicillin oral suspension 250 mg/5 mL. How many mL should the nurse administer per dose? (Round the answer to the nearest tenth. Use a leading zero if it applies. Do not use a trailing zero.)

USING RATIO AND PROPORTION

STEP 1: What is the unit of measurement the nurse should calculate?

mL

STEP 2: What is the dose the nurse should administer? Dose to administer = Desired

0.25 g

STEP 3: What is the dose available? Dose available = Have

250 mg

STEP 4: Should the nurse convert the units of measurement? Yes (g ≠ mg)

1 g = 1,000 mg (1 × 1,000)

0.25 g = 250 mg (0.25 × 1,000)

STEP 5: What is the quantity of the dose available? = Quantity

5 mL

STEP 6: Set up the equation and solve for X.

$$\frac{Have}{Quantity} = \frac{Desired}{X}$$

$$\frac{250 \text{ mg}}{5 \text{ mL}} = \frac{250 \text{ mg}}{X \text{ mL}}$$

$$X = 5$$

STEP 7: Round, if necessary.

STEP 8: Reassess to determine whether the amount to administer makes sense. If there are 250 mg/5 mL and the prescription reads 0.25 g (250 mg), it makes sense to administer 5 mL. The nurse should administer amoxicillin 5 mL PO every 8 hr.

USING DESIRED OVER HAVE

STEP 1: What is the unit of measurement the nurse should calculate?

mL

STEP 2: What is the dose the nurse should administer? Dose to administer = Desired

0.25 g

STEP 3: What is the dose available? Dose available = Have

250 mg

STEP 4: Should the nurse convert the units of measurement? Yes (g ≠ mg)

1 g = 1,000 mg (1 × 1,000)

0.25 g = 250 mg (0.25 × 1,000)

STEP 5: What is the quantity of the dose available? = Quantity

5 mL

STEP 6: Set up the equation and solve for X.

$$\frac{Desired \times Quantity}{Have} = X$$

$$\frac{250 \text{ mg} \times 5 \text{ mL}}{250 \text{ mg}} = X \text{ mL}$$

$$5 = X$$

STEP 7: Round, if necessary.

STEP 8: Reassess to determine whether the amount to administer makes sense. If there are 250 mg/5 mL and the prescription reads 0.25 g (250 mg), it makes sense to administer 5 mL. The nurse should administer amoxicillin 5 mL PO every 8 hr.

USING DIMENSIONAL ANALYSIS

STEP 1: What is the unit of measurement the nurse should calculate?

mL

STEP 2: What is the quantity of the dose available? = Quantity

5 mL

STEP 3: What is the dose available? Dose available = Have

250 mg

STEP 4: What is the dose the nurse should administer? Dose to administer = Desired

0.25 g

STEP 5: Should the nurse convert the units of measurement? Yes (g ≠ mg)

1,000 mg = 1 g

0.25 g = 250 mg (0.25 × 1,000)

STEP 6: Set up the equation and solve for X.

$$X = \frac{Quantity}{Have} \times \frac{Conversion\ (Have)}{Conversion\ (Desired)} \times Desired$$

$$X \text{ mL} = \frac{5 \text{ mL}}{250 \text{ mg}} \times \frac{1,000 \text{ mg}}{1 \text{ g}} \times 0.25 \text{ g}$$

$$X = 5$$

STEP 7: Round, if necessary.

STEP 8: Reassess to determine whether the amount to administer makes sense. If there are 250 mg/5 mL and the prescription reads 0.25 g (250 mg), it makes sense to administer 5 mL. The nurse should administer amoxicillin 5 mL PO every 8 hr.

Injectable dosage

Example: A nurse is preparing to administer heparin 8,000 units subcutaneously every 12 hr. Available is heparin injection 10,000 units/mL. How many mL should the nurse administer per dose? (Round the answer to the nearest tenth. Use a leading zero if it applies. Do not use a trailing zero.)

USING RATIO AND PROPORTION

STEP 1: What is the unit of measurement the nurse should calculate?

mL

STEP 2: What is the dose the nurse should administer? Dose to administer = Desired

8,000 units

STEP 3: What is the dose available? Dose available = Have

10,000 units

STEP 4: Should the nurse convert the units of measurement? No

STEP 5: What is the quantity of the dose available? = Quantity

1 mL

STEP 6: Set up the equation and solve for X.

$$\frac{Have}{Quantity} = \frac{Desired}{X}$$

$$\frac{10,000 \text{ units}}{1 \text{ mL}} = \frac{8,000 \text{ units}}{X \text{ mL}}$$

$$X = 0.8$$

STEP 7: Round, if necessary.

STEP 8: Reassess to determine whether the amount to administer makes sense. If there are 10,000 units/mL and the prescription reads 8,000 units, it makes sense to administer 0.8 mL. The nurse should administer heparin injection 0.8 mL subcutaneously every 12 hr.

USING DESIRED OVER HAVE

STEP 1: What is the unit of measurement the nurse should calculate?

mL

STEP 2: What is the dose the nurse should administer? Dose to administer = Desired

8,000 units

STEP 3: What is the dose available? Dose available = Have

10,000 units

STEP 4: Should the nurse convert the units of measurement? No

STEP 5: What is the quantity of the dose available? = Quantity

1 mL

STEP 6: Set up an equation and solve for X.

$$\frac{Desired \times Quantity}{Have} = X$$

$$\frac{8,000 \text{ units} \times 1 \text{ mL}}{10,000 \text{ units}} = X \text{ mL}$$

$$0.8 = X$$

STEP 7: Round, if necessary.

STEP 8: Reassess to determine whether the amount to administer makes sense. If there are 10,000 units/mL and the prescription reads 8,000 units, it makes sense to administer 0.8 mL. The nurse should administer heparin injection 0.8 mL subcutaneously every 12 hr.

USING DIMENSIONAL ANALYSIS

STEP 1: What is the unit of measurement the nurse should calculate?

mL

STEP 2: What is the quantity of the dose available? = Quantity

1 mL

STEP 3: What is the dose available? Dose available = Have

10,000 units

STEP 4: What is the dose the nurse should administer? Dose to administer = Desired

8,000 units

STEP 5: Should the nurse convert the units of measurement? No

STEP 6: Set up an equation and solve for X.

$$X = \frac{Quantity}{Have} \times \frac{Conversion\ (Have)}{Conversion\ (Desired)} \times Desired$$

$$X \text{ mL} = \frac{1 \text{ mL}}{10,000 \text{ units}} \times 8,000 \text{ units}$$

$$X = 0.8$$

STEP 7: Round, if necessary.

STEP 8: Reassess to determine whether the amount to administer makes sense. If there are 10,000 units/mL and the prescription reads 8,000 units, it makes sense to administer 0.8 mL. The nurse should administer heparin injection 0.8 mL subcutaneously every 12 hr.

Dosages by weight

Example: A nurse is preparing to administer cefixime 8 mg/kg/day PO to divide equally every 12 hr to a toddler who weighs 22 lb. Available is cefixime suspension 100 mg/5 mL. How many mL should the nurse administer per dose? (Round the answer to the nearest tenth. Use a leading zero if it applies. Do not use a trailing zero.)

STEP 1: What is the unit of measurement the nurse should calculate?

kg

STEP 2: Set up an equation and solve for X.

$$\frac{2.2 \text{ lb}}{1 \text{ kg}} = \frac{client's\ desired\ weight\ in\ lb}{X \text{ kg}}$$

$$\frac{2.2 \text{ lb}}{1 \text{ kg}} = \frac{22 \text{ lb}}{X \text{ kg}}$$

$$X = 10$$

STEP 3: Round, if necessary.

STEP 4: Reassess to determine whether the equivalent makes sense. If 1 kg = 2.2 lb, it makes sense that 22 lb = 10 kg.

STEP 5: What is the unit of measurement the nurse should calculate?

mg

STEP 6: Set up an equation and solve for X.

$$mg \times kg/day = X$$

$$\frac{8 \text{ mg} \times 10 \text{ kg}}{1 \text{ day}} = 80 \text{ mg}$$

STEP 7: Round, if necessary.

STEP 8: Reassess to determine whether the amount makes sense. If the prescription reads 8 mg/kg/day to divide equally every 12 hr and the toddler weighs 10 kg, it makes sense to give 80 mg/day, or 40 mg every 12 hr.

USING RATIO AND PROPORTION

STEP 9: What is the unit of measurement the nurse should calculate?

mL

STEP 10: What is the dose the nurse should administer? Dose to administer = Desired

40 mg

STEP 11: What is the dose available? Dose available = Have

100 mg

STEP 12: Should the nurse convert the units of measurement? No

STEP 13: What is the quantity of the dose available? = Quantity

5 mL

STEP 14: Set up the equation and solve for X.

$$\frac{Have}{Quantity} = \frac{Desired}{X}$$

$$\frac{100\ mg}{5\ mL} = \frac{40\ mg}{X\ mL}$$

$$X = 2$$

STEP 15: Round, if necessary.

STEP 16: Reassess to determine whether the amount to give makes sense. If there are 100 mg/5 mL and the prescription reads 40 mg, it makes sense to give 2 mL. The nurse should administer cefixime suspension 2 mL PO every 12 hr.

USING DESIRED OVER HAVE

STEP 9: What is the unit of measurement the nurse should calculate?

mL

STEP 10: What is the dose the nurse should administer? Dose to administer = Desired

40 mg

STEP 11: What is the dose available? Dose available = Have

100 mg

STEP 12: Should the nurse convert the units of measurement? No

STEP 13: What is the quantity of the dose available? = Quantity

5 mL

STEP 14: Set up an equation and solve for X.

$$\frac{Desired \times Quantity}{Have} = X$$

$$\frac{40\ mg \times 5\ mL}{100\ mg} = X\ mL$$

$$2 = X$$

STEP 15: Round, if necessary.

STEP 16: Reassess to determine whether the amount to give makes sense. If there are 100 mg/5 mL and the prescription reads 40 mg, it makes sense to give 2 mL. The nurse should administer cefixime suspension 2 mL PO every 12 hr.

USING DIMENSIONAL ANALYSIS

STEP 9: What is the unit of measurement the nurse should calculate?

mL

STEP 10: What is the quantity of the dose available? = Quantity

5 mL

STEP 11: What is the dose available? Dose available = Have

100 mg

STEP 12: What is the dose the nurse should administer? Dose to administer = Desired

40 mg

STEP 13: Should the nurse convert the units of measurement? No

STEP 14: Set up an equation and solve for X.

$$X = \frac{Quantity}{Have} \times \frac{Conversion\ (Have)}{Conversion\ (Desired)} \times Desired$$

$$X\ mL = \frac{5\ mL}{100\ mg} \times 40\ mg$$

$$X = 2$$

STEP 15: Round, if necessary.

STEP 16: Reassess to determine whether the amount to give makes sense. If there are 100 mg/5 mL and the prescription reads 40 mg, it makes sense to give 2 mL. The nurse should administer cefixime suspension 2 mL PO every 12 hr.

IV flow rates

Nurses calculate IV flow rates for large-volume continuous IV infusions and intermittent IV bolus infusions using electronic infusion pumps (mL/hr) and manual IV tubing (gtt/min).

IV INFUSIONS WITH ELECTRONIC INFUSION PUMPS

Infusion pumps control an accurate rate of fluid infusion. Infusion pumps deliver a specific amount of fluid during a specific amount of time. For example, an infusion pump can deliver 150 mL in 1 hr or 50 mL in 20 min.

> Example: A nurse is preparing to administer dextrose 5% in water (D_5W) 500 mL IV to infuse over 4 hr. The nurse should set the IV infusion pump to deliver how many mL/hr? (Round the answer to the nearest whole number. Use a leading zero if it applies. Do not use a trailing zero.)

STEP 1: What is the unit of measurement the nurse should calculate?

> mL/hr

STEP 2: What is the volume the nurse should infuse?

> 500 mL

STEP 3: What is the total infusion time?

> 4 hr

STEP 4: Should the nurse convert the units of measurement? No

STEP 5: Set up the equation and solve for X.

> $$\frac{Volume \text{ (mL)}}{Time \text{ (hr)}} = X \text{ mL/hr}$$
>
> $$\frac{500 \text{ mL}}{4 \text{ hr}} = X \text{ mL/hr}$$
>
> $$125 = X$$

STEP 6: Round, if necessary.

STEP 7: Reassess to determine whether the IV flow rate makes sense. If the prescription reads 500 mL to infuse over 4 hr, it makes sense to administer 125 mL/hr. The nurse should set the IV pump to deliver D_5W 500 mL IV at 125 mL/hr.

> Example: A nurse is preparing to administer cefotaxime 1 g intermittent IV bolus over 45 min. Available is cefotaxime 1 g in 100 mL 0.9% sodium chloride (0.9% NaCl). The nurse should set the IV infusion pump to deliver how many mL/hr? (Round the answer to the nearest whole number.)

STEP 1: What is the unit of measurement the nurse should calculate?

> mL/hr

STEP 2: Should the nurse convert the units of measurement? Yes (min ≠ hr) Yes (g ≠ mL)

> $$\frac{60 \text{ min}}{45 \text{ min}} = \frac{1 \text{ hr}}{X \text{ hr}} \qquad \frac{100 \text{ mL}}{1 \text{ g}} = \frac{X \text{ mL}}{1 \text{ g}}$$
>
> $$X = 0.75 \qquad\qquad X = 100$$

STEP 3: What is the total infusion time?

> 45 min

STEP 4: What is the volume the nurse should infuse?

> 100 mL

STEP 5: Set up an equation and solve for X.

> $$\frac{Volume \text{ (mL)}}{Time \text{ (hr)}} = X \text{ mL/hr}$$
>
> $$\frac{100 \text{ mL}}{0.75 \text{ hr}} = X \text{ mL/hr}$$
>
> $$133.3333 = X$$

STEP 6: Round, if necessary.

> $$133.3333 = 133$$

STEP 7: Reassess to determine whether the IV flow rate makes sense. If the prescription reads 100 mL to infuse over 45 min (0.75 hr), it makes sense to administer 133 mL/hr. The nurse should set the IV pump to deliver cefotaxime 1 g in 100 mL of 0.9% NaCl IV at 133 mL/hr.

MANUAL IV INFUSIONS

If an electronic infusion pump is not available, regulate the IV flow rate using the roller clamp on the IV tubing. When setting the flow rate, count the number of drops that fall into the drip chamber over 1 min. Then calculate the flow rate using the drop factor on the manufacturer's package containing the administration set. The drop factor is the number of drops per milliliter of solution.

> Example: A nurse is preparing to administer lactated Ringer's (LR) 1,500 mL IV to infuse over 10 hr. The drop factor of the manual IV tubing is 15 gtt/mL. The nurse should adjust the manual IV infusion to deliver how many gtt/min? (Round the answer to the nearest whole number. Use a leading zero if it applies. Do not use a trailing zero.)

USING RATIO AND PROPORTION AND DESIRED OVER HAVE

STEP 1: What is the unit of measurement the nurse should calculate?

gtt/min

STEP 2: What is the quantity of the drop factor that is available?

15 gtt/mL

STEP 3: What is the volume the nurse should infuse?

1,500 mL

STEP 4: What is the total infusion time?

10 hr

STEP 5: Should the nurse convert the units of measurement? No (mL = mL) Yes (hr ≠ min)

$$\frac{1 \text{ hr}}{60 \text{ min}} = \frac{10 \text{ hr}}{X \text{ min}}$$

$X = 600$ min

STEP 6: Set up the equation and solve for X.

$$\frac{Volume \text{ (mL)}}{Time \text{ (min)}} \times Drop\ factor \text{ (gtt/mL)} = X$$

$$\frac{1,500 \text{ mL}}{600 \text{ min}} \times 15 \text{ gtt/mL} = X \text{ gtt/min}$$

$37.5 = X$

STEP 7: Round, if necessary.

37.5 = 38

STEP 8: Reassess to determine whether the IV flow rate makes sense. If the prescription reads 1,500 mL to infuse over 10 hr (600 min), it makes sense to administer 38 gtt/min. The nurse should adjust the manual IV infusion to deliver LR 1,500 mL IV at 38 gtt/min.

USING DIMENSIONAL ANALYSIS

STEP 1: What is the unit of measurement the nurse should calculate?

gtt/min

STEP 2: What is the quantity of the drop factor that is available?

15 gtt/mL

STEP 3: What is the total infusion time?

10 hr

STEP 4: What is the volume the nurse should infuse?

1,500 mL

STEP 5: Should the nurse convert the units of measurement? No (mL = mL) Yes (hr ≠ min)

$$\frac{1 \text{ hr}}{60 \text{ min}} = \frac{10 \text{ hr}}{X \text{ min}}$$

$X = 600$ min

STEP 6: Set up the equation and solve for X.

$$X = \frac{Quantity}{1 \text{ mL}} \times \frac{Conversion\ (Have)}{Conversion\ (Desired)} \times \frac{Volume}{Time}$$

$$X \text{ gtt/min} = \frac{15 \text{ gtt}}{1 \text{ mL}} \times \frac{1 \text{ hr}}{60 \text{ min}} \times \frac{1,500 \text{ mL}}{10 \text{ hr}}$$

$X = 37.5$

STEP 7: Round, if necessary.

37.5 = 38

STEP 8: Reassess to determine whether the IV flow rate makes sense. If the prescription reads 1,500 mL to infuse over 10 hr (600 min), it makes sense to administer 38 gtt/min. The nurse should adjust the manual IV infusion to deliver LR 1,500 mL IV at 38 gtt/min.

Example: A nurse is preparing to administer ranitidine 150 mg by intermittent IV bolus. Available is ranitidine 150 mg in 100 mL of 0.9% sodium chloride (0.9% NaCl) to infuse over 30 min. The drop factor of the manual IV tubing is 10 gtt/mL. The nurse should adjust the manual IV infusion to deliver how many gtt/min? (Round the answer to the nearest whole number. Use a leading zero if it applies. Do not use a trailing zero.)

USING RATIO AND PROPORTION AND DESIRED OVER HAVE

STEP 1: What is the unit of measurement the nurse should calculate?

gtt/min

STEP 2: Should the nurse convert the units of measurement? Yes (mg ≠ mL)

$$\frac{150\ mg}{100\ mL} = \frac{150\ mg}{X\ mL}$$

$X = 100$

STEP 3: What is the total infusion time?

30 min

STEP 4: What is the quantity of the drop factor that is available?

10 gtt/mL

STEP 5: What is the volume the nurse should infuse?

100 mL

STEP 6: Set up an equation and solve for X.

$$\frac{Volume\ (mL)}{Time\ (min)} \times Drop\ factor\ (gtt/mL) = X$$

$$\frac{100\ mL}{30\ min} \times 10\ gtt/mL = X\ gtt/min$$

$33.3333 = X$

STEP 7: Round, if necessary.

33.3333 = 33

STEP 8: Reassess to determine whether the IV flow rate makes sense. If the amount prescribed is 100 mL to infuse over 30 min, it makes sense to administer 33 gtt/min. The nurse should adjust the manual IV infusion to deliver ranitidine 150 mg in 100 mL of 0.9% NaCl IV at 33 gtt/min.

USING DIMENSIONAL ANALYSIS

STEP 1: What is the unit of measurement to calculate?

gtt/min

STEP 2: What is the quantity of the drop factor that is available?

10 gtt/mL

STEP 3: What is the total infusion time?

30 min

STEP 4: Should the nurse convert the units of measurement? Yes (mg ≠ mL)

$$\frac{150\ mg}{100\ mL} = \frac{150\ mg}{X\ mL}$$

$X = 100$

STEP 5: What is the volume the nurse should infuse?

100 mL

STEP 6: Set up an equation and solve for X.

$$X = \frac{Quantity}{1\ mL} \times \frac{Conversion\ (Have)}{Conversion\ (Desired)} \times \frac{Volume}{Time}$$

$$X\ gtt/min = \frac{10\ gtt}{1\ mL} \times \frac{100\ mL}{30\ min}$$

$X = 33.3333$

STEP 7: Round, if necessary.

33.3333 = 33

STEP 8: Reassess to determine whether the IV flow rate makes sense. If the amount prescribed is 100 mL to infuse over 30 min, it makes sense to administer 33 gtt/min. The nurse should adjust the manual IV infusion to deliver ranitidine 150 mg in 100 mL of 0.9% NaCl IV at 33 gtt/min.

Application Exercises

1. A nurse is preparing to administer vancomycin 1 g by intermittent IV bolus. Available is vancomycin 1 g in 100 mL of dextrose 5% in water (D₅W) to infuse over 45 min. The drop factor of the manual IV tubing is 10 gtt/mL. The nurse should adjust the manual IV infusion to deliver how many gtt/min? (Round the answer to the nearest whole number. Do not use a trailing zero.)

2. A nurse is preparing to administer clindamycin 200 mg by intermittent IV bolus. The amount available is clindamycin injection 200 mg in 100 mL 0.9% sodium chloride (0.9% NaCl) to infuse over 30 min. The nurse should set the IV pump to deliver how many mL/hr? (Round the answer to the nearest whole number. Do not use a trailing zero.)

3. A nurse is preparing to administer furosemide 80 mg PO daily. The amount available is furosemide oral solution 10 mg/1 mL. How many mL should the nurse administer? (Round the answer to the nearest whole number. Do not use a trailing zero.)

4. A nurse is preparing to administer haloperidol 2 mg PO every 12 hr. The amount available is haloperidol 1 mg/tablet. How many tablets should the nurse administer? (Round the answer to the nearest whole number. Do not use a trailing zero.)

5. A nurse is preparing to administer amoxicillin 20 mg/kg/day PO to divide equally every 12 hr to a preschooler who weighs 44 lb. The amount available is amoxicillin suspension 250 mg/5 mL. How many mL should the nurse administer per dose? (Round the answer to the nearest whole number. Do not use a trailing zero.)

6. A nurse is preparing to administer heparin 15,000 units subcutaneously every 12 hr. The amount available is heparin injection 20,000 units/mL. How many mL should the nurse administer per dose? (Round the answer to the nearest tenth. Do not use a trailing zero.)

7. A nurse is preparing to administer acetaminophen 650 mg PO every 6 hr PRN for pain. The amount available is acetaminophen liquid 500 mg/5 mL. How many mL should the nurse administer per dose? (Round the answer to the nearest tenth. Use a leading zero if it applies. Do not use a trailing zero.)

8. A nurse is preparing to administer dextrose 5% in water (D₅W) 750 mL IV to infuse over 6 hr. The nurse should set the IV pump to deliver how many mL/hr? (Round the answer to the nearest whole number. Do not use a trailing zero.)

Application Exercises Key

1. **22** gtt/min

Using Ratio and Proportion and Desired Over Have

STEP 1: What is the unit of measurement the nurse should calculate? gtt/min

STEP 2: Should the nurse convert the units of measurement? Yes

$$\frac{1\,g}{100\,mL} \times \frac{1\,g}{X\,mL} = 100$$

STEP 3: What is the total infusion time? 45 min

STEP 4: What is the volume the nurse should infuse? 100 mL

STEP 5: What is the quantity of the drop factor that is available? 10 gtt/mL

STEP 6: Set up an equation and solve for X.

$$\frac{Volume\,(mL)}{Time\,(min)} \times Drop\,factor\,(gtt/mL) = X$$

$$\frac{100\,mL}{45\,min} \times 10\,gtt/mL = X\,gtt/mL$$

$$22.2222 = X$$

STEP 7: Round, if necessary. 22.2222 = 22

STEP 8: Reassess to determine whether the IV flow rate makes sense. If the amount prescribed is 100 mL to infuse over 45 min, it makes sense to administer 22 gtt/min. The nurse should adjust the manual IV infusion to deliver vancomycin 1 g in 100 mL of D₅W IV at 22 gtt/min.

Using Dimensional Analysis

STEP 1: What is the unit of measurement to calculate? gtt/min

STEP 2: What is the quantity of the drop factor that is available? 10 gtt/mL

STEP 3: What is the total infusion time? 45 min

STEP 4: Should the nurse convert the units of measurement? Yes

$$\frac{1\,g}{100\,mL} \times \frac{1\,g}{X\,mL} = 100$$

STEP 5: What is the volume the nurse should infuse? 100 mL

STEP 6: Set up an equation and solve for X.

$$X = \frac{Quantity}{1\,mL} \times \frac{Conversion\,(Have)}{Conversion\,(Desired)} \times \frac{Volume}{Time}$$

$$X\,gtt/min = \frac{10\,gtt}{1\,mL} \times \frac{100\,mL}{45\,min}$$

$$X = 22.2222$$

STEP 7: Round, if necessary. 22.2222 = 22

STEP 8: Reassess to determine whether the IV flow rate makes sense. If the amount prescribed is 100 mL to infuse over 45 min, it makes sense to administer 22 gtt/min. The nurse should adjust the manual IV infusion to deliver vancomycin 1 g in 100 mL of D₅W IV at 22 gtt/min.

Ⓝ *NCLEX® Connection: Pharmacological and Parenteral Therapies, Parenteral/Intravenous Therapies*

---

2. **200** mL/hr

STEP 1: What is the unit of measurement the nurse should calculate? mL/hr

STEP 2: Should the nurse convert the units of measurement? Yes (mg ≠ mL) Yes (min ≠ hr)

$$\frac{60\,min}{30\,min} = \frac{1\,hr}{X\,hr} \qquad \frac{200\,mg}{100\,mg} = \frac{200\,mg}{X\,mL}$$
$$X = 0.5 \qquad\qquad X = 100$$

STEP 3: What is the volume the nurse should infuse? 100 mL

STEP 4: What is the total infusion time? 30 min

STEP 5: Set up an equation and solve for X.

$$\frac{Volume\,(mL)}{Time\,(hr)} = X\,mL/hr \qquad \frac{100\,mL}{0.5\,hr} = X\,mL/hr$$
$$200 = X$$

STEP 6: Round, if necessary.

STEP 7: Reassess to determine whether the IV flow rate makes sense. If the prescription reads 100 mL to infuse over 30 min (0.5 hr), it makes sense to administer 200 mL/hr. The nurse should set the IV pump to deliver clindamycin 200 mg in 100 mL of 0.9% NaCl IV at 200 mL/hr.

Ⓝ *NCLEX® Connection: Pharmacological and Parenteral Therapies, Parenteral/Intravenous Therapies*

---

3. **8** mL

Using Ratio and Proportion

STEP 1: What is the unit of measurement the nurse should calculate? mL

STEP 2: What is the dose the nurse should administer? Dose to administer = Desired = 80 mg

STEP 3: What is the dose available? Dose available = Have = 10 mg

STEP 4: Should the nurse convert the units of measurement? No

STEP 5: What is the quantity of the dose available? = Quantity = 1 mL

STEP 6: Set up the equation and solve for X.

$$\frac{Have}{Quantity} = \frac{Desired}{X} \qquad \frac{10\,mg}{1\,mL} \times \frac{80\,mg}{X\,mL}$$
$$X = 8$$

STEP 7: Round, if necessary.

STEP 8: Reassess to determine whether the amount to administer makes sense. If there are 10 mg/1 mL and the prescription reads 80 mg, it makes sense to administer 8 mL. The nurse should administer furosemide 8 mL PO daily.

Using Desired Over Have

STEP 1: What is the unit of measurement the nurse should calculate? mL

STEP 2: What is the dose the nurse should administer? Dose to administer = Desired = 80 mg

STEP 3: What is the dose available? Dose available = Have = 10 mg

STEP 4: Should the nurse convert the units of measurement? No

STEP 5: What is the quantity of the dose available? = Quantity = 1 mL

STEP 6: Set up the equation and solve for X.

$$\frac{Desired \times Quantity}{Have} = X \qquad \frac{80\,mg \times 1\,mL}{10\,mg} = X\,mL$$
$$8 = X$$

STEP 7: Round, if necessary.

STEP 8: Reassess to determine whether the amount to administer makes sense. If there are 10 mg/1 mL and the prescription reads 80 mg, it makes sense to administer 8 mL. The nurse should administer furosemide 8 mL PO daily.

Using Dimensional Analysis

STEP 1: What is the unit of measurement the nurse should calculate? mL

STEP 2: What is the quantity of the dose available? = Quantity = 1 mL

STEP 3: What is the dose available? Dose available = Have = 10 mg

STEP 4: What is the dose the nurse should administer? Dose to administer = Desired = 80 mg

STEP 5: Should the nurse convert the units of measurement? No

STEP 6: Set up the equation and solve for X.

$$X = \frac{Quantity}{Have} \times \frac{Conversion\,(Have)}{Conversion\,(Desired)} \times Desired$$

$$X\,mL = \frac{1\,mL}{10\,mg} \times 80$$

$$X = 8$$

STEP 7: Round, if necessary.

STEP 8: Reassess to determine whether the amount to administer makes sense. If there are 10 mg/1 mL and the prescription reads 80 mg, it makes sense to administer 8 mL. The nurse should administer furosemide 8 mL PO daily.

Ⓝ *NCLEX® Connection: Pharmacological and Parenteral Therapies, Dosage Calculation*

4. **2** tablets

Using Ratio and Proportion

STEP 1: What is the unit of measurement the nurse should calculate? tablet

STEP 2: What is the dose the nurse should administer? Dose to administer = Desired = 2 mg

STEP 3: What is the dose available? Dose available = Have = 1 mg

STEP 4: Should the nurse convert the units of measurement? No

STEP 5: What is the quantity of the dose available? = Quantity = 1 tablet

STEP 6: Set up the equation and solve for X.

$$\frac{Have}{Quantity} = \frac{Desired}{X} \qquad \frac{1\ mg}{1\ tablet} \times \frac{2\ mg}{X\ tablets}$$

$X = 2$

STEP 7: Round, if necessary.

STEP 8: Reassess to determine whether the amount to administer makes sense. If there is 1 mg/tablet and the prescription reads 2 mg, it makes sense to administer 2 tablets. The nurse should administer haloperidol 2 tablets every 12 hr.

Using Desired Over Have

STEP 1: What is the unit of measurement the nurse should calculate? tablet

STEP 2: What is the dose the nurse should administer? Dose to administer = Desired = 2 mg

STEP 3: What is the dose available? Dose available = Have = 1 mg

STEP 4: Should the nurse convert the units of measurement? No

STEP 5: What is the quantity of the dose available? = Quantity = 1 tablet

STEP 6: Set up the equation and solve for X.

$$\frac{Desired \times Quantity}{Have} = X$$

$$\frac{2\ mg \times 1\ tablet}{1\ mg} = X\ tablets$$

$2 = X$

STEP 7: Round, if necessary.

STEP 8: Reassess to determine whether the amount to administer makes sense. If there is 1 mg/tablet and the prescription reads 2 mg, it makes sense to administer 2 tablets. The nurse should administer haloperidol 2 tablets every 12 hr.

Using Dimensional Analysis

STEP 1: What is the unit of measurement the nurse should calculate? tablets

STEP 2: What is the quantity of the dose available? = Quantity = 1 tablet

STEP 3: What is the dose available? Dose available = Have = 1 mg

STEP 4: What is the dose the nurse should administer? Dose to administer = Desired = 2 mg

STEP 5: Should the nurse convert the units of measurement? No

STEP 6: Set up the equation and solve for X.

$$X = \frac{Quantity}{Have} \times \frac{Conversion\ (Have)}{Conversion\ (Desired)} \times Desired$$

$$X\ tablets = \frac{1\ tablet}{1\ mg} \times 2\ mg$$

$X = 2$

STEP 7: Round, if necessary.

STEP 8: Reassess to determine whether the amount to administer makes sense. If there is 1 mg/tablet and the prescription reads 2 mg, it makes sense to administer 2 tablets. The nurse should administer haloperidol 2 tablets every 12 hr.

Ⓝ *NCLEX® Connection: Pharmacological and Parenteral Therapies, Dosage Calculation*

---

5. **4** mL

STEP 1: What is the unit of measurement the nurse should calculate? kg

STEP 2: Set up an equation and solve for X.

$$\frac{2.2\ lb}{1\ kg} = \frac{client's\ weight\ in\ lb}{X\ kg} \qquad \frac{2.2\ lb}{1\ kg} \times \frac{44\ lb}{X\ kg}$$

$X = 20$

STEP 3: Round, if necessary.

STEP 4: Reassess to determine whether the equivalent makes sense. If 1 kg = 2.2 lb, it makes sense that 44 lb = 20 kg.

STEP 5: What is the unit of measurement the nurse should calculate? mg

STEP 6: Set up an equation and solve for X. $mg \times kg/day = X$

$$\frac{20\ mg \times 20\ kg}{1\ day} = 400\ mg/day$$

STEP 7: Round, if necessary.

STEP 8: Reassess to determine whether the amount makes sense. If the prescription reads 20 mg/kg/day to divide equally every 12 hr and the preschooler weighs 20 kg, it makes sense to give 400 mg/day, or 200 mg every 12 hr.

Using Ratio and Proportion

STEP 9: What is the unit of measurement the nurse should calculate? mL

STEP 10: What is the dose the nurse should administer? Dose to administer = Desired = 200 mg

STEP 11: What is the dose available? Dose available = Have = 250 mg

STEP 12: Should the nurse convert the units of measurement? No

STEP 13: What is the quantity of the dose available? = Quantity = 5 mL

STEP 14: Set up the equation and solve for X.

$$\frac{Have}{Quantity} = \frac{Desired}{X} \qquad \frac{250\ mg}{5\ mL} \times \frac{200\ mg}{X\ mL}$$

$X = 4$

STEP 15: Round, if necessary.

STEP 16: Reassess to determine whether the amount to give makes sense. If there are 250 mg/5 mL and the prescription reads 200 mg, it makes sense to give 4 mL. The nurse should administer amoxicillin suspension 4 mL PO every 12 hr.

Using Desired Over Have

STEP 9: What is the unit of measurement the nurse should calculate? mL

STEP 10: What is the dose the nurse should administer? Dose to administer = Desired 200 mg

STEP 11: What is the dose available? Dose available = Have = 250 mg

STEP 12: Should the nurse convert the units of measurement? No

STEP 13: What is the quantity of the dose available? = Quantity = 5 mL

STEP 14: Set up an equation and solve for X.

$$\frac{Desired \times Quantity}{Have} = X \qquad \frac{200\ mg \times 5\ mL}{250\ mg} = X\ mL$$

$4 = X$

STEP 15: Round, if necessary.

STEP 16: Reassess to determine whether the amount to give makes sense. If there are 250 mg/5 mL and the prescription reads 200 mg, it makes sense to give 4 mL. The nurse should administer amoxicillin suspension 4 mL PO every 12 hr.

Using Dimensional Analysis

STEP 9: What is the unit of measurement the nurse should calculate? mL

STEP 10: What is the quantity of the dose available? = Quantity = 5 mL

STEP 11: What is the dose available? Dose available = Have = 250 mg

STEP 12: What is the dose the nurse should administer? Dose to administer = Desired = 200 mg

STEP 13: Should the nurse convert the units of measurement? No

STEP 14: Set up an equation and solve for X.

$$X = \frac{Quantity}{Have} \times \frac{Conversion\ (Have)}{Conversion\ (Desired)} \times Desired$$

$$X\ mL = \frac{5\ mL}{250\ mg} \times 200\ mg$$

$X = 4$

STEP 15: Round, if necessary.

STEP 16: Reassess to determine whether the amount to give makes sense. If there are 250 mg/5 mL and the prescription reads 200 mg, it makes sense to give 4 mL. The nurse should administer amoxicillin suspension 4 mL PO every 12 hr.

Ⓝ *NCLEX® Connection: Pharmacological and Parenteral Therapies, Dosage Calculation*

6. **0.8** mL

<table>
<tr><td>Using Ratio and Proportion</td><td>Using Desired Over Have</td><td>Using Dimensional Analysis</td></tr>
</table>

Using Ratio and Proportion

STEP 1: What is the unit of measurement the nurse should calculate?   mL

STEP 2: What is the dose the nurse should administer? Dose to administer = Desired = 15,000 units

STEP 3: What is the dose available? Dose available = Have = 20,000 units

STEP 4: Should the nurse convert the units of measurement?   No

STEP 5: What is the quantity of the dose available? = Quantity = 1 mL

STEP 6: Set up the equation and solve for X.

$$\frac{Have}{Quantity} = \frac{Desired}{X}$$

$$\frac{20{,}000\ units}{1\ mL} \times \frac{15{,}000\ units}{X\ mL}$$

$X = 0.75$

STEP 7: Round, if necessary.   0.75 = 0.8

STEP 8: Reassess to determine whether the amount to administer makes sense. If there are 20,000 units/mL and the prescription reads 15,000 units, it makes sense to administer 0.8 mL. The nurse should administer heparin injection 0.8 mL subcutaneously every 12 hr.

Using Desired Over Have

STEP 1: What is the unit of measurement the nurse should calculate?   mL

STEP 2: What is the dose the nurse should administer? Dose to administer = Desired = 15,000 units

STEP 3: What is the dose available? Dose available = Have = 20,000 units

STEP 4: Should the nurse convert the units of measurement?   No

STEP 5: What is the quantity of the dose available? = Quantity = 1 mL

STEP 6: Set up an equation and solve for X.

$$\frac{Desired \times Quantity}{Have} = X$$

$$\frac{15{,}000\ units \times 1\ mL}{20{,}000\ units} = X\ mL$$

$0.75 = X$

STEP 7: Round, if necessary.   0.75 = 0.8

STEP 8: Reassess to determine whether the amount to administer makes sense. If there are 10,000 units/mL and the prescription reads 8,000 units, it makes sense to administer 0.8 mL. The nurse should administer heparin injection 0.8 mL subcutaneously every 12 hr.

Using Dimensional Analysis

STEP 1: What is the unit of measurement the nurse should calculate?   mL

STEP 2: What is the quantity of the dose available? = Quantity = 1 mL

STEP 3: What is the dose available? Dose available = Have = 20,000 units

STEP 4: What is the dose the nurse should administer? Dose to administer = Desired = 15,000 units

STEP 5: Should the nurse convert the units of measurement?   No

STEP 6: Set up an equation and solve for X.

$$X = \frac{Quantity}{Have} \times \frac{Conversion\ (Have)}{Conversion\ (Desired)} \times Desired$$

$$X\ mL = \frac{1\ mL}{20{,}000\ units} \times 15{,}000\ units$$

$X = 0.75$

STEP 7: Round, if necessary.   0.75 = 0.8

STEP 8: Reassess to determine whether the amount to administer makes sense. If there are 10,000 units/mL and the prescription reads 8,000 units, it makes sense to administer 0.8 mL. The nurse should administer heparin injection 0.8 mL subcutaneously every 12 hr.

Ⓝ *NCLEX® Connection: Pharmacological and Parenteral Therapies, Dosage Calculation*

---

7. **6.5** mL

Using Ratio and Proportion

STEP 1: What is the unit of measurement the nurse should calculate?   mL

STEP 2: What is the dose the nurse should administer? Dose to administer = Desired = 650 mg

STEP 3: What is the dose available? Dose available = Have = 500 mg

STEP 4: Should the nurse convert the units of measurement?   No

STEP 5: What is the quantity of the dose available? = Quantity = 5 mL

STEP 6: Set up the equation and solve for X.

$$\frac{Have}{Quantity} = \frac{Desired}{X}$$

$$\frac{500\ mg}{5\ mL} \times \frac{650\ mg}{X\ mL}$$

$X = 6.5$

STEP 7: Round, if necessary.

STEP 8: Reassess to determine whether the amount to administer makes sense. If there are 500 mg/5 mL and the prescription reads 650 mg, it makes sense to administer 6.5 mL. The nurse should administer acetaminophen liquid 6.5 mL PO every 6 hr PRN for pain.

Using Desired Over Have

STEP 1: What is the unit of measurement the nurse should calculate?   mL

STEP 2: What is the dose the nurse should administer? Dose to administer = Desired = 650 mg

STEP 3: What is the dose available? Dose available = Have = 500 mg

STEP 4: Should the nurse convert the units of measurement?   No

STEP 5: What is the quantity of the dose available? = Quantity = 5 mL

STEP 6: Set up the equation and solve for X.

$$\frac{Desired \times Quantity}{Have} = X$$

$$\frac{650\ mg \times 5\ mL}{500\ mg} = X\ mL$$

$6.5 = X$

STEP 7: Round, if necessary.

STEP 8: Reassess to determine whether the amount to administer makes sense. If there are 500 mg/5 mL and the prescription reads 650 mg, it makes sense to administer 6.5 mL. The nurse should administer acetaminophen liquid 6.5 mL PO every 6 hr PRN for pain.

Using Dimensional Analysis

STEP 1: What is the unit of measurement the nurse should calculate?   mL

STEP 2: What is the quantity of the dose available? = Quantity = 5 mL

STEP 3: What is the dose available? Dose available = Have = 500 mg

STEP 4: What is the dose the nurse should administer? Dose to administer = Desired = 650 mg

STEP 5: Should the nurse convert the units of measurement?   No

STEP 6: Set up the equation and solve for X.

$$X = \frac{Quantity}{Have} \times \frac{Conversion\ (Have)}{Conversion\ (Desired)} \times Desired$$

$$X\ mL = \frac{5\ mL}{500\ mg} \times 650\ mg$$

$X = 6.5$

STEP 7: Round, if necessary.

STEP 8: Reassess to determine whether the amount to administer makes sense. If there are 500 mg/5 mL and the prescription reads 650 mg, it makes sense to administer 6.5 mL. The nurse should administer acetaminophen liquid 6.5 mL PO every 6 hr PRN for pain.

Ⓝ *NCLEX® Connection: Pharmacological and Parenteral Therapies, Dosage Calculation*

---

8. **125** mL/hr

STEP 1: What is the unit of measurement the nurse should calculate?   mL/hr

STEP 2: What is the volume the nurse should infuse?   750 mL

STEP 3: What is the total infusion time?   6 hr

STEP 4: Should the nurse convert the units of measurement?   No

STEP 5: Set up the equation and solve for X.

$$\frac{Volume\ (mL)}{Time\ (hr)} = X\ mL/hr \qquad \frac{750\ mL}{6\ hr} = X\ mL/hr$$

$125 = X$

STEP 6: Round, if necessary.

STEP 7: Reassess to determine whether the IV flow rate makes sense. If the prescription reads 750 mL to infuse over 6 hr, it makes sense to administer 125 mL/hr. The nurse should set the IV pump to deliver D₅W 750 mL IV at 125 mL/hr.

Ⓝ *NCLEX® Connection: Pharmacological and Parenteral Therapies, Parenteral/Intravenous Therapies*

CHAPTER 4

CHAPTER 4 *Intravenous Therapy*

Intravenous therapy involves administering fluids via an IV catheter to administer medications, supplement fluid intake, or give fluid replacement, electrolytes, or nutrients.

Nurses administer large-volume IV infusions on a continuous basis.

Nurses or pharmacists mix IV medication in a large volume of fluid to give as a continuous IV infusion or intermittently in a small amount of fluid. Nurses also administer medications as an IV bolus, giving the medication in a small amount of solution, concentrated or diluted, and injecting it over a short time (1 to 2 min or longer, depending on the medication).

DESCRIPTION OF PROCEDURE

The provider prescribes the type of IV fluid, the volume to infuse, and either the rate at which to infuse the IV fluid or the total amount of time it should take to infuse the fluid. The nurse regulates the IV infusion, either with an IV pump or manually, to be sure to deliver the right amount.

Nurses administer large-volume IV infusions on a continuous basis, such as 0.9% sodium chloride IV to infuse at 100 mL/hr or dextrose 5% in water 500 mL to infuse IV over 3 hr.

A fluid bolus is a large amount of IV fluid to give in a short time, usually less than 1 hr. It rapidly replaces fluid loss from dehydration, shock, hemorrhage, burns, or trauma.

A large-gauge IV catheter (18-gauge or larger) is essential for maintaining the rapid rate necessary to give a fluid bolus to an adult.

ADVANTAGES

- Rapid effects
- Precise amounts
- Less discomfort after initial insertion
- Constant therapeutic blood levels
- Less irritation to subcutaneous and muscle tissue

DISADVANTAGES

- Circulatory fluid overload is possible if the infusion is large or too rapid.
- Immediate absorption leaves little time to correct errors.
- IV fluid administration can irritate the lining of the vein.
- Failure to maintain surgical asepsis can lead to local and systemic infection.

WAYS TO ADMINISTER IV MEDICATIONS

Give the medication the pharmacist mixed in a large volume of fluid (500 to 1,000 mL) as a continuous IV infusion, such as potassium chloride and vitamins.

Deliver the medication in premixed solution bags from the medication's manufacturer.

Administer volume-controlled infusions.
- Give some medications, such as antibiotics, intermittently in a small amount of solution (25 to 250 mL) through a continuous IV fluid system or with saline or heparin lock systems.
- Infusing the medications for short periods of time and on a schedule
- Use a secondary ("piggyback") IV bag or bottle or tandem setup, a volume-control administration set, or a mini-infusion pump.

Give an IV bolus dose.
- Inject the medications in small amounts of solution, concentrated or diluted, over a short time (1 to 2 min or longer, depending on the medication).
- Administer medications directly into the peripheral IV or access port to achieve an immediate medication level in the bloodstream, such as with pain medication.
- Prepare medications in the correct concentration and at a safe rate (amount of medication per minute).
- Use extreme caution and observing for adverse reactions or complications (redness, burning, swelling, increasing pain) that indicate phlebitis, infiltration, or extravasation.

TYPES OF IV ACCESS

Peripheral vein via a catheter

Jugular or subclavian vein via a central venous access device through venipuncture (such as a peripherally inserted central catheter, or PICC), or by surgical intervention with implantation of access ports for long-term use

CONSIDERATIONS

PREPROCEDURE

EQUIPMENT

- Correct size catheter
  - 16-gauge for clients who have trauma, rapid fluid volume
  - 18- to 20-gauge for clients who are having surgery, rapid blood administration
  - 22- to 24-gauge for other clients (adults)
- Tubing
- Infusion pump
- Clean gloves
- Scissors or electric shaver for hair removal

NURSING ACTIONS

- Check the prescription (solution, rate).
- Assess for allergies to latex, tape, or iodine.
- Follow the rights of medication administration (including compatibilities of all IV solutions).
- Perform hand hygiene.
- Examine the IV solution for clarity, leaks, and expiration date.
- Prime the tubing.
- Don clean gloves before insertion.
- Assess extremities and veins.
- Clip hair at and around the insertion site with scissors or shave it with an electric shaver.

CLIENT EDUCATION

- Identify the client and explain the procedure.
- Place the client in a comfortable position.

INTRAPROCEDURE

NURSING ACTIONS

- **Select the vein by choosing**
  - Distal veins first on the nondominant hand
  - A site that is not painful or bruised and will not interfere with activity
  - A vein that is resilient and has a soft, bouncy feeling
- **Document in client's medical record**
  - Date and time of insertion
  - Insertion site and appearance
  - Catheter size
  - Type of dressing
  - IV fluid and rate
  - Number, locations, and conditions of previously attempted catheterizations
  - The client's response

  Sample documentation: 1/16/2016, 1423, Inserted 22-gauge IV catheter into right wrist cephalic vein (one attempt); applied sterile occlusive dressing. IV lactated Ringer's infusing at 100 mL/hr per infusion pump without redness or edema at the site. Tolerated without complications. L. Turner, RN

- Be sure to document thoroughly and accurately throughout the client's course of IV therapy.

POSTPROCEDURE

NURSING ACTIONS: Maintain the patency of IV access.

- Do not stop a continuous infusion or allow blood to back up into the catheter for any length of time. Clots can form at the tip of the needle or catheter and can lodge against the vein's wall, blocking the flow of fluid.
- Instruct clients not to manipulate flow rate device, change settings on IV pump, or lie on the tubing.
- Make sure the IV insertion site's dressing is not too tight.
- Flush intermittent IV catheters with the solution the facility specifies after every medication administration or every 8 to 12 hr when not in use.
- Monitor the site and infusion rate at least every hour.

GUIDELINES FOR SAFE IV MEDICATION ADMINISTRATION

- Use an infusion pump to administer medications, such as potassium chloride, that can cause serious adverse reactions. Never administer them by IV bolus. Double-check not only the dose of potassium the provider prescribed, but also the correct dilution or amount of fluid.
- Add medications to a new IV fluid container, not to an IV container that is already hanging.
- Never administer IV medications through tubing that is infusing blood, blood products, or parenteral nutrition solutions.
- Verify the compatibility of medications with IV solutions before infusing a medication through tubing that is infusing an IV solution.

Needlestick prevention

- Be familiar with IV insertion equipment.
- Do not use needles when needleless systems are available.
- Use protective safety devices when available.
- Dispose of needles immediately in designated puncture-resistant receptacles.
- Do not break, bend, or recap needles.

Specific considerations

- Older adult clients, clients who are taking anticoagulants, and clients who have fragile veins ⓖ
  - Avoid tourniquets. Use a blood pressure cuff to help visualize, but not overdistend, the veins to help prevent hematoma formation.
  - Do not slap the extremity to visualize veins.
  - Instruct the client to hold his hand below the level of his heart to help distend and thus visualize the veins.
  - Avoid using the back of the client's hand.
  - Avoid rigorous friction while cleaning the site.
- Edema in extremities
  - Apply digital pressure over the selected vein to displace edema.
  - Apply pressure with an alcohol pad.
  - Cannulate the vein quickly.
- Obese clients
- Use anatomical landmarks to find veins.

Preventing IV infections Qs

- Use standard precautions.
- Perform hand hygiene before and after handling IV systems.
- Change IV sites according to facility policy (usually 72 hr).
- Replace continuous and intermittent infusion tubing according to facility policy (usually every 24 or 48 hr).
- Remove catheters as soon as there is no clinical need for them.
- Replace catheters when suspecting any break in surgical aseptic technique, such as during emergency insertions.
- Use a sterile needle or catheter for each insertion attempt.
- Avoid writing on IV bags with pens or markers, because ink could seep through the bag and contaminate the solution.
- Replace the tubing immediately for potential or actual contamination.
- Do not allow fluids to hang for more than 24 hr unless it is a closed system (pressure bags for hemodynamic monitoring).
- Wipe all ports with alcohol or an antiseptic swab before connecting IV lines or inserting a syringe to prevent the introduction of micro-organisms into the system.
- Never disconnect tubing for convenience or to reposition the client.
- Do not allow ports to remain exposed to air.

COMPLICATIONS

Complications require notification of the provider and complete documentation. Use new tubing and catheters for restarting IV infusions after detecting complications.

Infiltration (infiltration of a nonvesicant solution)

FINDINGS: Pallor, local swelling at the site, decreased skin temperature around the site, damp dressing, slowed infusion

TREATMENT
- Stop the infusion and remove the catheter.
- Elevate the extremity.
- Encourage active range of motion.
- Apply a cold or warm compress depending on the type of solution that infiltrated the tissue.
- Check with the provider to determine whether the client still needs IV therapy. If so, restart the infusion proximal to the site or in another extremity.

PREVENTION
- Carefully select the site and catheter.
- Secure the catheter.

Extravasation (infiltration of a vesicant or tissue-damaging medication)

FINDINGS: Pain, burning, redness, swelling

TREATMENT
- Stop the infusion and notify the provider.
- Follow the facility's protocol, which may include infusing an antidote through the catheter before removal.

PREVENTION
- Closely monitor the IV site and dressing.
- Always use an infusion pump.

Hematoma

FINDINGS: Ecchymosis at the site

TREATMENT
- Do not apply alcohol.
- Apply pressure after IV catheter removal.
- Use a warm compress and elevation after bleeding stops.

PREVENTION
- Minimize tourniquet time.
- Remove the tourniquet before starting the IV infusion.
- Maintain pressure after IV catheter removal.

Catheter embolus

FINDINGS
- Missing catheter tip after discontinuation
- Severe pain at the site with migration, no symptoms if no migration

TREATMENT
- Place a tourniquet high on the extremity to limit venous flow.
- Prepare for removal under x-ray or via surgery.
- Save the catheter after removal to determine the cause.

PREVENTION: Do not reinsert the stylet needle into the catheter.

Phlebitis/thrombophlebitis

FINDINGS: Edema; throbbing, burning, or pain at the site; increased skin temperature; erythema; a red line up the arm with a palpable band at the vein site; slowed infusion

TREATMENT
- Promptly discontinue the infusion and remove the catheter.
- Elevate the extremity.
- Apply a cold compress to minimize the flow of blood, then apply a warm compress to increase circulation.
- Check with the provider to determine whether the client still needs IV therapy. If so, restart the infusion proximal to the site or in another extremity.
- Obtain a specimen for culture at the site and prepare the catheter for culture if drainage is present.

PREVENTION
- Rotate sites at least every 72 hr or sooner according to facility policy.
- Assess IV sites using a phlebitis scale.
- Avoid the lower extremities.
- Use hand hygiene.
- Use surgical aseptic technique.

Cellulitis

FINDINGS: Pain, warmth, edema, induration, red streaking, fever, chills, malaise

TREATMENT

- Promptly discontinue the infusion and remove the catheter.
- Elevate the extremity.
- Apply warm compresses three to four times/day.
- Obtain a specimen for culture at the site and prepare the catheter for culture if drainage is present.
- Administer:
  - Antibiotics
  - Analgesics
  - Antipyretics

PREVENTION

- Rotate sites at least every 72 hr or sooner according to the facility's policy.
- Avoid the lower extremities.
- Use hand hygiene.
- Use surgical aseptic technique.

Fluid overload

FINDINGS: Distended neck veins, increased blood pressure, tachycardia, shortness of breath, crackles in the lungs, edema, additional findings varying with the IV solution

TREATMENT

- Slow the IV rate or stop the infusion.
- Raise the head of the bed.
- Assess vital signs and oxygen saturation.
- Adjust the rate after correcting fluid overload.
- Anticipate administering diuretics.

PREVENTION

- Use an infusion pump.
- Monitor I&O.

Application Exercises

1. A nurse is assessing a client's IV infusion site. Which of the following findings should the nurse identify as an indication of phlebitis? (Select all that apply.)

   A. Pallor

   B. Dampness

   C. Erythema

   D. Coolness

   E. Pain

2. A nurse manager is reviewing the facility's policies for IV therapy with the members of his team. The nurse manager should remind the team that which of the following techniques helps minimize the risk of catheter embolism?

   A. Performing hand hygiene before and after IV insertion

   B. Rotating IV sites at least every 72 hr

   C. Minimizing tourniquet time

   D. Avoiding reinserting the needle into an IV catheter

3. A nurse is preparing to initiate IV therapy for an older adult client. Which of the following actions should the nurse plan to take?

   A. Use a disposable razor to remove excess hair on the extremity.

   B. Select the back of the client's hand to insert the IV catheter.

   C. Distend the veins by using a blood pressure cuff.

   D. Direct the client to raise his arm above his heart.

4. A nurse assessing a client's IV catheter insertion site notes a hematoma. Which of the following actions should the nurse take? (Select all that apply.)

   A. Stop the infusion.

   B. Apply alcohol to the insertion site.

   C. Apply warm compresses to the insertion site

   D. Elevate the client's arm.

   E. Obtain a specimen for culture at the insertion site.

PRACTICE Active Learning Scenario

A nurse on a medical-surgical unit is providing care for a group of clients who are receiving IV therapy. The nurse is assessing the clients for complications. Use the ATI Active Learning Template: Nursing Skill to complete this item.

INDICATIONS: Identify three indications for IV therapy.

POTENTIAL COMPLICATIONS: Identify four potential complications of IV therapy.

Application Exercises Key

1. A. Pallor at the insertion site is a manifestation of infiltration.

    B. Dampness at the insertion site indicates fluid leakage, which is a typical finding with infiltration.

    C. **CORRECT:** Erythema at the insertion site is a manifestation of phlebitis.

    D. Coolness at the insertion site is a manifestation of infiltration.

    E. **CORRECT:** Pain at the insertion site is a manifestation of phlebitis.

    Ⓝ NCLEX® Connection: Pharmacological and Parenteral Therapies, Parenteral/Intravenous Therapies

2. A. The nurse manager should remind the members of the team to perform hand hygiene to prevent infection, but this technique does not reduce the risk of catheter embolism.

    B. The nurse manager should remind the members of the team to rotate IV sites at least every 72 hr to help prevent phlebitis, but this technique does not minimize the risk of catheter embolism.

    C. The nurse manager should remind the members of the team to minimize tourniquet time, but this technique does not reduce the risk of catheter embolism.

    D. **CORRECT:** The nurse manager should remind the members of the team to avoid reinserting the stylet needle into an IV catheter. This action can result in severing the end of the catheter and consequently cause a catheter embolism.

    Ⓝ NCLEX® Connection: Pharmacological and Parenteral Therapies, Parenteral/Intravenous Therapies

3. A. The nurse should remove excess hair by clipping it with scissors. Shaving with a disposable razor can cause skin damage that can lead to infection.

    B. In most instances, the nurse inserts the IV catheter into a distal site, such as the back of the client's hand. However, when inserting an IV catheter for an older adult, the nurse should select a site on the arm because older adults typically have fragile veins in the back of their hands.

    C. **CORRECT:** The nurse should distend the veins using a blood pressure cuff to reduce overfilling of the vein, which can result in a hematoma.

    D. The nurse should direct the client to hold his arm below the level of his heart to distend the vein.

    Ⓝ NCLEX® Connection: Pharmacological and Parenteral Therapies, Parenteral/Intravenous Therapies

4. A. Hematoma formation is generally the result of an injury to blood vessels on insertion of an IV catheter. It does not affect the patency of the line or cause further injury unless the hematoma is expanding, so it is not necessary to stop the infusion. However, it is necessary to stop the bleeding if it is expanding.

    B. The nurse should not apply alcohol to the insertion site because it can be uncomfortable for the client and can increase capillary bleeding.

    C. **CORRECT:** Warm compresses can help promote healing of a hematoma.

    D. **CORRECT:** Elevation of the arm helps reduce edema, which can cause pressure and pain and additional bleeding in the area of the hematoma.

    E. A hematoma is not a result of infection, nor does it increase the risk for infection. Cultures are unnecessary.

    Ⓝ NCLEX® Connection: Pharmacological and Parenteral Therapies, Parenteral/Intravenous Therapies

PRACTICE Answer

Using the ATI Active Learning Template: Nursing Skill

INDICATIONS
- To administer medications
- To supplement fluid intake
- To replace electrolytes and nutrients

Ⓝ NCLEX® Connection: Pharmacological and Parenteral Therapies, Parenteral/Intravenous Therapies

POTENTIAL COMPLICATIONS
- Infiltration
- Extravasation
- Cellulitis
- Fluid overload
- Catheter embolus
- Hematoma
- Phlebitis, thrombophlebitis

UNIT 1 PHARMACOLOGICAL PRINCIPLES

CHAPTER 5 *Adverse Effects, Interactions, and Contraindications*

To ensure safe medication administration and prevent errors, the nurse must know why a medication is prescribed and its intended therapeutic effect. In addition, the nurse must be aware of potential side/adverse effects, interactions, contraindications, and precautions.

Every medication has the potential to cause side and adverse effects. Side effects occur when the medication is given at a therapeutic dose. Discontinuation of the medication is usually not warranted. Adverse effects are undesired, inadvertent, and unexpected severe responses to the medication. Adverse effects can occur at both therapeutic and higher-than-therapeutic doses. Providers will discontinue the medication immediately. Adverse effects are reported to the FDA using the MedWatch program.

Medications are chemicals that affect the body. When more than one medication is given, there is a potential for an interaction. In addition, medications can interact with foods, herbal medicines, or other unconventional remedies.

Contraindications and precautions of specific medications refer to client conditions that make it unsafe or potentially harmful to administer these medications.

Response to medications differs for individuals based on multiple factors, such as age, sex, disease process, and ethnic/genetic variations. These factors can be responsible for many expected and unexpected adverse effects.

ADVERSE MEDICATION EFFECTS

These effects can be classified according to body systems.

Central nervous system

Can result from central nervous system (CNS) stimulation (excitement) or CNS depression

NURSING CONSIDERATIONS
- If CNS stimulation is expected, clients can be at risk for seizures, and precautions should be taken.
- If CNS depression is likely, advise clients not to drive or participate in other activities that can be dangerous. Qs

Anticholinergic

- Effects that are a result of muscarinic receptor blockade.
- Most are seen in eyes, smooth muscle, exocrine glands, and the heart.

CLIENT EDUCATION: Teach clients how to manage these effects to minimize danger and discomfort.

> For example, dry mouth can be relieved by sipping on liquids; photophobia can be managed by use of sunglasses; and urinary retention can be reduced by urinating before taking the medication.

Cardiovascular

- Can involve blood vessels and the heart.
- Antihypertensives can cause orthostatic hypotension.

CLIENT EDUCATION: Instruct clients about signs of postural hypotension (lightheadedness, dizziness). If these occur, advise clients to sit or lie down. Postural hypotension can be minimized by getting up and changing position slowly.

Gastrointestinal (GI)

- Can result from local irritation of the GI tract.
- Stimulation of the vomiting center also results in adverse effects.

NURSING CONSIDERATIONS
- NSAIDs can cause GI upset. Advise clients to take these medications with food.
- Opioid analgesics slow peristalsis and can cause nausea and sedation. Advise clients taking opioids about methods to avoid constipation and GI irritation, and promote safety.

Hematologic

Relatively common and potentially life-threatening with some groups of medications.

NURSING CONSIDERATIONS: Bone marrow depression/suppression is generally associated with anticancer medications and hemorrhagic disorders with anticoagulants and thrombolytics.

CLIENT EDUCATION: Educate clients taking anticoagulants about bleeding (bruising, discolored urine/stool, petechiae, bleeding gums). Tell clients to notify the provider if these effects occur.

TOXICITY

- An adverse medication effect that is considered severe and can be life-threatening.
- It can be caused by an excessive dose, but it also can occur at therapeutic dose levels.

NURSING CONSIDERATIONS: Liver damage will occur with an acetaminophen (overdose. There is a greater risk of liver damage with chronic alcohol use. The antidote acetylcysteine (can be used to minimize liver damage.

Hepatotoxicity

- Can occur with many medications.
- Because most medications are metabolized in the liver, the liver is particularly vulnerable to drug-induced injury.
- Damage to liver cells can impair metabolism of many medications, causing medication accumulation in the body and producing adverse effects.
- Many medications can alter normal values of liver function tests with no obvious clinical signs of liver dysfunction.

NURSING CONSIDERATIONS

- When two or more medications that are hepatotoxic are combined, the risk for liver damage is increased.
- Liver function tests are indicated when clients start a medication known to be hepatotoxic and periodically thereafter.
- Monitor clients for manifestations of hepatotoxicity, such as nausea, vomiting, jaundice, dark urine, abdominal discomfort, and anorexia. Advise clients to monitor for these symptoms.

Nephrotoxicity

- Can occur with a number of medications, but it is primarily the result of certain antimicrobial agents and NSAIDs.
- Damage to the kidneys can interfere with medication excretion, leading to medication accumulation and adverse effects.

NURSING CONSIDERATIONS: Aminoglycosides injure cells in the renal tubules of the kidney. Monitor serum creatinine and BUN, as well as peak and trough medication levels for clients taking medication that is nephrotoxic.

ALLERGIC REACTION

- Occurs when an individual develops an immune response to a medication.
- The individual has been previously exposed to the medication and has developed antibodies.

NURSING CONSIDERATIONS

- Allergic reactions range from minor to serious. Mild rashes and hives can be treated with diphenhydramine
- Before administering any medications, obtain a complete medication history.

Anaphylactic reaction

A life-threatening, immediate allergic reaction that causes respiratory distress, severe bronchospasm, laryngeal edema, a quick drop in blood pressure, as well as cardiovascular collapse.

NURSING CONSIDERATIONS: Treat with epinephrine, bronchodilators, and antihistamines. Provide respiratory support, and inform the provider.

EXTRAPYRAMIDAL SYMPTOMS (EPSs)

- Abnormal body movements that can include involuntary fine-motor tremors, rigidity, uncontrollable restlessness, and acute dystonias (spastic movements and/or muscle rigidity affecting the head, neck, eyes, face, tongue, back, and limbs)
- Can occur within a few hours or take months to develop

NURSING CONSIDERATIONS

- EPSs are more often associated with medications affecting the CNS, such as those used to treat mental health disorders.
- Most EPSs can be treated with anticholinergic medications.

IMMUNOSUPPRESSION

Decreased or absent immune response.

NURSING CONSIDERATIONS

- Immunosuppressant medications, such as glucocorticoids, can mask the usual manifestations of infection, such as fever.
- Monitor clients taking an immunosuppressant, such as a glucocorticoid, for delayed wound healing and subtle manifestations of infection, such as sore throat.

CLIENT EDUCATION: Advise clients who take an immunosuppressant to avoid contact with anyone who has a communicable disease.

INTERACTIONS

DRUG-DRUG INTERACTIONS

Increased therapeutic effects

NURSING CONSIDERATIONS: Some medications can be given together to potentiate their action and increase therapeutic effects.

CLIENTS EDUCATION: Instruct clients who have asthma to use albuterol, a beta$_2$-adrenergic agonist inhaler, 5 min prior to using triamcinolone acetonide, a glucocorticoid inhaler, to increase the absorption of triamcinolone acetonide.

Increased adverse effects

NURSING CONSIDERATIONS: Clients can take two medications that have the same side/adverse effect. Taking these medications together increases the risk of potentiating these side effects. Diazepam and hydrocodone bitartrate 5 mg/acetaminophen 500 mg both have CNS depressant effects. When these medications are used together, clients have an increased risk for CNS depression.

Decreased therapeutic effects

NURSING CONSIDERATIONS: One medication can increase the metabolism or block the effects of a second medication and therefore decrease the serum level and effectiveness of the second medication.

> For example: Phenytoin increases hepatic medication-metabolizing enzymes that affect warfarin and thereby decreases the serum level and the effect of warfarin.

Decreased side/adverse effects

NURSING CONSIDERATIONS: One medication can be given to counteract the side/adverse effects of another medication. Ondansetron hydrochloride, an antiemetic, can be administered to counteract the side effects of nausea and vomiting for clients receiving chemotherapy.

Increased serum levels, leading to toxicity

NURSING CONSIDERATIONS: One medication can decrease the metabolism of a second medication and therefore increase the serum level of the second medication. This can lead to toxicity. Fluconazole inhibits hepatic medication-metabolizing enzymes that affect aripiprazole and thereby increases serum levels of this medication.

5.1 Over-the-counter (OTC) medication interactions

INTERACTIONS

Ingredients in OTC medications herbal supplements) can interact with other OTC or prescription medications.

Inactive ingredients, such as dyes, alcohol, or preservatives, can cause adverse reactions.

Potential for overdose exists because of the use of several preparations (including prescription medications and herbal supplements) with similar ingredients.

NURSING IMPLICATIONS

Obtain a complete medication history.

Instruct clients to follow the manufacturer's recommendation for dosage.

INTERACTION

Interactions of certain prescription and OTC medications can interfere with therapeutic effects.

NURSING IMPLICATIONS: Advise clients to use caution and to check with the provider before using any OTC preparations such as antacids, laxatives, decongestants, herbal supplements, or cough syrups. For example, antacids can interfere with the absorption of ranitidine) and other medications. Advise clients to take antacids 1 hr apart from other medications.

MEDICATION-FOOD INTERACTIONS

Food can alter medication absorption and/or can contain substances that react with certain medications.

EXAMPLES

- Consuming foods with tyramine while taking monoamine oxidase inhibitors (MAOIs) can lead to hypertensive crisis. Clients taking MAOIs should be aware of foods containing tyramine, such as cheese and processed meats, and avoid them.
- Vitamin K can decrease the therapeutic effects of warfarin (and place clients at risk for developing blood clots. Clients taking warfarin should include a consistent amount of vitamin K in their diet.
- Tetracycline can interact with a chelating agent, such as milk, and form an insoluble, unabsorbable compound. Instruct clients not to take tetracycline within 2 hr of consuming dairy products.
- Grapefruit juice seems to act by inhibiting medication metabolism in the small bowel, thus increasing the amount of medication available for absorption of certain oral medications. This increases either the therapeutic effects or the adverse reactions. Instruct clients to not drink grapefruit juice if they are taking such a medication. Q_{EBP}
- Food often decreases the rate of medication absorption. However, some foods increase the rate of absorption of certain medications.

CONTRAINDICATIONS AND PRECAUTIONS

- A specific medication can be contraindicated for a client based on the client's condition. For example, penicillins are contraindicated for a client who has an allergy to this medication.
- Precautions should be taken for a client who is more likely to have an adverse reaction than another client.

> Morphine depresses respiratory function, so it should be used with caution for clients who have asthma or impaired respiratory function.

CATEGORIES

The U.S. Food and Drug Administration places medications in categories based on risk to a fetus.

CATEGORY A: There is no evidence of risk to fetus during pregnancy based on adequate and well-controlled studies.

CATEGORY B: There is no evidence of risk to animal fetuses based on studies, but there are no adequate and well-controlled studies in pregnant women

CATEGORY C: Adverse effects have been demonstrated on animal fetuses. There are no adequate and well-controlled studies in pregnant women, but use of the medication during pregnancy can be warranted based on the potential benefits.

CATEGORY D: Adverse effects have been demonstrated on human fetuses based on data from investigational or marketing experience, but use of the medication during pregnancy can be warranted based on the potential benefits.

CATEGORY X: Adverse effects have been demonstrated on animal and human fetuses based on studies and data from investigational or marketing experience. The use of the medication is contraindicated during pregnancy because the risks outweigh the potential benefits.

Application Exercises

1. A nurse in a clinic is caring for a group of clients. The nurse should contact the provider about a potential contraindication to a medication for which of the following clients? (Select all that apply.)

    A. A client at 8 weeks of gestation who asks for an influenza immunization

    B. A client who takes prednisone and has a possible fungal infection

    C. A client who has chronic liver disease and is taking hydrocodone/acetaminophen

    D. A client who has peptic ulcer disease, takes sucralfate, and tells the nurse she has started taking OTC aluminum hydroxide

    E. A client who has a prosthetic heart valve, takes warfarin, and reports a suspected pregnancy

2. A nurse is preparing to administer an IM dose of penicillin to a client who has a new prescription. The client states she took penicillin 3 years ago and developed a rash. Which of the following actions should the nurse take?

    A. Administer the prescribed dose.

    B. Withhold the medication.

    C. Ask the provider to change the prescription to an oral form.

    D. Administer an oral antihistamine at the same time.

3. A nurse is providing discharge instructions for a client who has a new prescription for an antihypertensive medication. Which of the following statements should the nurse give?

    A. "Be sure to limit your potassium intake while taking the medication."

    B. "You should check your blood pressure every 8 hours while taking this medication."

    C. "Your medication dosage will be increased if you develop tachycardia."

    D. "Change positions slowly when you move from sitting to standing."

4. A nurse is reviewing a client's health record and notes that the client experiences permanent extrapyramidal effects caused by a previous medication. The nurse should recognize that the medication affected which of the following systems in the client?

    A. Cardiovascular

    B. Immune

    C. Central nervous

    D. Gastrointestinal

5. A nurse is caring for a client who is taking oral oxycodone The client states he is also taking ibuprofen in three recommended doses daily. The nurse should identify that an interaction between these two medications will cause which of the following findings?

    A. A decrease in serum levels of ibuprofen, possibly leading to a need for increased doses of this medication

    B. A decrease in serum levels of oxycodone, possibly leading to a need for increased doses of this medication

    C. An increase in the expected therapeutic effect of both medications

    D. An increase in expected adverse effects for both medications

---

PRACTICE Active Learning Scenario

A nurse is planning care for an older adult client who is receiving gentamicin IV bolus twice daily. The client has a history of musculoskeletal pain and takes naproxen daily for relief. What information should the nurse include in the client's plan of care? Use the ATI Active Learning Template: Medication to complete this item.

THERAPEUTIC USES: Describe the use of gentamicin.

COMPLICATIONS: Describe two adverse effects.

NURSING INTERVENTIONS:
• Describe two laboratory findings to monitor.
• Describe two nursing actions.

Application Exercises Key

1. A. The influenza vaccine is recommended for all clients older than 6 months of age and is not contraindicated for pregnant women.

    B. **CORRECT:** Glucocorticoids should not be taken by a client who has a possible systemic fungal infection. The nurse should recognize a contraindication and notify the provider.

    C. **CORRECT:** Acetaminophen is contraindicated due to toxicity for a client who has a liver disorder. The nurse should notify the provider, who can prescribe a medication that does not contain acetaminophen.

    D. There is no contraindication for a client who has peptic ulcer disease and takes sucralfate and also starts taking OTC aluminum hydroxide. The nurse should ensure that the client takes the two medications 30 min apart and verify that the provider knows what medications the client is taking.

    E. **CORRECT:** Warfarin is a Pregnancy Category X medication, which can cause severe birth defects to the fetus. The nurse should notify the provider about the suspected pregnancy.

    Ⓝ *NCLEX® Connection: Pharmacological and Parenteral Therapies, Adverse Effects/Contraindications/Side Effects/Interactions*

2. A. Administering the intramuscular penicillin in the prescribed dosage could cause a severe reaction and is not the appropriate action.

    B. **CORRECT:** The nurse should withhold the medication and notify the provider of the client's previous reaction to penicillin so that an alternative antibiotic can be prescribed. Allergic reactions to penicillin can range from mild to severe anaphylaxis, and prior sensitization should be reported to the provider.

    C. Administering the penicillin orally rather than intramuscularly would not prevent a reaction and is not the appropriate nursing action.

    D. Giving the penicillin along with an oral antihistamine would not prevent a reaction from occurring and is not the appropriate nursing action.

    Ⓝ *NCLEX® Connection: Pharmacological and Parenteral Therapies, Adverse Effects/Contraindications/Side Effects/Interactions*

3. A. Potassium can lower blood pressure, so clients who have hypertension should eat plenty of fruits and vegetables.

    B. Clients should check their blood pressure daily on a regular basis when taking an antihypertensive medication, but every 8 hr is unnecessary.

    C. Tachycardia is an adverse effect that would not warrant an increase in a dose of medication.

    D. **CORRECT:** Orthostatic hypotension is a common adverse effect of antihypertensive medications. The client should move slowly to a sitting or standing position and should be taught to sit or lie down if lightheadedness or dizziness occurs.

    Ⓝ *NCLEX® Connection: Pharmacological and Parenteral Therapies, Adverse Effects/Contraindications/Side Effects/Interactions*

4. A. Medications affecting the cardiovascular system generally do not cause extrapyramidal effects.

    B. Medications affecting the immune system generally do not cause extrapyramidal effects.

    C. **CORRECT:** The nurse should realize that extrapyramidal effects are movement disorders that can be caused by a number of central nervous system medications, such as typical antipsychotic medications.

    D. Medications affecting the gastrointestinal system generally do not cause extrapyramidal effects.

    Ⓝ *NCLEX® Connection: Pharmacological and Parenteral Therapies, Adverse Effects/Contraindications/Side Effects/Interactions*

5. A. Taking these medications together does not cause a decrease in serum levels of ibuprofen.

    B. Taking these medications together does not cause a decrease in serum levels of oxycodone.

    C. **CORRECT:** These medications work together to increase the pain-relieving effects of both medications. Oxycodone is a narcotic analgesic, and ibuprofen is an NSAID. They work by different mechanisms, but pain is better relieved when they are taken together.

    D. Adverse effects of oxycodone and ibuprofen are not increased when the medications are taken together.

    Ⓝ *NCLEX® Connection: Pharmacological and Parenteral Therapies, Adverse Effects/Contraindications/Side Effects/Interactions*

PRACTICE Answer

Using the ATI Active Learning Template: Medication

THERAPEUTIC USES: Gentamicin is a narrow-spectrum aminoglycoside antibiotic prescribed to treat serious infections caused by aerobic bacilli.

COMPLICATIONS
- Gentamicin can injure cells of the proximal renal tubules.
- Naproxen and other NSAIDs can cause renal insufficiency.
- The glomerular filtration rate of the kidneys decreases with advanced age, making this client at increased risk for nephrotoxicity.

NURSING INTERVENTIONS
- Laboratory Findings to Monitor
  ○ BUN
  ○ Serum creatinine
  ○ Peak and trough levels of gentamicin
  ○ Specific gravity of urine
  ○ Urinalysis
- Nursing Actions
  ○ Monitor intake and output.
  ○ Notify the provider of low urinary output.
  ○ Ensure that the client is adequately hydrated, and monitor for fluid overload.
  ○ Assess for manifestations of ototoxicity.

Ⓝ *NCLEX® Connection: Pharmacological and Parenteral Therapies, Adverse Effects/Contraindications/Side Effects Interactions*

UNIT 1   PHARMACOLOGICAL PRINCIPLES

CHAPTER 6 *Individual Considerations of Medication Administration*

Various factors affect how clients respond to medications. It is important for nurses to identify these factors to help them individualize nursing care when administering medications. Qᴘᴄᴄ

FACTORS AFFECTING MEDICATION DOSAGES AND RESPONSES

Body weight: Because body tissues absorb medications, individuals who have a greater body mass require larger doses. Because the percentage of body fat an individual has can alter the distribution of a medication, basing dosages on body surface area can be a more precise method of regulating an individual's response to a medication.

Age: Young children who have immature liver and kidney function, and older adults, often with reduced liver and kidney function, require proportionately smaller medication doses to compensate for their heightened sensitivities to medications. Ⓖ

Gender: Women respond differently to medications than men due to a higher proportion of body fat and the effects of female hormones.

Genetics: Genetic factors such as missing enzymes can alter the metabolism of certain medications, thus enhancing or reducing a medication's action. The usual effect is either fewer benefits from the medication or greater medication toxicity.

Biorhythmic cycles: Responses to some medications vary with the biologic rhythms of the body. For example, hypnotic medications work better when given at the usual sleep time than at other times.

Tolerance
- Reduced responsiveness to a medication clients take over time, such as morphine, is pharmacodynamic tolerance. Other medications, such as barbiturates, cause metabolic tolerance as metabolism of the medication increases over time and the effectiveness of the medication declines.
- Some clients develop cross-tolerance to another medication after they have become tolerant to a chemically similar medication.

Accumulation: Medication concentration in the body increases due to the inability to metabolize or excrete a medication rapidly enough, resulting in a toxic medication effect. For older adults, decreased kidney and liver function are the major causes of medication accumulation leading to toxicity. Ⓖ

Psychological factors: Emotional state and expectations can influence the effects of a medication. The placebo effect describes positive medication effects that psychological factors, not biochemical properties of the medication, influence.

Diet: Inadequate nutrition, such as starvation, can affect the protein-binding response of medications and subsequently increase the medication's response.

Medical problems
- Inadequate gastric acid inhibits the absorption of medications that require an acid medium to dissolve.
- Diarrhea causes oral medications to pass too quickly through the gastrointestinal tract for adequate absorption.
- Vascular insufficiency prevents distribution of a medication to affected tissue.
- Liver disease or failure impairs medication metabolism, which can cause toxicity.
- Kidney disease or failure prevents or delays medication excretion, which can cause toxicity.
- Prolonged gastric emptying time delays the absorption of medications in the intestines.

PHARMACOLOGY AND CHILDREN

Although most medications adults take are useful for children, the dosages are different. Providers base pediatric dosages on body weight or body surface area (BSA). Newborns and infants have immature liver and kidney function, alkaline gastric juices, and an immature blood-brain barrier, making them especially sensitive to medications that affect the CNS. Providers base some medication dosages on age due to a greater risk for decreased skeletal bone growth, acute cardiopulmonary failure, and hepatic toxicity.

ADDITIONAL PHARMACOKINETIC FACTORS SPECIFIC TO CHILDREN
- Decreased gastric acid production and slower gastric emptying time
- Decreased first-pass medication metabolism
- Increased absorption of topical medications (greater blood flow to the skin and thinner skin)
- Lower blood pressure (more blood flow to the liver and brain and less blood flow to the kidneys)
- Higher body water content (dilutes water-soluble medications)
- Decreased serum protein-binding sites (until 1 year of age). This can result in an increase in the serum level of protein-binding medications.
- Increased effects on the CNS system because the blood-brain barrier is not fully developed at birth
- Varying minimum effective concentration levels with IV and subcutaneous administration

NURSING CONSIDERATIONS WHEN ADMINISTERING MEDICATIONS TO CHILDREN Qs

- Check that dosages are accurate for weight or BSA.
- Be aware that most medications do not undergo testing on children.
- Initial pediatric dosages are an approximation.
- Some adult medication forms and concentrations require dilution, calculation, preparation, and administration of very small doses for administration to children.
- Limited sites exist for IV medication administration.
- Give written and verbal instructions to parents to promote adherence to medication regimens.

PHARMACOLOGY AND OLDER ADULTS (65+ YEARS)

PHYSIOLOGIC CHANGES WITH AGING THAT AFFECT PHARMACOKINETICS ⓖ

- Increased gastric pH (alkaline)
- Decreased gastrointestinal motility and gastric emptying time, resulting in a slower rate of absorption
- Decreased blood flow through cardiovascular system, liver, and kidneys
- Decreased hepatic enzyme function
- Decreased kidney function and glomerular filtration rate
- Decreased protein-binding sites, resulting in lower serum albumin levels
- Decreased body water, increased body fat, and decreased lean body mass

OTHER FACTORS AFFECTING MEDICATION THERAPY

- Multiple or severe illnesses
- Impaired memory or altered mental state
- Changes in vision and hearing
- Decreased mobility and dexterity
- Poor adherence
- Inadequate supervision of long-term therapy
- Limited financial resources
- Polypharmacy: The practice of taking several medications simultaneously (prescription and over-the-counter [OTC]) with diminished bodily functions and some medical problems can contribute to the potential for medication toxicity.

NURSING INTERVENTIONS

Decreasing the risk of adverse medication effects Qs

- Obtain a complete medication history, and include all OTC medications.
- Make sure medication therapy starts at the lowest possible dose.
- Assess and monitor for therapeutic and adverse effects.
- Monitor plasma medication levels to provide a rational basis for dosage adjustment.
- Assess and monitor for medication-medication and medication-food interactions.
- Document findings.
- Notify the provider of adverse effects.

PROMOTING ADHERENCE

- Give clear and concise instructions, verbally and in writing.
- Ensure that the dosage form is appropriate. Administer liquid forms to clients who have difficulty swallowing pills.
- Provide clearly marked containers that are easy to open.
- Assist the client with setting up a daily calendar with the use of pill containers.
- Discuss the availability of and access to local resources for obtaining and paying for medications.
- Suggest that the client obtain assistance from a friend, neighbor, or relative.
- Advise clients to dispose of medications they no longer take and those that have expired.

PHARMACOLOGY AND PREGNANCY AND LACTATION

Pregnancy: Any medication women who are pregnant ingest will affect the fetus.

- Most medications are potentially harmful to the fetus. Therefore, prescribers must weigh the benefits of maternal medication administration against possible fetal risk. Qs
- Medications women take during pregnancy include nutritional supplements (iron, vitamins, minerals) and medications that treat nausea, vomiting, gastric acidity, and mild discomforts. The U.S. Food and Drug Administration classifies medications in five categories that range from remote risk to proven risk of fetal harm.
- Due to the physiologic changes during pregnancy in the kidney, liver, and gastrointestinal tract, women might require a compensatory increase or decrease in medication dosage, depending on the specific medication.
- Providers manage chronic medical disorders such as diabetes mellitus and hypertension in conjunction with careful maternal-fetal monitoring. Pregnancy is a contraindication for live-virus vaccines (measles, mumps, polio, rubella, varicella, yellow fever) due to possible teratogenic effects, including gross malformations and neurobehavioral, congenital, and metabolic anomalies. The Advisory Committee on Immunization Practices recommends that women who are pregnant during influenza season receive the inactivated influenza vaccine.

Lactation: Most medications women who are lactating take enter breast milk. These women should avoid medications that have an extended half-life, are sustained-released, or are harmful to infants. For medications that are safe, give the medication immediately after breastfeeding to minimize the medication's concentration in the next feeding. Give the lowest effective dosage for the shortest possible time. QEBP

Application Exercises

1. A nurse is preparing to administer medications to a 4-month-old infant. Which of the following pharmacokinetic principles should the nurse consider when administering medications to this client? (Select all that apply.)

    A. Infants have a more rapid gastric emptying time.

    B. Infants have immature liver function.

    C. Infants' blood-brain barrier is poorly developed.

    D. Infants have an increased ability to absorb topical medications.

    E. Infants have an increased number of protein-binding sites.

2. A nurse in a provider's office is reviewing the medical record of a client who is pregnant and is at her first prenatal visit. Which of the following immunizations may the nurse administer safely to this client?

    A. Varicella vaccine

    B. Rubella vaccine

    C. Inactivated influenza vaccine

    D. Measles vaccine

3. A nurse on a medical-surgical unit administers a hypnotic medication to an older adult client at 2100. The next morning, the client is drowsy and wants to sleep instead of eating breakfast. Which of the following factors should the nurse identify as a possible reason for the client's drowsiness?

    A. Reduced cardiac function

    B. First-pass effect

    C. Reduced hepatic function

    D. Increased gastric motility

PRACTICE Active Learning Scenario

A nurse is preparing an in-service educational session about client-specific factors to consider when administering medications. Use the ATI Active Learning Template: Basic Concept to complete this item.

RELATED CONTENT: Identify four general factors that affect medication dosages and responses.

UNDERLYING PRINCIPLES: Identify three medical problems that affect medication dosages and responses.

Application Exercises Key

1. A. Gastric emptying is longer and inconsistent in infants. Medications the nurse administers orally remain in the stomach for a longer period of time, and absorption is more complete. Because gastric emptying is inconsistent, the time for therapeutic effects to occur is difficult to predict.

   B. **CORRECT:** Infants have immature liver function until 1 year of age. The nurse should administer medications the liver metabolizes in smaller dosages.

   C. **CORRECT:** Infants have a poorly developed blood-brain barrier, which places them at risk for adverse effects from medications that pass through the blood-brain barrier. The nurse should administer these medications in smaller dosages.

   D. **CORRECT:** Because infants have more blood flowing to the skin and their skin is thin, their medication absorption is increased, making them prone to toxicity from topical medications.

   E. Infants have limited protein-binding sites compared with adults, which makes them more vulnerable to increased effects of medications. Medication doses must be smaller during the first 12 months of life.

   (N) *NCLEX® Connection: Pharmacological and Parenteral Therapies, Expected Actions/Outcomes*

2. A. Pregnancy is a contraindication for vaccines that contain a live virus, including the varicella vaccine.

   B. Pregnancy is a contraindication for vaccines that contain a live virus, including the rubella vaccine.

   C. **CORRECT:** During influenza season, providers recommend the inactivated influenza vaccine for women who are pregnant.

   D. Pregnancy is a contraindication for vaccines that contain a live virus, including the measles vaccine.

   (N) *NCLEX® Connection: Pharmacological and Parenteral Therapies, Medication Administration*

3. A. Reduced cardiac function would not cause the client's medication to have a prolonged effect.

   B. The first-pass effect would cause faster metabolizing of the hypnotic medication, thus having a decreased effect.

   C. **CORRECT:** Older adults have reduced hepatic function, which can prolong the effects of medications the liver metabolizes. The client probably needs a lower dosage of the hypnotic medication.

   D. Increased gastric motility would cause a lesser effect of the medication, not an increased or prolonged effect.

   (N) *NCLEX® Connection: Pharmacological and Parenteral Therapies, Expected Actions/Outcomes*

PRACTICE Answer

Using the ATI Active Learning Template: Basic Concept

RELATED CONTENT: General factors

- Body weight
- Age
- Gender
- Genetics
- Biorhythmic cycles
- Tolerance
- Accumulation
- Psychological factors
- Diet

UNDERLYING PRINCIPLES: Medical problems

- Inadequate gastric acid inhibits the absorption of medications that require an acid medium to dissolve.
- Diarrhea causes oral medications to pass too quickly through the gastrointestinal tract for adequate absorption.
- Vascular insufficiency prevents distribution of a medication to affected tissue.
- Liver disease or failure impairs medication metabolism, which can cause toxicity.
- Kidney disease or failure prevents or delays medication excretion, which can cause toxicity.
- Prolonged gastric emptying time delays the absorption of medications in the intestines.

(N) *NCLEX® Connection: Pharmacological and Parenteral Therapies, Expected Actions/Outcomes*

When reviewing the following chapters, keep in mind the relevant topics and tasks of the NCLEX outline, in particular:

Client Needs: Psychosocial Integrity

CHEMICAL AND OTHER DEPENDENCIES/SUBSTANCE USE DISORDER: Plan and provide care to clients experiencing substance–related withdrawal or toxicity.

Client Needs: Pharmacological and Parenteral Therapies

ADVERSE EFFECTS/CONTRAINDICATIONS/SIDE EFFECTS/ INTERACTIONS: Assess the client for actual or potential side effects and adverse effects of medications.

EXPECTED ACTIONS/OUTCOMES: Obtain information on a client's prescribed medications.

MEDICATION ADMINISTRATION: Educate client about medications.

UNIT 2   MEDICATIONS AFFECTING THE NERVOUS SYSTEM

CHAPTER 7

Anxiety and Trauma- and Stressor-Related Disorders

Anxiety disorders include generalized anxiety disorder, panic disorder, obsessive-compulsive disorder, social anxiety disorder, and post-traumatic stress disorder. Persistent anxiety can become disabling and can require intervention with therapy, biofeedback, and relaxation techniques and/or the use of medications. Psychological manifestations of anxiety disorders can include fear and apprehension. Physical manifestations can include palpitations, tachycardia, and shortness of breath.

Sedative hypnotic anxiolytics: Benzodiazepines

SELECT PROTOTYPE MEDICATION: **Alprazolam**

OTHER MEDICATIONS
- Diazepam
- Lorazepam
- Chlordiazepoxide
- Clorazepate
- Oxazepam
- Clonazepam

PURPOSE

EXPECTED PHARMACOLOGICAL ACTION

Benzodiazepines enhance the inhibitory effects of gamma–aminobutyric acid (GABA) in the CNS. Relief from anxiety occurs rapidly following administration.

7.1 Medications at a glance

Major medications used to treat anxiety disorders

Benzodiazepine sedative hypnotic anxiolytics, such as lorazepam, alprazolam, and diazepam

Atypical anxiolytic/nonbarbiturate anxiolytics, such as buspirone

SELECTED ANTIDEPRESSANTS
- **Selective serotonin reuptake inhibitors (SSRIs):** paroxetine, sertraline, fluoxetine, citalopram, escitalopram, and fluvoxamine
- **Serotonin-norepinephrine reuptake inhibitors (SNRIs):** venlafaxine, duloxetine

OTHER ANTIDEPRESSANTS: **Tricyclic antidepressants (TCAs):** amitriptyline, imipramine, clomipramine

Other medications used less frequently
- Monoamine oxidase inhibitor (MAOI): phenelzine
- Mirtazapine
- Trazodone
- Antihistamines, such as hydroxyzine pamoate and hydroxyzine hydrochloride
- Beta-blockers, such as propranolol
- Alpha-blockers, such as prazosin
- Anticonvulsants, such as gabapentin

In addition to anxiety disorders, some of these medications are used to treat adjustment disorders, dissociative disorders, and depressive disorders.

THERAPEUTIC USES

Generalized anxiety disorder (GAD) and panic disorder

OTHER USES FOR BENZODIAZEPINES
- Trauma– and stressor-related disorders: Acute stress disorder (ASD) and post-traumatic stress disorder (PTSD)
- Hyperarousal manifestations of dissociative disorders
- Seizure disorders
- Insomnia
- Muscle spasm
- Alcohol withdrawal (for prevention and treatment of acute manifestations)
- Induction of anesthesia
- Amnesic prior to surgery or procedures

COMPLICATIONS

CNS depression

Sedation, lightheadedness, ataxia, decreased cognitive function

CLIENT EDUCATION
- Advise clients to observe for CNS depression. Instruct the client to notify the provider if effects occur.
- Advise clients to avoid activities that require alertness (driving, operating heavy equipment/machinery).
- Advise clients to avoid alcohol and other antianxiety medications due to potentiated depressant effects such as severe respiratory depression.

Anterograde amnesia

Difficulty recalling events that occur after dosing

CLIENT EDUCATION: Advise clients to observe for manifestations. Instruct clients to notify the provider if effects occur.

Toxicity

Acute toxicity

Oral toxicity: drowsiness, lethargy, confusion

IV toxicity: can lead to respiratory depression, severe hypotension, or cardiac/respiratory arrest
Benzodiazepines for IV use include
- Diazepam
- Lorazepam

NURSING CONSIDERATIONS
- For oral toxicity, gastric lavage is used, followed by the administration of activated charcoal or saline cathartics.
- Administer flumazenil for benzodiazepine overdose/toxicity to counteract sedation and reverse adverse effects.
- Monitor vital signs, maintain patent airway, and provide fluids to maintain blood pressure.
- Have resuscitation equipment available.

Paradoxical response

Insomnia, excitation, euphoria, anxiety, rage

CLIENT EDUCATION: Advise clients to watch for manifestations. Notify the provider if these occur.

Withdrawal effects

Include anxiety, insomnia, diaphoresis, tremors, lightheadedness, delirium, hypertension, muscle twitching, and seizures

CLIENT EDUCATION
- Advise clients that withdrawal effects are not common with short-term use.
- Advise clients who have been taking benzodiazepines regularly and in high doses to taper the dose over several weeks.

CONTRAINDICATIONS/PRECAUTIONS

- Benzodiazepines area Pregnancy Risk Category D medications and are avoided in women who are pregnant or breastfeeding.
- Benzodiazepines are classified under Schedule IV of the Controlled Substances Act.
- Benzodiazepines are contraindicated in clients who have sleep apnea, respiratory depression, or glaucoma.
- Use benzodiazepines cautiously in older adult clients and those who have liver disease or a history of mental illness or a substance use disorder.
- Benzodiazepines are generally used short-term due to the risk for dependence. Qs

INTERACTIONS

CNS depressants (alcohol, barbiturates, opioids) can result in respiratory depression. Anticonvulsants and antihistamines can cause increased CNS depression.
NURSING CONSIDERATIONS
- Advise clients to avoid alcohol and other substances that cause CNS depression.
- Advise clients to avoid activities that require alertness (driving, operating heavy equipment/machinery).

Grapefruit juice can reduce metabolism.
NURSING CONSIDERATIONS: Avoid the use of grapefruit juice.

High-fat meals can reduce absorption.
NURSING CONSIDERATIONS: Do not take with fatty foods.

NURSING ADMINISTRATION

- Advise clients to take the medication as prescribed and to avoid abrupt discontinuation of treatment to prevent withdrawal manifestations. Do not change the dosage or frequency without prior approval of prescriber.
- When discontinuing benzodiazepines that have been taken regularly for long periods and in higher doses, taper the dose over several weeks. QEBP
- Administer the medication with meals or snacks if gastrointestinal upset occurs.
- Administer the medication at bedtime if possible due to sedation.
- Advise clients to swallow sustained-release tablets and to avoid chewing or crushing the tablets.
- Inform clients about the possible development of dependency during and after treatment and to notify the provider if indications of withdrawal occur.
- Advise clients to keep benzodiazepines in a secure place due to their abuse potential.

Atypical anxiolytic/ nonbarbiturate anxiolytic

SELECT PROTOTYPE MEDICATION: Buspirone

PURPOSE

EXPECTED PHARMACOLOGICAL ACTION

- The exact antianxiety mechanism of this medication is unknown. This medication binds to serotonin and dopamine receptors. Dependency is much less likely than with other anxiolytics, and use of buspirone does not result in sedation or potentiate the effects of other CNS depressants.
- The major disadvantage is that antianxiety effects develop slowly. Initial responses take a week, and at least 2 to 6 weeks for it to reach its full effects. As a result of this pharmacological action, buspirone is taken on a scheduled basis, and is not suitable for PRN usage.

THERAPEUTIC USES

- Panic disorder
- Social anxiety disorder
- Obsessive-compulsive and related disorders
- Trauma- and stressor-related disorders, PTSD

COMPLICATIONS

Dizziness, nausea, headache, lightheadedness, agitation
CLIENT EDUCATION

- Advise the client to take with food to decrease nausea.
- Avoid activities that require alertness until effects are known.
- Instruct client that most adverse effects are self-limiting.

Constipation
CLIENT EDUCATION: Advise client to increase fiber and fluid.

Suicidal ideation
NURSING CONSIDERATIONS: Monitor and report manifestations of depression and thoughts of suicide.

CONTRAINDICATIONS/PRECAUTIONS

- Buspirone is Pregnancy Risk Category B.
- Buspirone is not recommended for use by women who are breastfeeding.
- Use buspirone cautiously in older adult clients and clients who have liver and/or renal dysfunction.
- Buspirone is contraindicated for concurrent use with MAOI antidepressants or for 14 days after MAOIs are discontinued. Hypertensive crisis can result. Qs

INTERACTIONS

Erythromycin, ketoconazole, St. John's wort, and grapefruit juice can increase the effects of buspirone.
NURSING CONSIDERATIONS

- Advise clients to avoid the use of these antimicrobial agents.
- Advise clients to avoid herbal preparations containing St. John's wort.
- Advise clients to avoid drinking grapefruit juice.

Increased risk for serotonin syndrome with SSRIs
NURSING CONSIDERATIONS: Monitor for serotonin syndrome, fever, tremor, diarrhea, and delirium. Avoid concurrent use.

NURSING ADMINISTRATION

- Advise clients to take the medication with meals to prevent gastric irritation.
- Advise clients that effects do not occur immediately. It can take a week to notice the first therapeutic effects and 2 to 6 weeks for the full benefit. Take on a regular basis and not PRN. QEBP
- Instruct clients that tolerance, dependence, or withdrawal effects are not an issue with this medication.
- Labeled for short-term treatment of anxiety, but has shown therapeutic benefit for as long as a year.

Selective serotonin reuptake inhibitors (SSRI antidepressants)

SELECT PROTOTYPE MEDICATION: Paroxetine

OTHER MEDICATIONS
- Sertraline
- Citalopram
- Escitalopram
- Fluoxetine
- Fluvoxamine

PURPOSE

EXPECTED PHARMACOLOGICAL ACTION

- Paroxetine selectively inhibits serotonin reuptake, allowing more serotonin to stay at the junction of the neurons.
- It does not block uptake of dopamine or norepinephrine.
- Paroxetine produces CNS stimulation, which can cause insomnia.
- The medication has a long effective half-life. A time frame of up to 4 weeks is necessary to produce therapeutic medication levels.

THERAPEUTIC USES

Paroxetine
- Generalized anxiety disorder (GAD)
- Panic disorder: Decreases both the frequency and intensity of panic attacks and also prevents anticipatory anxiety about attacks
- Obsessive-compulsive disorder (OCD): Reduces manifestations by increasing serotonin
- Social anxiety disorder
- Trauma- and stressor-related disorders
- Dissociative disorders
- Depressive disorders
- Adjustment disorders

Sertraline: indicated for panic disorder, OCD, social anxiety disorder, and PTSD.

Escitalopram: indicated for GAD and OCD.

Fluoxetine: used for panic disorder, OCD, and PTSD.

Fluvoxamine: used for OCD and social anxiety disorder.

COMPLICATIONS

Early adverse effects

First few days/weeks: nausea, diaphoresis, tremor, fatigue, drowsiness

CLIENT EDUCATION
- Instruct clients to report adverse effects to the provider.
- Instruct clients to take the medication as prescribed.
- Advise clients that these effects should soon subside.

Later adverse effects

After 5 to 6 weeks of therapy: sexual dysfunction (impotence, delayed or absent orgasm, delayed or absent ejaculation, decreased sexual interest)

CLIENT EDUCATION: Instruct clients to report problems with sexual function (managed with dose reduction, medication holiday, changing medications).

Weight gain

CLIENT EDUCATION: Advise clients to follow a well-balanced diet and exercise regularly.

GI bleeding

NURSING CONSIDERATIONS
- Use caution in clients who have a history of GI bleed or ulcers and in clients taking other medications that affect blood coagulation.
- Advise clients to report indications of bleeding such as dark stool or coffee ground emesis.

Hyponatremia

More likely in older adult clients taking diuretics

NURSING CONSIDERATIONS: Obtain baseline serum sodium, and monitor level periodically throughout treatment.

Serotonin syndrome

Agitation, confusion, disorientation, difficulty concentrating, anxiety, hallucinations, myoclonus (spastic, jerky muscle contractions), hyperreflexia, incoordination, tremors, fever, diaphoresis

NURSING CONSIDERATIONS
- Usually begins 2 to 72 hr after initiation of treatment
- Resolves when the medication is discontinued
- Watch for and advise clients to report any of these manifestations, which could indicate a lethal problem.

Bruxism

Grinding and clenching of teeth, usually during sleep

NURSING CONSIDERATIONS
- Report bruxism to the provider, who might switch the client to another class of medication.
- Treat bruxism with low-dose buspirone.
- Advise the client to use a mouth guard during sleep.

Withdrawal syndrome

Nausea, sensory disturbances, anxiety, tremor, malaise, unease

NURSING CONSIDERATIONS
- Minimized by tapering the medication slowly
- Advise clients that, after a long period of use, the medication is tapered slowly to avoid withdrawal syndrome.
- Advise clients not to discontinue use abruptly.

Postural hypotension

NURSING CONSIDERATIONS: Monitor for hypotension and advise client to change positions slowly.

Suicidal ideation

NURSING CONSIDERATIONS: Monitor and report manifestations of depression and thoughts of suicide.

CONTRAINDICATIONS/PRECAUTIONS

- Paroxetine is a Pregnancy Risk Category D medication.
- Paroxetine is contraindicated in clients taking MAOIs or a TCA.
- Clients taking paroxetine should avoid alcohol.
- Use paroxetine cautiously in clients who have liver and renal dysfunction, seizure disorders, or a history of GI bleeding. Qs

INTERACTIONS

Use of MAOI antidepressants or TCAs can cause serotonin syndrome.
NURSING CONSIDERATIONS: Educate the client about this combination. Avoid concurrent use.

Antiplatelet medications and anticoagulants can increase risk for bleeding
NURSING CONSIDERATIONS: Monitor for bleeding. Avoid concurrent use.

NURSING ADMINISTRATION

- Advise clients that medications can be taken with food. Sleep disturbances are minimized by taking medication in the morning.
- Instruct clients to take the medication on a daily basis to establish therapeutic plasma levels. Q EBP
- Assist with medication regimen adherence by informing clients that it can take up to 4 weeks to achieve therapeutic effects from an SSRI.

NURSING EVALUATION OF MEDICATION EFFECTIVENESS

Depending on therapeutic intent, effectiveness is evidenced by the following.
- Verbalizing feeling less anxious and more relaxed
- Description of improved mood
- Improved memory retrieval
- Maintaining regular sleep pattern
- Greater ability to participate in social and occupational interactions
- Improved ability to cope with manifestations and identified stressors

Application Exercises

1. A nurse working in an emergency department is caring for a client who has benzodiazepine toxicity due to an overdose. Which of the following actions is the nurse's priority?

   A. Administer flumazenil.

   B. Identify the client's level of orientation.

   C. Infuse IV fluids.

   D. Prepare the client for gastric lavage.

2. A nurse is teaching a client who has a new prescription for escitalopram for treatment of generalized anxiety disorder. Which of the following statements by the client indicates understanding of the teaching?

   A. "I should take the medication on an empty stomach."

   B. "I will follow a low-sodium diet while taking this medication."

   C. "I need to discontinue this medication slowly."

   D. "I should not crush this medication before swallowing."

3. A nurse is providing teaching to a client who has a new prescription for buspirone to treat anxiety. Which of the following information should the nurse include?

   A. "Take this medication on an empty stomach"

   B. "Expect optimal therapeutic effects within 24 hr."

   C. "Take this medication when needed for anxiety"

   D. "This medication has a low risk for dependency."

4. A nurse is teaching a client who has obsessive-compulsive disorder and has a new prescription for paroxetine. Which of the following instructions should the nurse include?

   A. "It can take several weeks before you feel like the medication is helping."

   B. "Take the medication just before bedtime to promote sleep."

   C. "You should take the medication when needed for obsessive urges."

   D. "Monitor for weight gain while taking this medication."

5. A nurse is caring for a client who takes paroxetine to treat posttraumatic stress disorder and reports that he grinds his teeth during the night. The nurse should identify which of the following interventions to manage bruxism? (Select all that apply.)

   A. Concurrent administration of buspirone

   B. Administration of a different SSRI

   C. Use of a mouth guard

   D. Changing to a different class of antidepressant medication

   E. Increasing the dose of paroxetine

PRACTICE Active Learning Scenario

A nurse is assessing a client 4 hr after receiving an initial dose of fluoxetine. The nurse is concerned that the client is developing serotonin syndrome. Use the ATI Active Learning Template: System Disorder and the Mental Health Nursing Review Module to complete this item.

ALTERATION IN HEALTH (DIAGNOSIS)

EXPECTED FINDINGS: Identify at least six.

RISK FACTORS: Describe at least one risk factor.

Application Exercises Key

1. A. The nurse should prepare to administer flumazenil to reverse the benzodiazepine toxicity. However, there is another action the nurse should take first.

   B. **CORRECT:** The first action the nurse should take when using the nursing process is to assess the client. Identifying the client's level of orientation is the priority action.

   C. The nurse should prepare to infuse IV fluids to support the client's blood pressure. However, there is another action the nurse should take first.

   D. The nurse should prepare to administer a gastric lavage to reverse the benzodiazepine toxicity. However, there is another action the nurse should take first.

   Ⓝ *NCLEX® Connection: Pharmacological and Parenteral Therapies, Adverse Effects/Contraindications/Side Effects/Interactions*

2. A. The client can take this medication with food for GI distress or without food.

   B. The client is at risk for hyponatremia while taking escitalopram.

   C. **CORRECT:** When discontinuing escitalopram, the client should taper the medication slowly according to a prescribed tapered dosing schedule to reduce the risk of withdrawal syndrome.

   D. The client can crush escitalopram before swallowing.

   Ⓝ *NCLEX® Connection: Pharmacological and Parenteral Therapies, Medication Administration*

3. A. The client can take this medication with food to reduce GI distress.

   B. Buspirone can take up to 3 to 6 weeks to obtain optimal therapeutic effects

   C. The client should take buspirone on a regular, not PRN, basis because therapeutic effects occur slowly.

   D. **CORRECT:** Buspirone has a low risk for physical or psychological dependence or tolerance.

   Ⓝ *NCLEX® Connection: Pharmacological and Parenteral Therapies, Medication Administration*

4. A. **CORRECT:** Paroxetine can take 1 to 4 weeks before the client reaches full therapeutic benefit.

   B. Take paroxetine in the morning to prevent insomnia.

   C. Take paroxetine on a regular basis rather than an as-needed basis.

   D. Paroxetine can cause decreased appetite and weight loss.

   Ⓝ *NCLEX® Connection: Pharmacological and Parenteral Therapies, Expected Actions/Outcomes*

5. A. **CORRECT:** Concurrent administration of a low dose of buspirone is an effective measure to manage the adverse effects of paroxetine.

   B. Other SSRIs also will have bruxism as an adverse effect. This is not an effective measure.

   C. **CORRECT:** Using a mouth guard during sleep can decrease the risk for oral damage resulting from bruxism.

   D. **CORRECT:** Changing to different class of antidepressant medication that does not have the adverse effect of bruxism is an effective measure.

   E. Increasing the dose of paroxetine can cause the adverse effect of bruxism to worsen. This is not an effective measure.

   Ⓝ *NCLEX® Connection: Pharmacological and Parenteral Therapies, Adverse Effects/Contraindications/Side Effects/Interactions*

PRACTICE Answer

Using the ATI Active Learning Template: System Disorder

ALTERATION IN HEALTH (DIAGNOSIS): Serotonin syndrome is a potentially lethal complication that usually begins 2 to 72 hr after initiation of treatment with an SSRI. The syndrome resolves when the medication is discontinued.

EXPECTED FINDINGS

- Agitation
- Confusion
- Disorientation
- Difficulty concentrating
- Anxiety
- Hallucinations
- Hyperreflexia
- Incoordination
- Tremors
- Fever
- Diaphoresis

RISK FACTORS

- Onset of treatment with an SSRI within the last 2 to 72 hr
- Concurrent use of an SSRI with an MAOI
- Concurrent use of an SSRI with a TCA

Ⓝ *NCLEX® Connection: Pharmacological and Parenteral Therapies, Adverse Effects/Contraindications/Side Effects/Interactions*

CHAPTER 8 *Depressive Disorders*

Depressive disorders are a widespread problem, ranking high among causes of disability. Clients who have major depression can require hospitalization with close observation and suicide precautions until antidepressant medications reach their peak effect.

Antidepressant medications are classified into five main groups: selective serotonin reuptake inhibitors (SSRIs), serotonin-norepinephrine reuptake inhibitors (SNRIs), atypical antidepressants, tricyclic antidepressants (TCAs), and monoamine oxidase inhibitors (MAOIs).

Selective serotonin reuptake inhibitors

SELECT PROTOTYPE MEDICATION: Fluoxetine

OTHER MEDICATIONS
- Citalopram
- Escitalopram
- Paroxetine
- Sertraline
- Fluvoxamine
- Vortioxetine

PURPOSE

EXPECTED PHARMACOLOGICAL ACTION
- SSRIs selectively block reuptake of the monoamine neurotransmitter serotonin in the synaptic space, thereby intensifying the effects of serotonin.
- SSRIs considered first-line treatment for depression. Can take 1 to 3 weeks or longer before pharmacological benefits take effect. Q EBP

THERAPEUTIC USES
- Major depression
- Obsessive-compulsive disorders
- Bulimia nervosa
- Premenstrual dysphoric disorders
- Panic disorders
- Posttraumatic stress disorder
- Social anxiety disorder
- Generalized anxiety disorder

COMPLICATIONS

Sexual dysfunction

Anorgasmia, impotence, decreased libido

NURSING CONSIDERATIONS
- Warn clients of possible adverse effects and to notify the provider if intolerable.
- Instruct client on ways to manage sexual dysfunction, which can include lowering dosage, discontinuing medication temporarily (medication holiday), and using adjunct medications to improve sexual function (e.g., sildenafil and buspirone)
- Inform clients that an atypical antidepressant such as bupropion has fewer sexual dysfunction adverse effects.

CNS stimulation

Inability to sleep, agitation, anxiety

NURSING CONSIDERATIONS
- Advise clients to notify the provider. Dose can need to be lowered.
- Advise clients to take dose in the morning.
- Advise clients to avoid caffeinated beverages.
- Teach relaxation techniques to promote sleep.

Weight loss early in therapy

Can be followed by weight gain with long-term treatment

NURSING CONSIDERATIONS
- Monitor the client's weight.
- Encourage clients to participate in regular exercise and to follow a healthy, well-balanced diet.

Serotonin syndrome

Can begin 2 to 72 hr after starting treatment and can be lethal. Qs

MANIFESTATIONS
- Mental confusion, delirium
- Fever
- Tachycardia
- Elevated blood pressure
- Abdominal pain, diarrhea
- Irritability, mood swings, agitation
- Anxiety, restlessness
- Incoordination, hyperreflexia
- Diaphoresis
- Tremors, muscle spasms
- Cardiovascular shock
- Seizures
- Death

NURSING CONSIDERATIONS
- Advise clients to observe for manifestations. If any occur, instruct the client to notify the provider and withhold the medication.
- Start symptomatic treatment (medications to create serotonin-receptor blockade and muscle rigidity, cooling blankets, anticonvulsants, artificial ventilation)

Withdrawal syndrome

Resulting in headache, nausea, visual disturbances, anxiety, dizziness, and tremors

NURSING CONSIDERATIONS: Instruct clients to taper dose gradually.

Hyponatremia

More likely in older adult clients taking diuretics

NURSING CONSIDERATIONS: Obtain baseline serum sodium, and monitor level periodically throughout treatment.

Rash

NURSING CONSIDERATIONS: Advise clients that a rash is treatable with an antihistamine or withdrawal of medication.

Sleepiness, faintness, lightheadedness

NURSING CONSIDERATIONS
- Advise clients that these adverse effects are not common, but can occur.
- Advise clients to avoid driving if these side effects occur.

Gastrointestinal bleeding

NURSING CONSIDERATIONS: Use caution in clients who have a history of GI bleed and ulcers, and those taking other medications that affect blood coagulation.

Bruxism

NURSING CONSIDERATIONS
- Advise clients to report to the provider.
- Advise clients to use a mouth guard.
- Changing to a different classification of antidepressants or adding a low dose of buspirone can decrease this adverse effect.

CONTRAINDICATIONS/PRECAUTIONS

- These medications are Pregnancy Risk Category C, except for paroxetine, which is Category D. **Qs**

  > Paroxetine increases the risk of birth defects. Therefore, other SSRIs are recommended. Late in pregnancy, use of SSRIs increases the risk of withdrawal symptoms or pulmonary hypertension in the newborn.

- SSRIs are contraindicated in clients taking MAOIs or TCAs. SSRIs need to be discontinued at least 2 weeks before initiating a MAOI.
- Use cautiously in clients who have liver and kidney dysfunction, cardiac disease, seizure disorders, diabetes, ulcers, and a history of GI bleeding.

INTERACTIONS

MAOIs, TCAs, and St. John's wort
MAOIs, TCAs, and St. John's wort increase the risk of serotonin syndrome.
NURSING CONSIDERATIONS
- MAOIs should be discontinued for 14 days prior to starting an SSRI. If already taking fluoxetine, the client should wait 5 weeks before starting an MAOI.
- Avoid concurrent use of TCAs and St. John's wort.

Warfarin
Fluoxetine can displace warfarin from bound protein and result in increased warfarin levels.
NURSING CONSIDERATIONS
- Monitor PT and INR levels.
- Assess for indications of bleeding and the need for dosage adjustment.

Tricyclic antidepressants and lithium
Fluoxetine can increase the levels of tricyclic antidepressants and lithium.
NURSING CONSIDERATIONS: Avoid concurrent use.

NSAIDs and anticoagulants
Fluoxetine suppresses platelet aggregation and thus increases the risk of bleeding when used concurrently with NSAIDs and anticoagulants.
NURSING CONSIDERATIONS: Advise clients to monitor for indications of bleeding (bruising, hematuria) and to notify the provider if they occur.

Serotonin-norepinephrine reuptake inhibitors

SELECT PROTOTYPE MEDICATION: Venlafaxine

OTHER MEDICATIONS
- Desvenlafaxine
- Duloxetine

PURPOSE

EXPECTED PHARMACOLOGICAL ACTION
SNRIs block reuptake of norepinephrine as well as serotonin with effects similar to the SSRIs.

THERAPEUTIC USES
- Major depression
- Generalized anxiety disorder
- Social anxiety disorder
- Panic disorder
- Pain due to fibromyalgia, osteoarthritis, low-back pain, diabetic neuropathy (duloxetine; unlabeled use for venlafaxine)

COMPLICATIONS

Nausea, anorexia, weight loss

NURSING CONSIDERATIONS: Monitor weight and food intake.

Headache, insomnia, anxiety

NURSING CONSIDERATIONS: Monitor for these findings.

Hypertension, tachycardia

NURSING CONSIDERATIONS: Monitor vital signs and report changes.

Dizziness, blurred vision

NURSING CONSIDERATIONS: Avoid driving, use of machinery until effects are known.

Withdrawal syndrome

Resulting in headache, nausea, visual disturbances, anxiety, dizziness, and tremors

NURSING CONSIDERATIONS: Instruct the client to withdraw from medication gradually.

Risk for suicide in children and adolescents

NURSING CONSIDERATIONS: Assess children/adolescents carefully for suicidal ideation, thought disorders. Qs

Sexual dysfunction

Anorgasmia, decreased libido, impotence, menstrual changes

NURSING CONSIDERATIONS
- Instruct clients to report sexual dysfunction to provider.
- Instruct clients on ways to manage sexual dysfunction, which can include lowering dosage, discontinuing medication temporarily (medication holiday), and using adjunct medications to improve sexual function (sildenafil, buspirone).
- Inform clients that an atypical antidepressant such as bupropion has fewer sexual dysfunction adverse effects.

Serotonin syndrome

See information under SSRIs (above)

Bronchitis, dyspnea

NURSING CONSIDERATIONS: Instruct client to report respiratory findings to provider

CONTRAINDICATIONS/PRECAUTIONS

- These medications are pregnancy category risk C. Avoid during the third trimester and avoid breastfeeding while taking an SNRI.
- SNRIs are contraindicated in clients taking SSRIs, MAOIs, or TCAs. SNRIs need to be discontinued at least 2 weeks before initiating an MAOI. Qs
- Precautions are needed for older adults, and clients who have bipolar disorder, mania, seizure disorder, recent MI, or interstitial lung disease.

INTERACTIONS

Neuroleptic malignant syndrome if given concurrently with MAOIs
NURSING CONSIDERATIONS: Stop MAOI at least 14 days before beginning a SNRI.

NSAIDs, anticoagulants increase risk for bleeding with venlafaxine
NURSING CONSIDERATIONS: Review client's medications with provider, including over-the-counter medications.

Alcohol and other medications affecting the CNS increase risk for CNS effects
NURSING CONSIDERATIONS: Avoid alcohol and other CNS depressants.
Use caution when driving or using machinery. Qs

Kava, Valerian increase risk for CNS depression; St. John's wort can cause serotonin syndrome.
NURSING CONSIDERATIONS: Instruct client to avoid these supplements.

Atypical antidepressants

SELECT PROTOTYPE MEDICATION: Bupropion

OTHER MEDICATIONS
- Vilazodone
- Mirtazapine
- Reboxetine
- Trazodone

PURPOSE

EXPECTED PHARMACOLOGICAL ACTION
Bupropion acts by inhibiting norepinephrine and dopamine uptake, and is referred to as a norepinephrine-dopamine reuptake inhibitor.

THERAPEUTIC USES
- Treatment of depression
- Alternative to SSRIs and SNRIs for clients unable to tolerate sexual dysfunction side effects of these antidepressants
- Aid for smoking cessation
- Prevention of seasonal pattern depression
- Alternative treatment choice for attention-deficit disorder

COMPLICATIONS

Headache, dry mouth, GI distress, constipation, increased heart rate, hypertension, restlessness, and insomnia

NURSING CONSIDERATIONS
- Advise clients to observe for effects and to notify the provider if intolerable.
- Treat headache with mild analgesic.
- Advise clients to sip on fluids to treat dry mouth and to increase dietary fiber to prevent constipation.

Nausea, vomiting, anorexia, weight loss

NURSING CONSIDERATIONS: Monitor weight and food intake.

Seizures

NURSING CONSIDERATIONS
- Avoid administering to clients at risk for seizures, such as a clients who have head injuries.
- Monitor for seizures, and treat accordingly.

CONTRAINDICATIONS/PRECAUTIONS

- Bupropion is a Pregnancy Risk Category B. Qs
- Contraindicated in clients taking MAOIs
- Contraindicated for clients who have seizure disorders or eating disorders

INTERACTIONS

MAOIs such as phenelzine increase the risk of toxicity.
NURSING CONSIDERATIONS: MAOIs should be discontinued 2 weeks prior to beginning treatment with bupropion.

Other atypical antidepressants

Vilazodone

PHARMACOLOGICAL ACTION: Both blocks serotonin and works as a serotonin agonist at receptor sites (first medication to work in this way)

NURSING CONSIDERATIONS
- Contraindicated with SSRIs and SNRIs (serotonin syndrome), and other serotonin receptor agonists, such as buspirone and phenothiazines. Stop MAOI at least 14 days before starting vilazodone.
- Teach manifestations of serotonin syndrome to client and instruct when to notify provider.
- Monitor for suicidal ideation
- Instruct clients to avoid grapefruit juice while taking vilazodone.
- Many adverse effects are similar to those of SSRIs and SNRIs.
- Take with food to help increase absorption.

Mirtazapine

PHARMACOLOGICAL ACTION: Referred to as a serotonin–norepinephrine disinhibitor. It increases the release of serotonin and norepinephrine by blocking presynaptic receptors, and thereby increases the amount of neurotransmitters available for impulse transmission.

NURSING CONSIDERATIONS
- Therapeutic effects can occur sooner with less sexual dysfunction than with SSRIs.
- Mirtazapine is generally well tolerated. Clients can experience sleepiness that can be exacerbated by other CNS depressants (alcohol, benzodiazepines), weight gain, and elevated cholesterol.
- Advise client to take at bedtime; can be used as a sleep aid.

Reboxetine

PHARMACOLOGICAL ACTION: Selectively inhibits the reuptake of norepinephrine, thereby increasing the amount of neurotransmitters available for impulse transmission.

NURSING CONSIDERATIONS
- Similar results as with SSRIs.
- Generally well tolerated, but clients can experience dry mouth, decreased blood pressure, constipation, sexual dysfunction, and urinary hesitancy or retention.
- Weight gain and sleepiness do not occur.
- This medication should not be combined with an MAOI.

Trazodone

PHARMACOLOGICAL ACTION: Moderate selective blockade of serotonin receptors, which allows more serotonin to be available for impulse transmission.

NURSING CONSIDERATIONS
- Usually used with another antidepressant agent.
- Sedation is a potential problem; can be indicated for a client who has insomnia.
- Priapism is a potential adverse effect. Instruct clients to seek medical attention immediately if this occurs.

Tricyclic antidepressants

SELECT PROTOTYPE MEDICATION: Amitriptyline

OTHER MEDICATIONS
- Imipramine
- Doxepin
- Nortriptyline
- Amoxapine
- Trimipramine
- Desipramine
- Clomipramine

PURPOSE

EXPECTED PHARMACOLOGICAL ACTION
- These medications block reuptake of norepinephrine and serotonin in the synaptic space, thereby intensifying the effects of these neurotransmitters.
- It can take 10 to 14 days or longer before TCAs begin to work, and maximum effects might be not seen until 4 to 8 weeks.

THERAPEUTIC USES
- Depression
- Depressive episodes of bipolar disorders

OTHER USES
- Neuropathic pain
- Fibromyalgia
- Anxiety disorders
- Obsessive-compulsive disorder
- Insomnia
- Attention-deficit/hyperactivity disorder (ADHD)

COMPLICATIONS

Orthostatic hypotension

NURSING CONSIDERATIONS
- Instruct clients about the effects of postural hypotension (lightheadedness, dizziness). If these occur, advise the client to sit or lie down. Orthostatic hypotension is minimized by changing positions slowly.
- Monitor blood pressure and heart rate for clients in the hospital for orthostatic changes before administration and 1 hr after. If a significant decrease in blood pressure or increase in heart rate is noted, do not administer the medication, and notify the provider.

Anticholinergic effects

- Dry mouth
- Blurred vision
- Photophobia
- Urinary hesitancy or retention
- Constipation
- Tachycardia

NURSING CONSIDERATIONS
- Instruct clients on ways to minimize anticholinergic effects.
  - Chewing sugarless gum
  - Sipping on water
  - Wearing sunglasses when outdoors
  - Eating foods high in fiber
  - Participating in regular exercise
  - Increasing fluid intake to at least 2 to 3 L a day from beverages and food sources
  - Voiding just before taking medication
- Advise the client to notify the provider if effects persist.

Sedation

This effect usually diminishes over time.

NURSING CONSIDERATIONS
- Advise clients to avoid hazardous activities such as driving if sedation is excessive.
- Advise clients to take medication at bedtime to minimize daytime sleepiness and to promote sleep.

Toxicity

Resulting in cholinergic blockade and cardiac toxicity evidenced by dysrhythmias, mental confusion, and agitation, followed by seizures, coma, and possible death

NURSING CONSIDERATIONS
- Obtain baseline ECG.
- Monitor vital signs frequently.
- Monitor signs of toxicity.
- Notify the provider if signs of toxicity occur.

Decreased seizure threshold

NURSING CONSIDERATIONS: Monitor clients who have seizure disorders.

Excessive sweating

NURSING CONSIDERATIONS: Inform clients of adverse effects. Assist clients with frequent linen changes.

CONTRAINDICATIONS/PRECAUTIONS

- TCAs are Pregnancy Risk Category C.
- Contraindicated in clients who have seizure disorders or who have recently experienced a myocardial infarction.
- Use cautiously in clients who are elderly or who have coronary artery disease; diabetes, liver, kidney, or respiratory disorders; urinary retention or obstruction; angle-closure glaucoma; benign prostatic hyperplasia; and hyperthyroidism. Ⓒ
- Clients at an increased risk for suicide should receive a 1-week supply of medication at a time due to the lethality of an overdose. Qs

INTERACTIONS

Concurrent use with MAOIs or St. John's wort can lead to serotonin syndrome.
NURSING CONSIDERATIONS: Avoid concurrent use.

Antihistamines and other anticholinergic agents have additive anticholinergic effects.
NURSING CONSIDERATIONS: Avoid concurrent use.

Increased effects of epinephrine, dopamine (direct-acting sympathomimetics) occur because uptake into the nerve terminals is blocked by TCAs, and they remain for a longer amount of time in the synaptic space.
NURSING CONSIDERATIONS: Avoid concurrent use.

TCAs decrease the effects of ephedrine, amphetamine (indirect-acting sympathomimetics) because uptake into the nerve terminals is blocked, and they are unable to reach their site of action.
NURSING CONSIDERATIONS: Avoid concurrent use.

Alcohol, benzodiazepines, opioids, and antihistamines cause additive CNS depression when used concurrently.
NURSING CONSIDERATIONS: Advise clients to avoid other CNS depressants.

8.1 Medications used to treat depression, but not classified as antidepressants

Atypical antipsychotics

ARIPIPRAZOLE: used as an augmenting antidepressant agent in conjunction with SSRIs

QUETIAPINE: approved for treatment of depression and bipolar depression

Monoamine oxidase inhibitors

SELECT PROTOTYPE MEDICATION: Phenelzine

OTHER MEDICATIONS
- Isocarboxazid
- Tranylcypromine
- Selegiline (transdermal MAOI)

PURPOSE

EXPECTED PHARMACOLOGICAL ACTION: These medications block MAO in the brain, thereby increasing the amount of norepinephrine, dopamine, serotonin, and tyramine available for transmission of impulses. An increased amount of these neurotransmitters at nerve endings intensifies responses and relieves depression. However, the increase in tyramine can cause heightened blood pressure or hypertensive crisis if dietary and medication restrictions are not implemented.
- Onset of therapeutic action is not immediate, and usually takes 2 to 4 weeks.
- Less frequently used in comparison to other antidepressants due to food/drug interactions and side effects.

THERAPEUTIC USES
- Depression
- Bulimia nervosa
- Panic disorder
- Social anxiety disorder
- Generalized anxiety disorder
- Obsessive-compulsive disorder
- Posttraumatic stress disorder

COMPLICATIONS

CNS stimulation

Anxiety, agitation, mania, or hypomania

NURSING CONSIDERATIONS: Advise clients to observe for effects and notify the provider if they occur.

Orthostatic hypotension

NURSING CONSIDERATIONS: Monitor blood pressure and heart rate for orthostatic changes. Hold medication and notify the provider of significant changes. Instruct the client to change positions slowly.

Hypertensive crisis, severe hypertension, headache, nausea, increased heart rate, and increased blood pressure

- Hypertensive crisis resulting from intake of dietary tyramine, which could lead to a cerebral vascular accident
- Severe hypertension as a result of intensive vasoconstriction and stimulation of the heart
- Headache, nausea, and increased heart rate and blood pressure

NURSING CONSIDERATIONS
- Administer phentolamine IV (a rapid-acting alpha-adrenergic blocker) or nifedipine SL.
- Provide continuous cardiac monitoring and respiratory support as indicated.

Local rash with transdermal preparation

NURSING CONSIDERATIONS
- Choose a clean, dry area for each application.
- Apply a topical glucocorticoid on the affected area.

CONTRAINDICATIONS/PRECAUTIONS

- MAOIs are Pregnancy Risk Category C. **Qs**
- Contraindicated in clients taking SSRIs and in those who have pheochromocytoma, heart failure, cardiovascular and cerebral vascular disease, and severe renal insufficiency.
- Use cautiously in clients who have diabetes and seizure disorders or those taking TCAs.
- Transdermal selegiline is contraindicated for clients taking carbamazepine or oxcarbazepine, which can increase blood levels of the MAOI.

INTERACTIONS

Indirect-acting sympathomimetic medications (ephedrine, amphetamine) promote the release of norepinephrine and can lead to hypertensive crisis.
NURSING CONSIDERATIONS: Instruct clients to avoid over-the-counter decongestants and cold remedies, which frequently contain medications with sympathomimetic action.

Use of tricyclic antidepressants can lead to hypertensive crisis.
NURSING CONSIDERATIONS: Use MAOIs and TCAs cautiously.

Use of SSRIs can lead to serotonin syndrome.
NURSING CONSIDERATIONS: Avoid concurrent use.

Antihypertensives have an additive hypotensive effect.
NURSING CONSIDERATIONS
- Monitor blood pressure.
- Notify the provider if there is a significant drop in blood pressure. A reduced dosage of antihypertensive can be indicated.

Use of meperidine can lead to hyperpyrexia.
NURSING CONSIDERATIONS: Use an alternative analgesic.

Tyramine-rich foods can lead to hypertensive crisis.
- Clients will most likely experience headache, nausea, increased heart rate, and increased blood pressure
- Tyramine-rich foods include aged cheese, pepperoni, salami, avocados, figs, bananas, smoked fish, protein dietary supplements, soups, soy sauce, some beers, and red wine.
- The MAOI transdermal patch does not seem to affect tyramine sensitivity at its low dose, but tyramine restriction is recommended at higher doses.

NURSING CONSIDERATIONS
- Assess for ability to follow strict adherence to dietary restrictions.
- Inform clients of manifestations and to notify the provider if they occur.
- Provide clients with written instructions regarding foods and beverages to avoid.
- Advise clients to avoid taking any medications without approval of the provider.
- Advise clients that dietary and medication restrictions should be continued for 2 weeks after the MAOI has been discontinued.

Concurrent use of vasopressors (phenylethylamine, caffeine) can result in hypertension.
NURSING CONSIDERATIONS: Advise clients to avoid foods that contain these agents (caffeinated beverages, chocolate, fava beans, ginseng).

General anesthetics
NURSING CONSIDERATIONS: Advise clients that MAOIs should not be used within 10 to 14 days before or after surgery

---

For all medications in this chapter

NURSING ADMINISTRATION

- Instruct clients to take these medications as prescribed on a daily basis to establish therapeutic plasma levels.
- Assist with medication regimen adherence by informing clients that it can take 1 to 3 weeks to begin experiencing therapeutic effects. Full therapeutic effects can take 2 to 3 months. Q**PCC**
- Instruct clients to continue therapy after achieving therapeutic effects. Sudden discontinuation of medication can result in relapse.
- Advise clients that therapy usually continues for 6 months after resolution of symptoms and can continue for a year or longer.
- Assess for suicide risk. Antidepressant medications can increase a client's risk for suicide, particularly during initial treatment. Antidepressant-induced suicide is mainly associated with clients younger than age 25. Q**s**

SSRIs and SNRIs

- Advise clients to take medication in the morning to minimize sleep disturbances.
- Advise clients to take medications with food to minimize GI disturbances.
- Advise clients about potential sexual side effects.
- Avoid use of MAOIs.
- Obtain baseline sodium levels for older adult clients taking diuretics, and monitor periodically. Ⓖ

Atypical antidepressants

- For all atypical antidepressant medications, avoid use with MAOIs.
- Advise clients taking bupropion for prevention of seasonal pattern depression to take medication beginning in the autumn each year and gradually taper dose and discontinue by spring.

TCAs

- Monitor for toxicity manifested by cardiac dysrhythmias.
- Administer at bedtime due to sedation and risk for orthostatic hypotension.
- Monitor for clients "cheeking" or hoarding TCAs due to potential lethality in overdose.

MAOIs

- Give clients a list of tyramine-rich foods so hypertensive crises can be avoided.
- Advise the client to avoid taking any other prescription or nonprescription medications unless approved by the provider.

NURSING EVALUATION OF MEDICATION EFFECTIVENESS

Depending on therapeutic intent, effectiveness is evidenced by the following.
- Verbalizing improvement in mood
- Increased hopefulness and will to live
- Ability to perform ADLs
- Improved sleeping and eating habits
- Increased interaction with peers

Application Exercises

1. A nurse is caring for a client who has a new prescription for phenelzine for the treatment of depression. Which of the following indicates that the client has developed an adverse effect of this medication?

   A. Orthostatic hypotension

   B. Hearing loss

   C. Gastrointestinal bleeding

   D. Weight loss

2. A nurse is providing teaching to a client who has a new prescription for amitriptyline for treatment of depression. Which of the following should the nurse include in the teaching? (Select all that apply.)

   A. Expect therapeutic effects in 24 to 48 hr.

   B. Discontinue the medication after a week of improved mood.

   C. Change positions slowly to minimize dizziness.

   D. Decrease dietary fiber intake to control diarrhea.

   E. Chew sugarless gum to prevent dry mouth.

3. A nurse is providing discharge teaching to a client who has a new prescription for fluoxetine for posttraumatic stress disorder. Which of the following statements should the nurse include in the teaching?

   A. "You may have a decreased desire for intimacy while taking this medication."

   B. "You should take this medication at bedtime to help promote sleep."

   C. "You will have fewer urinary adverse effects if you urinate just before taking this medication."

   D. "You'll need to wear sunglasses when outdoors due to the light sensitivity caused by this medication."

4. A nurse is caring for a client who has depression and a new prescription for venlafaxine. For which of the following adverse effects should the nurse monitor this client? (Select all that apply)

   A. Cough

   B. Dizziness

   C. Decreased libido

   D. Alopecia

   E. Hypotension

5. A nurse is caring for a client who has been taking sertraline for the past 2 days. Which of the following assessment findings should alert the nurse to the possibility that the client is developing serotonin syndrome?

   A. Bruising

   B. Fever

   C. Abdominal pain

   D. Rash

PRACTICE Active Learning Scenario

A nurse in an emergency department is caring for a client who is experiencing hypertensive crisis. The client reports taking tranylcypromine for the treatment of depression and that he ate pepperoni pizza shortly before the manifestations began. Use the ATI Active Learning Template: System Disorder and the ATI Mental Health Review Module to complete this item.

ALTERATION IN HEALTH (DIAGNOSIS)

EXPECTED FINDINGS: Identify at least three.

MEDICATIONS: Identify at least one medication appropriate for treatment.

CLIENT EDUCATION: Identify four dietary sources of tyramine the client should avoid.

Application Exercises Key

1. A. **CORRECT:** Orthostatic hypotension is an adverse of effect of MAOIs, including phenelzine.

   B. Phenelzine is more likely to cause blurred vision than hearing loss.

   C. Clients taking phenelzine are at risk for multiple adverse effects. However, these do not include GI bleeding.

   D. Clients taking phenelzine are at risk for weight gain rather than weight loss.

   Ⓝ *NCLEX® Connection: Pharmacological and Parenteral Therapies, Adverse Effects/Contraindications/Side Effects/Interactions*

2. A. Therapeutic effects are expected after several weeks of taking amitriptyline.

   B. Stopping amitriptyline abruptly can result in relapse.

   C. **CORRECT:** Changing positions slowly helps prevent orthostatic hypotension, which is an adverse effect of amitriptyline.

   D. Clients should increase dietary fiber to prevent constipation, which is an adverse effect of amitriptyline.

   E. **CORRECT:** Chewing sugarless gum can minimize dry mouth, which is an adverse effect of amitriptyline.

   Ⓝ *NCLEX® Connection: Pharmacological and Parenteral Therapies, Medication Administration*

3. A. **CORRECT:** Decreased libido is a potential adverse effect of fluoxetine and other SSRIs.

   B. Clients should take fluoxetine in the morning due to CNS stimulation.

   C. Clients taking a TCA, rather than fluoxetine, should void prior to taking the medication due to the potential for urinary hesitancy or retention.

   D. Clients taking a TCA, rather than fluoxetine, should wear sunglasses when outdoors due to the potential for photophobia.

   Ⓝ *NCLEX® Connection: Pharmacological and Parenteral Therapies, Medication Administration*

4. A. **CORRECT:** Cough and dyspnea can indicate that the client has developed bronchitis, which is an adverse effect of venlafaxine.

   B. **CORRECT:** Dizziness is a common adverse effect of venlafaxine.

   C. **CORRECT:** Sexual dysfunction, such as decreased libido, decreased orgasm, impotence, and menstrual changes are adverse effects of venlafaxine.

   D. Alopecia is not an adverse effect of venlafaxine.

   E. Hypertension and tachycardia are adverse effects of venlafaxine.

   Ⓝ *NCLEX® Connection: Pharmacological and Parenteral Therapies, Adverse Effects/Contraindications/Side Effects/Interactions*

5. A. Bleeding can result if an SSRI is administered with warfarin. However, this is not an indication of serotonin syndrome.

   B. **CORRECT:** Fever is a manifestation of serotonin syndrome, which can result from taking an SSRI such as sertraline.

   C. Abdominal pain is not an indication of serotonin syndrome.

   D. A localized rash is associated with transdermal preparation. However, it is not an indication of serotonin syndrome.

   Ⓝ *NCLEX® Connection: Pharmacological and Parenteral Therapies, Adverse Effects/Contraindications/Side Effects/Interactions*

PRACTICE Answer

Using the ATI Active Learning Template: System Disorder

ALTERATION IN HEALTH (DIAGNOSIS):
Hypertensive crisis results from intensive vasoconstriction due to the intake of dietary tyramine while taking an MAOI.

EXPECTED FINDINGS
- Severe hypertension
- Headache
- Nausea
- Increased heart rate

MEDICATIONS
- Phentolamine IV, a rapid-acting alpha-adrenergic blocker
- Nifedipine, a calcium channel blocker

CLIENT EDUCATION
- Aged cheeses
- Smoked or preserved fish or meats, such as pepperoni and salami
- Avocados
- Figs
- Bananas
- Protein dietary supplements
- Soups containing meat extracts
- Soy sauce
- Some beers
- Red wine

Ⓝ *NCLEX® Connection: Pharmacological and Parenteral Therapies, Medication Administration*

CHAPTER 9 *Bipolar Disorders*

Bipolar disorders are primarily managed with mood-stabilizing medications such as lithium carbonate. Other medications used to treat bipolar disorders include antiepileptic drugs (AEDs), such as valproic acid, carbamazepine, lamotrigine, oxcarbazepine, and topiramate.

Atypical antipsychotics, such as olanzapine, can be useful in early treatment to promote sleep and to decrease anxiety and agitation. These medications also demonstrate mood-stabilizing properties

Anxiolytics, such as clonazepam and lorazepam, can be useful in treating acute mania and managing the psychomotor agitation often seen in mania.

Antidepressant medications, such as bupropion and sertraline, can be useful during the depressive phase, but need to be used with caution, so as to not trigger a manic cycle. These are typically prescribed in combination with a mood stabilizer to prevent rebound mania.

Mood stabilizer

SELECT PROTOTYPE MEDICATION: Lithium carbonate

PURPOSE

EXPECTED PHARMACOLOGICAL ACTION
- Lithium produces neurochemical changes in the brain, including serotonin receptor blockade.
- There is evidence that the use of lithium can show a decrease in neuronal atrophy and/or an increase in neuronal growth.

THERAPEUTIC USES: Lithium is used in the treatment of bipolar disorders. Lithium controls episodes of acute mania, and helps prevent the return of mania or depression.

COMPLICATIONS

Effects with therapeutic lithium levels (some resolve within a few weeks)

Gastrointestinal (GI) distress

Nausea, diarrhea, abdominal pain

NURSING CONSIDERATIONS
- Advise clients that effects are usually transient.
- Administer medication with meals or milk.

Fine hand tremors

Can interfere with purposeful motor skills and can be exacerbated by factors such as stress and caffeine

NURSING CONSIDERATIONS
- Administer beta-adrenergic blocking agents such as propranolol.
- Adjust to the lowest possible dosage, give in divided doses, or use long-acting formulations.
- Advise clients to report an increase in tremors.

Polyuria, mild thirst

NURSING CONSIDERATIONS
- Use a potassium-sparing diuretic, such as spironolactone.
- Instruct clients to maintain adequate fluid intake by consuming 2,000 to 3,000 mL fluid from beverages and food sources.

Weight gain

NURSING CONSIDERATIONS: Assist clients to follow a healthy diet and regular exercise regimen.

Renal toxicity

NURSING CONSIDERATIONS
- Monitor I&O.
- Adjust dosage, and keep dose low.
- Assess baseline kidney function, and monitor kidney function periodically.

Goiter and hypothyroidism

With long-term treatment

NURSING CONSIDERATIONS
- Obtain baseline T_3, T_4, and TSH levels prior to starting treatment, and then annually.
- Advise clients to monitor for manifestations of hypothyroidism (cold, dry skin; decreased heart rate; weight gain).
- Administer levothyroxine to manage hypothyroid effects.

Bradydysrhythmia, hypotension, and electrolyte imbalances

NURSING CONSIDERATIONS: Encourage clients to maintain adequate fluid and sodium intake.

Lithium toxicity

Early indications
LITHIUM LEVEL: Below 1.5 mEq/L
- MANIFESTATIONS: Diarrhea, nausea, vomiting, thirst, polyuria, muscle weakness, fine hand tremor, slurred speech, lethargy
- NURSING CONSIDERATIONS
  - Advise clients to withhold medication and notify the provider.
  - Administer new dosage based on serum lithium levels.

Advanced indications
LITHIUM LEVEL: 1.5 to 2.0 mEq/L
- MANIFESTATIONS: Ongoing gastrointestinal distress, including nausea, vomiting, and diarrhea; mental confusion; poor coordination; coarse tremors; sedation
- NURSING CONSIDERATIONS
  - Advise clients to withhold medication and notify the provider.
  - Administer new dosage based on serum lithium levels.
  - If manifestations are severe, it can be necessary to promote excretion.

Severe toxicity
- LITHIUM LEVEL: 2.0 to 2.5 mEq/L
  - MANIFESTATIONS: Extreme polyuria of dilute urine, tinnitus, involuntary extremity movements, blurred vision, ataxia, seizures, severe hypotension leading to coma and possibly death from respiratory complications
  - NURSING CONSIDERATIONS
    - Administer an emetic to clients who are alert.
    - Perform gastric lavage or administer urea, mannitol, or aminophylline to increase the rate of excretion.
- LITHIUM LEVEL: Greater than 2.5 mEq/L
  - MANIFESTATIONS: Oliguria, seizures, rapid progression of symptoms leading to coma and death
  - NURSING CONSIDERATIONS: Hemodialysis

CONTRAINDICATIONS/PRECAUTIONS

- Lithium is Pregnancy Risk Category D. This medication is teratogenic, especially during the first trimester. Qs
- Discourage clients from breastfeeding if lithium therapy is necessary. QEBP
- Use cautiously in clients who have renal dysfunction, heart disease, sodium depletion, or dehydration.

INTERACTIONS

Diuretics

Sodium is excreted with the use of diuretics. Reduced serum sodium decreases lithium excretion, which can lead to toxicity.

NURSING CONSIDERATIONS
- Monitor for indications of toxicity.
- Advise clients to observe for indications of toxicity and to notify the provider.
- Encourage clients to maintain a diet adequate in sodium, and to drink 2,000 mL to 3,000 mL of water each day from food and beverage sources.

NSAIDs (ibuprofen and celecoxib)

Concurrent use will increase renal reabsorption of lithium, leading to toxicity.

NURSING CONSIDERATIONS
- Avoid use of NSAIDs.
- Use aspirin as a mild analgesic.

Anticholinergics

Antihistamines and tricyclic antidepressants can induce urinary retention and polyuria, leading to abdominal discomfort.

NURSING CONSIDERATIONS: Advise clients to avoid medications with anticholinergic effects.

NURSING ADMINISTRATION

- Monitor plasma lithium levels during treatment.
  - At initiation of treatment, monitor levels at least 5 days after starting lithium therapy and after any dosage change, until therapeutic level has been achieved; then every 1 to 3 months, depending on length of treatment and stability. QEBP
  - Older adult clients often require more frequent monitoring. G
  - Lithium blood levels should be obtained in the morning, usually 12 hr after the last dose.
  - During initial treatment of a manic episode, levels should be between 0.8 to 1.4 mEq/L.
  - Maintenance level range is between 0.4 to 1.0 mEq/L.
  - Plasma levels at or greater than 1.5 mEq/L can result in toxicity.
- Care for clients who have a toxic plasma lithium level in an acute care setting, and provide supportive measures. Hemodialysis can be indicated.
- Monitor CBC, serum electrolytes, renal function tests, and thyroid function tests during lithium therapy.
- Advise clients that effects begin within 7 to 14 days.
- Advise clients to take lithium as prescribed. Lithium must be administered in 2 to 3 doses daily due to a short half-life. Taking lithium with food will help decrease GI distress.
- Encourage clients to adhere to laboratory appointments needed to monitor lithium effectiveness and adverse effects. Emphasize the high risk of toxicity due to the narrow therapeutic range.
- Provide nutritional counseling. Stress the importance of adequate fluid and sodium intake. QPCC
- Instruct clients to monitor for manifestations of toxicity and when to contact the provider. Clients should withhold medication and seek medical attention if experiencing diarrhea, vomiting, or excessive sweating.
- Conditions that cause dehydration, such as exercising in hot weather or diarrhea, put client at risk for lithium toxicity.

Mood-stabilizing antiepileptic drugs

SELECT PROTOTYPE MEDICATIONS
- Carbamazepine
- Valproic acid
- Lamotrigine

Oxcarbazepine and topiramate are less frequently used and recommended for maintenance treatment of bipolar disorder.

PURPOSE

EXPECTED PHARMACOLOGICAL ACTION: AEDs help treat and manage bipolar disorders by various mechanisms.
- Slowing the entrance of sodium and calcium back into the neuron and, thus, extending the time it takes for the nerve to return to its active state.
- Potentiating the inhibitory effects of gamma butyric acid (GABA).
- Inhibiting glutamic acid (glutamate), which in turn suppresses CNS excitation.

THERAPEUTIC USES: Treatment and prevention of relapse of mania and depressive episodes. Especially useful for clients who have mixed mania and rapid cycling bipolar disorders.

COMPLICATIONS

CARBAMAZEPINE

CNS effects

Cognitive function is minimally affected, but CNS effects can include nystagmus, double vision, vertigo, staggering gait, and headache.

NURSING CONSIDERATIONS
- Administer low doses initially, then gradually increase dosage.
- Instruct clients to avoid driving and other activities that require alertness at the beginning of treatment. Qs
- Advise clients that CNS effects should subside within a few weeks.
- Administer dose at bedtime.

Blood dyscrasias

Leukopenia, anemia, thrombocytopenia

NURSING CONSIDERATIONS
- Obtain baseline CBC and platelets, and perform ongoing monitoring.
- Observe for indications of bruising and bleeding of gums.
- Monitor for sore throat, fatigue, or other indications of infection.

Teratogenesis

NURSING CONSIDERATIONS: Advise clients to avoid use in pregnancy.

Hypo-osmolality

Promotes secretion of ADH, which inhibits water excretion by the kidneys and places older adult clients who have heart failure at risk for fluid overload Ⓖ

NURSING CONSIDERATIONS
- Monitor serum sodium.
- Monitor for edema, decrease in urine output, and hypertension.

Skin disorders

Dermatitis, rash, and Stevens-Johnson syndrome, which is potentially life-threatening

NURSING CONSIDERATIONS
- Treat mild reactions with anti-inflammatory or antihistamine medications.
- Advise clients to wear sunscreen.
- Instruct clients to notify the provider if Stevens-Johnson syndrome rash occurs and to withhold medication.

Hepatotoxicity

Evidenced by anorexia, nausea, vomiting, fatigue abdominal pain, and jaundice

NURSING CONSIDERATIONS
- Assess baseline liver function, and monitor liver function regularly.
- Advise clients to observe for indications and to notify the provider if they occur.
- Avoid using in children younger than 2 years old.
- Administer lowest effective dose.

LAMOTRIGINE

Double or blurred vision, dizziness, headache, nausea, and vomiting

NURSING CONSIDERATIONS: Caution clients about performing activities requiring concentration.

Serious skin rashes

Include Stevens-Johnson syndrome

NURSING CONSIDERATIONS: Instruct clients to withhold medication and notify provider if rash occurs.

VALPROIC ACID

GI effects

Nausea, vomiting, indigestion

NURSING CONSIDERATIONS
- Advise clients that manifestations are usually self-limiting.
- Advise clients to take medication with food or switch to enteric-coated pills.

Hepatotoxicity

Evidenced by anorexia, nausea, vomiting, fatigue abdominal pain, jaundice

NURSING CONSIDERATIONS
- Assess baseline liver function, and monitor liver function regularly.
- Advise clients to observe for indications and to notify the provider if they occur.
- Avoid using in children younger than 2 years old.
- Administer lowest effective dose.

Pancreatitis

Evidenced by nausea, vomiting, and abdominal pain

NURSING CONSIDERATIONS
- Advise clients to observe for indications and to notify the provider immediately if they occur.
- Monitor amylase levels.
- Discontinue medication if pancreatitis develops.

Thrombocytopenia

NURSING CONSIDERATIONS
- Advise clients to observe for manifestations, such as bruising, and to notify the provider if these occur.
- Monitor platelet counts.

Teratogenesis

NURSING CONSIDERATIONS: Advise clients to avoid use in pregnancy.

Weight gain

NURSING CONSIDERATIONS: Advise clients to follow a healthy low-calorie diet, engage in regular exercise, and monitor weight.

CONTRAINDICATIONS/PRECAUTIONS

- These medications are Pregnancy Risk Category D and can result in birth defects. Lamotrigine is Pregnancy Risk Category C, but can cause cleft lip and palate if taken during the first trimester.
- Carbamazepine is contraindicated in clients who have bone marrow suppression or bleeding disorders. Qs
- Valproic acid is contraindicated in clients who have liver disorders.
- Monitor plasma valproic acid and carbamazepine levels while undergoing treatment.

INTERACTIONS

CARBAMAZEPINE

Oral contraceptives, warfarin

Concurrent use causes a decrease in the effects of these medications due to stimulation of hepatic drug-metabolizing enzymes.

NURSING CONSIDERATIONS
- Advise clients to use an alternate form of birth control.
- Monitor for therapeutic effects of warfarin.
- Dosages can need to be adjusted.

Grapefruit juice

Inhibits metabolism, thus increasing carbamazepine levels.

NURSING CONSIDERATIONS: Advise clients to avoid intake of grapefruit juice.

Phenytoin and phenobarbital

Decrease the effects of carbamazepine by stimulating metabolism.

NURSING CONSIDERATIONS
- Monitor phenytoin and phenobarbital levels.
- Adjust dosage of medications as prescribed.

LAMOTRIGINE

Carbamazepine, phenytoin, and phenobarbital

These promote liver drug-metabolizing enzymes, thereby decreasing the effect of lamotrigine.

NURSING CONSIDERATIONS
- Monitor for therapeutic effects.
- Adjust dosage of medications as prescribed.

Valproic acid

Inhibits medication-metabolizing enzymes and thus increases the half-life of lamotrigine.

NURSING CONSIDERATIONS
- Monitor for adverse effects.
- Adjust dosage of medications as prescribed.

VALPROIC ACID

Phenytoin and phenobarbital

Serum levels of these medications are increased when used concurrently with valproic acid.

NURSING CONSIDERATIONS
- Monitor phenytoin and phenobarbital levels.
- Adjust dosage of medications as prescribed.

NURSING EVALUATION OF MEDICATION EFFECTIVENESS

Depending on therapeutic intent, effectiveness is evidenced by the following.
- Relief of acute manic symptoms (flight of ideas, excessive talking, agitation) or depressive symptoms (fatigue, poor appetite, psychomotor retardation)
- Mood stability
- Ability to perform ADLs
- Improved sleeping and eating habits
- Appropriate interaction with peers

PRACTICE Active Learning Scenario

A nurse is reviewing discharge instructions with a client who has a new diagnosis of bipolar disorder. The client has a new prescription for lithium carbonate 600 mg PO three times a day. Use the ATI Active Learning Template: Medication to complete this item.

CLIENT EDUCATION: Include three side/adverse effects the nurse should include in the teaching.

Application Exercises

1. A nurse is reviewing laboratory findings and notes that a client's plasma lithium level is 2.1 mEq/L. Which of the following is an appropriate action by the nurse?
   - A. Perform immediate gastric lavage.
   - B. Prepare the client for hemodialysis.
   - C. Administer an additional oral dose of lithium.
   - D. Request a stat repeat of the laboratory test.

2. A nurse is caring for a client who has a new prescription for lithium carbonate. When teaching the client about ways to prevent lithium toxicity, the nurse should advise the client to do which of the following?
   - A. Avoid the use of acetaminophen for headaches.
   - B. Restrict intake of foods rich in sodium.
   - C. Decrease fluid intake to less than 1,500 mL daily
   - D. Limit aerobic activity in hot weather.

3. A nurse is assessing a client who takes lithium carbonate for the treatment of bipolar disorder. The nurse should recognize which of the following findings as a possible indication of toxicity to this medication?
   - A. Severe hypertension
   - B. Coarse tremors
   - C. Constipation
   - D. Muscle spasms

4. A nurse is caring for a client who has a new prescription for valproic acid. The nurse should instruct the client that while taking this medication he will need to have which of the following laboratory tests completed periodically? (Select all that apply.)
   - A. Thrombocyte count
   - B. Hematocrit
   - C. Amylase
   - D. Liver function tests
   - E. Potassium

5. A nurse is preparing a teaching plan for a female client who has bipolar disorder and a new prescription for carbamazepine. Which of the following instructions should the nurse include in the teaching?
   - A. "This medication can safely be taken during pregnancy."
   - B. "Eliminate grapefruit juice from your diet."
   - C. "You will need to have a complete blood count and carbamazepine levels drawn periodically."
   - D. "Notify your provider if you develop a rash."
   - E. "Avoid driving for the first few days after starting this medication."

1. A. **CORRECT:** Gastric lavage is appropriate for a client who has severe toxicity, as evidenced by a plasma lithium level of 2.1 mEq/L. This action will lower the client's lithium level.

   B. Hemodialysis is appropriate for a client who has a plasma lithium level greater than 2.5 mEq/L.

   C. Administering an additional dose of lithium will worsen the level of toxicity.

   D. There is no indication that the client needs another laboratory test, and this action can delay needed treatment.

   Ⓝ *NCLEX® Connection: Pharmacological and Parenteral Therapies, Adverse Effects/Contraindications/Side Effects/Interactions*

2. A. The client should use acetaminophen, rather than NSAIDs such as ibuprofen, for headaches because NSAIDs interact with lithium and can cause increased blood levels of lithium.

   B. The client should increase, rather than decrease, sodium intake to reduce the risk for toxicity.

   C. The client should increase, rather than decrease, fluid intake to reduce the risk for toxicity.

   D. **CORRECT:** The client should avoid activities that have the potential to cause sodium/water depletion, which can increase the risk for toxicity.

   Ⓝ *NCLEX® Connection: Pharmacological and Parenteral Therapies, Adverse Effects/Contraindications/Side Effects/Interactions*

3. A. Severe hypotension, rather than hypertension, is an indication of toxicity.

   B. **CORRECT:** Coarse tremors are an indication of toxicity.

   C. Diarrhea, rather than constipation, is an indication of toxicity.

   D. Muscle weakness, rather than muscle spasm, is an indication of lithium toxicity.

   Ⓝ *NCLEX® Connection: Pharmacological and Parenteral Therapies, Adverse Effects/Contraindications/Side Effects/Interactions*

4. A. **CORRECT:** Treatment with valproic acid can result in thrombocytopenia. The client's thrombocyte count should be monitored periodically.

   B. Treatment with valproic acid is not known to have an effect on a client's hematocrit.

   C. **CORRECT:** Treatment with valproic acid can result in pancreatitis. The client's amylase should be monitored periodically.

   D. **CORRECT:** Treatment with valproic acid can result in hepatotoxicity. The client's liver function should be monitored periodically.

   E. Treatment with valproic acid is not known to have an effect on a client's potassium.

   Ⓝ *NCLEX® Connection: Pharmacological and Parenteral Therapies, Expected Actions/Outcomes*

5. A. Carbamazepine is a Pregnancy Category Risk D medication. The client should be instructed to avoid pregnancy while taking carbamazepine.

   B. **CORRECT:** Grapefruit juice affects carbamazepine metabolism and should be avoided.

   C. **CORRECT:** Carbamazepine blood levels and the CBC should be monitored during therapy. The client is at risk for bone marrow depression while taking carbamazepine and should notify the provider for a sore throat or other manifestations of an infection.

   D. **CORRECT:** Carbamazepine can cause Stevens-Johnson syndrome, which can be fatal. The client should notify the provider promptly if a rash occurs.

   E. **CORRECT:** CNS effects such as drowsiness or dizziness can occur early in treatment with carbamazepine and the client should avoid activities requiring alertness until these effects subside.

   Ⓝ *NCLEX® Connection: Pharmacological and Parenteral Therapies, Medication Administration*

PRACTICE Answer

Using the ATI Active Learning Template: Medication

CLIENT EDUCATION

- Gastrointestinal distress: nausea, diarrhea, abdominal pain
- Fine hand tremors
- Polyuria
- Mild thirst
- Weight gain
- Renal toxicity
- Goiter and hypothyroidism
- Bradydysrhythmias
- Hypotension
- Electrolyte imbalances

Ⓝ *NCLEX® Connection: Pharmacological and Parenteral Therapies, Medication Administration*

Schizophrenia spectrum disorders are the primary reason for the administration of antipsychotic medications. The clinical course of schizophrenia usually involves acute exacerbations with intervals of semi-remission.

Medications are used to treat positive symptoms related to behavior, thought, perception, and speech (agitation, bizarre behavior, delusions, hallucinations, flight of ideas, illogical thinking patterns, tangential speech patterns) and negative symptoms (social withdrawal, lack of emotion, lack of energy [anergia], flattened affect, decreased motivation, decreased pleasure in activities).

The goals of psychopharmacological treatment for schizophrenia spectrum and other psychotic disorders include suppressing acute episodes, preventing acute recurrence, and maintaining the highest possible level of functioning. Q̊EBP

Antipsychotics: First-generation (conventional)

These medications control mainly positive symptoms of psychotic disorders, such as hallucinations, delusions, and bizarre behavior.

SELECT PROTOTYPE MEDICATION:
Chlorpromazine: low potency

OTHER MEDICATIONS
- Haloperidol: high potency
- Fluphenazine: high potency
- Thiothixene: high potency
- Perphenazine: medium potency
- Thioridazine: low potency

PURPOSE

EXPECTED PHARMACOLOGICAL ACTION
- Block dopamine (D_2), acetylcholine, histamine, and norepinephrine receptors in the brain and periphery.
- Inhibition of psychotic manifestations, believed to be a result of D_2 blockade in the brain.

THERAPEUTIC USES
- Acute and chronic psychotic disorders
- Schizophrenia spectrum disorders
- Bipolar disorders (primarily the manic phase)
- Tourette syndrome
- Agitation
- Prevention of nausea/vomiting through blocking of dopamine in the chemoreceptor trigger zone of the medulla
- Indications
- These medications are reserved for clients who are:
- Using them successfully and can tolerate the adverse effects.
- Violent or particularly aggressive.

COMPLICATIONS

EXTRAPYRAMIDAL SIDE EFFECTS (EPSs)

Acute dystonia

The client experiences severe spasms of tongue, neck, face, or back. This is a crisis situation, which requires rapid treatment. Q̊s

NURSING CONSIDERATIONS
- Monitor for acute dystonia between 5 hr to 5 days after administration of the first dose.
- Treat with anticholinergic agents, such as benztropine or diphenhydramine. Use oral doses for less acute effects and IM or IV doses for serious effects.

Parkinsonism

Findings include bradykinesia, rigidity, shuffling gait, drooling, and tremors.

NURSING CONSIDERATIONS
- Observe for parkinsonism within 1 month of initiation of therapy.
- Treat with benztropine, diphenhydramine, or amantadine. Discontinue these medications to determine if they are still needed. If manifestations return, administer atypical antipsychotic as prescribed.

Akathisia

The client is unable to stand still or sit, and is continually pacing and agitated.

NURSING CONSIDERATIONS
- Observe for akathisia within 2 months of the initiation of treatment.
- Manage effects with beta-blocker, benzodiazepine, or anticholinergic medication.

Tardive dyskinesia (TD)

- Manifestations include involuntary movements of the tongue and face, such as lip-smacking, which cause speech and/or eating disturbances.
- Can also include involuntary movements of arms, legs, or trunk.

NURSING CONSIDERATIONS
- TD is a late EPS that can occur months to years after the start of therapy, and can improve following medication change or can be permanent.
- Administer the lowest dosage possible to control manifestations.
- Evaluate the client after 12 months of therapy and then every 3 months. If indications of TD appear, dosage should be lowered or the client should be switched to an atypical agent.

OTHER ADVERSE EFFECTS

Neuroleptic malignant syndrome

! Life-threatening medical emergency.

Manifestations include sudden high-grade fever, blood pressure fluctuations, dysrhythmias, muscle rigidity, diaphoresis, drooling, and change in level of consciousness developing into coma. Qs

NURSING CONSIDERATIONS
- Stop antipsychotic medication.
- Monitor vital signs.
- Apply cooling blankets.
- Administer antipyretics (aspirin, acetaminophen).
- Increase fluid intake.
- Administer diazepam to control anxiety.
- Administer dantrolene and bromocriptine to induce muscle relaxation.
- Wait 2 weeks before resuming therapy. Consider switching to an atypical agent.

Anticholinergic effects

- Dry mouth
- Blurred vision
- Photophobia
- Urinary hesitancy/retention
- Constipation
- Tachycardia

NURSING CONSIDERATIONS
Suggest strategies to decrease anticholinergic effects.
- Chewing sugarless gum
- Sipping water
- Avoiding hazardous activities
- Wearing sunglasses when outdoors
- Eating foods high in fiber
- Participating in regular exercise
- Maintaining fluid intake of 2 to 3 L water daily from food and beverage sources
- Voiding just before taking medication

Neuroendocrine effects

Effects include gynecomastia (breast enlargement), galactorrhea, and menstrual irregularities.

NURSING CONSIDERATIONS: Advise clients to observe for manifestations and to notify the provider if these occur.

Seizures

The greatest risk for developing seizures is existing seizure disorders.

NURSING CONSIDERATIONS
- Advise clients to report seizure activity to the provider.
- An increase in antiseizure medication can be necessary.

Skin effects

Effects include photosensitivity resulting in severe sunburn, and contact dermatitis from handling medications.

NURSING CONSIDERATIONS
- Advise clients to avoid excessive exposure to sunlight, use sunscreen, and wear protective clothing.
- Advise clients to avoid direct contact with medication.

Orthostatic hypotension

NURSING CONSIDERATIONS
- Clients should develop tolerance in 2 to 3 months.
- In the hospital setting, monitor blood pressure and heart rate for orthostatic changes. If a significant decrease in blood pressure or increase in heart rate is noted, do not administer the medication, and notify the provider.
- Instruct clients about the signs of postural hypotension (lightheadedness, dizziness). If these occur, advise the client to sit or lie down. Orthostatic hypotension can be minimized by getting up or changing positions slowly.

Sedation

NURSING CONSIDERATIONS
- Inform clients that effects should diminish within a few weeks.
- Clients can take this medication at bedtime to avoid daytime sleepiness.
- Advise clients not to drive until sedation has subsided. Q_S

Sexual dysfunction

Common in men and women

NURSING CONSIDERATIONS
- Advise clients of possible adverse effects.
- Encourage clients to report adverse effects to the provider.
- Client can need a lower dosage or to be switched to a high-potency agent.

Agranulocytosis

NURSING CONSIDERATIONS
- Advise clients to observe for indications of infection (fever, sore throat), and to notify the provider if these occur.
- If indications of infection appear, obtain a baseline WBC. Medication should be discontinued if laboratory tests indicate the presence of infection.

Severe dysrhythmias

NURSING CONSIDERATIONS
- Obtain baseline ECG and potassium level prior to treatment and periodically throughout the treatment period.
- Avoid concurrent use with other medications that prolong QT interval.

Liver impairment

NURSING CONSIDERATIONS
- Assess baseline liver function, and monitor liver function regularly
- Advise clients to observe for indications (anorexia, nausea, vomiting, fatigue, abdominal pain, jaundice) and to notify the provider

CONTRAINDICATIONS/PRECAUTIONS

- Contraindicated in clients in a coma, and clients who have severe depression, Parkinson's disease, prolactin-dependent cancer of the breast, and severe hypotension.
- Contraindicated in older clients who have dementia. Ⓖ
- Use cautiously in clients who have glaucoma, paralytic ileus, prostate enlargement, heart disorders, liver or kidney disease, and seizure disorders.

INTERACTIONS

Anticholinergic agents

Concurrent use with other anticholinergic medications will increase anticholinergic effects.

NURSING CONSIDERATIONS: Advise clients to avoid over-the-counter medications that contain anticholinergic agents, such as sleep aids.

CNS depressants

Alcohol, opioids, and antihistamines have additive CNS depressant effects.

NURSING CONSIDERATIONS
- Advise clients to avoid alcohol and other medications that cause CNS depression.
- Advise clients to avoid hazardous activities, such as driving.

Levodopa

By activating dopamine receptors, levodopa counteracts the effects of antipsychotic agents.

NURSING CONSIDERATIONS: Avoid concurrent use of levodopa and other direct dopamine receptor agonists.

NURSING ADMINISTRATION

- Use the Abnormal Involuntary Movement Scale (AIMS) to screen for the presence of EPS. Q_{EBP}
- Assess clients to differentiate between EPSs and worsening of psychotic disorder.
- Administer anticholinergics, beta-blockers, and benzodiazepines to control early EPSs. If adverse effects are intolerable, the client can be switched to a low-potency or an atypical antipsychotic agent.
- Advise clients that antipsychotic medications do not cause addiction.
- Advise clients to take medication as prescribed and on a regular schedule.
- Advise clients that some therapeutic effects can be noticeable within a few days, but significant improvement can take 2 to 4 weeks, and possibly several months for full effects.
- Consider depot preparations administered IM once every 2 to 4 weeks for clients who have difficulty maintaining medication regimen. Inform the client that lower doses can be used with depot preparations, which will decrease the risk of adverse effects and the development of tardive dyskinesia. Q_{PCC}
- Start oral administration with twice-a-day dosing, then switch to daily dosing at bedtime to decrease daytime drowsiness and promote sleep.

Antipsychotics: Second- and third-generation (atypical)

These agents are often chosen as first-line treatment for schizophrenia. They are medications of choice for clients receiving initial treatment and for treating breakthrough episodes in clients on conventional medication therapy, because they are more effective with fewer adverse effects.

SELECT PROTOTYPE MEDICATION:
Risperidone (second-generation antipsychotic)

OTHER MEDICATIONS (10.1)
- Olanzapine
- Quetiapine
- Ziprasidone
- Clozapine
- Asenapine
- Lurasidone
- Paliperidone
- Iloperidone
- Aripiprazole (third-generation)

PURPOSE

EXPECTED PHARMACOLOGICAL ACTION:
Second-generation antipsychotic agents work mainly by blocking serotonin, and to a lesser degree, dopamine receptors. These medications also block receptors for norepinephrine, histamine, and acetylcholine. The third-generation medication (aripiprazole) works by stabilizing the dopamine system as both an agonist and antagonist.

THERAPEUTIC USES
- Schizophrenia spectrum disorders (negative and positive symptoms)
- Psychotic episodes induced by levodopa therapy
- Bipolar disorders
- Impulse control disorders

10.1 Other atypical antipsychotic agents

Olanzapine
FORMULATIONS: Tablets, orally disintegrating tablets, short-acting injectable, extended-release injection

COMPLICATIONS
- Low risk of EPS
- High risk for diabetes mellitus, weight gain, and dyslipidemia
- Other adverse effects: sedation, orthostatic hypotension, anticholinergic effects

Quetiapine
FORMULATIONS: Tablets, extended-release tablets

COMPLICATIONS
- Low risk of EPS
- Moderate risk for diabetes mellitus, weight gain, and dyslipidemia
- Other effects: cataracts, sedation, orthostatic hypotension, anticholinergic effects
- Clients should have screening eye exam and then every 6 months.

Ziprasidone
Affects both dopamine and serotonin; can be used for clients who have concurrent depression

FORMULATIONS: Capsules, short-acting injectable

COMPLICATIONS
- Low risk of EPS, diabetes mellitus, weight gain, dyslipidemia
- Other effects: sedation, orthostatic hypotension, anticholinergic effects, rash
- ECG changes and QT prolongation can lead to torsades de pointes.

Clozapine
The first atypical antipsychotic developed. Despite its effectiveness for schizophrenia spectrum disorders, it is no longer considered a first-line medication because of its serious adverse effects.

FORMULATIONS: Tablets, orally disintegrating tablets

COMPLICATIONS
- Low risk of EPS
- High risk of weight gain, diabetes mellitus, dyslipidemia
- Agranulocytosis can occur. Obtain baseline WBC and monitor weekly, bi-weekly, to monthly per protocol.
- Monitor for indications of infection (fever, sore throat, lesions in mouth), and notify the provider if manifestations occur. **Qs**
- Other adverse effects: sedation, hypersalivation, orthostatic hypotension, and anticholinergic effects
- Pregnancy Risk Category B

Asenapine
FORMULATION: Sublingual tablets

COMPLICATIONS
- Drowsiness, prolonged QT interval, EPS (higher doses)
- Causes temporary numbing of the mouth
- Low risk of diabetes mellitus, weight gain, dyslipidemia, anticholinergic effects

Lurasidone
FORMULATION: Tablets

COMPLICATIONS
- Common adverse effects: sedation, akathisia, parkinsonism, agitation, anxiety
- Low risk for diabetes mellitus, weight gain, dyslipidemia
- Does not cause anticholinergic effects
- Pregnancy Risk Category B

Paliperidone
FORMULATIONS: Extended-release tablets, extended-release injections

COMPLICATIONS
- High risk for diabetes mellitus, weight gain, dyslipidemia
- Other adverse effects: sedation, prolonged QT interval, orthostatic hypotension, anticholinergic effects, mild EPS

Iloperidone
FORMULATION: Tablets

COMPLICATIONS
- Common adverse effects: dry mouth, sedation, fatigue, nasal congestion
- Significant risk for weight gain, prolonged QT interval, orthostatic hypotension
- Advise clients to follow titration schedule during initial therapy to minimize hypotension.
- Low risk for diabetes mellitus, dyslipidemia, EPS

Aripiprazole (third-generation antipsychotic)
FORMULATIONS: Tablets, orally disintegrating tablets, oral solution, sustained-release injectable

COMPLICATIONS: Bleeding and cardiovascular effects

ADVANTAGES
- Relief of both the positive and negative symptoms of the disease
- Decrease in affective manifestations (depression, anxiety) and suicidal behaviors
- Improvement of neurocognitive deficits, such as poor memory
- Fewer or no EPSs, including TD, because of less dopamine blockade
- Fewer anticholinergic adverse effects because most atypical antipsychotics, with the exception of clozapine, cause little or no blockade of cholinergic receptors
- Less relapse

FORMULATIONS
- Tablets
- Quick-dissolving tablets
- Oral solution
- IM depot preparations

COMPLICATIONS

Diabetes mellitus

New onset of diabetes mellitus or loss of glucose control in clients who have diabetes (referred to as metabolic syndrome and also includes weight gain and dyslipidemia)

NURSING CONSIDERATIONS
- Obtain baseline fasting blood glucose and monitor throughout treatment.
- Instruct client to report indications (increased thirst, urination, and appetite).

Weight gain

NURSING CONSIDERATIONS: Advise client to follow a healthy low-calorie diet, engage in regular exercise, and monitor weight gain.

Hypercholesterolemia

With increased risk for hypertension and other cardiovascular disease

NURSING CONSIDERATIONS: Monitor cholesterol, triglycerides, and blood glucose if weight gain is more than 14 kg (30 lb).

Orthostatic hypotension

NURSING CONSIDERATIONS: Monitor blood pressure and heart rate for orthostatic changes. Instruct clients to change positions slowly.

Anticholinergic effects

Include urinary hesitancy or retention, and dry mouth

NURSING CONSIDERATIONS
- Monitor for effects and report occurrence to the provider.
- Educate clients about measures to relieve dry mouth, such as sipping fluids.

Agitation, dizziness, sedation, sleep disruption

NURSING CONSIDERATIONS
- Monitor for effects and report to the provider if they occur.
- Administer alternative medication if prescribed.

Mild EPSs, such as tremor or akathisia

NURSING CONSIDERATIONS
- Monitor for and teach clients to recognize EPSs.
- Use AIMS assessment to screen for EPSs.

Elevated prolactin levels

NURSING CONSIDERATIONS
- Advise clients to observe for galactorrhea, gynecomastia, amenorrhea and to notify the provider if these occur.
- Obtain prolactin level if indicated.

Sexual dysfunction (anorgasmia, impotence, low libido)

NURSING CONSIDERATIONS
- Advise clients to observe for possible sexual side effects and notify the provider if they are intolerable.
- Instruct client on ways to manage sexual dysfunction, which can include using adjunct medications to improve sexual function (e.g., sildenafil).

CONTRAINDICATIONS/PRECAUTIONS

- Risperidone and most other atypical antipsychotics are Pregnancy Risk Category C.
- Lurasidone and clozapine are Category B.
- Contraindicated for clients who have dementia. All atypical antipsychotic medications can cause death related to cerebrovascular accident or infection. Ⓖ
- Clients should avoid use of alcohol.
- Use cautiously in clients who have cardiovascular or cerebrovascular disease, seizures, or diabetes mellitus. Obtain a fasting blood glucose for clients who have diabetes mellitus, and monitor blood glucose carefully.

INTERACTIONS

Immunosuppressive medications

Immunosuppressants, such as anticancer medications, can further suppress immune function in clients taking clozapine.

NURSING CONSIDERATIONS: Avoid use in clients taking clozapine.

Alcohol, opioids, and antihistamines

Have additive CNS depressant effects.

NURSING CONSIDERATIONS
- Advise clients to avoid alcohol and medications that cause CNS depression.
- Advise clients to avoid hazardous activities, such as driving.

Antipsychotic agents

By activating dopamine receptors, levodopa counteracts the effects of antipsychotic agents.

NURSING CONSIDERATIONS: Avoid concurrent use of levodopa and other direct dopamine receptor agonists.

Tricyclic antidepressants, amiodarone, and clarithromycin

Prolong QT interval and thus increase the risk of cardiac dysrhythmias in clients taking ziprasidone.

NURSING CONSIDERATIONS: Atypical antipsychotics that prolong the QT interval should not be used concurrently with other medications that have the same effect.

Barbiturates and phenytoin

Stimulate hepatic medication-metabolizing enzymes and thereby decrease drug levels of aripiprazole, quetiapine, and ziprasidone.

NURSING CONSIDERATIONS: Monitor medication effectiveness.

Fluconazole

Inhibits hepatic medication-metabolizing enzymes and thereby increases levels of aripiprazole, quetiapine, and ziprasidone

NURSING CONSIDERATIONS: Monitor for adverse effects or toxicity.

NURSING ADMINISTRATION

- Administer by oral or IM route. Risperidone is also available as a depot injection administered IM once every 2 weeks, and the long-acting injectable of paliperidone is administered every 28 days. Aripiprazole also has a long-acting injectable, which is administered on a monthly basis. Use for clients who have difficulty adhering to medication regimen. Therapeutic effect occurs up to several weeks following the first depot injection. Clients often require oral preparations until effectiveness is achieved. Advise clients that low doses of medication are given initially and are then gradually increased. Qpcc
- Use oral disintegrating tablets for clients who might attempt to "cheek" (or pocket) tablets or have difficulty swallowing them.
- Advise clients taking asenapine to avoid eating or drinking for 10 min after each dose.
- Administer lurasidone and ziprasidone with food (at least 350 calories) to increase absorption.
- The cost of antipsychotic medications can be a factor for some clients. Assess the need for case management intervention. Qtc

NURSING EVALUATION OF MEDICATION EFFECTIVENESS

- Depending on therapeutic intent, effectiveness can be evidenced by improvement in the following.
- Positive and negative manifestations (prevention of acute psychotic manifestations, absence of hallucinations, delusions, anxiety, and hostility)
- Ability to perform ADLs
- Ability to interact socially with peers
- Sleeping and eating habits

Application Exercises

1. A nurse is teaching a client who has schizophrenia strategies to cope with anticholinergic effects of fluphenazine. Which of the following should the nurse suggest to the client to minimize anticholinergic effects?

   A. Take the medication in the morning to prevent insomnia.

   B. Chew sugarless gum to moisten the mouth.

   C. Use cooling measures to decrease fever.

   D. Take an antacid to relieve nausea.

2. A nurse is assessing a male client who recently began taking haloperidol. Which of the following findings is the highest priority to report to the provider?

   A. Shuffling gait

   B. Neck spasms

   C. Drowsiness

   D. Impotence

3. A nurse is providing discharge teaching to a client who has a new prescription for clozapine. Which of the following statements should the nurse include in the teaching?

   A. "You should have a high-carbohydrate snack between meals and at bedtime."

   B. "You are likely to develop hand tremors if you take this medication for a long period of time."

   C. "You may experience temporary numbness of your mouth after each dose."

   D. "You should have your white blood cell count monitored every week."

4. A nurse is providing teaching for a male client who has schizophrenia and is taking risperidone. Which of the following instructions should the nurse include in the teaching?

   A. "Add extra snacks to your diet to prevent weight loss."

   B. "Notify the provider if you develop breast enlargement."

   C. "You may begin to have mild seizures while taking this medication."

   D. "This medication is likely to increase your libido."

5. A nurse is preparing to perform a follow-up assessment on a client who takes chlorpromazine for the treatment of schizophrenia. The nurse should expect to find the greatest improvement in which of the following manifestations? (Select all that apply.)

   A. Disorganized speech

   B. Bizarre behavior

   C. Impaired social interactions

   D. Hallucinations

   E. Decreased motivation

PRACTICE Active Learning Scenario

A nurse caring for a client who has neuroleptic malignant syndrome.

Use the ATI Active Learning Template: System Disorder to complete this item to include the following sections.

DESCRIPTION OF DISORDER/DISEASE PROCESS

ASSESSMENT: Identify at least four expected objective findings.

MEDICATIONS: Identify two medications appropriate for treatment and their purpose.

NURSING CARE: Identify at least three appropriate interventions.

Application Exercises Key

1. A. Insomnia is not an anticholinergic effect.

   B. **CORRECT:** Chewing sugarless gum can help the client cope with dry mouth, a potential anticholinergic effect of fluphenazine.

   C. Fever is not an anticholinergic effect.

   D. Nausea is not an anticholinergic effect.

   Ⓝ *NCLEX® Connection: Pharmacological and Parenteral Therapies, Medication Administration*

2. A. Shuffling gait is an indication of parkinsonism and should be reported to the provider. However, this is not the greatest risk to the client and is therefore not the priority finding.

   B. **CORRECT:** Neck spasms are an indication of acute dystonia which is a crisis situation requiring rapid treatment. This is the greatest risk to the client and is therefore the priority finding.

   C. Drowsiness is an adverse effect of haloperidol and should be reported to the provider. However, this is not the greatest risk to the client and is therefore not the priority finding.

   D. Sexual dysfunction is an adverse effect of haloperidol and should be reported to the provider. However, this is not the greatest risk to the client and is therefore not the priority finding.

   Ⓝ *NCLEX® Connection: Pharmacological and Parenteral Therapies, Adverse Effects/Contraindications/Side Effects/Interactions*

3. A. Clozapine increases the client's risk of developing diabetes mellitus and weight gain. It is not appropriate to increase carbohydrate intake.

   B. Clozapine has a low risk of EPS such as hand tremors.

   C. Asenapine, rather than clozapine, causes temporary numbing of the mouth.

   D. **CORRECT:** Due to the risk for fatal agranulocytosis weekly monitoring of the client's WBC count is recommended while taking clozapine.

   Ⓝ *NCLEX® Connection: Pharmacological and Parenteral Therapies, Adverse Effects/Contraindications/Side Effects/Interactions*

4. A. Risperidone and other atypical antidepressants cause weight gain and the client should be taught to maintain a lower-calorie balanced diet.

   B. **CORRECT:** Gynecomastia (breast enlargement) and galactorrhea can occur due to an increase in prolactin levels while taking risperidone. The client should inform the provider if these manifestations occur.

   C. Seizures are not an adverse effect of risperidone.

   D. Sexual dysfunction, causing decreased libido and impotence are adverse effects of risperidone.

   Ⓝ *NCLEX® Connection: Pharmacological and Parenteral Therapies, Medication Administration*

5. A. **CORRECT:** A client who takes a conventional antipsychotic medication, such as chlorpromazine, should have the greatest improvement in positive symptoms such as disorganized speech.

   B. **CORRECT:** A client who takes a conventional antipsychotic medication, such as chlorpromazine, should have the greatest improvement in positive symptoms such as bizarre behavior.

   C. Conventional antipsychotic medications, such as chlorpromazine, have less effect on negative symptoms such as impaired social interactions.

   D. **CORRECT:** A client who takes a conventional antipsychotic medication, such as chlorpromazine, should have the greatest improvement in positive symptoms such as hallucinations.

   E. Conventional antipsychotic medications, such as chlorpromazine, have less effect on negative symptoms such as decreased motivation.

   Ⓝ *NCLEX® Connection: Pharmacological and Parenteral Therapies, Expected Actions/Outcomes*

PRACTICE Answer

Using the ATI Active Learning Template: System Disorders

DESCRIPTION OF DISORDER/DISEASE PROCESS: Neuroleptic malignant syndrome is a potential adverse effect of first-generation (conventional) antipsychotic medications that most commonly occurs within the first 2 weeks of treatment.

ASSESSMENT
- Sudden high fever
- Blood pressure fluctuations
- Drooling
- Diaphoresis
- Dysrhythmias
- Muscle rigidity
- Changes in level of consciousness
- Coma

MEDICATIONS
- Aspirin: antipyretic
- Acetaminophen: antipyretic
- Dantrolene: induces muscle relaxation
- Bromocriptine: induces muscle relaxation

NURSING CARE
- Notify the provider immediately.
- Withhold the conventional antipsychotic medication.
- Monitor vital signs.
- Apply cooling blankets.
- Increase fluid intake.
- Discuss with the provider the need to wait 2 weeks before resuming therapy.
- Discuss with the provider the possible need to switch to an atypical agent.

Ⓝ *NCLEX® Connection: Pharmacological and Parenteral Therapies, Expected Actions/Outcomes*

UNIT 2   MEDICATIONS AFFECTING THE NERVOUS SYSTEM

CHAPTER 11

Medications for Children and Adolescents Who Have Mental Health Issues

Various medications are used to manage behavioral disorders in children and adolescents, including attention deficit-hyperactivity disorder, conduct disorder, intermittent explosive disorder, and autism spectrum disorders. Parents should understand that pharmacological management is most effective when accompanied by techniques to modify behavior.

Central nervous system stimulants

11.1 Select prototypes and other medications

	SHORT-ACTING	INTERMEDIATE-ACTING	LONG-ACTING
Methylphenidate	3 to 5 hr	6 to 8 hr	8 to 12 hr
Dexmethylphenidate	4 to 5 hr	n/a	12 hr
Dextroamphetamine	4 to 6 hr	n/a	6 to 10 hr
Amphetamine mixture	4 to 6 hr	n/a	10 to 12 hr
Lisdexamfetamine dimesylate	n/a	n/a	10 to 12 hr

PURPOSE

EXPECTED PHARMACOLOGICAL ACTION: Raise the levels of norepinephrine and dopamine in the central nervous system (CNS).

THERAPEUTIC USES
- ADHD
- Conduct disorder
- Narcolepsy
- Obesity

COMPLICATIONS

CNS stimulation

Insomnia, restlessness

NURSING CONSIDERATIONS
- Advise clients to observe for effects and notify the provider if they occur.
- Administer the last dose before 4 p.m. Q EBP

Decreased appetite, weight loss, growth suppression

NURSING CONSIDERATIONS
- Monitor the client's weight and compare to baseline height and weight.
- Administer medication immediately during or after meals.
- Promote good nutrition in children.
- Encourage children to eat at regular meal times and avoid unhealthy foods for snacks.
- Consult with prescriber about possible "drug holidays."

Cardiovascular effects

Dysrhythmias, chest pain, high blood pressure

NURSING CONSIDERATIONS
- These medications can increase the risk of sudden death in clients who have heart abnormalities.
- Monitor vital signs and ECG.
- Advise clients to observe for effects (shortness of breath, chest pain, dizziness) and to notify the provider if they occur.

Development of psychotic manifestations

Such as hallucinations and paranoia

CLIENT EDUCATION: Instruct clients to report manifestations immediately and to discontinue the medication if they occur.

Physical tolerance and withdrawal reaction

Headache, nausea, vomiting, and muscle weakness, depression

CLIENT EDUCATION: Advise clients to not stop taking medication suddenly. Doing so can lead to depression and severe fatigue. Withdraw medication gradually.

Hypersensitivity skin reaction to transdermal methylphenidate

Hives, papules

NURSING CONSIDERATIONS: Remove the patch and notify the provider.

Toxicity

Dizziness, palpitations, hypertension, hallucinations, seizures

NURSING CONSIDERATIONS
- Treat hallucinations with chlorpromazine.
- Treat seizures with diazepam.
- Administer fluids.

CONTRAINDICATIONS/PRECAUTIONS

- Use with caution in clients who are pregnant (Pregnancy Risk Category C), breastfeeding, or have hypertension or depression.
- These medications are contraindicated in clients who have a history of substance use disorder, hypertension, hyperthyroidism, cardiovascular disorders, glaucoma, severe anxiety, and psychosis.

INTERACTIONS

Concurrent use of MAOIs can cause hypertensive crisis.
NURSING CONSIDERATIONS: Avoid concurrent use. Do not use within 14 days of MAOIs.

Concurrent use of caffeine can increase CNS stimulant effects.
NURSING CONSIDERATIONS: Instruct clients to avoid foods and beverages that contain caffeine.

Methylphenidate inhibits metabolism of phenytoin warfarin and phenobarbital, leading to increased serum levels.
NURSING CONSIDERATIONS
- Monitor clients for adverse effects (CNS depression, toxicity, indications of bleeding).
- Concurrent use of these medications is done with caution.

OTC cold and decongestant medications with sympathomimetic action can increase CNS stimulant effects.
NURSING CONSIDERATIONS: Instruct clients to avoid use of OTC medications.

NURSING ADMINISTRATION

- Advise clients to swallow sustained-release tablets whole and to not chew or crush the tablets.
- Teach clients the importance of administering the medication on a regular schedule.
- Teach clients who use transdermal medication to place the patch on one hip daily in the morning and leave it in place no longer than 9 hr. Alternate hips daily.
- Instruct parents and clients that ADHD is not cured by medication. Management with an overall treatment plan that includes family therapy and cognitive-behavioral therapy will improve outcomes. Q**EBP**
- Instruct parents that these medications have specific handling procedures controlled by federal law. Handwritten prescriptions are required for medication refills.
- Instruct parents in safety and storage of medications.
- Advise parents that these medications have a high potential for development of a substance use disorder, especially in adolescents. Instruct clients to use strictly as prescribed.
- Advise clients to avoid activities that require alertness until medication effects are known.

NURSING EVALUATION OF MEDICATION EFFECTIVENESS

Depending on therapeutic intent, effectiveness is evidenced by the following.
- Improvement of manifestations of ADHD, such as increased ability to focus and complete tasks, interact with peers, and manage impulsivity
- Improved ability to stay awake

Norepinephrine selective reuptake inhibitors

SELECT PROTOTYPE MEDICATION: Atomoxetine

OTHER MEDICATION: Bupropion

PURPOSE

EXPECTED PHARMACOLOGICAL ACTION
- Block reuptake of norepinephrine at synapses in the CNS. Atomoxetine is not a stimulant medication.
- Bupropion blocks the synaptic reuptake of norepinephrine and dopamine. It is considered a second-line medication for ADHD.

THERAPEUTIC USES
- ADHD
- Depression

COMPLICATIONS

Atomoxetine is usually tolerated well with minimal adverse effects.

Appetite suppression, weight loss, growth suppression

NURSING CONSIDERATIONS
- Monitor the client's weight and compare to baseline height and weight.
- Administer medication with or without meals.
- Encourage children to eat at regular meal times and avoid unhealthy foods for snacks.

GI effects

Nausea and vomiting

CLIENT EDUCATION: Advise clients to take with food if these occur.

Suicidal ideation

In children and adolescents

NURSING CONSIDERATIONS
- Monitor for indications of depression.
- Advise clients to report change in mood, excessive sleeping, agitation, and irritability. Q**s**

Hepatotoxicity

CLIENT EDUCATION: Advise clients to report indications of liver damage (flu-like manifestations, yellowing skin, abdominal pain).

Seizure activity

NURSING CONSIDERATIONS: Use low doses, and monitor for seizure activity. Do not use in clients who have a seizure disorder.

CONTRAINDICATIONS/PRECAUTIONS

- Use cautiously in clients who have cardiovascular, hepatic, disorders, and hypo/hypertension.
- Atomoxetine is contraindicated in clients who have angle-closure glaucoma, heart failure, and jaundice.
- Bupropion increases seizure risk at high dosages. It is contraindicated in clients who have seizure risk factors and eating disorders.

INTERACTIONS

Concurrent use of MAOIs can cause hypertensive crisis.
NURSING CONSIDERATIONS: Avoid concurrent use. Do not use within 14 days of MAOIs.

Paroxetine, fluoxetine, and quinidine gluconate inhibit hepatic metabolizing enzymes, thereby increasing levels of atomoxetine.
NURSING CONSIDERATIONS
- Teach clients to watch for and report increased adverse reactions of atomoxetine.
- Reduce dosage of atomoxetine if used concurrently with these medications.

NURSING ADMINISTRATION

- Note any changes in the child's behavior related to dosing and timing of medications.
- Administer the medication in a daily dose in the morning, or in two divided doses (morning and afternoon), with or without food.
- Instruct clients that therapeutic effects can take 1 to 3 weeks to fully develop.

NURSING EVALUATION OF MEDICATION EFFECTIVENESS

Depending on therapeutic intent, effectiveness is evidenced by improvement of manifestations of ADHD such as increase in ability to focus and complete tasks, interact with peers, and manage impulsivity.

Tricyclic antidepressants

SELECT PROTOTYPE MEDICATION: Desipramine

OTHER MEDICATIONS
- Imipramine
- Clomipramine

PURPOSE

EXPECTED PHARMACOLOGICAL ACTION: These medications block reuptake of the monoamine neurotransmitters norepinephrine and serotonin in the synaptic space, thereby intensifying the effects that these neurotransmitters produce.

THERAPEUTIC USES IN CHILDREN
- Depression
- Autism spectrum disorder
- ADHD (considered less effective than CNS stimulants and used as second-line treatment for ADHD)
- Panic, social phobia, separation anxiety disorder
- Obsessive compulsive disorder (OCD)

COMPLICATIONS

Orthostatic hypotension

NURSING CONSIDERATIONS: Monitor blood pressure with first dose. Instruct client to change positions slowly. Qs

Anticholinergic effects

Dry mouth, blurred vision, photophobia, urinary hesitancy or retention, constipation, tachycardia

CLIENT EDUCATION
- Instruct clients about ways to minimize anticholinergic effects.
  - Chewing sugarless gum
  - Sipping on water
  - Avoiding activities that require alertness
  - Wearing sunglasses when outdoors
  - Eating foods high in fiber
  - Participating in regular exercise
  - Increasing fluid intake to at least 2 to 3 L/day from beverages or food sources
  - Voiding just before taking medication
- Advise clients to notify the provider if anticholinergic effects are intolerable.

Weight gain

NURSING CONSIDERATIONS
- Monitor client weight.
- Encourage clients to participate in regular exercise and to follow a healthy, low-calorie diet.

Sedation

CLIENT EDUCATION
- Advise clients that this adverse effect usually diminishes over time.
- Advise clients to avoid activities that require alertness, such as driving if sedation is excessive.
- Advise clients to take medication at bedtime to minimize daytime sleepiness and to promote sleep.

Toxicity

Resulting in cholinergic blockade and cardiac toxicity evidenced by dysrhythmias, mental confusion, and agitation, followed by seizures and coma

NURSING CONSIDERATIONS
- Give clients who are acutely ill a 1-week supply of medication.
- Obtain baseline ECG.
- Monitor vital signs frequently.
- Monitor for toxicity and notify the provider if indications of toxicity occur.

Decreased seizure threshold

NURSING CONSIDERATIONS: Monitor clients who have seizure disorders.

Excessive sweating

CLIENT EDUCATION: Inform clients of this adverse effect and assist with frequent linen changes.

CONTRAINDICATIONS/PRECAUTIONS

- Use cautiously in clients who have seizure disorders; diabetes mellitus; liver, kidney and respiratory disorders; and hyperthyroidism.
- Contraindicated in clients who have closed-angle glaucoma, and acute MI.

INTERACTIONS

Concurrent use of monoamine oxidase inhibitors (MAOIs) causes hypertension.
NURSING CONSIDERATIONS
- Avoid concurrent use.
- Do not use within 14 days of MAOIs.

Antihistamines and other anticholinergic agents have additive anticholinergic effects.
NURSING CONSIDERATIONS: Avoid concurrent use.

Tricyclic antidepressants (TCAs) block uptake of epinephrine and NE (direct-acting sympathomimetics) in the synaptic space, leading to decreased intensity of their effects.
NURSING CONSIDERATIONS: Avoid concurrent use.

TCAs inhibit uptake of ephedrine and amphetamine (indirect-acting sympathomimetics) and reduce their ability to get to the site of action in the nerve terminal, leading to decreased responses to these medications.
NURSING CONSIDERATIONS: Avoid concurrent use.

Alcohol, benzodiazepines, opioids, and antihistamines cause additive CNS depression when used concurrently.
NURSING CONSIDERATIONS: Advise clients to avoid concurrent use with CNS depressants.

NURSING ADMINISTRATION

- Instruct the client's parents to administer this medication as prescribed on a daily basis to establish therapeutic plasma levels.
- Assist with medication regimen compliance by informing clients and parents that it can take 2 to 3 weeks to experience therapeutic effects. Full therapeutic effects can take 2 to 3 months.
- Instruct clients and parents the importance of continuing therapy after improvement in manifestations. Sudden discontinuation of the medication can result in relapse.
- Take medication at bedtime to prevent daytime drowsiness.
- Give only 1 week worth of medication at a time for an acutely ill client. Tricyclics have high lethality in overdosage. Qs

NURSING EVALUATION OF MEDICATION EFFECTIVENESS

Depending on therapeutic intent, effectiveness is evidenced by the following.

For depression
- Verbalizing improvement in mood
- Improved sleeping and eating habits
- Increased interaction with peers

For autism spectrum disorder: Decreased anger, agitation, and compulsive behavior

For ADHD: Less hyperactivity, greater ability to pay attention

Alpha₂-adrenergic agonists

SELECT PROTOTYPE MEDICATION: Guanfacine

OTHER MEDICATION: Clonidine

PURPOSE

EXPECTED PHARMACOLOGICAL ACTION: The action of alpha₂-adrenergic agonists is not completely understood. However, they are known to activate presynaptic alpha₂-adrenergic receptors within the brain.

THERAPEUTIC USES: ADHD

COMPLICATIONS

CNS effects

Sedation, drowsiness, fatigue

NURSING CONSIDERATIONS
- Monitor for these adverse effects and report their occurrence to the provider.
- Advise clients to avoid activities that require alertness.

Cardiovascular effects

Hypotension, bradycardia

NURSING CONSIDERATIONS
- Monitor blood pressure and pulse especially during initial treatment.
- Advise client not to abruptly discontinue medication which can cause rebound hypertension.

Weight gain

NURSING CONSIDERATIONS
- Monitor client weight.
- Encourage clients to participate in regular exercise and to follow a healthy, well-balanced diet.

CONTRAINDICATIONS/PRECAUTIONS

- Extended-release clonidine is contraindicated for children younger than 6 years old.
- Use cautiously in clients who have cardiac disease, cerebrovascular disease, kidney or liver impairment, and older adults.

INTERACTIONS

CNS depressants, including alcohol, can increase CNS effects.
NURSING CONSIDERATIONS: Avoid concurrent use.

Antihypertensives can worsen hypotension.
NURSING CONSIDERATIONS: Avoid concurrent use.

Foods with high-fat content will increase guanfacine absorption.
NURSING CONSIDERATIONS: Advise clients to avoid taking medication with a high-fat meal. Ⓠ EBP

NURSING ADMINISTRATION

- Assess use of alcohol and CNS depressants, especially with adolescent clients.
- Instruct clients to not chew, crush, or split extended-release preparations.
- Monitor blood pressure and pulse at baseline, with initial treatment, and with each dosage change.
- Advise clients to avoid abrupt discontinuation of medication, which can result in rebound hypertension. Medication should be tapered according to a prescribed dosage schedule when discontinuing treatment.

NURSING EVALUATION OF MEDICATION EFFECTIVENESS

Depending on therapeutic intent, effectiveness is evidenced by improvement of manifestations of ADHD, such as increase in ability to focus and complete tasks, interact with peers, and manage impulsivity.

Antipsychotics: Atypical

SELECT PROTOTYPE MEDICATION: Risperidone

OTHER MEDICATIONS
- Olanzapine
- Quetiapine
- Aripiprazole

PURPOSE

EXPECTED PHARMACOLOGICAL ACTION
- Second-generation antipsychotic agents (risperidone, olanzapine, quetiapine) work mainly by blocking serotonin, and to a lesser degree, dopamine receptors. These medications also block receptors for norepinephrine, histamine, and acetylcholine.
- Aripiprazole is a third-generation antipsychotic and acts as a dopamine system stabilizer. It not only blocks dopamine and serotonin receptors, it also is a partial agonist at these receptors. Thus, net effects on receptor activity will depend on how much dopamine and serotonin is present.

THERAPEUTIC USES
- Autism spectrum disorder
- Conduct disorder
- Posttraumatic stress disorder (PTSD)
- Relief of psychotic manifestations
- Intermittent explosive disorder

COMPLICATIONS

Diabetes mellitus

New onset of diabetes mellitus or loss of glucose control in clients who have diabetes (referred to as metabolic syndrome, along with the risk of weight gain, and dyslipidemia)

NURSING CONSIDERATIONS
- Obtain baseline fasting blood glucose and monitor periodically throughout treatment.
- Instruct clients to report indications such as increased thirst, urination, and appetite.

Weight gain

CLIENT EDUCATION: Advise clients to follow a healthy, low-caloric diet, engage in regular exercise, and monitor weight gain.

Hypercholesterolemia

With increased risk for hypertension and other cardiovascular disease

NURSING CONSIDERATIONS: Monitor cholesterol, triglycerides, and blood glucose if weight gain is more than 14 kg (30 lb).

Orthostatic hypotension

NURSING CONSIDERATIONS: Monitor blood pressure with first dose. Instruct client to change positions slowly.

Anticholinergic effects

Urinary hesitancy or retention, dry mouth

NURSING CONSIDERATIONS
- Monitor for these adverse effects and report their occurrence to the provider.
- Encourage client to use measures to relieve dry mouth such as sipping fluids throughout the day.

Agitation, dizziness, sedation, sleep disruption

NURSING CONSIDERATIONS
- Monitor for these adverse effects and report their occurrence to the provider. Avoid activities that require alertness until effects are known.
- Administer an alternative medication if prescribed.

Mild extrapyramidal adverse effects, such as tremor

NURSING CONSIDERATIONS: Monitor for and teach clients to recognize extrapyramidal adverse effects. These are usually dose-related.

Agranulocytosis, neutropenia

NURSING CONSIDERATIONS: Monitor WBC periodically and advise clients to monitor and report manifestations of an infection, such as a sore throat. Qs

Hyperprolactinemia

NURSING CONSIDERATIONS: Monitor and report gynecomastia and amenorrhea.

CONTRAINDICATIONS/PRECAUTIONS

- Be aware of possible alcohol use in the adolescent client. Instruct clients to avoid the use of alcohol.
- Use cautiously in clients who have cardiovascular disease, seizures, dehydration, kidney/hepatic disease, or diabetes mellitus. Obtain a baseline fasting glucose for clients who have diabetes mellitus and monitor carefully.

INTERACTIONS

Alcohol, opioids, and antihistamines cause additive CNS depressant effects.
NURSING CONSIDERATIONS
- Advise clients to avoid alcohol and other medications that cause CNS depression.
- Advise clients to avoid hazardous activities, such as driving.

By activating dopamine receptors, levodopa counteracts effects of antipsychotic agents.
NURSING CONSIDERATIONS: Avoid concurrent use of levodopa and other direct dopamine receptor agonists.

Tricyclic antidepressants, amiodarone and clarithromycin prolong QT interval and thus increase the risk of cardiac dysrhythmias.
NURSING CONSIDERATIONS: Avoid concurrent use.

Barbiturates promote hepatic medication-metabolizing enzymes, thereby decreasing medication levels of quetiapine.
NURSING CONSIDERATIONS: Monitor medication effectiveness.

Medications that inhibit CYP3A4, such as fluconazole inhibit hepatic medication-metabolizing enzymes, thereby increasing medication levels of aripiprazole, quetiapine, and ziprasidone.
NURSING CONSIDERATIONS: Monitor for adverse effects.

NURSING ADMINISTRATION

- Administer by oral or IM route.
  - Risperidone is available in an oral solution and quick-dissolving tablets for ease in administration.
  - Olanzapine is available in an orally disintegrating tablet for ease in administration.
- Advise clients that low doses of medication are given initially and are then gradually increased.

NURSING EVALUATION OF MEDICATION EFFECTIVENESS

Depending on therapeutic intent, effectiveness is evidenced by the following.

For autism spectrum disorder: reduction of hyperactivity, agitation, and improvement in mood

For conduct disorder: decrease in aggressiveness

For ADHD: reduction in hyperactivity and impulsivity

Selective serotonin reuptake inhibitors

SELECT PROTOTYPE MEDICATION: Fluoxetine

OTHER MEDICATION: Sertraline

PURPOSE

EXPECTED PHARMACOLOGICAL ACTION: Selectively blocks the reuptake of serotonin, intensifying monoamine effects in the CNS.

THERAPEUTIC USES
- Autism spectrum disorder
- Obsessive compulsive disorder
- Major depressive disorder
- Intermittent explosive disorder
- Bulimia nervosa

COMPLICATIONS

Serotonin syndrome

Agitation, confusion, hallucinations

NURSING CONSIDERATIONS: Do not use within 14 days of MAOIs. Monitor for effects and discontinue.

Weight gain

NURSING CONSIDERATIONS: Advise clients to follow a healthy, low-caloric diet, engage in regular exercise, and monitor weight gain.

Withdrawal syndrome

Dizziness, nausea, tremors

NURSING CONSIDERATIONS: Do not discontinue abruptly.

Suicidal ideation

NURSING CONSIDERATIONS: Monitor and report any thoughts of suicide.

Extrapyramidal effects

Ataxia, tremors

NURSING CONSIDERATIONS: Monitor and report manifestations.

Dizziness, fatigue, insomnia, agitation

NURSING CONSIDERATIONS: Advise clients to avoid activities that require alertness until effects are known. Reduce dosage if needed.

Sexual dysfunction

Impotence, decreased libido

NURSING CONSIDERATIONS: Advise clients about this possible adverse effect.

Dysrhythmias

NURSING CONSIDERATIONS: Monitor for dysrhythmias. Reduce dosage as needed.

CONTRAINDICATIONS/PRECAUTIONS

- Pregnancy Risk Category C: Can cause abstinence syndrome and pulmonary hypertension in the newborn.
- Use cautiously in clients who are breastfeeding and clients who have narrow-angle glaucoma.

INTERACTIONS

Concurrent use of MAOIs and other medications that can cause serotonin syndrome (SNRIs, buspirone, phenothiazines) increases the risk for serotonin syndrome.
NURSING CONSIDERATIONS
- Avoid concurrent use.
- Do not use within 14 days of MAOIs.

Elevation of plasma levels of TCAs and lithium
NURSING CONSIDERATIONS
- Avoid concurrent use.
- Monitor for toxicity.

Antiplatelet medications and anticoagulants increase risk for bleeding.
NURSING CONSIDERATIONS
- Avoid concurrent use.
- Monitor for bleeding.

NURSING ADMINISTRATION

- Administer orally with or without meals.
- Therapeutic effects can take 1 to 4 weeks.
- Notify provider if pregnancy is suspected.

NURSING EVALUATION OF MEDICATION EFFECTIVENESS

Depending on therapeutic intent, effectiveness is evidenced by the following.

Improvement in mood, decreased manifestations of obsessive compulsive disorder, decrease in aggressiveness

For depression
- Verbalizing improvement in mood
- Improved sleeping and eating habits
- Increased interaction with peers

For autism spectrum disorder, intermittent explosive disorder: Decreased anger, agitation, and compulsive behavior

Application Exercises

1. A nurse is teaching the parents of a child who has a new prescription for desipramine. The nurse should instruct the parents that which of the following adverse effects is the priority to report to the provider?

    A. Constipation
    B. Suicidal thoughts
    C. Photophobia
    D. Dry mouth

2. A nurse is teaching an adolescent client who has a new prescription for clomipramine for OCD. Which of the following instructions should the nurse include to minimize an adverse effect of his medication?

    A. Wear sunglasses when outdoors.
    B. Check your temperature daily.
    C. Take this medication in the morning.
    D. Add extra calories to your diet.

3. A nurse is caring for a school-age child who has a new prescription for atomoxetine. The nurse should monitor the client for which of the following adverse effects of this medication?

    A. Kidney toxicity
    B. Liver damage
    C. Seizure activity
    D. Adrenal insufficiency

4. A nurse is teaching the parents of a school-age child about transdermal methylphenidate. Which of the following instructions should the nurse include?

    A. Apply one patch twice per day.
    B. Leave the patch on for 9 hr.
    C. Apply the patch to the child's waist.
    D. Use opened tray within 6 months.

5. A nurse is teaching a school-age child and his parents about a new prescription for lisdexamfetamine. Which of the following information should the nurse include in the teaching? (Select all that apply.)

    A. An adverse effect of this medication is CNS stimulation.
    B. Administer the medication before bedtime.
    C. Monitor blood pressure while taking this medication.
    D. Therapeutic effects of this medication will take 1 to 3 weeks to fully develop.
    E. This medication raises the levels of dopamine in the brain.

Application Exercises Key

1. A. The client is at risk for constipation because of the anticholinergic effects of desipramine. The client should increase fluid intake to reduce the risk of constipation. However, another adverse effect is the priority.

   B. **CORRECT:** The greatest risk to this client is injury from a suicide attempt; therefore, this is the priority. Desipramine can cause suicidal thoughts and behaviors which puts the client at risk. The parents should monitor and report any indication of increased depression or thoughts of suicidal behavior.

   C. The client is at risk for photophobia, because of the anticholinergic effects of desipramine. The client should wear sun glasses when exposed to sunlight. However, another adverse effect is the priority.

   D. The client is at risk for dry mouth because of the anticholinergic effects of desipramine. The client should increase fluids and use hard candy to reduce dry mouth. However, another adverse effect is the priority.

   Ⓝ *NCLEX® Connection: Pharmacological and Parenteral Therapies, Adverse Effects/Contraindications/Side Effects/Interactions*

2. A. **CORRECT:** Wearing sunglasses when outdoors will decrease photophobia, an anticholinergic effect associated with TCA use.

   B. Checking the client's temperature daily is not necessary while taking a TCA.

   C. The client should take this medication at bedtime rather than in the morning to prevent daytime sleepiness.

   D. Following a low-calorie diet plan will help prevent weight gain, an adverse effect of TCAs.

   Ⓝ *NCLEX® Connection: Pharmacological and Parenteral Therapies, Adverse Effects/Contraindications/Side Effects/Interactions*

3. A. Atomoxetine can cause urinary retention, but not kidney toxicity.

   B. **CORRECT:** Liver damage is an adverse effect of atomoxetine. The nurse should monitor for manifestations such as jaundice, upper abdominal tenderness, darkening of urine, and elevated liver enzymes.

   C. Bupropion increases seizure risk at high dosages. Seizure activity is not an adverse effect of atomoxetine.

   D. Atomoxetine can cause suicidal ideation and mood swings. Adrenal insufficiency is not an adverse effect of atomoxetine.

   Ⓝ *NCLEX® Connection: Pharmacological and Parenteral Therapies, Adverse Effects/Contraindications/Side Effects/Interactions*

4. A. Transdermal methylphenidate is administered once per day.

   B. **CORRECT:** Transdermal methylphenidate is administered for 9 hr/day.

   C. Transdermal methylphenidate is applied to the child's hip.

   D. Use the opened tray of transdermal methylphenidate within 2 months.

   Ⓝ *NCLEX® Connection: Pharmacological and Parenteral Therapies, Medication Administration*

5. A. **CORRECT:** An adverse effect of lisdexamfetamine is CNS stimulation such as insomnia and restlessness.

   B. Administer lisdexamfetamine daily in the morning to reduce insomnia.

   C. **CORRECT:** The nurse should instruct the client to monitor his blood pressure due to potential cardiovascular effects of lisdexamfetamine.

   D. Therapeutic effects of lisdexamfetamine begin immediately and last 10 to 12 hrs.

   E. **CORRECT:** Lisdexamfetamine, a CNS stimulant, works by raising the levels of norepinephrine and dopamine in the CNS.

   Ⓝ *NCLEX® Connection: Pharmacological and Parenteral Therapies, Medication Administration*

PRACTICE Active Learning Scenario

A nurse working in a pediatric mental health clinic is caring for a client who has a new prescription for risperidone for the treatment of conduct disorder. Use the ATI Active Learning Template: Medication to complete this item.

COMPLICATIONS: Identify at least four adverse effects of this medication.

NURSING INTERVENTIONS: Identify at least four nursing interventions to prevent or minimize the adverse effects of this medication.

PRACTICE Answer

Using the ATI Active Learning Template: Medication

COMPLICATIONS
- New onset of diabetes mellitus or loss of glucose control in clients who have diabetes
- Weight gain
- Hypercholesterolemia
- Orthostatic hypotension
- Anticholinergic effects (urinary hesitancy or retention, dry mouth)
- Agitation
- Dizziness
- Sedation
- Sleep disruption
- Tremors
- Agranulocytosis, neutropenia
- Hyperprolactinemia

NURSING INTERVENTIONS
- Obtain the client's fasting blood glucose prior to and periodically throughout treatment.
- Instruct the client to report indications of diabetes mellitus including increased thirst, urination, and appetite.
- Advise clients to follow a healthy, low-caloric diet.
- Recommend regular exercise.
- Monitor weight throughout treatment.
- Monitor cholesterol and triglycerides, especially if weight gain is more than 30 lb.
- Monitor blood pressure with first dose and instruct client to change positions slowly.
- Encourage the client to sip fluids throughout the day.
- Monitor and report manifestations of an infection, such as a sore throat.
- Monitor and report gyneocomastia, and amenorrhea.

Ⓝ *NCLEX® Connection: Pharmacological and Parenteral Therapies, Adverse Effects/Contraindications/Side Effects/Interactions*

CHAPTER 12

CHAPTER 12　*Substance Use Disorders*

Abstinence syndrome occurs when clients abruptly withdraw from a substance to which they are physically dependent.

Clients who have a substance use disorder can experience tolerance and withdrawal. Tolerance requires increased amounts of the substance to achieve the desired effect. Withdrawal is physiological manifestations that occur when the concentration of the substance in the client's bloodstream declines.

Withdrawing from a substance that has the potential to cause physical dependence can cause abstinence syndrome. The client can experience distressing manifestations that can lead to coma and death.

Major substances associated with substance use disorder include alcohol, caffeine, cannabis, hallucinogens, inhalants, opioids, sedatives/hypnotics/anxiolytics, stimulants, tobacco, and other (or unknown) substances, such as anabolic steroids, betel nut, and unidentified black market substances.

Substance withdrawal varies depending on the substance and can produce a variety of manifestations, including gastrointestinal distress, neurological and behavioral changes, cardiovascular changes, and seizures.

Medications to support withdrawal/abstinence from alcohol

- Effects of withdrawal usually start within 4 to 12 hr of the last intake of alcohol and can continue 5 to 7 days.
- Manifestations include nausea; vomiting; tremors; restlessness and inability to sleep; depressed mood or irritability; increased heart rate, blood pressure, respiratory rate, and temperature; diaphoresis; and tonic-clonic seizures. Illusions are also common.
- Alcohol withdrawal delirium can occur 2 to 3 days after cessation of alcohol, and is considered a medical emergency. Findings include severe disorientation, psychotic manifestations (auditory or visual hallucinations), severe hypertension, and cardiac dysrhythmias that can progress to death. Qs

WITHDRAWAL

Benzodiazepines

First-line treatment for treatment of alcohol withdrawal

EXAMPLES: Chlordiazepoxide, diazepam, lorazepam, clorazepate, oxazepam

INTENDED EFFECTS
- Maintenance of vital signs within expected limits.
- Decrease in the risk of seizures.
- Decrease in the intensity of withdrawal manifestations
- Substitution therapy during alcohol withdrawal.

NURSING CONSIDERATIONS
- Administer around the clock or PRN.
- Obtain baseline vital signs.
- Monitor vital signs and neurological status on an ongoing basis.
- Provide seizure precautions.

Adjunct medications to treatment with benzodiazepines

EXAMPLES: Carbamazepine, clonidine, propranolol and atenolol

INTENDED EFFECTS
- Decrease in seizures: carbamazepine
- Depression of autonomic response (decrease in blood pressure, heart rate): clonidine, propranolol, and atenolol
- Decrease in craving: propranolol and atenolol

NURSING CONSIDERATIONS
- Provide seizure precautions.
- Obtain baseline vital signs, and continue to monitor on an ongoing basis.
- Check heart rate prior to administration of propranolol and withhold if less than 60/min.

ABSTINENCE MAINTENANCE (FOLLOWING WITHDRAWAL)

Disulfiram

INTENDED EFFECTS

- Disulfiram is a daily oral medication that is a type of aversion (behavioral) therapy.
- Disulfiram used concurrently with alcohol will cause acetaldehyde syndrome to occur.
- Effects include nausea, vomiting, weakness, sweating, palpitations, and hypotension.
- Acetaldehyde syndrome can progress to respiratory depression, cardiovascular suppression, seizures, and death.

NURSING CONSIDERATIONS

- Inform clients of the dangers and potentially fatal reaction of drinking any alcohol.
- Advise clients to avoid any products that contain alcohol (cough syrups, sauces, mouthwash, aftershave lotion, colognes, and hand sanitizer).
- Monitor liver function tests to detect hepatotoxicity.
- Encourage clients to wear a medical alert bracelet.
- Encourage clients to participate in a 12-step self-help program.
- Advise clients that medication effects (potential for acetaldehyde syndrome with alcohol ingestion) persist for 2 weeks following discontinuation of disulfiram.

Naltrexone

INTENDED EFFECTS: Naltrexone is a pure opioid antagonist that suppresses the craving and pleasurable effects of alcohol (also used for opioid withdrawal).

NURSING CONSIDERATIONS

- Take an accurate history to determine whether clients are also dependent on opioids. Concurrent use of naltrexone and opiates increases the risk for an opiate overdose. **Qs**
- Clients must abstain from alcohol before starting naltrexone.
- Advise clients to take the medication with meals to decrease gastrointestinal distress.
- Suggest monthly IM injections of depot naltrexone for clients who have difficulty adhering to an oral treatment regimen.

Acamprosate

INTENDED EFFECTS: Acamprosate decreases unpleasant effects resulting from abstinence (dysphoria, anxiety, restlessness).

CLIENT EDUCATION

- Inform clients that diarrhea can result.
- Advise clients to maintain adequate fluid intake and to receive adequate rest.
- Advise clients to take medication three times a day with meals.
- Advise clients to avoid use in pregnancy.

Medications to support withdrawal/abstinence from opioids

- Characteristic withdrawal syndrome occurs within 1 hr to several days after cessation of substance use.
- Findings include agitation, insomnia, flu-like manifestations, rhinorrhea, yawning, sweating, piloerection, abdominal cramping, and diarrhea.
- Manifestations are non-life-threatening, although suicidal ideation can occur.

Methadone substitution

INTENDED EFFECTS

- Methadone substitution is an oral opioid agonist that replaces the opioid to which the client has a physical dependence.
- This will prevent abstinence syndrome from occurring and remove the need for the client to obtain illegal substances.
- It is used for withdrawal and long-term maintenance.
- Dependence will be transferred from the illegal opioid to methadone.

NURSING CONSIDERATIONS

- Observe the client to make sure the dosage is adequate to suppress withdrawal. (Client's report of prior opiate usage can be unreliable).
- Inform clients that the methadone dose must be slowly tapered to produce withdrawal.
- Encourage clients to participate in a 12-step self-help program. **Qpcc**
- Inform clients that medication must be administered from an approved treatment center.

Clonidine

INTENDED EFFECTS

- Clonidine assists with withdrawal effects related to autonomic hyperactivity (diarrhea, nausea, vomiting).
- Clonidine therapy does not reduce the craving for opioids.

NURSING CONSIDERATIONS

- Obtain baseline vital signs.
- Advise clients to avoid activities that require mental alertness until drowsiness subsides.
- Encourage clients to chew sugarless gum or suck on hard candy and to sip small amounts of water or suck on ice chips to treat dry mouth.

Buprenorphine

INTENDED EFFECTS

- Buprenorphine is an agonist-antagonist opioid used for withdrawal and maintenance.
- It is substituted for the opioid to which the client has a physical dependence and prevents withdrawal manifestations.
- Decreases feelings of craving and can be effective in maintaining adherence.
- Considered safer than methadone due to a decreased risk for respiratory depression and potential for dependence.

NURSING CONSIDERATIONS: Unlike methadone, a primary care provider can prescribe and dispense buprenorphine. Administer sublingually (tablets or films)

Medications to support withdrawal/abstinence from nicotine

Abstinence syndrome is evidenced by irritability, nervousness, restlessness, insomnia, and difficulty concentrating.

Bupropion

INTENDED EFFECTS: Bupropion decreases nicotine craving and manifestations of withdrawal.

NURSING CONSIDERATIONS

- To treat dry mouth, encourage clients to chew sugarless gum or suck on hard candy and to sip small amounts of water or suck on ice chips.
- Advise clients to avoid caffeine and other CNS stimulants to control insomnia.
- Avoid use in clients who have an increased risk for seizures.

Nicotine replacement therapy

INTENDED EFFECTS

- These nicotine replacements are pharmaceutical product substitutes for the nicotine in cigarettes or chewing tobacco.
- The use of nicotine replacement therapy approximately doubles the success rate of smoking cessation.

NURSING CONSIDERATIONS

- Clients should avoid using any nicotine products while pregnant or breastfeeding.
- **Nicotine lozenge**
  ○ Instruct clients to allow the lozenge to slowly dissolve in the mouth (20 to 30 min).
  ○ Avoid oral intake 15 min prior to or during lozenge use.
  ○ Follow product directions for dosage strength and recommended titration.
  ○ Advise the client to limit lozenge use to five in a 6 hr period or a maximum of 20/day.
- **Nicotine gum**
  ○ Use of nicotine gum is not recommended for longer than 6 months.
  ○ Advise clients to chew gum slowly and intermittently over 30 min.
  ○ Advise clients to avoid eating or drinking 15 min prior to and while chewing the gum.
- **Nicotine patch**
  ○ Clients should apply a nicotine patch to an area of clean, dry skin each day.
  ○ Advise clients to avoid using any nicotine products while the patch is on.
  ○ Follow product directions for dosage times.
  ○ Advise clients to stop using patches and to notify the provider if local skin reactions occur.
  ○ Remove the patch prior to MRI scan, and replace when the scan is completed.

- **Nicotine nasal spray**
  ○ Provides pleasurable effects of smoking due to rapid rise of nicotine in the client's blood level.
  ○ One spray in each nostril delivers the amount of nicotine in one cigarette.
  ○ Advise client to follow product instructions for dosage frequency.
  ○ Not recommended for clients who have disorders affecting the upper respiratory system such as chronic sinus problems, allergies, or asthma.
- **Nicotine inhaler**
  ○ Simulates smoking by puffing on the inhaler, which delivers nicotine.
  ○ Contains menthol, which creates sensation in the back of the throat similar to smoking.
  ○ Advise clients to gradually taper use over 2 to 3 months and then discontinue. Ⓠ EBP
  ○ Avoid in clients who have asthma.

Varenicline

INTENDED EFFECTS

- Varenicline is a nicotinic receptor agonist that promotes the release of dopamine to simulate the pleasurable effects of nicotine.
- Reduces cravings for nicotine as well as the severity of withdrawal manifestations.
- Reduces the incidence of relapse by blocking the desired effects of nicotine.

NURSING CONSIDERATIONS

- Instruct client to take medication after a meal.
- Monitor blood pressure during treatment.
- Monitor clients who have diabetes mellitus for loss of glycemic control.
- Follow instructions for titration to minimize adverse effects.
- Advise client to notify the provider if nausea, vomiting, insomnia, new-onset depression, or suicidal thoughts occur. Can cause neuropsychiatric effects such as unpredictable behavior, mood changes, and thoughts of suicide. Due to potential adverse effects, varenicline is banned for use in clients who are commercial truck or bus drivers, air traffic controllers, or airplane pilots. Ⓠ s

---

For all medication classifications in this chapter.

NURSING EVALUATION OF MEDICATION EFFECTIVENESS

Depending on therapeutic intent, effectiveness is evidenced by the following.
- Absence of injury
- Decreased cravings for substance
- Abstinence from substance
- Regular attendance at self-help group
- Improved coping skills to replace substance usage

Application Exercises

1. A nurse is providing teaching for a client who is withdrawing from alcohol and has a new prescription for propranolol. Which of the following information should the nurse to include in the teaching?

   A. Increases the risk for seizure activity

   B. Provides a form of aversion therapy

   C. Decreases cravings

   D. Results in mild hypertension

2. A charge nurse is planning a staff education session to discuss medications used during the care of a client experiencing alcohol withdrawal. Which of the following medications should the charge nurse include in the discussion? (Select all that apply.)

   A. Lorazepam

   B. Diazepam

   C. Disulfiram

   D. Naltrexone

   E. Acamprosate

3. A nurse is providing teaching to a client who has a new prescription for clonidine to assist with maintenance of abstinence from opioids. The nurse should instruct the client to monitor for which of the following adverse effects?

   A. Diarrhea

   B. Dry mouth

   C. Insomnia

   D. Hypertension

4. A nurse is teaching a female client who has tobacco use disorder about nicotine replacement therapy. Which of the following statements by the client indicates understanding of the teaching?

   A. "I should avoid eating right before I chew a piece of nicotine gum."

   B. "I will need to stop using the nicotine gum after 1 year."

   C. "I know that nicotine gum is a safe alternative to smoking if I become pregnant."

   D. "I must chew the nicotine gum quickly for about 15 minutes."

5. A nurse in an acute mental health facility is caring for a client who is experiencing withdrawal from opioid use and has a new prescription for clonidine. Which of the following actions should the nurse identify as the priority?

   A. Administer the clonidine on the prescribed schedule.

   B. Provide ice chips at the client's bedside.

   C. Educate the client on the effects of clonidine.

   D. Obtain baseline vital signs.

PRACTICE Active Learning Scenario

A nurse is teaching a client who has tobacco use disorder about a new prescription for varenicline to promote smoking cessation. Use the ATI Active Learning Template: Medication to complete this item.

EXPECTED PHARMACOLOGICAL ACTION

THERAPEUTIC USES

COMPLICATIONS: Identify at least three adverse effects.

CLIENT EDUCATION: Identify at least two teaching points.

EVALUATION OF MEDICATION EFFECTIVENESS: Identify a client outcome to indicate medication effectiveness.

Application Exercises Key

1. A. Seizure activity is a potential effect of alcohol withdrawal. However, propranolol does not increase this risk.

   B. Disulfiram, rather than propranolol, provides a form of aversion therapy.

   C. **CORRECT:** Propranolol is an adjunct medication used during withdrawal to decrease the client's craving for alcohol.

   D. Propranolol is an antihypertensive medication that can result in hypotension rather than hypertension.

   Ⓝ *NCLEX® Connection: Pharmacological and Parenteral Therapies, Medication Administration*

2. A. **CORRECT:** Lorazepam is a benzodiazepine used during alcohol withdrawal to decrease anxiety and reduce the risk for seizures.

   B. **CORRECT:** Diazepam is a benzodiazepine used during alcohol withdrawal to decrease anxiety and reduce the risk for seizures.

   C. Disulfiram is administered to assist the client in maintaining abstinence from alcohol following withdrawal.

   D. Naltrexone is administered to assist the client in maintaining abstinence from alcohol following withdrawal.

   E. Acamprosate decreases unpleasant effects, such as anxiety or restlessness, resulting from abstinence.

   Ⓝ *NCLEX® Connection: Pharmacological and Parenteral Therapies, Expected Actions/Outcomes*

3. A. Constipation, rather than diarrhea, is a common adverse effect associated with clonidine use.

   B. **CORRECT:** Dry mouth is a common adverse effect associated with clonidine use.

   C. Sedation, rather than insomnia, is a common adverse effect associated with clonidine use.

   D. Clonidine is more likely to cause hypotension than hypertension.

   Ⓝ *NCLEX® Connection: Pharmacological and Parenteral Therapies, Adverse Effects/Contraindications/Side Effects/Interactions*

4. A. **CORRECT:** The client should avoid eating or drinking 15 min prior to and while chewing the nicotine gum.

   B. The client should not use nicotine gum for longer than 6 months.

   C. The client should avoid all nicotine products, including nicotine gum, while pregnant or breastfeeding.

   D. The client should chew the nicotine gum slowly and intermittently over 30 min.

   Ⓝ *NCLEX® Connection: Pharmacological and Parenteral Therapies, Medication Administration*

5. A. Administering clonidine as prescribed is an important nursing action. However, it is not the priority action.

   B. Providing ice chips is an important nursing action. However, it is not the priority action.

   C. Educating the client about the medication is an important nursing action. However, it is not the priority action.

   D. **CORRECT:** Assessment is the initial step of the nursing process. Obtaining the client's baseline vital signs is the priority nursing action.

   Ⓝ *NCLEX® Connection: Pharmacological and Parenteral Therapies, Medication Administration*

PRACTICE Answer

Using the ATI Active Learning Template: Medication

EXPECTED PHARMACOLOGICAL ACTION: Varenicline is a nicotinic receptor agonist that promotes the release of dopamine to simulate the pleasurable effects of nicotine.

THERAPEUTIC USES: Varenicline is indicated to reduce nicotine cravings and block the desired effects of nicotine in clients who have tobacco use disorder.

COMPLICATIONS	CLIENT EDUCATION	EVALUATION OF MEDICATION EFFECTIVENESS
• New-onset hypertension • Loss of glycemic control in clients who have diabetes mellitus • Nausea • Vomiting • Insomnia • New-onset depression • Suicidal thoughts	• Clients who are commercial truck or bus drivers, airplane pilots, or air traffic controllers should not take varenicline. • Take medication after a meal. • Titrate as prescribed to minimize adverse effects. • Notify the provider if adverse effects occur.	• The client will maintain smoking cessation. • The client will report reduced cravings for nicotine.

Ⓝ *NCLEX® Connection: Pharmacological and Parenteral Therapies, Medication Administration*

Chronic neurologic disorders include Parkinson's disease and seizure disorders. Medications administered for chronic neurologic disorders are used to manage manifestations and improve quality of life.

Cholinesterase inhibitors

Cholinesterase inhibitors are known as anticholinesterase agents and have two categories.

Irreversible inhibitors (e.g., echothiophate): Therapeutic effect is for a long duration and is used to treat glaucoma. Pralidoxime is used to reverse the effect of echothiophate.

Reversible inhibitors: Therapeutic effect lasts for a moderate duration (2 to 4 hr) and is used to treat Alzheimer's disease and Parkinson's disease, and reverse the effects of nondepolarizing neuromuscular blocking agents.

SELECT PROTOTYPE MEDICATION:
Neostigmine (reversible inhibitor)

OTHER MEDICATIONS
• Physostigmine
• Edrophonium
• Donepezil

PURPOSE

EXPECTED PHARMACOLOGICAL ACTION

Cholinesterase inhibitors prevent the enzyme cholinesterase from inactivating acetylcholine (ACh), thereby increasing the amount of ACh available at receptor sites. Transmission of nerve impulses is increased at all sites responding to ACh as a transmitter.

THERAPEUTIC USES

13.1 Therapeutic uses for cholinesterase inhibitors	NEOSTIGMINE	ECHOTHIOPHATE	PHYSOSTIGMINE	EDROPHONIUM	DONEPEZIL
Reversal of muscarinic antagonists			✓		
Treatment of glaucoma		✓			
Reversal of nondepolarizing neuromuscular blocking agents	✓			✓	
Treatment of Alzheimer's disease					✓
Treatment of Parkinson's disease					✓

COMPLICATIONS

Excessive muscarinic stimulation

As evidenced by increased gastrointestinal (GI) motility, increased GI secretions, diaphoresis, increased salivation, bradycardia, and urinary urgency

NURSING CONSIDERATIONS
• Advise the client of potential adverse effects. If effects become intolerable, instruct the client to notify the provider.
• Treat severe adverse effects with atropine.

Cholinergic crisis

Excessive muscarinic stimulation and respiratory depression from neuromuscular blockade

NURSING CONSIDERATIONS
• Provide respiratory support through mechanical ventilation and oxygen, and administer atropine to reverse muscarinic stimulation. Qs
• Have resuscitation equipment available.

CONTRAINDICATIONS/PRECAUTIONS

• Pregnancy Risk Category C
• Obstruction of GI and renal system
• Use cautiously in clients who have seizure disorders, hyperthyroidism, peptic ulcer disease, asthma, bradycardia, and hypotension.

INTERACTIONS

Atropine counteracts the effects of cholinesterase inhibitors.
• Atropine is used to treat toxicity from cholinesterase inhibitors (increased muscarinic stimulation and respiratory depression).
• NURSING CONSIDERATIONS: Monitor the client closely and provide mechanical ventilation until the client has regained full muscle function.

Neostigmine and edrophonium reverse neuromuscular blockade caused by nondepolarizing neuromuscular blocking agents after surgical procedures and overdose.
NURSING CONSIDERATIONS: Monitor for return of respiratory function. Support respiratory function as necessary. If used to treat overdose, provide mechanical ventilation until the client has regained full muscle function.

Succinylcholine is a depolarizing short-acting neuromuscular blocker used for surgical procedures.
• Cholinesterase inhibitors increase the neuromuscular blockage of depolarizing neuromuscular blockers.
• NURSING CONSIDERATIONS: Avoid concurrent use.

NURSING ADMINISTRATION

- Neostigmine can be given PO, IM, IV, or subcutaneously.
- Advise clients that dosage is very individualized, starts at very low doses, and is titrated until desired muscle function is achieved.
- Advise clients to wear a medical alert bracelet.

NURSING EVALUATION OF MEDICATION EFFECTIVENESS

Depending on therapeutic intent, effectiveness is evidenced by the following.
- Recovery of muscle strength
- Improved cognition and slow disease progression

Anti-Parkinson's medications

SELECT PROTOTYPE MEDICATIONS

Dopaminergic medications promote dopamine synthesis, activate dopamine receptors, prevent dopamine breakdown, promote dopamine release, or block the degradation of levodopa.
- **Dopamine synthesis medications** (levodopa) are prepared in combination with a dopamine agonist (carbidopa), or listed as levodopa/carbidopa.
  - Levodopa crosses the blood-brain barrier, whereas dopamine alone cannot cross this barrier and has a very short half-life. Levodopa is taken up by dopaminergic nerve terminals and converted to dopamine (DA). This newly synthesized DA is released into the synaptic space and causes stimulation of DA receptors.
  - Carbidopa is used to augment levodopa by decreasing the amount of levodopa that is converted to DA in the intestine and periphery. This results in larger amounts of levodopa reaching the CNS.

Dopamine agonists activate dopamine receptors: pramipexole; bromocriptine; ropinirole, a first-line supplement to levodopa. Apomorphine is a rescue medication for "off" times.
- Catecholamine-O-methyltransferase (COMT) inhibitor enhances the effect of levodopa by blocking its breakdown: entacapone, tolcapone
- Monoamine oxidase-B (MAO-B) prevents dopamine breakdown: selegiline, rasagiline
- Dopamine releaser prevents dopamine reuptake: amantadine
- Anticholinergic medications block the muscarinic receptors, which assist in maintaining balance between dopamine and acetylcholine receptors in the brain.
- Dopamine agonists, COMT inhibitors, MAO-B inhibitors, dopamine releasers, and centrally acting anticholinergic antagonists are used concurrently to increase the beneficial effects of levodopa/carbidopa.

PURPOSE

EXPECTED PHARMACOLOGICAL ACTION

These medications do not halt the progression of Parkinson's disease (PD). However, they do offer relief from dyskinesias (bradykinesia, resting tremors, and muscle rigidity) and an increase in the ability to perform ADLs by maintaining the balance between dopamine and acetylcholine in the extrapyramidal nervous system.

THERAPEUTIC USES

Levodopa/carbidopa

- Most effective for PD treatment, but the beneficial effects diminish by the end of year five.
- "Wearing off" times occur at the end of the dose cycle or can occur at any time even at high dose levels, lasting minutes to several hours.

Dopamine agonist

Pramipexole, ropinirole, apomorphine
- Administered as monotherapy in early-stage PD and used in conjunction with levodopa/carbidopa in late-stage PD to allow for lower dosage of levodopa/carbidopa.
- Administered more often in younger clients who are better able to tolerate daytime drowsiness and postural hypotension.

Bromocriptine, an ergot derivative, is poorly tolerated and has a high incidence of valvular heart injury. This medication is administered less frequently.

Dopamine releaser

Amantadine releases dopamine where it is stored in the neurons, prevents dopamine reuptake, and can block cholinergic and glutamate receptors.

COMT inhibitors

Beneficial in combination with levodopa/carbidopa to inhibit the metabolism of levodopa in the intestines and peripheral tissues: entacapone, tolcapone.

MAO-B inhibitors

MAO-B is a first-line medication in combination with levodopa/carbidopa to decrease the "wear-off" effect.

Selegiline can preserve dopamine produced from levodopa, and prolong the effects of levodopa but only up to one or two years.

Rasagiline preserves dopamine in the brain and is not converted into amphetamine or methamphetamine like selegiline does.

Centrally acting anticholinergics

Centrally acting anticholinergic antagonists diminish cholinergic effect (neuron excitability) due to decreased dopamine: benztropine, trihexyphenidyl.

ADVERSE EFFECTS

Levodopa/carbidopa

Usually dose-dependent

Nausea and vomiting, drowsiness
NURSING CONSIDERATIONS
- Administer with food, in small doses, at the start of treatment and if GI effects occur.
- Avoid administering with foods high in protein because absorption is delayed and reduces the therapeutic effect causing an "off" episode. Q EBP
- Advise clients to eat protein in several small portions during the day.
- Advise clients to avoid vitamin preparations and foods containing pyridoxine (wheat germ, green vegetables, bananas, whole-grain cereals, liver, legumes), which reduce the therapeutic effects of levodopa/carbidopa.
- Carbidopa can reduce nausea and vomiting.

Dyskinesias
- Head bobbing, tics, grimacing, tremors
- NURSING CONSIDERATIONS
  ○ Decrease the dosage. The decrease can result in resumption of PD manifestations.
  ○ Administer amantadine (releases and uptakes DA) to decrease dyskinesias.
  ○ Surgical or electrical stimulation.

Orthostatic hypotension
NURSING CONSIDERATIONS
- Monitor blood pressure.
- Instruct clients about indications of postural hypotension (lightheadedness, dizziness) and to avoid sudden changes of position.

Cardiovascular effects from beta$_1$ stimulation
- Tachycardia, palpitations, irregular heartbeat
- NURSING CONSIDERATIONS
  ○ Monitor vital signs.
  ○ Monitor ECG.
  ○ Notify the provider if manifestations occur.
  ○ Use cautiously in clients who have cardiovascular disorders.

Psychosis
- Visual hallucinations, nightmares, paranoid ideation
- NURSING CONSIDERATIONS
  ○ Administer second-generation antipsychotic medications, such as clozapine, as prescribed to decrease psychotic effects without increasing the manifestations of Parkinson's disease.
  ○ Second-generation antipsychotic medications do not block dopamine receptors in the striatum.
  ○ Avoid concurrent use of conventional antipsychotic agents, such as haloperidol, which block dopamine receptors.
  ○ Assess for the concurrent use of antidepressant MAOI medications, which can result in hypertensive crisis. Do not use levodopa/carbidopa within 2 weeks of MAOI use.

Discoloration of sweat and urine
NURSING CONSIDERATIONS: Advise the client that this finding is harmless.

Activation of malignant melanoma
NURSING CONSIDERATIONS: Avoid use of medication in clients who have skin lesions that have not been diagnosed.

Dopamine agonist

Sudden inability to stay awake
NURSING CONSIDERATIONS: Advise clients to notify the provider immediately if this occurs.

Daytime sleepiness
NURSING CONSIDERATIONS
- Advise clients of the potential for drowsiness and to avoid activities that require alertness.
- Advise clients to avoid other CNS depressants such as alcohol.

Orthostatic hypotension
NURSING CONSIDERATIONS: Instruct clients about the manifestations of postural hypotension (lightheadedness, dizziness) and to avoid sudden changes of position.

Psychosis
- Visual hallucinations, nightmares, especially in older adults Ⓖ
- NURSING CONSIDERATIONS: Administer second-generation antipsychotic medications, such as clozapine, if manifestations occur.

Impulse control disorder
- Gambling, shopping, binge eating, and hypersexuality
- NURSING CONSIDERATIONS
  ○ Manifestations appear 9 months after initial dose. Manifestations subside when medication is discontinued.
  ○ Screen for compulsive behavior before initiating therapy.

Dyskinesias
- Head bobbing, tics, grimacing, tremors
- NURSING CONSIDERATIONS: Decrease dosage of medication.

Nausea
NURSING CONSIDERATIONS: Advise clients to take medication with food (slows absorption of medication).

Dopamine releaser

CNS effects
- Confusion, dizziness, restlessness
- NURSING CONSIDERATIONS: Advise the client to avoid activities that require alertness while taking the medication.

Atropine-like effects
- Dry mouth, blurred vision, mydriasis (dilated pupils), urinary hesitancy or retention, constipation
- NURSING CONSIDERATIONS
  - Advise the client to observe for manifestations and notify the provider.
  - Monitor I&O, and assess the client for hesitancy or urinary retention.
  - Advise the client to chew sugarless gum, eat high-fiber foods, and increase fluid intake to 2 to 3 L/day from beverage and food.

Discoloration of skin, also called livedo reticularis
NURSING CONSIDERATIONS: Advise the client that discoloration of the skin will subside when the medication is discontinued.

COMT inhibitors

Same as for pramipexole when administered with levodopa/carbidopa
NURSING CONSIDERATIONS: Interventions are the same as for pramipexole when administered with levodopa/carbidopa.

GI: vomiting, diarrhea, constipation
NURSING CONSIDERATIONS: Treat adverse effects according to manifestations.

Discoloration of urine to a yellow-orange
NURSING CONSIDERATIONS: Assure the client that the urine color is harmless.

Rhabdomyolysis: muscle pain, tendon weakness
NURSING CONSIDERATIONS: Advise client to monitor and report manifestations to provider.

Liver failure
NURSING CONSIDERATIONS
- Monitor liver function periodically.
- Monitor for manifestations of liver failure (nausea, fatigue, jaundice, abdominal pain).
- Use with caution if hepatic function is impaired.

MAO-B inhibitors

Insomnia (selegiline)
NURSING CONSIDERATIONS: Administer selegiline no later than noon.

Hypertensive crisis triggered from foods containing tyramine
NURSING CONSIDERATIONS: Advise the client to avoid eating foods that contain tyramine (avocados, soybeans, figs, smoked meats, dried or cured fish, cheese, yeast products, beer, chianti wine, chocolate, caffeinated beverages).

Hypertensive crisis and death from some medications
NURSING CONSIDERATIONS: Provide a list of medications to avoid (e.g., meperidine, fluoxetine, MAO inhibitors, antidepressants, and sympathomimetics).

Nausea, diarrhea
NURSING CONSIDERATIONS: Take with meals and limit protein intake to increase absorption

Centrally acting anticholinergics

Nausea, vomiting
NURSING CONSIDERATIONS: Advise clients to take medication with food but to avoid high-protein snacks.

Atropine-like effects
- Dry mouth, blurred vision, mydriasis (dilated pupils), urinary retention, constipation
- NURSING CONSIDERATIONS
  - Advise clients to observe for manifestations and notify the provider if they occur.
  - Monitor I&O and assess clients for urinary retention.
  - Advise clients to chew sugarless gum, eat foods high in fiber, and increase fluid intake to 2 to 3 L/day from beverage and food sources.
  - Advise the client to schedule periodic eye exam to measure for increased intraocular pressure that can result in glaucoma.

Antihistamine effects (sedation, drowsiness)
- NURSING CONSIDERATIONS
  - Advise the client to avoid activities that require alertness while taking the medication.
  - Avoid administering to older adult client due to CNS adverse effects (sedation, confusion, delusions and hallucinations).

CLIENT EDUCATION

- Instruct family members to assist clients with the medication at home.
- Instruct the client about the possible sudden loss of the effects of medication and to notify the provider if manifestations occur.
- Inform the client that effects might not be noticeable for several weeks to several months.
- Medication "holidays" must be monitored in a hospital setting.
- Advise clients to avoid high-protein meals and snacks.
- Advise client, if applicable, to avoid pregnancy when taking levodopa or pramipexole.
- Advise clients the use of pramipexole with cimetidine can increase the amount of pramipexole in blood levels.
- Advise clients not to discontinue medications abruptly.

NURSING EVALUATION OF MEDICATION EFFECTIVENESS

Depending on therapeutic intent, effectiveness is evidenced by the following.
- Improvement of manifestations as demonstrated by absence of tremors, and reduction of irritability and stiffness
- Increase in ability to perform ADLs

Antiepileptics (AEDs)

TRADITIONAL ANTIEPILEPTIC MEDICATIONS
- Phenobarbital
- Primidone
- Phenytoin
- Carbamazepine: administered also for bipolar disorder, trigeminal and glossopharyngeal neuralgias
- Valproic acid: can be used for bipolar disorder and migraine headaches
- Ethosuximide

NEWER ANTIEPILEPTIC MEDICATIONS
- Lamotrigine
- Levetiracetam
- Topiramate
- Oxcarbazepine
- Gabapentin
- Pregabalin
- Tiagabine
- Zonisamide
- Lacosamide
- Vigabatrin
- Ezogabine

OTHER MEDICATIONS: Benzodiazepines used for status epilepticus (acute prolonged seizure)
- Diazepam
- Lorazepam

PURPOSE

EXPECTED PHARMACOLOGICAL ACTION

AEDs control seizure disorders by various mechanisms. **(13.2)**
- Slowing the entrance of sodium and calcium back into the neuron, thus extending the time it takes for the nerve to return to its active state and slows the frequency of neuron firing.
- Suppressing neuronal firing, which decreases seizure activity and prevents propagation of seizure activity into other areas of the brain
- Decreasing seizure activity by enhancing the inhibitory effects of gamma butyric acid (GABA).

COMPLICATIONS

TRADITIONAL ANTIEPILEPTIC MEDICATIONS

Barbiturates: phenobarbital, primidone

CNS effects
- In adults, manifest as drowsiness, sedation, and depression, and in the older adult can cause confusion and anxiety.
- In children, CNS effects manifest as irritability and hyperactivity.
- NURSING CONSIDERATIONS
  - Advise the client to observe for manifestations and to notify the provider if they occur.
  - Advise the client to avoid activities that require alertness, such as driving.
  - Never administer primidone with phenobarbital because phenobarbital is an active metabolic (stimulates medication metabolism cell porphyria).
  - Primidone is generally administered with phenytoin or carbamazepine.
  - Avoid administering other CNS depressants (alcohol, benzodiazepines, opioids).

13.2 Antiepileptic medications

	Traditional antiepileptic medications	PHENOBARBITAL	PRIMIDONE	PHENYTOIN	CARBAMAZEPINE	VALPROIC ACID	ETHOSUXIMIDE	Newer antiepileptic medications	LAMOTRIGINE	LEVETIRACETAM	TOPIRAMATE	OXCARBAZEPINE	GABAPENTIN	PREGABALIN	TIAGABINE	ZONISAMIDE	LACOSAMIDE	VIGABATRIN	EZOGABINE
Simple partial, complex partial, secondarily generalized seizures		✓	✓	✓	✓	✓			✓	✓	✓	✓	✓	✓	✓	✓	✓	✓	✓
Primary generalized seizures	Tonic-clonic	✓	✓	✓	✓	✓			✓	✓	✓								
	Absence					✓	✓		✓										
	Myoclonic					✓			✓	✓	✓								

Toxicity

- Nystagmus, ataxia, respiratory depression, coma, pinpoint pupils, hypotension, death
- NURSING CONSIDERATIONS
  - Stop medication. Administer oxygen and maintain respiratory function with ventilatory support. Qs
  - Monitor vital signs.
  - Have resuscitation equipment available.

Decrease synthesis of vitamins K and D, and decreased effectiveness of warfarin

NURSING CONSIDERATIONS: Monitor laboratory values (INR, calcium, vitamin D).

Hydantoins: phenytoin

CNS effects

- Nystagmus, sedation, ataxia, double vision, cognitive impairment
- NURSING CONSIDERATIONS: Monitor for manifestations of CNS effects, and notify the provider if they occur.

Gingival hyperplasia

- Softening and overgrowth of gum tissue, tenderness, and bleeding gums
- NURSING CONSIDERATIONS: Advise clients to maintain good oral hygiene (dental flossing, massaging gums). Folic acid supplements can decrease the occurrence.

Skin rash

NURSING CONSIDERATIONS: Stop medication if rash develops.

Cardiovascular effects: dysrhythmias, hypotension

NURSING CONSIDERATIONS

- Administer at slow IV rate (no faster than 50 mg/min) and in dilute solution to prevent adverse cardiovascular effects.
- Avoid administering to a client who has sinus bradycardia, sinoatrial block, or Stokes-Adams syndrome.

Endocrine and other effects

- Coarsening of facial features, hirsutism, and interference with vitamin D metabolism
- NURSING CONSIDERATIONS
  - Instruct the client to report changes.
  - Encourage the client to consume adequate amounts of calcium and vitamin D.

Interference with vitamin K-dependent clotting factors causing bleeding in newborns

NURSING CONSIDERATIONS: Administer prophylactic vitamin K to the mother for 1 month before the infant is delivered.

Carbamazepine

CNS effects

- Nystagmus, double vision, vertigo, staggering gait, and headache can occur, but cognitive function is minimally affected.
- NURSING CONSIDERATIONS
  - Administer in low doses initially and then gradually increase dosage.
  - Administer dose at bedtime.

Blood dyscrasias

- Leukopenia, anemia, thrombocytopenia
- NURSING CONSIDERATIONS
  - Obtain baseline CBC and platelets. Perform ongoing monitoring of CBC and platelets.
  - Observe for manifestations of bruising and bleeding of gums, sore throat, fever, pallor, weakness, and infection.
  - Avoid administering to a client who has bone marrow suppression or bleeding disorders.

Hypo-osmolarity

- Carbamazepine promotes secretion of ADH, which inhibits water excretion by the kidneys and places clients who have heart failure at risk for fluid overload.
- NURSING CONSIDERATIONS
  - Monitor serum sodium periodically.
  - Monitor for edema, decrease in urine output, and hypertension.

Skin disorders

- Dermatitis, rash, Stevens-Johnson syndrome
- NURSING CONSIDERATIONS
  - Treat mild reactions with anti-inflammatory or antihistamine medications.
  - Medication should be discontinued if there is a severe reaction.

Valproic acid

GI effect

- Nausea, vomiting, indigestion
- NURSING CONSIDERATIONS: Advise the client to take medication with food. Enteric-coated formulation can decrease manifestations.

Hepatotoxicity

- Anorexia, abdominal pain, jaundice
- NURSING CONSIDERATIONS
  - Assess baseline liver function and monitor liver function periodically.
  - Advise the client to observe for manifestations of hepatotoxicity such as anorexia, nausea, vomiting, abdominal pain, and jaundice, and to notify the provider if they occur.
  - This medication should not be used for children younger than 2 years old.
  - Medication should be prescribed in lowest effective dose.
  - Avoid administering to a client who has liver disease.

Pancreatitis
NURSING CONSIDERATIONS
- As evidenced by nausea, vomiting, and abdominal pain
- Advise the client to observe for manifestations and to notify the provider immediately if these occur.
- Monitor amylase levels.
- Medication should be discontinued if pancreatitis develops.

Thrombocytopenia
NURSING CONSIDERATIONS
- Advise the client to observe for manifestations such as bruising, and to notify the provider if these occur.
- Monitor platelet counts and bleeding time.

CNS effects from hyperammonemia
- Vomiting, lethargy, impaired cognitive alertness
- NURSING CONSIDERATIONS
  - Monitor blood ammonia levels periodically.
  - Discontinue the medication.

Ethosuximide

GI effects
- Nausea, vomiting
- NURSING CONSIDERATIONS: Administer with food.

CNS effects
- Sleepiness, lightheadedness, fatigue
- NURSING CONSIDERATIONS
  - Administer low initial dosage.
  - Advise clients to avoid hazardous activities, such as driving.

  Note: Ethosuximide is indicated only for absence seizures.

NEWER ANTIEPILEPTIC MEDICATIONS

Lamotrigine

CNS effects
- CNS effects include dizziness, somnolence, aphasia, double or blurred vision, headache, nausea or vomiting, depression
- NURSING CONSIDERATIONS
  - Avoid activities that require alertness until effects are stabilized.
  - Discontinue medication if manifestations are severe.
  - Monitor for suicidal ideation.

Aseptic meningitis
- Aseptic meningitis effects include headache, fever, stiff neck, nausea, vomiting, rash, sensitivity to light
- NURSING CONSIDERATIONS
  - Monitor for and report manifestations to the provider.
  - Discontinue medication.

Skin disorders
- Can include life-threatening rashes (Stevens-Johnson syndrome and toxic epidermal necrolysis).
- NURSING CONSIDERATIONS
  - Treat mild reactions with anti-inflammatory or antihistamine medications.
  - Discontinue medication if there is a severe reaction.
  - Concurrent use with valproic acid increases risk of skin disorder development.

Levetiracetam

CNS effects
- Dizziness, asthenia (loss of strength, weakness) agitation, anxiety, depression, suicidal ideation
- NURSING CONSIDERATIONS
  - Discontinue medication if there is a severe reaction.
  - Monitor for suicidal ideation.

Topiramate

CNS effects
- Somnolence, dizziness, ataxia, nervousness, diplopia, confusion, impaired cognitive function
- NURSING CONSIDERATIONS: Discontinue medication if there is a severe reaction.

Reduced sweating and increased body temperature
NURSING CONSIDERATIONS: Advise clients to monitor amount of strenuous activity while taking medication.

Metabolic acidosis
NURSING CONSIDERATIONS
- Monitor serum bicarbonate levels.
- Advise the client to report hyperventilation, fatigue, anorexia.
- Discontinue medication or reduce the dosage as prescribed by the provider.

Angle-closure glaucoma
NURSING CONSIDERATIONS
- Inform the client of manifestations of glaucoma (ocular pain, redness, blurring of vision).
- Advise the client to have periodic eye exams to measure intraocular pressure.

Oxcarbazepine

CNS effects
- Dizziness, drowsiness, double vision, nystagmus, headache, nausea, vomiting, and ataxia
- NURSING CONSIDERATIONS
  - Administer low initial dosage.
  - Advise the client to avoid activities that require alertness, such as driving.
  - Monitor serum sodium levels if having nausea and vomiting.

Skin disorders
- Can include life-threatening rashes (Stevens-Johnson syndrome and toxic epidermal necrolysis
- NURSING CONSIDERATIONS
  - Treat mild reactions with anti-inflammatory or antihistamine medications.
  - Discontinue medication if there is a severe reaction.

Hyponatremia
- Nausea, drowsiness, headache, and confusion
- NURSING CONSIDERATIONS
  - Monitor serum sodium laboratory values.
  - Use caution when the client is administered diuretic medication.

Multiorgan hypersensitivity reactions
- Fever and rash with some of the following: lymphadenopathy, hepatorenal syndrome, hematologic abnormalities
- NURSING CONSIDERATIONS: Discontinue medication if manifestations develop or are suspected.

Gabapentin

CNS effects
- Somnolence, dizziness, ataxia, fatigue, nystagmus, and peripheral edema diminish in time.
- NURSING CONSIDERATIONS: Advise the client to avoid driving if experiencing a high degree of drowsiness.

Pregabalin

CNS effects
- Somnolence, dizziness, adverse cognitive effect, headache
- NURSING CONSIDERATIONS
  - Advise the client to avoid driving if experiencing a high degree of drowsiness.
  - Discontinue medication if there is a severe reaction.

Weight gain, peripheral edema, dry mouth
NURSING CONSIDERATIONS
- Monitor daily weight, and report significant increase to the provider.
- Advise the client to chew gum or suck on hard candy to increase salivation.

Hypersensitivity reactions (angioedema)
NURSING CONSIDERATIONS: Advise client to immediately discontinue use and contact provider if manifestations develop.

CONTRAINDICATIONS/PRECAUTIONS

TRADITIONAL ANTIEPILEPTIC MEDICATIONS

Barbiturates: phenobarbital, primidone

Phenobarbital not recommended during pregnancy due to increased risk of fetus developing malformations
NURSING CONSIDERATIONS: Inform the client of the potential risk of pregnancy and to consult with the provider.

Hydantoins: phenytoin

Pregnancy
- Teratogenic: Cleft palate, heart defects, developmental deficiencies
- Pregnancy Risk Category D: Administer only if the benefits outweigh the risks.

Carbamazepine

Pregnancy
- Birth defects: Associated with spina bifida, neural tube defect, and delays in growth.
- Pregnancy Risk Category D: Administer only if the benefits outweigh the risks.

Valproic acid

Pregnancy
- Teratogenic: Cleft palate, heart defects
- Pregnancy Risk Category D: Administer only if the benefits outweigh the risks.

NEWER ANTIEPILEPTIC MEDICATIONS

Lamotrigine

Pregnancy
- Teratogenic: Cleft palate, heart defects are low risk.
- Pregnancy Risk Category C: Administer only if the benefits outweigh the risks.

Topiramate

Pregnancy
- Teratogenic: Cleft lip, cleft palate, heart defects
- Pregnancy Risk Category D: Administer only if the benefits outweigh the risks.

Oxcarbazepine

Pregnancy
- Teratogenic: Cleft palate, heart defects
- Pregnancy Risk Category C: Administer only if the benefits outweigh the risks.

Pregabalin

Pregnancy
- Birth defects: Can cause skeletal and visceral malformations.
- Pregnancy Risk Category C: Administer only if the benefits outweigh the risks.

INTERACTIONS

TRADITIONAL ANTIEPILEPTIC MEDICATIONS

Barbiturates: phenobarbital, primidone

Decreased effectiveness of oral contraceptives
NURSING CONSIDERATIONS: Advise the client to consider other forms of contraceptives.

Hydantoins: phenytoin

Phenytoin causes a decrease in the effects of oral contraceptives, warfarin, and glucocorticoids due to stimulation of hepatic medication-metabolizing enzymes.
NURSING CONSIDERATIONS
- Dose of oral contraceptives may need to be adjusted, or an alternative form of birth control used.
- Monitor for therapeutic effects of warfarin and glucocorticoids (INR, blood glucose levels). Adjust dosage as needed.

Alcohol (when used acutely), diazepam, cimetidine, and valproic acid increase phenytoin levels.
NURSING CONSIDERATIONS
- Advise clients to avoid alcohol use.
- Monitor serum levels.

Carbamazepine, phenobarbital, and chronic alcohol use decrease phenytoin levels.
NURSING CONSIDERATIONS: Encourage the client to avoid use of alcohol.

Additive CNS depressant effects can occur with concurrent use of CNS depressants (barbiturates, alcohol).
NURSING CONSIDERATIONS: Advise clients to avoid concurrent use of alcohol and other CNS depressants.

Carbamazepine

Carbamazepine causes a decrease in the effects of oral contraceptives and warfarin due to stimulation of hepatic medication-metabolizing enzymes.
NURSING CONSIDERATIONS
- Adjust dose of oral contraceptives or use an alternative form of birth control.
- Monitor for therapeutic effects of warfarin with PT and INR.
- Adjust dose as needed.

Grapefruit juice inhibits metabolism, and thus increases carbamazepine levels.
NURSING CONSIDERATIONS: Advise the client to avoid intake of grapefruit juice.

Phenytoin and phenobarbital decrease effects of carbamazepine.
NURSING CONSIDERATIONS: Concurrent use is not recommended.

Valproic acid

Concurrent use of valproic acid increases levels of phenytoin and phenobarbital.
NURSING CONSIDERATIONS
- Monitor phenytoin and phenobarbital levels.
- Adjust dosage of medications as prescribed.

NEWER ANTIEPILEPTIC MEDICATIONS

Topiramate

Phenytoin and carbamazepine can decrease topiramate level. Topiramate can increase phenytoin levels.
NURSING CONSIDERATIONS: Consult provider before administering phenytoin or carbamazepine with topiramate.

Oxcarbazepine

Decreases oral contraceptive levels.
NURSING CONSIDERATIONS: Advise the client to use alternate form of contraception.

Phenytoin levels increase when administered with oxcarbazepine
NURSING CONSIDERATIONS: Consult provider before administering with phenytoin.

Depresses CNS if alcohol is consumed
NURSING CONSIDERATIONS: Advise the client to avoid alcohol.

Pregabalin

Benzodiazepines, alcohol, and opioids intensify CNS effects
NURSING CONSIDERATIONS: Advise the client to avoid medications that affect the CNS.

CLIENT EDUCATION

- Inform the client that monitoring therapeutic plasma levels is recommended as prescribed by the provider.
- Monitor therapeutic plasma levels for medications prescribed and be aware of therapeutic levels for each medication. Notify the provider of results.
- Advise the client taking antiepileptic medications that treatment provides for control of seizures, not cure of disorder.
- Encourage the client to keep a seizure frequency diary to monitor effectiveness of therapy.
- Advise the client to take medications as prescribed and not to stop medications without consulting the provider. Sudden cessation of medication can trigger seizures.
- Advise the client to avoid activities that require alertness (driving, operating heavy machinery) until seizures are fully controlled and medication effects are known.
- Advise the client who is traveling to carry extra medication to avoid interruption of treatment.
- Advise the client of childbearing age to avoid pregnancy, because medications can cause birth defects and congenital abnormalities.
- Advise the client that phenytoin doses must be individualized. Dosing usually starts twice a day and can be switched to once-a-day dosing with an extended-release form when maintenance dose has been established.
- Advise the client that phenytoin has a narrow therapeutic range, and strict adherence to the medication regimen is imperative to prevent toxicity or therapeutic failure.

NURSING EVALUATION OF MEDICATION EFFECTIVENESS

Depending on therapeutic intent, effectiveness is evidenced by:
- Absence or decreased occurrence of seizures
- Ability to perform ADLs
- Absence of injury

Application Exercises

1. A nurse in the post-anesthesia recovery unit is caring for a client who received a nondepolarizing neuromuscular blocking agent and has muscle weakness. The nurse should anticipate a prescription for which of the following medications?

   A. Neostigmine

   B. Naloxone

   C. Dantrolene

   D. Vecuronium

2. A nurse is providing information to a client who has early Parkinson's disease and a new prescription for pramipexole. The nurse should instruct the client to monitor for which of the following adverse effects of this medication?

   A. Hallucinations

   B. Increased salivation

   C. Diarrhea

   D. Discoloration of urine

3. A nurse is teaching a client who has a new prescription for levodopa/carbidopa for Parkinson's disease. Which of the following instructions should the nurse include?

   A. Increase intake of protein-rich foods.

   B. Expect muscle twitching to occur.

   C. Take this medication with food.

   D. Anticipate relief of manifestations in 24 hr.

4. A nurse is preparing to administer a medication to a client who has absence seizures. The nurse should anticipate administering which of the following medications to the client? (Select all that apply.)

   A. Phenytoin

   B. Ethosuximide

   C. Gabapentin

   D. Carbamazepine

   E. Valproic acid

   F. Lamotrigine

5. A nurse is reviewing a new prescription for oxcarbazepine with a female client who has partial seizures. Which of the following instructions should the nurse include? (Select all that apply.)

   A. "Use caution if given a prescription for a diuretic medication."

   B. "Consider using an alternate form of contraception if you are using oral contraceptives."

   C. "Chew gum to increase saliva production."

   D. "Avoid driving until you see how the medication affects you."

   E. "Notify your provider if you develop a skin rash."

PRACTICE Active Learning Scenario

A nurse is planning care for a client who has tonic-clonic seizures and a new prescription for phenytoin. Considering the adverse effects and nursing interventions, what should the nurse include in the plan of care?

Use the ATI Active Learning Template: Medication to complete this item to include the following:

THERAPEUTIC USES: Describe.

COMPLICATIONS: Describe two adverse effects and two medication interactions.

NURSING INTERVENTIONS: Include two interventions that relate to the two adverse effects, and two interventions that relate to the two medication interactions.

Application Exercises Key

1. A. **CORRECT:** Neostigmine is a cholinesterase inhibitor used to reverse the effects of nondepolarizing neuromuscular blockers.

   B. Naloxone is used to reverse the effects of opioids.

   C. Dantrolene acts on skeletal muscles to reduce metabolic activity and treat malignant hyperthermia.

   D. Vecuronium is an intermediate-acting nondepolarizing neuromuscular blocker.

   Ⓝ *NCLEX® Connection: Pharmacological and Parenteral Therapies, Medication Administration*

2. A. **CORRECT:** Pramipexole can cause hallucinations within 9 months of the initial dose and might require discontinuation.

   B. Increased salivation is an adverse effect of cholinesterase inhibitors. Dry mouth is an adverse effect of pramipexole.

   C. Constipation is an adverse effect of pramipexole.

   D. Discoloration of urine is an adverse effect of COMT inhibitors and not an adverse effect of pramipexole.

   Ⓝ *NCLEX® Connection: Pharmacological and Parenteral Therapies, Adverse Effects/Contraindications/Side Effects/Interactions*

3. A. The client should avoid protein-rich foods, which can result in decreased therapeutic effects of levodopa.

   B. The client should monitor and report muscle twitching which can indicate toxicity.

   C. **CORRECT:** The client should take this medication with food to reduce GI effects.

   D. The client should anticipate relief of manifestations to take several weeks to months.

   Ⓝ *NCLEX® Connection: Pharmacological and Parenteral Therapies, Adverse Effects/Contraindications/Side Effects/Interactions*

4. A. Phenytoin is prescribed for partial seizures and tonic-clonic seizures and has no therapeutic effect for a client who has absence seizures.

   B. **CORRECT:** Ethosuximide's only mechanism of action is to treat a client who has absence seizures.

   C. Gabapentin is prescribed for partial seizures and tonic-clonic seizures and has no therapeutic effect for a client who has absence seizures.

   D. Carbamazepine is prescribed for partial seizures and tonic-clonic seizures and has no therapeutic effect for a client who has absence seizures.

   E. **CORRECT:** Valproic acid has a therapeutic effect when treating a client who has absence seizures and all other forms of seizures.

   F. **CORRECT:** Lamotrigine has a therapeutic effect when treating a client who has absence seizures and all other forms of seizures.

   Ⓝ *NCLEX® Connection: Pharmacological and Parenteral Therapies, Expected Actions/Outcomes*

5. A. **CORRECT:** Diuretic medications are administered with caution because of the high risk for hyponatremia when taking oxcarbazepine.

   B. **CORRECT:** An alternate form of contraception is recommended for clients taking oral contraceptives because oxcarbazepine decreases oral contraceptive levels.

   C. Chewing gum to increase salivation is not indicated because the medication does not cause dry mouth.

   D. **CORRECT:** The client should avoid driving if CNS effects of dizziness, drowsiness, and double vision develop.

   E. **CORRECT:** The client should notify the provider if a skin rash occurs because life-threatening skin disorders can develop.

   Ⓝ *NCLEX® Connection: Pharmacological and Parenteral Therapies, Medication Administration*

PRACTICE Answer

Using the ATI Active Learning Template: Medication

THERAPEUTIC USES: Phenytoin is a hydantoin medication that suppresses partial seizure and primary generalized seizure activity in the affected neurons.

COMPLICATIONS

- CNS effects
- Gingival hyperplasia
- Teratogenic birth defects
- Decreases effectiveness of oral contraceptives, warfarin, and glucocorticoids
- Causes stimulation of hepatic medication-metabolizing enzymes
- Alcohol (acute use), diazepam, cimetidine, and valproic acid increase phenytoin levels.
- Carbamazepine, phenobarbital, and chronic alcohol use decrease phenytoin levels.
- Additive CNS depressant effects can occur with concurrent use of CNS depressants.

NURSING INTERVENTIONS

- Instruct the client to refrain from alcohol and other medications that cause CNS depression (e.g., barbiturates).
- Encourage the client to use dental floss and massage gums daily.
- Instruct the client to avoid pregnancy and use an alternate form of contraception.
- Monitor INR if on warfarin and blood glucose levels if taking a glucocorticoid.
- Monitor therapeutic effects of warfarin and glucocorticoids.
- Never abruptly discontinue antiepileptic medications.
- Advise clients to avoid use of alcohol and other CNS depressants
- Monitor serum phenytoin levels

Ⓝ *NCLEX® Connection: Pharmacological and Parenteral Therapies, Adverse Effects/Contraindications/Side Effects/Interactions*

UNIT 2   MEDICATIONS AFFECTING THE NERVOUS SYSTEM

CHAPTER 14 *Eye and Ear Disorders*

Eye disorders

Glaucoma is a frequent cause of blindness. Damage to the optic nerve occurs when aqueous humor does not exit from the anterior chamber of the eye. This results in the buildup of aqueous humor, increased intraocular pressure (IOP), and loss of vision.

TYPES OF GLAUCOMA

Primary open-angle glaucoma (POAG)

- POAG is the most common form of glaucoma.
- Peripheral vision is lost gradually, with central visual field loss occurring if damage to the optic nerve continues.
- Clients typically do not experience manifestations until there is widespread damage. Manifestations can include halos seen around lights, loss of peripheral vision, and headaches.
- The expected reference range for IOP is 10 to 21 mm Hg. IOP greater than 21 mm Hg is a major risk factor for POAG. However, it can occur at therapeutic IOP levels.
- Treatment includes medication therapy to reduce IOP. Surgical intervention is indicated if IOP cannot be reduced by medications.
- POAG is treated with the following medications:
  - Beta-adrenergic blockers
  - Alpha$_2$-adrenergic agonists
  - Prostaglandin analogs
  - Cholinergic agonists
  - Carbonic anhydrase inhibitors

Angle-closure (narrow-angle) glaucoma

- This is an acute disorder with a sudden onset, resulting in irreversible blindness within 1 to 2 days without emergency treatment.
- Findings include acute onset of ocular pain, seeing halos around lights, brow pain, nausea, blurred vision, and photophobia. The optic nerve is damaged when the aqueous humor builds up as a result of displacement of the iris.
- Treatment includes medication therapy to reduce IOP, with subsequent corrective surgery for restoration of the iris.
- Although several other classes of glaucoma medications are used to treat angle-closure glaucoma, osmotic agents are first-line medications used to control the condition until corrective surgery can be implemented.

Beta-adrenergic blockers

NONSELECTIVE BETA BLOCKERS (which have both beta$_1$ and beta$_2$ properties)
- Timolol
- Carteolol
- Metipranolol
- Levobunolol

CARDIOSELECTIVE BETA$_1$ BLOCKERS: Betaxolol

PURPOSE

EXPECTED PHARMACOLOGICAL ACTION

Beta blockers decrease IOP by decreasing the amount of aqueous humor produced.

THERAPEUTIC USES

- Topical beta blockers are used primarily to treat POAG. They can be prescribed in combination with other topical medications to lower IOP.
- These medications are occasionally used to treat acute closed-angle glaucoma on an emergency basis.

COMPLICATIONS

Stinging discomfort

Reports of temporary stinging discomfort in the eye immediately after drop is instilled

NURSING CONSIDERATIONS: Educate clients that this effect is transient.

Occasional conjunctivitis, blurred vision, photophobia, dry eyes

NURSING CONSIDERATIONS: Instruct clients to report these effects to the provider.

Systemic effects of beta blockade on heart and lungs

NURSING CONSIDERATIONS
- Warn clients that overdose could cause or increase the chance of systemic effects.
- When taking beta$_1$ blockers, clients should monitor for bradycardia. Inform client to notify the provider for heart rate less than 58/min.

CONTRAINDICATIONS/PRECAUTIONS

- Do not use beta$_2$ blockers for clients who have chronic respiratory disease because they can constrict airway and cause bronchospasms. Use beta$_1$ blockers with caution in clients who have chronic respiratory disease.
- Do not use beta blockers for clients who have sinus bradycardia, or AV heart block and use with caution in clients who have heart failure.

INTERACTIONS

Oral beta blockers and calcium channel blockers can increase cardiovascular and respiratory effects.
NURSING CONSIDERATIONS: Instruct clients to inform the provider if they are taking any of these medications.

Beta blockers can interfere with some effects of insulin.
NURSING CONSIDERATIONS: Advise clients who have diabetes to monitor their blood glucose.

NURSING ADMINISTRATION

- Instill one drop in the affected eye once or twice daily.
- Review the proper method of instilling eye drops, and provide instruction to a family member if indicated. Qpcc
- Use sterile technique when handling the applicator portion of the container. Avoid touching any part of the applicator, and keep the lid in place when not in use.
- Hold gentle pressure on the nasolacrimal duct for 30 to 60 seconds immediately after instilling the drop(s) to prevent or minimize any expected systemic effect.
- Monitor pulse rate/rhythm as indicated for beta blocker. Qs

Alpha₂-adrenergic agonists

SELECT PROTOTYPE MEDICATION: Brimonidine

OTHER MEDICATION: Apraclonidine

ALPHA₂-AGONIST/BETA BLOCKER COMBINATION: Brimonidine and timolol

PURPOSE

EXPECTED PHARMACOLOGICAL ACTION

Brimonidine decreases production and can also increase outflow of aqueous humor to lower IOP.

THERAPEUTIC USES

- Brimonidine is used as a first-line medication for long-term topical treatment of POAG.
- Apraclonidine is a short-term therapy for POAG only and is also used preoperatively for laser eye surgeries.

COMPLICATIONS

Stinging discomfort, pruritus

- Localized stinging discomfort and pruritus of conjunctiva
- Sensation that a foreign body is in the eye

NURSING CONSIDERATIONS: Advise clients not to rub their eyes.

Dilated pupils, blurred vision, headache, dry mouth

NURSING CONSIDERATIONS: Instruct clients to report these effects.

Reddened sclera

Caused by blood–vessel engorgement

NURSING CONSIDERATIONS: Inform clients of the possibility of this effect.

Hypotension, drowsiness

Brimonidine crosses the blood–brain barrier

NURSING CONSIDERATIONS: Advise clients to use caution with driving and other tasks, and to inform the provider if dizziness and/or weakness occur.

CONTRAINDICATIONS/PRECAUTIONS

Advise clients who wear soft contact lenses to administer brimonidine with lenses removed. Delay insertion of the lens at least 15 min after administration to prevent absorption of medication into the lens. Qpcc

INTERACTIONS

Antihypertensive medications can intensify hypotension caused by brimonidine.
NURSING CONSIDERATIONS: Instruct clients to inform the provider if they are taking any antihypertensive medications.

MAO inhibitors can decrease effects of brimonidine and cause hypertensive crisis.
NURSING CONSIDERATIONS: Instruct clients to inform the provider if they are taking MAO inhibitors.

NURSING ADMINISTRATION

- Review proper method of administering eye drops and minimizing systemic effects.
- Monitor blood pressure for hypotension or hypertension.

Prostaglandin analogs

SELECT PROTOTYPE MEDICATION: Latanoprost

OTHER MEDICATIONS
- Travoprost
- Bimatoprost

PURPOSE

EXPECTED PHARMACOLOGICAL ACTION

Latanoprost reduces IOP by increasing aqueous humor outflow through relaxation of ciliary muscle.

THERAPEUTIC USES

These agents are topical first-line medications for clients who have POAG and ocular hypertension. **(14.1)**

COMPLICATIONS

Bulging of ocular blood vessels

NURSING CONSIDERATIONS: Inform clients about the possibility of this effect.

Increased pigmentation

Permanent increased brown pigmentation, usually occurring in individuals with brown-colored iris (can also cause pigmentation of lids, lashes)

NURSING CONSIDERATIONS: Inform clients about the possibility of this effect.

Stinging, burning, reddened conjunctiva

NURSING CONSIDERATIONS: Instruct clients to not rub their eyes.

Blurred vision

NURSING CONSIDERATIONS: Instruct clients to report to the provider.

Migraine

Rare adverse effect

NURSING CONSIDERATIONS: Instruct clients to report to the provider.

Osmotic agents

SELECT PROTOTYPE MEDICATION: Mannitol

PURPOSE

EXPECTED PHARMACOLOGICAL ACTION

Osmotic agents decrease intraocular pressure by making the plasma hypertonic, thus drawing fluid from the anterior chamber of the eye.

THERAPEUTIC USES

These agents treat the rapid progression of closed-angle glaucoma to prevent blindness.

COMPLICATIONS

Adverse effects include headache, nausea, and vomiting

Carbonic anhydrase inhibitor (systemic)

SELECT PROTOTYPE MEDICATION: Acetazolamide

OTHER MEDICATIONS: Methazolamide

PURPOSE

EXPECTED PHARMACOLOGICAL ACTION

Reduces production of aqueous humor by causing diuresis through renal effects.

THERAPEUTIC USES

- Quickly lower IOP in clients for whom other medications have been ineffective.
- Acetazolamide, a nonantimicrobial sulfonamide, can be used as an emergency medication prior to surgery for acute angle-closure glaucoma and as a second-line medication for treatment of POAG.
- Acetazolamide may also be used to treat acute altitude sickness, seizures, and heart failure (as a diuretic).

COMPLICATIONS

Severe allergic reactions

- Severe allergic reactions (anaphylaxis)
- Possible cross-sensitivity with sulfonamides

NURSING CONSIDERATIONS
- Educate clients about effects and to notify provider.
- Ask about sulfonamide allergy.

Serious blood disorders

Rare serious blood disorders, such as bone marrow depression

NURSING CONSIDERATIONS: Educate clients to recognize and immediately report effects.

14.1 Second-line topical medications for glaucoma

Direct-acting cholinergic (muscarinic) agonist
PROTOTYPE: Pilocarpine

PURPOSE
- Second-line treatment for POAG; lowers IOP indirectly through ciliary contraction.
- Also used to treat closed-angle glaucoma.

ADVERSE EFFECTS
- Retinal detachment
- Parasympathetic effects, such as bradycardia, increase in saliva, sweating, flushing, pupil constriction
- Decreased visual acuity

Carbonic anhydrase inhibitor
PROTOTYPE: Dorzolamide

Also available in combination with timolol

PURPOSE
- Second-line treatment for POAG, which decreases aqueous humor production.
- Timolol/dorzolamide combination produces increased effect of both medications.

ADVERSE EFFECTS
- Localized allergic reactions in up to 15%
- Blurred vision, dryness, photophobia
- Can absorb into soft contacts

Gastrointestinal side effects

Gastrointestinal (GI) side effects (nausea and diarrhea)

NURSING CONSIDERATIONS: Report GI adverse effects and weight loss to provider.

Electrolyte depletion (sodium and potassium), dehydration, altered liver function

NURSING CONSIDERATIONS: Prepare clients for the need to obtain regular laboratory testing. Weigh daily, monitor for postural hypotension, increase fluid intake to 2 to 3 L/day, unless contraindicated.

Generalized flu-like symptoms

Headache, fever, body aches

NURSING CONSIDERATIONS: Educate client about possible reactions.

Central nervous system disturbances

Paresthesias of extremities, fatigue, sleepiness, rarely seizures

NURSING CONSIDERATIONS
- Educate client about possible reactions.
- Medication may be discontinued.

Glucose disturbances

In clients who have diabetes mellitus

NURSING CONSIDERATIONS: Teach clients who have diabetes to closely monitor blood glucose and watch for indications of hypo- or hyperglycemia.

CONTRAINDICATIONS/PRECAUTIONS

- Acetazolamide is Pregnancy Risk Category C (teratogenic).
- Use during lactation only after evaluation by the provider.

INTERACTIONS

Serious effects, such as metabolic acidosis, can occur in clients using high-dose aspirin.
NURSING CONSIDERATIONS: Question clients about aspirin use, and notify the provider.

Acetazolamide can increase the risk of toxic effects of quinidine.
NURSING CONSIDERATIONS: Instruct clients to notify the provider of concurrent use and to watch for indications of toxicity, such as decreased heart rate.

Acetazolamide can decrease blood levels of lithium.
NURSING CONSIDERATIONS: Teach clients taking lithium to watch for increased indications of mania. Monitor lithium levels regularly.

Acetazolamide can increase osteomalacia, an adverse effect of phenytoin.
NURSING CONSIDERATIONS: Teach clients taking phenytoin to watch for bone pain or weakness and report symptoms to the provider.

Sodium bicarbonate increases the risk of kidney stones.
NURSING CONSIDERATIONS: Question clients about the use of sodium bicarbonate and other over-the-counter antacids.

NURSING ADMINISTRATION

Acetazolamide is available orally as a tablet or a capsule. It is also available for parenteral administration.

NURSING EVALUATION OF MEDICATION EFFECTIVENESS

Depending on therapeutic intent, effectiveness can be evidenced by the following.
- Reduced IOP
- Safe self-administration of medication
- Prevention or minimization of systemic effects

Ear disorders

Acute otitis media

- This condition occurs most often in young children.
- A bacterial or a viral infection causes a buildup of fluid in the middle ear (middle ear effusion).
- The major indication is acute onset of pain. Objective findings include erythema, bulging of the tympanic membrane, and fever. Diagnosis is confirmed when there is acute onset of symptoms, middle-ear effusion, and middle-ear inflammation.
- Treatment for bacterial infection, especially in infants and young children, is an antibiotic. Treatment for viral infection is symptomatic.

  Because of the increase in antibiotic-resistant bacteria, the current trend is to administer medications for pain relief (acetaminophen, ibuprofen), observe children over age 2 for 48 to 72 hr, and prescribe antibiotics if the condition does not resolve or worsens over several days.

- Medications for treating otitis media
  - Oral penicillins
  - Other antimicrobials, oral or parenteral
  - Pain medication
- Incidence of acute otitis media in infants and children can be reduced by yearly influenza vaccination and vaccination with pneumococcal conjugate vaccine.

Otitis externa

- This condition, also known as swimmer's ear, is caused by a bacterial infection of the external auditory canal.
- Any object that abrades or leaves moisture in the canal facilitates colonization of bacteria and the onset of otitis externa.
- Manifestations include acute onset of pain, especially with movement of the pinna, itching, diminished hearing, and purulent discharge.
- Treatment usually resolves infection within 10 days.
- Otitis externa is usually treated by topical antimicrobial/anti-inflammatory combination.

Antimicrobials

SELECT PROTOTYPE MEDICATION: Amoxicillin

OTHER MEDICATION: Amoxicillin/clavulanate PO

Antibiotics used to treat acute otitis media in clients who have a type 11 penicillin allergy (mild) or penicillin-resistant otitis media
- Ceftriaxone IM, IV (severe illness)
- Cefdinir PO
- Cefuroxime PO, IM, IV
- Cefpodoxime PO

Antibiotics used to treat acute otitis media in clients who have a type 1 penicillin allergy (severe)
- Ceftriaxone IM, IV (severe illness)
- Azithromycin PO, IV
- Clindamycin PO, IM, IV (macrolide antibiotic)

PURPOSE

EXPECTED PHARMACOLOGICAL ACTION

Eradication of infection

THERAPEUTIC USES

Used to treat otitis media and various other bacterial infections throughout the body.

COMPLICATIONS

Possible allergic reaction

Most common risk when taking penicillin

NURSING CONSIDERATIONS
- Question the client and family regarding the presence of penicillin or other antibiotic allergy.
- The client might need alternative medication.
- A skin test may be used to test for sensitivity.

GI upset

Usually less with amoxicillin than with ampicillin

NURSING CONSIDERATIONS: Educate family to inform the provider of severe diarrhea, especially in an infant or young child.

Suprainfection

With other microbes, such as oral candidiasis

NURSING CONSIDERATIONS: Report indications of new infection to the provider.

CONTRAINDICATIONS/PRECAUTIONS

- Amoxicillin is contraindicated for clients who have an allergy to penicillin,
- Use amoxicillin with caution in clients who have an allergy to cephalosporins.
- Use cautiously in infants younger than 3 months of age due to immature renal system and increased risk for toxicity.

NURSING ADMINISTRATION

- Amoxicillin is usually prescribed 3 times daily PO.
- Amoxicillin can be taken with meals.
- As with all antibiotics, instruct the client to take the full course of medication.

NURSING EVALUATION OF MEDICATION EFFECTIVENESS

Depending on therapeutic intent, effectiveness can be evidenced by
- Reduction of symptoms (e.g., fever, earache)
- Absence of infection
- Absence of recurrence of infection

Fluoroquinolone antibiotic plus steroid medication

SELECT PROTOTYPE MEDICATION: Ciprofloxacin plus hydrocortisone otic drops

OTHER MEDICATIONS
- Acetic acid 2% solution otic drops
- Ciprofloxacin plus dexamethasone otic drops
- Ofloxacin otic drops

PURPOSE

EXPECTED PHARMACOLOGICAL ACTION

The bactericidal effect of ciprofloxacin and anti-inflammatory effect of hydrocortisone should decrease pain, edema, and erythema in the ear canal.

THERAPEUTIC USES

Topical medications to treat otitis externa

COMPLICATIONS

CNS effects

Dizziness, lightheadedness, tremors, restlessness, convulsions

NURSING CONSIDERATIONS: Instruct clients to inform the provider if any of these occur.

Rash

NURSING CONSIDERATIONS: Question the client/family about allergies to fluoroquinolone antibiotics or to steroids such as dexamethasone or cortisone.

NURSING ADMINISTRATION

- Review the method for instilling otic drops.
- Inform clients that movement of the tragus or pinna may be very painful when instilling otic drops.
- Warm the medication by gently rolling the container between hands before instilling drops. Cold drops can cause dizziness. Gently shake medication that is in suspension form.
- Place the client on the unaffected side.
- Keep clients in a side-lying position for 5 min with the affected ear up after instilling drops. Place a small piece of cotton in the ear. Avoid packing it tightly. Remove cotton after 15 min.
- Instruct client/family to prevent otic medications from being placed in the eye or ingested orally. Qs
- Teach client/family to prevent otitis externa by
  - Keeping foreign bodies, such as cotton swabs, out of the ear canal, and avoiding the use of manual measures to remove cerumen
  - Drying the ear canal after bathing or swimming, using a towel, and tilting the head to promote drainage
  - Avoiding the use of earplugs, except for swimming

NURSING EVALUATION OF MEDICATION EFFECTIVENESS

Depending on therapeutic intent, effectiveness can be evidenced by the following.
- Subsiding of manifestations
- Use of measures to prevent reinfection

Application Exercises

1. A nurse is instructing a client who has a new prescription for timolol how to insert eye drops. The nurse should instruct the client to press on which of the following areas to prevent systemic absorption of the medication?

   A. Bony orbit

   B. Nasolacrimal duct

   C. Conjunctival sac

   D. Outer canthus

2. A nurse is teaching a client who has a new prescription for brimonidine ophthalmic drops and wears soft contact lenses. Which of the following instructions should the nurse include in the teaching?

   A. "This medication can stain your contacts."

   B. "This medication can cause your pupils to constrict."

   C. "This medication can absorb into your contacts."

   D. "This medication can slow your heart rate."

3. A nurse in an emergency unit is reviewing the medical record of a client who is being evaluated for angle-closure glaucoma. Which of the following findings are indicative of this condition?

   A. Insidious onset of painless loss of vision

   B. Gradual reduction in peripheral vision

   C. Severe pain around eyes

   D. Intraocular pressure 12 mm Hg

4. A nurse is teaching a client about preventing otitis externa. Which of the following instructions should the nurse include?

   A. Clean the ear with a cotton-tipped swab daily.

   B. Place earplugs in the ears when sleeping at night.

   C. Use a cool water irrigation solution to remove earwax.

   D. Tip the head to the side to remove water from the ears after showering.

5. A nurse in a provider's office is instructing a parent of a toddler how to administer ear drops. Which of the following instructions should the nurse include? (Select all that apply.)

   A. "Place the child on his unaffected side when you are ready to administer the medication."

   B. "Warm the medication by gently rolling it between your hands for a few minutes."

   C. "Gently shake medication that is in suspension form."

   D. "Keep the child on his side for 5 minutes after instillation of the ear drops."

   E. "Tightly pack the ear with cotton after instillation of the ear drops."

PRACTICE Active Learning Scenario

A nurse in a provider's office is teaching a client who has a prescription for ciprofloxacin/hydrocortisone about the medication and how to prevent otitis externa. Use the ATI Active Learning Template: Medication to complete this item.

THERAPEUTIC USES: Identify two therapeutic effects of the medication.

MEDICATION ADMINISTRATION: Identify two actions to prevent otitis externa.

Application Exercises Key

1. A. Pressing on the bony orbit will not prevent systemic absorption of the medication.

    B. **CORRECT:** Pressing on the nasolacrimal duct blocks the lacrimal punctum and prevents systemic absorption of the medication.

    C. Pressing on the conjunctival sac will not prevent systemic absorption of the medication.

    D. Pressing on the outer canthus will not prevent systemic absorption of the medication.

    Ⓝ *NCLEX® Connection: Pharmacological and Parenteral Therapies, Medication Administration*

2. A. Rifampin can stain soft contact lenses. Brimonidine does not stain contacts.

    B. Brimonidine can cause mydriasis or dilated pupils.

    C. **CORRECT:** Brimonidine can absorb into soft contact lenses. The client should remove his contacts then instill the medication and wait at least 15 min before putting in his contacts back in.

    D. Beta-adrenergic blockers, such as timolol, can slow the heart rate. Brimonidine can cause hypertension or hypotension.

    Ⓝ *NCLEX® Connection: Pharmacological and Parenteral Therapies, Medication Administration*

3. A. Acute-angle glaucoma is painful and has a sudden onset.

    B. Gradual loss of peripheral vision is a manifestation of primary open-angle glaucoma.

    C. **CORRECT:** Severe pain around eyes that radiates over the face is a manifestation of acute angle-closure glaucoma.

    D. An IOP of 12 mm Hg is within the expected reference range. Elevated IOP is a manifestation of angle-closure glaucoma.

    Ⓝ *NCLEX® Connection: Pharmacological and Parenteral Therapies, Adverse Effects/Contraindications/Side Effects/Interactions*

4. A. The client should not insert anything in the ear because this can push cerumen into the eardrum, damage the epithelium, or puncture the eardrum.

    B. The client should wear earplugs only when swimming to reduce the risk for otitis externa.

    C. The client should not use cool water irrigation solution to remove cerumen. Cool fluid can cause vertigo, dizziness, and nausea. The client should not remove cerumen from the ear to reduce the risk for otitis externa.

    D. **CORRECT:** The client should remove water from the ear after showering or swimming to reduce the risk for otitis externa.

    Ⓝ *NCLEX® Connection: Pharmacological and Parenteral Therapies, Medication Administration*

5. A. **CORRECT:** The parent should have the child on his unaffected side to allow access to the affected ear and to promote drainage of the medication by gravity into the ear.

    B. **CORRECT:** The parent should warm the medication by rolling it between his hands. Administering the medication cold can cause dizziness.

    C. **CORRECT:** The parent should gently shake medication that is in suspension form to evenly- disperse the medication.

    D. **CORRECT:** The parent should keep the child on his side to promote drainage of the medication by gravity into the ear.

    E. The parent should loosely pack the child's ear with cotton.

    Ⓝ *NCLEX® Connection: Pharmacological and Parenteral Therapies, Medication Administration*

PRACTICE Answer

Using ATI Active Learning Template: Medication

THERAPEUTIC USES: The bactericidal effects of ciprofloxacin and the anti-inflammatory effect of hydrocortisone decreases pain, edema, and erythema in the ear.

MEDICATION ADMINISTRATION
- Keep foreign bodies out of ear canal.
- Avoid manual measures to remove cerumen.
- Dry ear canal after bathing or swimming using a towel.
- Avoid use of ear plugs except for swimming.

Ⓝ *NCLEX® Connection: Pharmacological and Parenteral Therapies, Medication Administration*

CHAPTER 15
Miscellaneous Central Nervous System Medications

Neuromuscular blocking agents have various uses, including causing muscle relaxation during general anesthesia, control of seizures during electroconvulsive therapy, and suppression of gag reflex during endotracheal intubation. Medications include succinylcholine and vecuronium.

Muscle relaxants and antispasmodic agents can affect both the central and peripheral nervous systems. These agents are used for spasticity related to muscle injury, cerebral palsy, spinal cord injury, and multiple sclerosis. Agents include diazepam, baclofen, and dantrolene. Bethanechol, a **muscarinic agonist**, is used for urinary retention. Oxybutynin, a **muscarinic antagonist**, is used for neurogenic bladder.

Neuromuscular blocking agents

SELECT PROTOTYPE MEDICATION
- **Depolarizing** neuromuscular blockers: Succinylcholine
- **Nondepolarizing** neuromuscular blockers: Pancuronium

OTHER MEDICATIONS: Nondepolarizing neuromuscular blockers
- Atracurium
- Cisatracurium
- Rocuronium
- Vecuronium

PURPOSE

EXPECTED PHARMACOLOGICAL ACTION

Nondepolarizing neuromuscular blocking agents block acetylcholine (ACh) at the neuromuscular junction, resulting in muscle relaxation and hypotension. They do not cross the blood-brain barrier, so complete paralysis is achieved without loss of consciousness or decreased pain sensation.

Succinylcholine

- Mimics ACh by binding with cholinergic receptors at the neuromuscular junction. This agent fills the cholinergic receptors, preventing ACh from binding with them, and causes sustained depolarization of the muscle, resulting in muscle paralysis.
- Short duration of action because of degradation by the plasma enzyme pseudocholinesterase.

Pancuronium, atracurium, vecuronium

- Block ACh from binding with cholinergic receptors at the motor end plate. Muscle paralysis occurs because of inhibited nerve depolarization and skeletal muscle contraction.
- Reversal agent: neostigmine

THERAPEUTIC USES

- Neuromuscular blocking agents are used as adjuncts to general anesthesia to promote muscle relaxation.
- These agents are used to control spontaneous respiratory movements in clients receiving mechanical ventilation.
- These agents are used as seizure control during electroconvulsive therapy.
- Neuromuscular blocking agents are used during endotracheal intubation and endoscopy.

COMPLICATIONS

Respiratory arrest

From paralyzed respiratory muscles

NURSING CONSIDERATIONS
- Maintain continuous cardiac and respiratory monitoring.
- Have equipment ready for resuscitation and mechanical ventilation.
- Monitor for return of respiratory function when medication is discontinued.
- Administer a cholinesterase inhibitor, neostigmine, to reverse the action of nondepolarizing neuromuscular blocking agents as needed.

ATRACURIUM

Hypotension

Possible with atracurium

NURSING CONSIDERATIONS: Monitor for decreased blood pressure. Administer antihistamine if indicated.

SUCCINYLCHOLINE

Prolonged apnea

Low pseudocholinesterase activity can lead to prolonged apnea.

NURSING CONSIDERATIONS
- Test blood or administer a small test dose for clients suspected of having low levels of pseudocholinesterase.
- Withhold medication if pseudocholinesterase activity is low.

Malignant hyperthermia

Manifestations include muscle rigidity accompanied by increased temperature, as high as 43° C (109.4° F).

NURSING CONSIDERATIONS
- Monitor vital signs.
- Stop succinylcholine and other anesthetics.
- Administer oxygen at 100%.
- Initiate cooling measures including administration of iced 0.9% sodium chloride, applying a cooling blanket, and placing ice bags in groin and other areas.
- Administer dantrolene to decrease metabolic activity of skeletal muscle.

Muscle pain

After 12 to 24 hr postoperative, clients can experience muscle pain in the upper body and back.

NURSING CONSIDERATIONS
- Advise clients that this response is not unusual and eventually will subside.
- Notify the provider to consider short-term use of muscle relaxant.

Hyperkalemia

NURSING CONSIDERATIONS
- Monitor potassium levels.
- Observe for manifestations of hyperkalemia.
- Do not use succinylcholine for clients who have severe burns, multiple trauma, or upper motor neuron injury.

CONTRAINDICATIONS/PRECAUTIONS

- **Pregnancy Risk Category C**
- Succinylcholine is contraindicated in clients who have risk of hyperkalemia (major trauma, severe burns).
- Use cautiously in clients who have myasthenia gravis, respiratory dysfunction, or fluid and electrolyte imbalances.

> Note that neuromuscular blocker medications are not anesthetics and therefore have no effect on hearing, thinking, or ability to feel pain.

INTERACTIONS

General anesthetics are often used concurrently in surgery.
NURSING CONSIDERATIONS: Reduce dosage of neuromuscular blocker to prevent extreme neuromuscular blockade.

Aminoglycosides and tetracyclines can increase the effects of neuromuscular blockade.
NURSING CONSIDERATIONS: Take complete medication history of clients who are to receive neuromuscular blockade. Monitor for prolonged neuromuscular blockage.

Neostigmine and other cholinesterase inhibitors increase the effects of depolarizing neuromuscular blockers, such as succinylcholine.
NURSING CONSIDERATIONS: Monitor clients during neuromuscular blockade reversal after surgery.

NURSING ADMINISTRATION

- Clients must receive continuous cardiac and respiratory monitoring during therapy. **Qs**
- Monitor clients following administration of a neuromuscular blocker for respiratory depression. Have life support equipment available.
- Continue to carefully monitor for return of respiratory function.
- Have a cholinesterase inhibitor available to reverse nondepolarizing neuromuscular blocking agents.

NURSING EVALUATION OF MEDICATION EFFECTIVENESS

Depending on therapeutic intent, effectiveness can be evidenced by
- Muscle relaxation during surgery
- No spontaneous respiratory movements in clients receiving mechanical ventilation
- Absence of seizures in clients receiving electroconvulsive therapy
- Successful endotracheal intubation

Muscle relaxants and antispasmodics

SELECT PROTOTYPE MEDICATION
- **Centrally acting muscle relaxants:** Diazepam
- **Peripherally acting muscle relaxants:** Dantrolene

OTHER MEDICATIONS: Centrally acting muscle relaxants
- Baclofen
- Cyclobenzaprine
- Tizanidine

PURPOSE

Diazepam

EXPECTED PHARMACOLOGICAL ACTION: Acts in the CNS to enhance GABA and produce sedative effects and depress spasticity of muscles.

THERAPEUTIC USES
- Muscle spasm related to muscle injury and spasticity
- Anxiety and panic disorders
- Insomnia
- Status epilepticus
- Alcohol withdrawal
- Anesthesia induction

Cyclobenzaprine, tizanidine

EXPECTED PHARMACOLOGICAL ACTION: Act in the CNS to enhance GABA and produce sedative effects and depress spasticity of muscles. They have no direct muscle relaxant action and so do not decrease muscle strength.

THERAPEUTIC USES: Relief of muscle spasm related to muscle injury

Baclofen

EXPECTED PHARMACOLOGICAL ACTION: Acts in the CNS to enhance GABA, produce sedative effects, and depress hyperactive spasticity of muscles. There are no direct effects on skeletal muscles.

THERAPEUTIC USES: Relief of spasticity related to cerebral palsy, spinal cord injury, and multiple sclerosis

Dantrolene

EXPECTED PHARMACOLOGICAL ACTION: A peripherally acting muscle relaxant that acts directly on spastic muscles and inhibits muscle contraction by preventing release of calcium in skeletal muscles.

THERAPEUTIC USES
- Relief of spasticity related to cerebral palsy, spinal cord injury, and multiple sclerosis
- Treatment of malignant hyperthermia

COMPLICATIONS

CNS depression

Sleepiness, lightheadedness, fatigue

NURSING CONSIDERATIONS
- Start at low doses.
- Inform clients of potential adverse effects.
- Advise clients to avoid hazardous activities, such as driving and concurrent use of other CNS depressants, including alcohol.
- Can occur with all muscle relaxants and antispasmodic medications.

DIAZEPAM, CYCLOBENZAPRINE, TIZANIDINE

Hepatic toxicity with tizanidine

Anorexia, nausea, vomiting, abdominal pain, jaundice

NURSING CONSIDERATIONS
- Obtain baseline liver function and perform periodic follow-up liver function tests.
- Observe for indications of toxicity and notify the provider if they occur.
- Start at a low dose.

Physical dependence from chronic long-term use

NURSING CONSIDERATIONS: Advise clients not to discontinue the medication abruptly.

BACLOFEN

Nausea, constipation, urinary retention

NURSING CONSIDERATIONS
- Advise clients of adverse effects and to notify the provider if they occur.
- Advise clients to take with meals to reduce gastric upset.
- Monitor I&O.
- Advise clients to increase intake of high-fiber foods.

Seizures

NURSING CONSIDERATIONS
- Advise clients of adverse effects and to notify the provider if they occur.
- Monitor for seizure activity

DANTROLENE

Hepatic toxicity

Anorexia, nausea, vomiting, abdominal pain, jaundice

NURSING CONSIDERATIONS
- Obtain baseline liver function studies and perform periodic follow-up liver function tests.
- Observe for indications of toxicity and notify the provider if they occur.
- Start at low doses.

Muscle weakness

NURSING CONSIDERATIONS: Monitor effectiveness of the medication.

CONTRAINDICATIONS/PRECAUTIONS

BACLOFEN AND DANTROLENE: Pregnancy Risk Category C

DIAZEPAM
- Controlled Substance (Schedule IV)
- Pregnancy Risk Category D

  Use both of these medications cautiously in clients who have impaired liver and renal function.

INTERACTIONS

CNS depressants (alcohol, opioids, antihistamines) have additive CNS depressant effects.
NURSING CONSIDERATIONS: Advise clients to avoid concurrent use.

NURSING ADMINISTRATION

- Instruct clients to take medications as prescribed.
- Advise clients not to stop taking the medication abruptly to avoid withdrawal reaction.
- Advise clients to avoid CNS depressants while using these medications.
- Provide assistance as needed in self-administration of medication and performance of ADLs. Qpcc

NURSING EVALUATION OF MEDICATION EFFECTIVENESS

Depending on therapeutic intent, effectiveness can be evidenced by:
- Absence of muscle rigidity and spasms, good range of motion
- Absence of pain
- Increased ability to perform ADLs

Muscarinic agonists

SELECT PROTOTYPE MEDICATION: Bethanechol

OTHER MEDICATIONS
- Cevimeline
- Pilocarpine
- Acetylcholine

PURPOSE

EXPECTED PHARMACOLOGICAL ACTION: Stimulation of muscarine receptors of the GU tract, thereby causing relaxation of the trigone and sphincter muscles and contraction of the detrusor muscle to increase bladder pressure and excretion of urine

THERAPEUTIC USES
- Nonobstructive urinary retention, usually postoperatively or postpartum
- On an investigational basis to treat gastroesophageal reflux

COMPLICATIONS

Extreme muscarinic stimulation can result in increased gastric acid secretion, abdominal cramps, diarrhea, sweating, tearing, urinary urgency, bradycardia and hypotension; bronchoconstriction

NURSING CONSIDERATIONS
- Instruct clients to report adverse effects if they occur. Monitor for bradycardia and hypotension.
- Administer on an empty stomach to reduce effects.

CONTRAINDICATIONS/PRECAUTIONS

Contraindicated in clients who have urinary or gastrointestinal obstruction, peptic ulcer disease, coronary insufficiency, asthma and hyperthyroidism.

NURSING ADMINISTRATION

- Administer by oral route, 1 hr before or 2 hr after meals to minimize nausea and vomiting.
- Monitor I&O.

NURSING EVALUATION OF MEDICATION EFFECTIVENESS

Depending on therapeutic intent, effectiveness can be evidenced by relief of urinary retention.

Muscarinic antagonists

SELECT PROTOTYPE MEDICATION: M_3 receptor selective: oxybutynin

OTHER MEDICATIONS
- **M_3 receptor selective:** Darifenacin, solifenacin
- **Nonselective:** Tolterodine, fesoterodine, trospium

PURPOSE

EXPECTED PHARMACOLOGICAL ACTION: Inhibit muscarinic receptors of the detrusor muscle of the bladder, which prevents contractions of the bladder and the urge to void

THERAPEUTIC USES: Overactive bladder

COMPLICATIONS

Anticholinergic effects

Constipation, dry mouth, blurred vision, photophobia, dry eyes, tachycardia)

NURSING CONSIDERATIONS: Instruct clients to increase dietary fiber, consume 2 to 3 L/day fluid from beverage and food sources, sip fluids, and avoid driving or other hazardous activities if vision is impaired.

CNS, cardiovascular effects

CNS effects: hallucinations, confusion, insomnia, nervousness)

Cardiovascular effects: prolonged QT interval

NURSING CONSIDERATIONS
- Instruct clients to report manifestations to the provider. Discontinue medication.
- Avoid use in older adult clients.
- Monitor ECG.

CONTRAINDICATIONS/PRECAUTIONS

- Contraindicated in clients who have glaucoma, myasthenia gravis, paralytic ileus, GI or GU obstruction, or urinary retention.
- Use cautiously in children and older adults.
- Use cautiously in clients who have gastroesophageal reflux disease, heart failure, or kidney or liver impairment.

INTERACTIONS

Antihistamines, tricyclic antidepressants, or phenothiazines used concurrently can result in extreme muscarinic blockage.

NURSING CONSIDERATIONS: Concurrent use is not recommended.

NURSING ADMINISTRATION

- Oral formulations are available as syrup, immediate-release (IR) tablets, and also extended-release (ER) tablets, which minimize anticholinergic effects. QPCC
- Advise clients to swallow ER tablets whole and to avoid chewing or crushing the tablets.
- Instruct clients that the shell of ER tablets will be eliminated whole in the stool.
- The transdermal patch is administered two times per week. Instruct clients to apply to dry skin of the hip, abdomen, or buttock and to rotate sites.

NURSING EVALUATION OF MEDICATION EFFECTIVENESS

Depending on therapeutic intent, effectiveness can be evidenced by a decrease in urinary urgency and frequency, nocturia, and urge incontinence.

PRACTICE Active Learning Scenario

A nurse manager in a surgical center is reviewing nursing responsibilities regarding administration of succinylcholine. Use the ATI Active Learning Template: Medication to complete this item.

THERAPEUTIC USES: Identify two common indications for use.

MEDICATION ADMINISTRATION: Identify two nursing responsibilities regarding the use of succinylcholine.

Application Exercises

1. A nurse in the operating room is caring for a client who received a dose of succinylcholine. During the operation, the client suddenly develops rigidity, and his body temperature begins to rise. The nurse should anticipate a prescription for which of the following medications?

   A. Neostigmine

   B. Naloxone

   C. Dantrolene

   D. Vecuronium

2. A nurse in the post-anesthesia care unit is caring for a client who is experiencing malignant hyperthermia. Which of the following actions should the nurse take? (Select all that apply.)

   A. Place a cooling blanket on the client.

   B. Administer oxygen at 100%.

   C. Administer iced 0.9% sodium chloride.

   D. Administer potassium chloride IV.

   E. Monitor core body temperature.

3. A nurse is teaching a client who has a new prescription for baclofen to treat muscle spasms. Which of the following statements by the client indicates an understanding of the teaching? (Select all that apply.)

   A. "I will stop taking this medication right away if I develop dizziness."

   B. "I know the doctor will gradually increase my dose of this medication for a while."

   C. "I should increase fiber to prevent constipation from this medication."

   D. "I won't be able to drink alcohol while I'm taking this medication."

   E. "I should take this medication on an empty stomach each morning."

4. A nurse is reviewing the health care record of a client who reports urinary incontinence and asks about a prescription for oxybutynin. The nurse should recognize that oxybutynin is contraindicated in the presence of which of the following conditions?

   A. Bursitis

   B. Sinusitis

   C. Depression

   D. Glaucoma

5. A nurse is caring for a client who has a prescription for bethanechol to treat urinary retention. The nurse should recognize that which of the following findings is a manifestation of muscarinic stimulation?

   A. Dry mouth

   B. Hypertension

   C. Excessive perspiration

   D. Fecal impaction

1. A. Neostigmine is a cholinesterase inhibitor used to reverse the effects of nondepolarizing neuromuscular blockers. It can delay inactivation of succinylcholine, a depolarizing neuromuscular blocker.

   B. Naloxone is used to reverse the effects of opioids. It is not used to treat malignant hyperthermia.

   C. **CORRECT:** Muscle rigidity and a sudden rise in temperature is a manifestation of malignant hyperthermia. Dantrolene acts on skeletal muscles to reduce metabolic activity and treat malignant hyperthermia.

   D. Vecuronium is an intermediate-acting nondepolarizing neuromuscular blocker. It is not useful in treating malignant hyperthermia.

   Ⓝ *NCLEX® Connection: Pharmacological and Parenteral Therapies, Expected Actions/Outcomes*

2. A. **CORRECT:** The nurse should apply a cooling blanket and apply ice to the axilla and groin.

   B. **CORRECT:** The nurse should administer oxygen at 100% to treat decreased oxygen saturation.

   C. **CORRECT:** The nurse should take action to decrease the client's body temperature by administering iced IV fluids.

   D. A client who has malignant hyperthermia is at risk for hyperkalemia.

   E. **CORRECT:** The nurse should monitor core body temperature to prevent hypothermia and to determine progress with treatment measures.

   Ⓝ *NCLEX® Connection: Pharmacological and Parenteral Therapies, Parenteral/Intravenous Therapies*

3. A. Abrupt withdrawal from baclofen can result in a number of adverse effects, including visual hallucinations and seizures.

   B. **CORRECT:** The provider starts the client on a low dose, and the dose is increased gradually to prevent CNS depression.

   C. **CORRECT:** The client should increase fluids and fiber to reduce the risk for constipation.

   D. **CORRECT:** The intake of alcohol and other CNS depressants can exacerbate the CNS depressant effects of baclofen. Therefore, the client is instructed to avoid CNS depressants while taking baclofen.

   E. The client should take baclofen with meals to reduce gastric upset.

   Ⓝ *NCLEX® Connection: Pharmacological and Parenteral Therapies, Medication Administration*

4. A. Oxybutynin is contraindicated in clients who have unstable cardiovascular disease, not bursitis.

   B. Oxybutynin is contraindicated in clients who have urinary retention, not sinusitis.

   C. Oxybutynin is contraindicated in clients who have myasthenia gravis, not depression.

   D. **CORRECT:** Oxybutynin is an anticholinergic and can increase intraocular pressure. It is contraindicated for clients who have glaucoma.

   Ⓝ *NCLEX® Connection: Pharmacological and Parenteral Therapies, Adverse Effects/Contraindications/Side Effects/Interactions*

5. A. Increased salivation is a manifestation of muscarinic stimulation.

   B. Hypotension is a manifestation of muscarinic stimulation.

   C. **CORRECT:** Bethanechol is a muscarinic agonist. Muscarinic stimulation can result in sweating.

   D. Diarrhea is an adverse effect of bethanechol.

   Ⓝ *NCLEX® Connection: Pharmacological and Parenteral Therapies, Adverse Effects/Contraindications/Side Effects/Interactions*

PRACTICE Answer

Using the Active Learning Template: Medication

THERAPEUTIC USES
- Endotracheal intubation
- Electroconvulsive therapy
- Endoscopy
- Adjunct to mechanical ventilation
- Muscle relaxation during surgery

MEDICATION ADMINISTRATION
- Clients must receive continuous cardiac and respiratory monitoring during therapy.
- Monitor clients following administration of a neuromuscular blocker for respiratory depression and have life support equipment available.
- Continue to carefully monitor for return of respiratory function.
- Succinylcholine is contraindicated for clients at risk for hyperkalemia (trauma, severe burns).

Ⓝ *NCLEX® Connection: Pharmacological and Parenteral Therapies, Adverse Effects/Contraindications/Side Effects/Interactions*

CHAPTER 16

CHAPTER 16 *Sedative-Hypnotics*

Sedatives are CNS depressants that induce a sense of calm and decrease anxiety. Hypnotics are CNS depressants that induce sleep.

The three types of sedative-hypnotics are **benzodiazepines, barbiturates,** and **benzodiazepine-like medications.** The most commonly used are benzodiazepines and benzodiazepine-like medications because barbiturates cause tolerance and dependence, have multiple interactions, and are powerful respiratory depressants.

IV anesthetics usually are administered during induction of general anesthesia. Most have a quick onset of action and short duration. These medications can be nonopioids or opioids.

Benzodiazepines

SELECT PROTOTYPE MEDICATION: Diazepam

OTHER MEDICATIONS
- Alprazolam
- Lorazepam
- Midazolam
- Temazepam
- Triazolam
- Clonazepam
- Oxazepam
- Chlordiazepoxide

PURPOSE

EXPECTED PHARMACOLOGICAL ACTION: Enhance the action of gamma-aminobutyric acid (GABA) in the CNS.

THERAPEUTIC USES Q EBP
- Anxiety disorders (alprazolam, chlordiazepoxide, diazepam, lorazepam, oxazepam)
- Seizure disorders (clonazepam, diazepam, lorazepam)
- Insomnia (triazolam, temazepam)
- Muscle spasm (diazepam)
- Alcohol withdrawal (chlordiazepoxide, diazepam, lorazepam, oxazepam)
- Panic disorder (alprazolam, clonazepam, lorazepam)
- Induction of anesthesia/preoperative sedation (diazepam, midazolam, lorazepam)

COMPLICATIONS

CNS depression

Lightheadedness, drowsiness, incoordination

NURSING CONSIDERATIONS
- Advise clients to observe for manifestations and notify the provider if they occur.
- Advise clients to avoid hazardous activities such as driving or operating heavy equipment/machinery.

Paradoxical response

Such as insomnia, excitation, euphoria, anxiety, rage

NURSING CONSIDERATIONS: Advise clients to observe for manifestations. If manifestations occur, instruct clients to notify the provider and stop the medication.

Nausea, vomiting, anorexia

Nursing considerations: Clients can take with food

Respiratory depression

Especially with IV administration

NURSING CONSIDERATIONS
- Monitor vital signs.
- Have resuscitation equipment available.

Physical dependence

- Withdrawal following short-term therapy manifests as anxiety, insomnia, tremors and dizziness.
- Withdrawal following long-term therapy manifests as delirium, paranoia, panic, hypertension and seizures.

NURSING CONSIDERATIONS: Discontinue medication slowly by tapering dose over weeks to months.

Acute toxicity

- Oral: drowsiness, lethargy, confusion
- IV: respiratory depression, cardiac arrest

NURSING CONSIDERATIONS
- Oral: Gastric lavage can be used, followed by the administration of activated charcoal or saline cathartics.
- IV: Administer flumazenil to counteract sedation and reverse adverse effects.
- Monitor vital signs, maintain patent airway, and provide fluids to maintain blood pressure.
- Have resuscitation equipment available.

TEMAZEPAM, TRIAZOLAM

Anterograde amnesia and sleep-related behaviors

Sleep driving, sleep eating

NURSING CONSIDERATIONS: Advise clients to observe for manifestations and notify the provider if they occur.

CONTRAINDICATIONS/PRECAUTIONS

- Most benzodiazepines are Pregnancy Risk Category D. Triazolam and temazepam are Pregnancy Risk Category X. ⓠs
- Contraindicated in clients who have sleep apnea, respiratory depression, and organic brain disease, or who are breastfeeding.
- Use cautiously in clients who have a history of substance use disorder, liver dysfunction, and kidney failure.
- Older adults can require decreased dosages. Precautions should be taken when administering benzodiazepines to older adult clients because memory difficulties can result. ⓖ

INTERACTIONS

CNS depressants such as alcohol, barbiturates, and opioids cause additive CNS depressant effects with concurrent use.

NURSING CONSIDERATIONS

- Take complete medication history to identify concurrent use of other CNS depressants.
- Advise clients to avoid alcohol and other CNS depressants.

NURSING ADMINISTRATION

- Ensure proper route of administration.
  - All agents may be given by oral route.
  - IV administration is acceptable with diazepam, midazolam, and lorazepam.
  - Lorazepam is the agent of choice for IM injection.
- Advise clients to take the medication as prescribed and to avoid abrupt discontinuation of treatment to prevent manifestations of medication withdrawal. ⓠs
- When discontinuing benzodiazepines, taper dose over several weeks.
- Administer medication with meals. Advise clients to swallow sustained-release tablets and to avoid chewing or crushing the tablet.
- For insomnia, take 15 to 20 minutes before bedtime. Limit continuous use to 7 to 10 days. Teach client nonpharmacologic strategies to facilitate sleep. ⓠPCC
- Inform clients about possible development of dependency during and after treatment, and to notify the provider if manifestations occur.

NURSING EVALUATION OF MEDICATION EFFECTIVENESS

Depending on therapeutic intent, effectiveness can be evidenced by improvement of well-being as evidenced by absence of panic attacks, decrease or absence of anxiety, normal sleep pattern, absence of seizures, absence of withdrawal manifestations from alcohol, and relaxation of muscles.

Nonbenzodiazepines

SELECT PROTOTYPE MEDICATION: Zolpidem

OTHER MEDICATIONS
- Zaleplon
- Eszopiclone

PURPOSE

EXPECTED PHARMACOLOGICAL ACTION: Enhance the action of GABA in the CNS. This results in prolonged sleep duration and decreased awakenings. These medications do not function as antianxiety, muscle relaxant, or antiepileptic agents. There is a low risk of tolerance, substance use disorder, and dependence.

THERAPEUTIC USES: Management of insomnia

COMPLICATIONS

Daytime sleepiness and lightheadedness, headache

NURSING CONSIDERATIONS
- Administer medication at bedtime.
- Advise clients to take medication allowing for at least 8 hr of sleep.
- Advise clients that more rapid absorption occurs when the medication is taken when the stomach is empty.

CONTRAINDICATIONS/PRECAUTIONS

- Pregnancy Risk Category C.
- Precautions are necessary for clients who are breastfeeding.
- Zolpidem has been associated with sleep-related complex behaviors similar to the benzodiazepines.
- Use cautiously in older adult clients and in clients who have impaired kidney, liver, or respiratory function. ⓠs

INTERACTIONS

CNS depressants such as alcohol, barbiturates, opioids cause additive CNS depression.
NURSING CONSIDERATIONS: Advise clients to avoid alcohol and other CNS depressants.

NURSING ADMINISTRATION

- Advise clients to take the medication just before bedtime.
- Administer all agents by oral or sublingual route.

NURSING EVALUATION OF MEDICATION EFFECTIVENESS

Depending on therapeutic intent, effectiveness can be evidenced by effective sleep pattern.

Melatonin agonist

SELECT PROTOTYPE MEDICATION: Ramelteon

PURPOSE

EXPECTED PHARMACOLOGICAL ACTION: Activation of melatonin receptors

THERAPEUTIC USES: Management of insomnia

COMPLICATIONS

Sleepiness, dizziness, fatigue

NURSING CONSIDERATIONS
- Ramelteon is generally well tolerated. Instruct clients to notify the provider if manifestations occur.
- Advise clients to avoid activities such as driving if manifestations occur.

Hormonal effects

Amenorrhea, decreased libido, infertility, and galactorrhea caused by increased levels of prolactin

NURSING CONSIDERATIONS: Instruct clients to notify the provider if manifestations occur. Medication may be discontinued.

CONTRAINDICATIONS/PRECAUTIONS

- Pregnancy Risk Category C.
- Contraindicated in lactation, severe forms of liver disease, depression, apnea, and COPD.
- Use cautiously in clients who have moderate liver disease and older adults. ©

INTERACTIONS

High-fat meals can prolong absorption of ramelteon.
NURSING CONSIDERATIONS
- Avoid high-fat meals before taking the medication.
- Take medication on an empty stomach for rapid onset.

Concurrent use of fluvoxamine can increase levels of ramelteon.
NURSING CONSIDERATIONS: Avoid concurrent use.

CNS depressants such as opioids, alcohol can cause additive CNS depression.
NURSING CONSIDERATIONS: Avoid concurrent use.

NURSING ADMINISTRATION

- Administer by oral route.
- Instruct clients to take medication 30 min prior to bedtime.
- Instruct clients to take medication on an empty stomach and to avoid high-fat foods before taking ramelteon.
- Instruct clients the purpose of ramelteon is to induce sleep; it is not prescribed for sleep maintenance.

NURSING EVALUATION OF MEDICATION EFFECTIVENESS

Depending on therapeutic intent, effectiveness can be evidenced by improvement in sleep patterns.

Intravenous anesthetics

Intravenous nonopioid agents

SELECT PROTOTYPE MEDICATIONS
- **Barbiturates:** Pentobarbital sodium
- **Benzodiazepines** (used for preoperative sedation): Midazolam, diazepam, lorazepam
- **Other medications:** Propofol, ketamine

Intravenous opioid agents

SELECT PROTOTYPE MEDICATION: Fentanyl

OTHER MEDICATIONS
- Alfentanil
- Sufentanil
- Morphine sulfate

PURPOSE

EXPECTED PHARMACOLOGICAL ACTION: Loss of consciousness and elimination of response to painful stimuli

THERAPEUTIC USES
- Induction and maintenance of anesthesia
- Moderate (conscious) sedation (usually an IV nonopioid agent combined with an opioid agent)
- Intubation and mechanical ventilation

COMPLICATIONS

Respiratory and cardiovascular depression with high risk for hypotension

NURSING CONSIDERATIONS
- Provide continuous monitoring of vital signs and ECG.
- Maintain mechanical ventilation during procedure.
- Have equipment ready for resuscitation. Qs

PROPOFOL

Bacterial infection

NURSING CONSIDERATIONS
- Use opened vials within 6 hr.
- Monitor for indications of infection such as fever, malaise after surgery.

KETAMINE

Psychological reactions

- Hallucinations, mental confusion
- Children less than 15 years of age and adults older than 65 years of age at higher risk

NURSING CONSIDERATIONS
- Avoid use in clients who have a history of mental illness.
- Maintain a quiet, low-stimulus environment during recovery.
- Give diazepam or midazolam prior to ketamine.

CONTRAINDICATIONS/PRECAUTIONS

- Avoid use in clients who have a history of mental illness.
- Use cautiously in clients who have respiratory and cardiovascular disease.
- Midazolam is contraindicated in clients who have glaucoma. Precautions should be taken in children, older adults, and clients who have kidney or hepatic failure, status asthmaticus, or alcohol intoxication.
- Pentobarbital and midazolam are Pregnancy Risk Category D.

INTERACTIONS

Additive CNS depression
- Created by CNS depressants (alcohol, barbiturates, opioids)
- NURSING CONSIDERATIONS
  - Clients can require lower dose.
  - Provide continuous monitoring of vital signs and ECG.
  - Have equipment ready for resuscitation.

Additive CNS stimulation
- Created by CNS stimulants (amphetamines, cocaine)
- NURSING CONSIDERATIONS
  - Clients can require higher doses.
  - Provide continuous monitoring of vital signs and ECG.
  - Have equipment ready for resuscitation.

NURSING ADMINISTRATION

- For moderate (conscious) sedation or for neonatal anesthesia, administer slowly over 2 min.
- Monitor carefully during and after moderate sedation or anesthesia for respiratory arrest or hypotension.
- Inject propofol into large vein to decrease pain at injection site.
- Instruct clients to arrange for a ride home following outpatient procedure. Qpcc

NURSING EVALUATION OF MEDICATION EFFECTIVENESS

Depending on therapeutic intent, effectiveness can be evidenced by
- Surgical procedure occurs with loss of consciousness and elimination of pain.
- Postoperative recovery as demonstrated by
  - Vital signs return to baseline.
  - Client is oriented to time, place, and person.
  - Bowel sounds return.
  - Voiding occurs within 8 hr.
  - Nausea and vomiting are controlled.

Application Exercises

1. A nurse is providing instructions to a client who has been experiencing insomnia and has a new prescription for temazepam. The nurse should inform the client that which of the following manifestations are adverse effects of temazepam? (Select all that apply.)

   A. Incoordination

   B. Hypertension

   C. Pruritus

   D. Sleep driving

   E. Amnesia

2. A nurse is caring for a client who is receiving moderate sedation with diazepam IV. The client is oversedated. Which of the following medications should the nurse anticipate administering to this client?

   A. Ketamine

   B. Naltrexone

   C. Flumazenil

   D. Fluvoxamine

3. A nurse is teaching a client who has a new prescription for ramelteon. The nurse should instruct the client to avoid which of the following foods while taking this medication?

   A. Baked potato

   B. Fried chicken

   C. Whole-grain bread

   D. Citrus fruits

4. A nurse is caring for a client who is admitted to undergo a surgical procedure. Which of the following preexisting conditions can be a contraindication for the use of ketamine as an intravenous anesthetic?

   A. Peptic ulcer disease

   B. Breast cancer

   C. Diabetes mellitus

   D. Schizophrenia

5. A nurse is providing instructions to a female client who has a new prescription for zolpidem. Which of the following instructions should the nurse include?

   A. "Notify the provider if you plan to become pregnant."

   B. "Take the medication 1 hr before you plan to go to sleep."

   C. "Allow at least 6 hr for sleep when taking zolpidem."

   D. "To increase the effectiveness of zolpidem, take it with a bedtime snack."

PRACTICE Active Learning Scenario

A nurse manager is preparing an educational session to review client use of benzodiazepines for the nurses on her unit. Use the ATI Active Learning Template: Medication to complete this item.

THERAPEUTIC USES: Identify five therapeutic uses for benzodiazepines.

CONTRAINDICATIONS/PRECAUTIONS: Identify four contraindications for taking benzodiazepines.

Application Exercises Key

1. A. **CORRECT:** Due to CNS depression, incoordination is an adverse effect of temazepam.

   B. Hypotension is an adverse effect of temazepam.

   C. Pruritus is not an adverse effect of temazepam.

   D. **CORRECT:** Sleep driving (driving after taking the medication without memory of doing so) is an adverse effect of temazepam.

   E. **CORRECT:** Retrograde amnesia, the inability to remember the events that occurred after taking the medication, can occur as an adverse effect of temazepam.

   Ⓝ *NCLEX® Connection: Pharmacological and Parenteral Therapies, Adverse Effects/Contraindications/Side Effects/Interactions*

2. A. Ketamine is an anesthetic agent.

   B. Naltrexone is an opioid antagonist used to treat opioid overdose and alcohol use disorders.

   C. **CORRECT:** Flumazenil is a competitive benzodiazepine antagonist used to reverse the sedation and other effects of benzodiazepines.

   D. Fluvoxamine is a selective serotonin reuptake inhibitor used to treat depression.

   Ⓝ *NCLEX® Connection: Pharmacological and Parenteral Therapies, Adverse Effects/Contraindications/Side Effects/Interactions*

3. A. A baked potato does not affect absorption of ramelteon.

   B. **CORRECT:** High-fat foods, such as fried chicken prolong the absorption of ramelteon and should be avoided.

   C. Whole-grain breads do not affect the absorption of ramelteon.

   D. Citrus fruits do not affect the absorption of ramelteon.

   Ⓝ *NCLEX® Connection: Pharmacological and Parenteral Therapies, Adverse Effects/Contraindications/Side Effects/Interactions*

4. A. Peptic ulcer disease is not a contraindication for the use of ketamine.

   B. Breast cancer is not a contraindication for the use of ketamine.

   C. Diabetes mellitus is not a contraindication for the use of ketamine.

   D. **CORRECT:** Ketamine can produce psychological effects, such as hallucinations. Therefore, schizophrenia can be a contraindication for the use of ketamine.

   Ⓝ *NCLEX® Connection: Pharmacological and Parenteral Therapies, Adverse Effects/Contraindications/Side Effects/Interactions*

5. A. **CORRECT:** Zolpidem is Pregnancy Risk Category C. The client should notify the provider if she plans to become pregnant.

   B. Zolpidem should be taken at bedtime.

   C. The client should allow at least 8 hr for sleep when taking zolpidem.

   D. Zolpidem is absorbed best on an empty stomach.

   Ⓝ *NCLEX® Connection: Pharmacological and Parenteral Therapies, Medication Administration*

PRACTICE Answer

Using the ATI Active Learning Template: Medication

THERAPEUTIC USES

- Anxiety disorders
- Seizure disorders
- Insomnia
- Muscle spasms
- Alcohol withdrawal
- Panic disorder
- Induction of anesthesia

CONTRAINDICATIONS/PRECAUTIONS

- Pregnancy: Benzodiazepines are Pregnancy Risk Category D (a high risk to the fetus)
- Sleep apnea
- Respiratory depression
- Organic brain disease
- Lactation
- Cautious use in clients who have a history of substance use disorders, liver dysfunction, and kidney failure

Ⓝ *NCLEX® Connection: Pharmacological and Parenteral Therapies, Medication Administration*

NCLEX® Connections

When reviewing the following chapters, keep in mind the relevant topics and tasks of the NCLEX outline, in particular:

Client Needs: Pharmacological and Parenteral Therapies

ADVERSE EFFECTS/CONTRAINDICATIONS/SIDE EFFECTS/ INTERACTIONS: Provide information to the client on common side effects/adverse effects/potential interactions of medications and inform the client when to notify the primary health care provider.

EXPECTED ACTIONS/OUTCOMES: Use clinical decision making/critical thinking when addressing expected effects/outcomes of medications.

MEDICATION ADMINISTRATION: Educate the client on medication self-administration procedures.

UNIT 3   MEDICATIONS AFFECTING THE
RESPIRATORY SYSTEM

CHAPTER 17 *Airflow Disorders*

Asthma is a chronic inflammatory disorder of the airways. It is an intermittent and reversible airflow obstruction that affects the bronchioles. The obstruction occurs either by inflammation or airway hyper-responsiveness leading to bronchoconstriction.

Medication management usually addresses both inflammation and bronchoconstriction. These same medications can also be used to treat the manifestations of chronic obstructive pulmonary disease (COPD).

Medications include bronchodilator agents, such as beta$_2$-adrenergic agonists, methylxanthines, inhaled anticholinergics, and anti-inflammatory agents, such as glucocorticoids, mast cell stabilizers, and leukotriene modifiers.

Beta$_2$-adrenergic agonists

SELECT PROTOTYPE MEDICATION: Albuterol

OTHER MEDICATIONS
- Formoterol
- Levalbuterol
- Salmeterol
- Terbutaline

PURPOSE

EXPECTED PHARMACOLOGICAL ACTION

Beta$_2$-adrenergic agonists act by selectively activating the beta$_2$-receptors in the bronchial smooth muscle, resulting in bronchodilation. As a result of this:
- Bronchospasm is relieved.
- Histamine release is inhibited.
- Ciliary motility is increased.

THERAPEUTIC USES

Albuterol, levalbuterol

ROUTE
- Inhaled, short-acting
- Oral, long-acting (albuterol)

THERAPEUTIC USES
- Prevention of asthma episode (exercise-induced)
- Inhaled, short-acting, used for prevention of asthma
- Treatment for bronchospasm
- Long-term control of asthma

Formoterol, salmeterol

ROUTE: Inhaled, long-acting

THERAPEUTIC USES: Long-term control of asthma

Terbutaline

ROUTE: Oral, long-acting

THERAPEUTIC USES: Long-term control of asthma

COMPLICATIONS

Tachycardia, angina

Oral agents can cause tachycardia and angina due to activation of alpha$_1$ receptors in the heart.

NURSING CONSIDERATIONS
- Advise clients to observe for chest, jaw, or arm pain or palpitations and to notify the provider if they occur.
- Instruct clients to check pulse and to report an increase of greater than 20 to 30 beats/min.
- Advise clients to avoid caffeine.
- Dosage might need to be reduced.

Tremors

Caused by activation of beta$_2$ receptors in skeletal muscle

NURSING CONSIDERATIONS
- Tremors usually resolve with continued medication use.
- Dosage might need to be reduced.

CONTRAINDICATIONS/PRECAUTIONS

- Pregnancy Risk Category C Q̈s
- Contraindicated in clients who have tachydysrhythmia.
- Use cautiously in clients who have diabetes mellitus, hyperthyroidism, heart disease, hypertension, and angina.

INTERACTIONS

Use of beta-adrenergic blockers can negate effects of both medications.
NURSING CONSIDERATIONS: Beta-adrenergic blockers should not be used concurrently.

MAOIs and tricyclic antidepressants can increase the risk of tachycardia and angina.
NURSING CONSIDERATIONS: Instruct clients to report changes in heart rate and chest pain.

NURSING ADMINISTRATION

- Instruct clients to follow manufacturer's instructions for use of metered-dose inhaler (MDI), dry-powder inhaler (DPI), and nebulizer.
- When a client has prescriptions for an inhaled beta$_2$-agonist and an inhaled glucocorticoid, advise the client to inhale the beta$_2$-agonist before inhaling the glucocorticoid. The beta$_2$-agonist promotes bronchodilation and enhances absorption of the glucocorticoid.
- Advise clients not to exceed prescribed dosages.
- Ensure that clients know the dosage schedule (if the medication is to be taken on a fixed or as-needed schedule).
- Formoterol and salmeterol are long-acting beta$_2$-agonist inhalers. These inhalers are used every 12 hr for long-term control and are not used to abort an asthma attack, or exacerbation. These long-acting agents are not used alone but are prescribed in combination with an inhaled glucocorticoid.

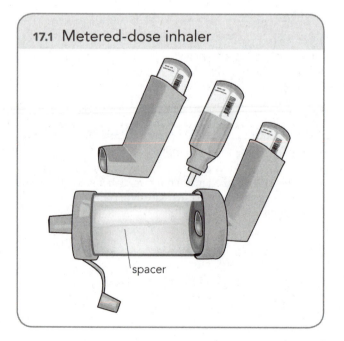

17.1 Metered-dose inhaler

spacer

- A short-acting beta$_2$-agonist is used to treat an acute episode.
- Advise clients to observe for indications of an impending asthma episode and to keep a log of the frequency and intensity of exacerbations.
- Instruct clients to notify the provider if there is an increase in the frequency and intensity of asthma exacerbations.

NURSING EVALUATION OF MEDICATION EFFECTIVENESS

Depending on therapeutic intent, effectiveness is evidenced by
- Long-term control of asthma
- Prevention of exercise-induced asthma
- Resolution of asthma exacerbations as evidenced by absence of shortness of breath, clear breath sounds, absence of wheezing, and return of respiratory rate to baseline

Methylxanthines

SELECT PROTOTYPE MEDICATION: Theophylline

PURPOSE

EXPECTED PHARMACOLOGICAL ACTION
- Relaxation of bronchial smooth muscle, resulting in bronchodilation
- Once the first-line medication for asthma, now used infrequently because newer medications are safer and more effective

THERAPEUTIC USES: Oral theophylline is used for long-term control of chronic asthma or COPD.

ROUTE OF ADMINISTRATION: oral or IV (emergency use only)

COMPLICATIONS

Mild toxicity reaction can include GI distress and restlessness.

More severe reactions can occur with higher therapeutic levels and can include **dysrhythmias** and **seizures**.

NURSING CONSIDERATIONS
- Monitor theophylline serum levels to keep within therapeutic range (5 to 15 mcg/mL). Adverse effects are unlikely to occur at levels less than 20 mcg/mL.
- If manifestations occur, stop the medication. Activated charcoal is used to decrease absorption, lidocaine is used to treat dysrhythmias, and diazepam is used to control seizures.
- Instruct client that periodic monitoring of blood levels is needed. Advise client to report nausea, diarrhea, or restlessness, which are indicative of toxicity.

CONTRAINDICATIONS/PRECAUTIONS

- Pregnancy Risk Category C Qs
- Use cautiously in clients who have heart disease, hypertension, liver and kidney dysfunction, and diabetes mellitus.
- Use cautiously in children and older adults. Ⓒ

INTERACTIONS

Caffeine
- Caffeine increases CNS and cardiac adverse effects of theophylline.
- Caffeine can increase theophylline levels.
- NURSING CONSIDERATIONS: Advise clients to avoid consuming caffeinated beverages (coffee, caffeinated colas).

Phenobarbital, phenytoin, and rifampin decrease theophylline levels.
NURSING CONSIDERATIONS: When theophylline is used concurrently with these medications, increase the dosage of theophylline.

Cimetidine, ciprofloxacin, and other fluoroquinolone antibiotics increase theophylline levels.
NURSING CONSIDERATIONS: When theophylline is used concurrently with these medications, decrease the dosage of theophylline.

NURSING ADMINISTRATION

- Advise clients to take the medication as prescribed. If a dose is missed, the following dose should not be doubled.
- Instruct clients to not chew or crush sustained-release preparations. These medications should be swallowed whole.

NURSING EVALUATION OF MEDICATION EFFECTIVENESS

Depending on therapeutic intent, effectiveness is evidenced by long-term control of asthma and COPD.

Inhaled anticholinergics

SELECT PROTOTYPE MEDICATION: Ipratropium

OTHER MEDICATIONS: Tiotropium

PURPOSE

EXPECTED PHARMACOLOGICAL ACTION: Block muscarinic receptors of the bronchi, resulting in bronchodilation

THERAPEUTIC USES
- Relieve bronchospasm associated with COPD
- Allergen-induced and exercise-induced bronchospasm

ROUTE OF ADMINISTRATION: inhalation

COMPLICATIONS

Local anticholinergic effects

Dry mouth, hoarseness

NURSING CONSIDERATIONS: Advise clients to sip fluids and suck on sugar-free hard candies to control dry mouth.

CONTRAINDICATIONS/PRECAUTIONS

- Pregnancy Risk Category B Qs
- Contraindicated in clients who have an allergy to peanuts because the medication preparations can contain soy lecithin.
- Use cautiously in clients who have narrow-angle glaucoma and benign prostatic hyperplasia (due to anticholinergic effects).

NURSING ADMINISTRATION

- Advise clients to rinse the mouth after inhalation to decrease unpleasant taste.
- Usual adult dosage is 2 puffs. Instruct clients to wait the length of time directed between puffs.
- If two inhaled medications are prescribed, instruct clients to wait at least 5 min between medications.
- Advise clients not to swallow tiotropium capsules. An inhalation device is used for administration of the capsule.

NURSING EVALUATION OF MEDICATION EFFECTIVENESS

Depending on therapeutic intent, effectiveness is evidenced by the following.
- Control of bronchospasm in clients who have COPD
- Prevention of allergen-induced and exercise-induced bronchospasm

Glucocorticoids

SELECT PROTOTYPE MEDICATIONS
- Inhalation: beclomethasone
- Oral: prednisone

OTHER MEDICATIONS
- Inhalation
  - Budesonide
  - Budesonide and formoterol
  - Fluticasone and salmeterol
  - Fluticasone
  - Mometasone and formoterol
- Oral: prednisolone
- IV
  - Hydrocortisone
  - Methylprednisolone

PURPOSE

EXPECTED PHARMACOLOGICAL ACTION
- Prevent inflammation, suppress airway mucus production, and promote responsiveness of beta$_2$ receptors in the bronchial tree
- Reduction in airway mucosa edema

> The use of glucocorticoids does not provide immediate effects, but rather promotes decreased frequency and severity of exacerbations and acute attacks.

THERAPEUTIC USES
- Short-term IV agents are used for status asthmaticus.
- Inhaled agents are used for long-term prophylaxis of asthma.
- Short-term oral therapy is used to treat manifestations following an acute asthma episode.
- Long-term oral therapy is used to treat chronic, severe asthma.
- Promote lung maturity and decrease respiratory distress in fetuses at risk for preterm birth.

COMPLICATIONS

BECLOMETHASONE

Difficulty speaking, hoarseness, and candidiasis

NURSING CONSIDERATIONS
- Advise clients to rinse mouth or gargle with water after use.
- Advise clients to monitor for redness, sores, or white patches and to report to provider if they occur. Treat candidiasis with nystatin oral suspension.

PREDNISONE

Prednisone when used for 10 days or more can result in:

Suppression of adrenal gland function

Such as a decrease in the ability of the adrenal cortex to produce glucocorticoids (can occur with inhaled agents and oral agents)

NURSING CONSIDERATIONS
- Administer oral glucocorticoid on an alternate-day dosing schedule.
- Monitor blood glucose levels.
- Taper the dose. Do not stop abruptly.

Bone loss

Can occur with inhaled agents and oral agents

NURSING CONSIDERATIONS
- Advise clients to perform weight-bearing exercises.
- Advise clients to consume a diet with sufficient calcium and vitamin D intake.
- Use the lowest dose possible to control manifestations.
- Oral medications should be given on an alternate-day dosing schedule.

Hyperglycemia and glycosuria

NURSING CONSIDERATIONS
- Clients who have diabetes should have their blood glucose monitored.
- Clients might need an increase in insulin dosage.

Myopathy

As evidenced by muscle weakness

NURSING CONSIDERATIONS
- Instruct clients to report signs of muscle weakness.
- Medication dosage should be decreased.

Peptic ulcer disease

NURSING CONSIDERATIONS
- Advise clients to avoid NSAIDs.
- Advise clients to report black, tarry stools. Check stool for occult blood periodically.
- Administer with food or meals.

Infection

NURSING CONSIDERATIONS: Advise clients to notify the provider if early manifestations of infection occur (sore throat, weakness, malaise).

Disturbances of fluid and electrolytes

Fluid retention as evidenced by weight gain, and edema and hypokalemia as evidenced by muscle weakness

NURSING CONSIDERATIONS: Instruct clients to observe for manifestations and report to the provider.

CONTRAINDICATIONS/PRECAUTIONS

- Pregnancy Risk Category C **Qs**
- Contraindicated in clients who have received a live virus vaccine and those who have systemic fungal infections.
- Use cautiously in children, and in clients who have diabetes mellitus, hypertension, heart failure, peptic ulcer disease, osteoporosis, and/or kidney dysfunction.

INTERACTIONS

Prednisone

Concurrent use of potassium-depleting diuretics increases the risk of hypokalemia.
NURSING CONSIDERATIONS: Monitor potassium level and administer supplements as needed.

Concurrent use of NSAIDs increases the risk of GI ulceration.
NURSING CONSIDERATIONS: Advise clients to avoid use of NSAIDs. If GI distress occurs, instruct clients to notify the provider.

Concurrent use of glucocorticoids and hypoglycemic agents (oral and insulin) counteract the effects.
NURSING CONSIDERATIONS: Clients should notify the provider if hyperglycemia occurs. The client might need increased dosage of insulin or oral hypoglycemics.

NURSING ADMINISTRATION

- Instruct clients to use glucocorticoid inhalers on a regular, fixed schedule for long-term therapy of asthma. Glucocorticoids are not to be used to treat an acute episode.
- Administer using an MDI device, DPI, or nebulizer.
- Glucocorticoid MDIs using chlorofluorocarbons (CFCs) as a propellant are being withdrawn from the market. The new devices using hydroflouroalkane (HFA) no longer require a spacer to increase drug delivery.
- When a client is prescribed an inhaled beta$_2$-agonist and an inhaled glucocorticoid, advise the client to inhale the beta$_2$-agonist before inhaling the glucocorticoid. The beta$_2$-agonist promotes bronchodilation and enhances absorption of the glucocorticoid.
- Oral glucocorticoids are used short-term, 3 to 10 days following an acute asthma exacerbation.
- If client is on long-term oral therapy, additional dosages of oral glucocorticoids are required in times of stress (infection, trauma).
- Clients who discontinue oral glucocorticoid medications or switch from oral to inhaled agents require additional doses of oral or IV glucocorticoids during periods of stress.

NURSING EVALUATION OF MEDICATION EFFECTIVENESS

Depending on therapeutic intent, effectiveness is evidenced by the following.
- Long-term control of asthma
- Resolution of acute exacerbation as demonstrated by absence of shortness of breath, clear breath sounds, absence of wheezing, and return of respiratory rate to baseline

Leukotriene modifiers

SELECT PROTOTYPE MEDICATION: Montelukast

OTHER MEDICATIONS
- Zileuton
- Zafirlukast

PURPOSE

EXPECTED PHARMACOLOGICAL ACTION: Leukotriene modifiers suppress the effects of leukotrienes, thereby reducing inflammation, bronchoconstriction, airway edema, and mucus production.

THERAPEUTIC USES: Long-term therapy of asthma in adults and children, and to prevent exercise-induced bronchospasm
- Montelukast is used in children as young as 12 months of age.
- Zafirlukast is used in children age 5 years and up.
- Zileuton is used in adolescents and adults.

ROUTE OF ADMINISTRATION: oral

COMPLICATIONS

Depression, suicidal ideation

NURSING CONSIDERATIONS: Monitor for behavior changes and report to provider.

Liver injury with use of zileuton and zafirlukast

NURSING CONSIDERATIONS
- Obtain baseline liver function tests and monitor periodically.
- Advise clients to monitor for indications of liver damage (nausea, anorexia, abdominal pain).
- Instruct clients to notify the provider if manifestations occur.

CONTRAINDICATIONS/PRECAUTIONS

- Montelukast and zafirlukast are Pregnancy Category B. Zileuton is Pregnancy Category C. **Qs**
- Use cautiously in clients who have liver dysfunction.

INTERACTIONS

Zileuton and zafirlukast inhibit metabolism of warfarin leading to increased warfarin levels.

NURSING CONSIDERATIONS

- Advise clients to observe for indications of bleeding and to notify the provider.
- Monitor prothrombin time (PT) and INR levels.

Zileuton and zafirlukast inhibit metabolism of theophylline, leading to increased theophylline levels.

NURSING CONSIDERATIONS

- Monitor theophylline levels.
- Advise clients to observe for manifestations of theophylline toxicity (nausea, vomiting, seizures), and to notify the provider.

Montelukast used concurrently with phenytoin can inhibit effects of montelukast.

NURSING CONSIDERATIONS: Advise client to observe for therapeutic effects of montelukast.

NURSING ADMINISTRATION

- Advise clients to take zileuton as prescribed, 1 hr before or after a meal.
- Advise clients to avoid taking zafirlukast with food.
- Advise clients to take montelukast once daily at bedtime. For exercise-induced bronchospasm, take 2 hr before exercise. Instruct clients taking daily montelukast to not take an additional dose for exercise induced bronchospasm.

NURSING EVALUATION OF MEDICATION EFFECTIVENESS

Depending on therapeutic intent, effectiveness is evidenced by long-term control of asthma.

Application Exercises

1. A nurse is teaching a client who has a new prescription for beclomethasone. Which of the following instructions should the nurse include?

   A. "Rinse your mouth after each use of this medication."

   B. "Limit fluid intake while taking this medication."

   C. "Increase your intake of vitamin B$_{12}$ while taking this medication."

   D. "You can take the medication as needed."

2. A nurse is providing instructions to a client who has a new prescription for albuterol and beclomethasone inhalers for the control of asthma. Which of the following instructions should the nurse include in the teaching?

   A. Take the albuterol at the same time each day.

   B. Administer the albuterol inhaler prior to using the beclomethasone inhaler.

   C. Use beclomethasone if experiencing an acute episode.

   D. Avoid shaking the beclomethasone before use.

3. A nurse is providing instructions to the parent of an adolescent client who has a new prescription for albuterol, PO. Which of the following instructions should the nurse include?

   A. "You can take this medication to abort an acute asthma attack."

   B. "Tremors are an adverse effect of this medication."

   C. "Prolonged use of this medication can cause hyperglycemia."

   D. "This medication can slow skeletal growth rate."

4. A nurse is teaching a client who has a prescription for long-term use of oral prednisone for treatment of chronic asthma. The nurse should instruct the client to monitor for which of the following adverse effects of this medication?

   A. Weight gain

   B. Nervousness

   C. Bradycardia

   D. Constipation

PRACTICE Active Learning Scenario

A nurse is instructing a client who has a new prescription for albuterol PO. What should the nurse include in the teaching? Use the ATI Active Learning Template: Medication to complete this item.

THERAPEUTIC USES

COMPLICATIONS: List two adverse effects.

1. A. **CORRECT:** The client should rinse her mouth after each use to reduce the risk of oral fungal infections.

   B. A client who has asthma should increase fluid intake to liquefy secretions, unless contraindicated by another condition.

   C. Glucocorticoids place the client at risk for bone loss. There is no need for the client to increase her intake of vitamin B_{12}. The client should ensure an adequate intake of calcium and vitamin D.

   D. Beclomethasone is an inhaled glucocorticoid and is taken on a fixed schedule.

   Ⓝ *NCLEX® Connection: Pharmacological and Parenteral Therapies, Medication Administration*

2. A. Albuterol is a short acting inhaled $beta_2$-agonist and used for short term relief of bronchospasm.

   B. **CORRECT:** When a client is prescribed an inhaled $beta_2$-agonist (such as albuterol) and an inhaled glucocorticoid (such as beclomethasone), the client should take the $beta_2$-agonist first. The $beta_2$-agonist promotes bronchodilation and enhances absorption of the glucocorticoid.

   C. Beclomethasone is administered on a fixed schedule. It is not used to treat an acute attack.

   D. The client should shake the metered dose inhaler well before administration.

   Ⓝ *NCLEX® Connection: Pharmacological and Parenteral Therapies, Medication Administration*

3. A. Inhaled albuterol is used to abort an acute asthma episode.

   B. **CORRECT:** Tremors can occur due to excessive stimulation of $beta_2$ receptors of skeletal muscles.

   C. Prolonged use of glucocorticoids can cause hyperglycemia.

   D. Glucocorticoids slow skeletal growth rate in children and adolescents. However, height when the child reaches adulthood is not reduced.

   Ⓝ *NCLEX® Connection: Pharmacological and Parenteral Therapies, Medication Administration*

4. A. **CORRECT:** Weight gain and fluid retention are adverse effects of oral prednisone due to the effect of sodium and water retention.

   B. Nervousness and insomnia are adverse effects of beta agonists, not glucocorticoids.

   C. Tachycardia are adverse effects of prednisone and beta agonists.

   D. Diarrhea is an adverse effect of prednisone. Constipation is an adverse effect of tiotropium.

   Ⓝ *NCLEX® Connection: Pharmacological and Parenteral Therapies, Adverse Effects/Contraindications/Side Effects/Interactions*

PRACTICE Answer

Using the ATI Active Learning Template: Medication

THERAPEUTIC USES: $Beta_2$-adrenergic agonists act by selectively activating the $beta_2$-receptors in the bronchial smooth muscle, resulting in bronchodilation. They also suppress histamine release and promote ciliary motility.

COMPLICATIONS
- Oral agents can cause tachycardia and angina due to activation of $alpha_1$ receptors in the heart.
- Activation of $beta_2$ receptors in skeletal muscle causes tremors.

Ⓝ *NCLEX® Connection: Pharmacological and Parenteral Therapies, Medication Administration*

CHAPTER 18 *Upper Respiratory Disorders*

The medications in this section work on the CNS, nasal passages, or other parts of the respiratory system to treat the effects of allergic or nonallergic rhinitis or coughs from the common cold, influenza, and other disorders.

Antihistamines, often prescribed for allergic rhinitis, are also used to treat nausea, motion sickness, allergic reactions, and insomnia.

Medications in this section are frequently combined for increased effectiveness. For example, an antitussive is combined with an expectorant to reduce a cough.

Antitussives: Opioids

SELECT PROTOTYPE MEDICATION: Codeine

OTHER MEDICATION: Hydrocodone

PURPOSE

EXPECTED PHARMACOLOGICAL ACTION: Codeine suppresses cough through its action on the central nervous system to increase cough threshold.

THERAPEUTIC USES: Codeine is used for chronic nonproductive cough to decrease the frequency and intensity.

COMPLICATIONS

CNS effects

Dizziness, lightheadedness, drowsiness, respiratory depression

NURSING CONSIDERATIONS
- Obtain baseline vital signs.
- Monitor clients when ambulating.
- Advise clients to change position slowly and to lie down if feeling lightheaded.
- Observe for manifestations respiratory depression, such as respirations less than 12/min. Stimulate the client to breathe if respiratory depression occurs. It can be necessary to stop the medication and administer naloxone. Qs
- Advise clients to avoid activities that require alertness, such as driving, while taking codeine.

GI distress (nausea, vomiting, constipation)

CLIENT EDUCATION
- Instruct clients to take oral codeine with food.
- Advise clients to increase fluids and dietary fiber.

Opioid use disorder

NURSING CONSIDERATIONS
- Advise clients of the potential for abuse.
- Use for a short duration.

CONTRAINDICATIONS/PRECAUTIONS

- Codeine is Pregnancy Risk Category C. Qs
- Codeine used alone is in the Schedule II class of the Controlled Substances Act. Codeine that is mixed with other antitussives is classified as Schedule V.
- This medication is contraindicated in clients who have respiratory depression, acute asthma, head trauma, liver and renal dysfunction, and acute alcohol use disorder.
- Use cautiously in children, older adults, and clients who have a history of substance use disorder. ©

NURSING ADMINISTRATION

- Advise clients to avoid activities that require alertness, such as driving, while taking codeine.
- Advise clients to change positions slowly and to lie down if feeling dizzy.
- Advise clients to avoid alcohol and other CNS depressants while taking codeine.

Antitussives: Nonopioids

SELECT PROTOTYPE MEDICATION: Dextromethorphan (found in many different products for cough)

OTHER MEDICATIONS
- Benzonatate
- Diphenhydramine

PURPOSE

EXPECTED PHARMACOLOGICAL ACTION:
Dextromethorphan suppresses cough through its action on the CNS. Although not an opioid, it is derived from opioids.

THERAPEUTIC USES
- Cough suppression
- Can reduce pain when combined with an opioid

COMPLICATIONS

- This medication has few adverse effects.
- Some mild nausea, dizziness, and sedation can occur.
- There is some potential for abuse as the medication can instill euphoria in high doses.

CONTRAINDICATIONS/PRECAUTIONS

Pregnancy Category Risk C **Qs**

INTERACTIONS

Can cause high fever when used within 2 weeks of MAOI antidepressants.

NURSING ADMINISTRATION

- Some formulations contain alcohol and/or sucrose.
- Available forms include capsules, lozenges (for clients older than 12 years), liquids, and syrups.

NURSING EVALUATION OF MEDICATION EFFECTIVENESS

Depending on therapeutic intent, effectiveness is evidenced by absence or decreased episodes of coughing.

Expectorants

SELECT PROTOTYPE MEDICATION: Guaifenesin

PURPOSE

EXPECTED PHARMACOLOGICAL ACTION: Guaifenesin promotes increased cough production by increasing and thinning mucous secretions. These actions allow clients to decrease chest congestion by coughing out secretions.

THERAPEUTIC USES: Although guaifenesin is available as an expectorant alone, it is often combined with antitussives (either opioid or nonopioid) or a decongestant for treating manifestations of colds, allergic or nonallergic rhinitis, or for cough caused by lower respiratory disorders.

COMPLICATIONS

GI upset

CLIENT EDUCATION: Take with food if GI upset occurs.

Drowsiness, dizziness

CLIENT EDUCATION: Do not take prior to driving or activities that require alertness, if these reactions occur.

Allergic reaction (rash)

CLIENT EDUCATION: Stop taking guaifenesin and obtain medical care if rash or other manifestations of allergy occur.

CONTRAINDICATIONS/PRECAUTIONS

- Guaifenesin is Pregnancy Risk Category C. **Qs**
- Advise clients who are breastfeeding to talk to the provider before taking medications containing guaifenesin.
- Depending on the formulation and medication combinations, preparations containing guaifenesin might be contraindicated for children.

NURSING ADMINISTRATION

- Advise clients to increase fluid intake when taking guaifenesin, in order to promote liquefying secretions.
- This medication is available in tablets (which should not be crushed) and capsules, which can be opened to sprinkle on foods.
- Advise clients to read over-the-counter labels carefully to discover what medications have been combined in the preparation used. Guaifenesin is frequently combined with other medications (antitussives, decongestants) as a liquid or syrup (for example, guaifenesin is combined with the sympathomimetic decongestant, pseudoephedrine).
- Report a cough lasting longer than 1 week to the provider.

NURSING EVALUATION OF MEDICATION EFFECTIVENESS

Depending on therapeutic intent, effectiveness is evidenced by the following.
- Cough is more productive and mucous is easier to expectorate.
- Chest congestion is decreased.

Mucolytics

SELECT PROTOTYPE MEDICATION: Acetylcysteine

OTHER MEDICATION: Hypertonic saline

PURPOSE

EXPECTED PHARMACOLOGICAL ACTION: Mucolytics thin and enhance the flow of secretions in the respiratory passages.

THERAPEUTIC USES
- Mucolytics are used in clients who have acute and chronic pulmonary disorders exacerbated by large amounts of secretions.
- Mucolytics are used in clients who have cystic fibrosis.
- Acetylcysteine is the antidote for acetaminophen poisoning.

COMPLICATIONS

Aspiration and bronchospasm when administered orally

NURSING CONSIDERATIONS: Monitor clients for manifestations of aspiration and bronchospasm. Stop medication immediately and notify the provider.

Dizziness, drowsiness, hypotension, tachycardia

NURSING CONSIDERATIONS: Monitor vital signs. Advise client to change position slowly, and avoid activities that require alertness.

Hepatotoxicity

NURSING CONSIDERATIONS: Monitor liver function tests.

CONTRAINDICATIONS/PRECAUTIONS

- Acetylcysteine is Pregnancy Risk Category B. Qs
- This medication should not be used in clients who are hypersensitive to acetylcysteine.
- Use cautiously in clients who have hypothyroidism, CNS depression, renal, liver disease, and seizure disorders.
- Due to the potential for bronchospasm, acetylcysteine should be used cautiously in clients who have asthma.

NURSING ADMINISTRATION

- Advise clients that acetylcysteine has an odor that smells like rotten eggs.
- Acetylcysteine is administered by inhalation to liquefy nasal and bronchial secretions and facilitate coughing.
- The medication is administered orally or IV for acetaminophen overdose.
- Be prepared to suction clients if aspiration occurs with oral administration.
- Monitor liver function tests, PT, BUN, creatinine, glucose, electrolytes and acetaminophen levels in clients who have acetaminophen toxicity.

NURSING EVALUATION OF MEDICATION EFFECTIVENESS

Depending on therapeutic intent, effectiveness is evidenced by improvement of manifestations as demonstrated by regular respiratory rate, clear lung sounds, and increased ease of expectoration.

Decongestants

SELECT PROTOTYPE MEDICATION: Phenylephrine

OTHER MEDICATIONS
- Ephedrine
- Naphazoline
- Pseudoephedrine

PURPOSE

EXPECTED PHARMACOLOGICAL ACTION: Sympathomimetic decongestants stimulate $alpha_1$–adrenergic receptors, causing reduction in the inflammation of the nasal membranes.

THERAPEUTIC USES
- This medication can be used to treat allergic or nonallergic rhinitis by relieving nasal stuffiness.
- Acts as a decongestant for clients who have sinusitis and the common cold.

COMPLICATIONS

Rebound congestion

Secondary to prolonged use of topical agents

NURSING CONSIDERATIONS
- Advise clients to use for short-term therapy, no more than 3 to 5 days.
- Taper use and discontinue medication using one nostril at a time.

CNS stimulation

Agitation, nervousness, uneasiness

NURSING CONSIDERATIONS
- CNS stimulation is rare with the use of topical agents.
- Advise clients to observe and report manifestations of CNS stimulation.
- Stop medication.

Vasoconstriction

CLIENT EDUCATION: Advise clients who have hypertension, cerebrovascular disease, dysrhythmias, and coronary artery disease to avoid using these medications.

CONTRAINDICATIONS/PRECAUTIONS

- These medications are contraindicated in clients who have closed-angle glaucoma. Qs
- Use cautiously in clients who have coronary artery disease, hypertension, cerebrovascular disease, and dysrhythmias.

NURSING ADMINISTRATION

- When administering nasal drops, instruct clients to be in the lateral, head-low position to increase the desired effect and to prevent swallowing the medication.
- Drops are preferred for children because they can be administered precisely and toxicity can be prevented.
- When nasal spray preparations are prescribed, teach clients their proper use.
- Educate clients in the differences between topical and oral agents.
  - Topical agents are usually more effective and work faster.
  - Topical agents have a shorter duration.
  - Vasoconstriction and CNS stimulation are uncommon with topical agents, but are a concern with oral agents.
  - Oral agents do not lead to rebound congestion.
- Advise clients to use topical decongestants for no longer than 3 to 5 days to avoid rebound congestion.
- Instruct clients not to exceed recommended doses.
- Pseudoephedrine and ephedrine can produce effects similar to amphetamine and are easily converted into amphetamine. These medications are available without a prescription. However, they must be purchased with identification.

NURSING EVALUATION OF MEDICATION EFFECTIVENESS

Depending on therapeutic intent, effectiveness is evidenced by improvement of manifestations (relief of congestion, increased ease of breathing).

Antihistamines

SELECT PROTOTYPE MEDICATIONS

1st generation H₁ antagonists
- Diphenhydramine
- Promethazine
- Dimenhydrinate

2nd generation H₁ antagonists
- Loratadine
- Cetirizine
- Fexofenadine
- Desloratadine

Intranasal antihistamines
- Azelastine
- Olopatadine

PURPOSE

EXPECTED PHARMACOLOGICAL ACTION: Antihistamine action is on the H_1 receptors, which results in the blocking of histamine release in the small blood vessels, capillaries, and nerves during allergic reactions. These medications relieve itching, sneezing, and rhinorrhea, but do not relieve nasal congestion. First generation antihistamines produce cholinergic effects and drowsiness.

THERAPEUTIC USES
- Mild allergic reactions (seasonal allergic rhinitis, urticaria, mild transfusion reaction)
- Anaphylaxis (hypotension, acute laryngeal edema, bronchospasm)
- Motion sickness
- Insomnia
- Often used in combination with sympathomimetics to provide a nasal decongestant effect

COMPLICATIONS

Sedation

Common with 1st generation H_1 antagonists

NURSING CONSIDERATIONS
- Advise clients to take the medication at night to minimize daytime sedative effect.
- Avoid driving, or other activities that require alertness, consumption of alcohol, and other CNS depressant medications (barbiturates, benzodiazepines, opioids).

Anticholinergic effects

- Dry mouth, constipation
- More common with 1st generation agents

NURSING CONSIDERATIONS: Advise clients to take sips of water, suck on sugarless candies, and maintain 2 to 3 L of water each day from food and beverage sources.

Gastrointestinal discomfort

Nausea, vomiting, constipation

NURSING CONSIDERATIONS: Advise clients to take antihistamine with meals.

Acute toxicity, excitation, hallucinations, incoordination, and seizures in children

Flushed face, high fever, tachycardia, dry mouth, urinary retention, pupil dilation

NURSING CONSIDERATIONS
- Advise clients to notify the provider if effects occur.
- Administer activated charcoal and cathartic to decrease absorption of antihistamine.
- Administer acetaminophen for fever.
- Apply ice packs or sponge baths.

Respiratory depression and local tissue injury at intravenous site

Promethazine

NURSING CONSIDERATIONS:
- Monitor client for manifestations of respiratory distress, and have resuscitation equipment available.
- IM administration is the preferred route. If unavailable, administer through a large-bore IV in concentrations of 25 mg/mL or less.
- Monitor for manifestations of extravasation, and advise clients to report any pain or burning sensations.

CONTRAINDICATIONS/PRECAUTIONS

- Antihistamines are contraindicated during the third trimester of pregnancy, for mothers who are breastfeeding, and for newborns. Newborns are sensitive to the adverse effects, such as sedation, of these medications. Qs
- Promethazine is Pregnancy Category C. It is contraindicated in clients who have cardiac dysrhythmias, hepatic diseases, and those on MAOI therapy. Promethazine is also contraindicated in clients under 2 years of age.
- Use cautiously in children and older adults (impact of adverse effects, especially respiratory depression). ©
- Use cautiously in clients who have asthma, seizure disorder, cardiac disease, renal disease, urinary retention, open-angle glaucoma, hypertension, and prostate hypertrophy (impact of anticholinergic medications).

INTERACTIONS

CNS depressants/alcohol cause additive CNS depression.

NURSING CONSIDERATIONS: Advise clients to avoid alcohol and medications causing CNS depression (opioids, barbiturates, and benzodiazepines).

NURSING ADMINISTRATION

Advise clients taking 1st generation medications to be aware of sedating effects.

NURSING EVALUATION OF MEDICATION EFFECTIVENESS

Depending on therapeutic intent, effectiveness is evidenced by the following.
- Improvement of allergic reaction (absence of rhinitis, urticaria)
- Relief of motion sickness (decreased nausea and vomiting)

Nasal glucocorticoids

SELECT PROTOTYPE MEDICATION: Mometasone

OTHER MEDICATIONS
- Fluticasone
- Triamcinolone
- Budesonide

PURPOSE

EXPECTED PHARMACOLOGICAL ACTION: Nasal glucocorticoids decrease inflammation associated with allergic rhinitis. They are the first line of treatment for nasal congestion.

THERAPEUTIC USE: To reduce the effects of allergic rhinitis including sneezing, nasal itching, runny nose.

COMPLICATIONS

Sore throat, nosebleed, headache, burning in the nose

NURSING CONSIDERATIONS: Contact provider if adverse effects occur.

CONTRAINDICATIONS/PRECAUTIONS

Pregnancy Risk Category C.

NURSING CONSIDERATIONS
- Advise client that a metered-dose spray device is used to administer the medication.
- Advise client to administer dose daily, not just when manifestations occur.
- Advise clients who have seasonal allergic rhinitis it can take 7 days or more to get the maximum relief.
- Advise clients who have perennial allergic rhinitis it can take as long as 21 days to get the maximum relief.
- Advise clients to clear blocked nasal passages with a topical decongestant prior to glucocorticoid administration.

Application Exercises

1. A nurse is caring for a client who states she has been taking phenylephrine nasal drops for the past 10 days for sinusitis. The nurse should assess the client for which of the following adverse effects of this medication?

    A. Sedation

    B. Nasal congestion

    C. Productive cough

    D. Constipation

2. A nurse is teaching a client who has a new prescription for dextromethorphan to suppress a cough. The nurse should instruct the client to monitor for which of the following adverse effects of this medication?

    A. Diarrhea

    B. Anxiety

    C. Sedation

    D. Palpitations

3. A nurse is teaching the family of a child who has cystic fibrosis and a new prescription for acetylcysteine. Which of the following information should the nurse include in the instructions?

    A. "Expect this medication to suppress your cough."

    B. "Expect this medication to smell like rotten eggs."

    C. "Expect this medication to cause euphoria."

    D. "Expect this medication to turn your urine orange."

4. A nurse is teaching a client who has a new prescription for diphenhydramine for allergic rhinitis. The nurse should instruct the client to monitor for which of the following adverse reactions of this medication? (Select all that apply.)

    A. Dry mouth

    B. Nonproductive cough

    C. Skin rash

    D. Drowsiness

    E. Urinary hesitation

5. A nurse is teaching a client about the use of fluticasone to treat perennial rhinitis. Which of the following statements by the client indicates an understanding of the teaching?

    A. "I should use the spray every 4 hours while I am awake."

    B. "It can take as long as 3 weeks before the medication takes a maximum effect."

    C. "This medication can also be used to treat motion sickness."

    D. "I can use this medication when my nasal passages are blocked."

PRACTICE Active Learning Scenario

A nurse in a provider's office is providing teaching for a client who has a new prescription for guaifenesin. Use the ATI Active Learning Template: Medication to complete this item.

COMPLICATIONS: Identify two adverse effects of this medication.

EVALUATION OF MEDICATION EFFECTIVENESS: Identify two findings that indicate that the medication is effective.

Application Exercises Key

1. A. Insomnia, rather than sedation, is an adverse effect of this medication.

    B. **CORRECT:** When used for over 5 days, rebound nasal congestion can occur when taking nasal sympathomimetic medications, such as phenylephrine.

    C. Phenylephrine can cause a headache, but productive cough is not an adverse effect of this medication.

    D. Constipation is an adverse effect of first generation antihistamines, but is not caused by sympathomimetic medications such as phenylephrine.

    Ⓝ *NCLEX® Connection: Pharmacological and Parenteral Therapies, Adverse Effects/Contraindications/Side Effects/Interactions*

2. A. Dextromethorphan can cause nausea.

    B. Phenylephrine can cause anxiety and irritability.

    C. **CORRECT:** Dextromethorphan can cause sedation. Advise the client to avoid activities that require alertness.

    D. Phenylephrine can cause tachycardia and palpitations.

    Ⓝ *NCLEX® Connection: Pharmacological and Parenteral Therapies, Adverse Effects/Contraindications/Side Effects/Interactions*

3. A. Acetylcysteine can stimulate a cough. Dextromethorphan suppresses a cough.

    B. **CORRECT:** Acetylcysteine has a sulfur content that causes a rotten-egg odor.

    C. Dextromethorphan can cause euphoria at high doses. Acetylcysteine can cause drowsiness.

    D. Discoloration of urine is an adverse effect of COMT inhibitors. Acetylcysteine can cause diarrhea.

    Ⓝ *NCLEX® Connection: Pharmacological and Parenteral Therapies, Medication Administration*

4. A. **CORRECT:** Dry mouth is an anticholinergic manifestation that can occur when a client takes diphenhydramine.

    B. Cough is not an adverse reaction to this medication. Diphenhydramine is prescribed to treat nonproductive cough.

    C. Skin rash is not an adverse reaction to this medication. Diphenhydramine is sometimes prescribed for skin rash caused by allergies.

    D. **CORRECT:** Drowsiness is an adverse reaction of this medication. Diphenhydramine is administered to treat insomnia.

    E. **CORRECT:** Urinary retention is an anticholinergic manifestation that can occur when a client takes diphenhydramine.

    Ⓝ *NCLEX® Connection: Pharmacological and Parenteral Therapies, Adverse Effects/Contraindications/Side Effects/Interactions*

5. A. The client should use the medication once a day.

    B. **CORRECT:** The client can see some benefits of the medication within a few hours, but the maximum benefits can take up to 3 weeks.

    C. Diphenhydramine is used to treat motion sickness.

    D. The client should blow his nose to clear the nasal passages or use a topical decongestant, prior to use of the medication.

    Ⓝ *NCLEX® Connection: Pharmacological and Parenteral Therapies, Medication Administration*

PRACTICE Answer

Using the ATI Active Learning Template: Medication

COMPLICATIONS
- GI upset
- Dizziness
- Drowsiness
- Rash

EVALUATION OF MEDICATION EFFECTIVENESS
- Cough is more productive, mucous is easier to expectorate.
- Chest congestion is decreased.

Ⓝ *NCLEX® Connection: Pharmacological and Parenteral Therapies, Medication Administration*

When reviewing the following chapters, keep in mind the relevant topics and tasks of the NCLEX outline, in particular:

Client Needs: Pharmacological and Parenteral Therapies

ADVERSE EFFECTS/CONTRAINDICATIONS/ SIDE EFFECTS/INTERACTIONS: Notify the primary health care provider of side effects, adverse effects, and contraindications of medications and parenteral therapy.

DOSAGE CALCULATION: Use clinical decision making/ critical thinking when calculating dosages.

EXPECTED ACTIONS/OUTCOMES: Evaluate client response to medication.

MEDICATION ADMINISTRATION: Titrate dosage of medication based on assessment and ordered parameters.

UNIT 4 MEDICATIONS AFFECTING THE CARDIOVASCULAR SYSTEM

CHAPTER 19 *Medications Affecting Urinary Output*

Indications for medications that affect urinary output include management of blood pressure; excretion of edematous fluid related to heart failure and kidney and liver disease; and prevention of kidney failure.

Medications include high-ceiling loop diuretics, thiazide diuretics, potassium-sparing diuretics, and osmotic diuretics.

High-ceiling loop diuretics

SELECT PROTOTYPE MEDICATION: Furosemide

OTHER MEDICATIONS
- Ethacrynic acid
- Bumetanide
- Torsemide

PURPOSE

EXPECTED PHARMACOLOGICAL ACTION

High-ceiling loop diuretics work in the ascending limb of loop of Henle.
- Block reabsorption of sodium and chloride and prevents reabsorption of water
- Causes extensive diuresis even with severe renal impairment

THERAPEUTIC USES

High-ceiling loop diuretics are used when there is an emergent need for rapid mobilization of fluid.
- Pulmonary edema caused by heart failure
- Conditions not responsive to other diuretics, such as edema caused by liver, cardiac, or kidney disease; or hypertension

UNLABELED USE: Hypercalcemia

ROUTE OF ADMINISTRATION: Oral, IV, IM

COMPLICATIONS

Dehydration, hyponatremia, hypochloremia

NURSING CONSIDERATIONS
- Assess/monitor for manifestations of dehydration: dry mouth, increased thirst, minimal urine output, and weight loss.
- Monitor electrolytes.
- Report urine output less than 30 mL/hr. Stop medication and notify the provider.
- If headache or chest, calf, or pelvic pain occur, notify the provider. This can indicate thrombosis or embolism.
- Minimize the risk for dehydration by starting clients on low doses and monitoring daily weights.

Hypotension

NURSING CONSIDERATIONS
- Monitor blood pressure.
- Instruct clients about manifestations of postural hypotension (lightheadedness, dizziness). If these occur, advise clients to sit or lie down.
- Advise clients to avoid sudden changes of position and arise slowly from lying down or sitting.

Ototoxicity

Transient with furosemide and irreversible with ethacrynic acid

NURSING CONSIDERATIONS
- Advise clients to notify the provider of tinnitus, which can indicate ototoxicity.
- Avoid use with other ototoxic medications, such as aminoglycoside antibiotics (gentamicin).

Hypokalemia

K+ less than 3.5 mEq/L

NURSING CONSIDERATIONS
- Monitor cardiac status and potassium levels.
- Report a decrease in potassium level (K+ less than 3.5 mEq/L).
- Teach clients to consume high–potassium foods (e.g., bananas, potatoes, dried fruits, nuts, spinach, and citrus fruit).
- Teach clients manifestations of hypokalemia, such as nausea, vomiting, fatigue, leg cramps, and general weakness.

Other adverse effects

Hyperglycemia, hyperuricemia, hypocalcemia, hypomagnesemia, decrease in HDL cholesterol levels, increase in LDL cholesterol levels

NURSING CONSIDERATIONS
- Monitor blood glucose, uric acid, calcium, magnesium, and lipid levels.
- Report levels outside of the expected reference range.
- Instruct clients to observe for manifestations of low magnesium levels (e.g., weakness, muscle twitching, and tremors).

CONTRAINDICATIONS/PRECAUTIONS

- Avoid using these medications during pregnancy unless absolutely required.
- Contraindicated in clients who have anuria (no urine output).
- Use cautiously in clients who have cardiovascular disease, diabetes mellitus, dehydration, electrolyte depletion, and gout. Use cautiously in clients taking digoxin, lithium, ototoxic medications, NSAIDs, or antihypertensives.

INTERACTIONS

Digoxin toxicity (ventricular dysrhythmias) can occur in the presence of hypokalemia.
NURSING CONSIDERATIONS
- Monitor cardiac status and potassium and digoxin levels.
- Potassium-sparing diuretics often are used in conjunction with loop diuretics to reduce the risk of hypokalemia.
- Administer potassium supplements as prescribed by the provider.

Concurrent use of antihypertensives can have additive hypotensive effect.
NURSING CONSIDERATIONS: Monitor blood pressure.

Lithium carbonate serum levels can increase, which can lead to toxicity, if hyponatremia occurs due to the loop diuretic.
NURSING CONSIDERATIONS: Monitor lithium levels. Adjust dosage if needed.

NSAIDs decrease blood flow to the kidneys, which reduces the diuretic effect.
NURSING CONSIDERATIONS: Watch for a decrease in the effectiveness of the diuretic, such as a decrease in urine output.

NURSING ADMINISTRATION

- Obtain baseline data, including orthostatic blood pressure, weight, electrolytes, and location and extent of edema.
- Weigh clients at the same time each day with same amount of clothing and bed linen (if using a bed scale), usually upon awakening.
- Monitor blood pressure and I&O.
- Avoid administering the medication late in the day to prevent nocturia. Usual dosing time is 0800 and 1400.
- Administer furosemide orally, IV bolus dose, or continuous IV infusion. Infuse IV doses at 20 mg/min or slower to avoid abrupt hypotension and hypovolemia.
- If potassium level drops below 3.5 mEq/L, monitor the ECG, and notify the provider because the client might require a potassium supplement.
- If the medication is used for hypertension, teach clients to self-monitor blood pressure and weight by keeping a log.
- Advise clients to get up slowly to minimize postural hypotension and monitor blood pressure, and to assess for hypovolemia. If faintness or dizziness occurs, instruct clients to sit or lie down.

- Teach clients to report significant weight loss, lightheadedness, dizziness, GI distress, or general weakness to the provider. These can indicate hypokalemia or hypovolemia.
- Encourage clients to consume foods high in potassium.
- Instruct clients who have diabetes to monitor for elevated blood glucose levels.
- Instruct clients to observe for manifestations of low magnesium levels (e.g., weakness, muscle twitching, and tremors).
- Instruct clients to observe for manifestations of low calcium levels (muscle twitching, muscle cramps, tingling in hands and feet).
- Instruct client to report manifestations of ototoxicity, such as tinnitus or hearing loss.

NURSING EVALUATION OF MEDICATION EFFECTIVENESS

Depending on therapeutic intent, effectiveness is evidenced by the following.
- Decrease in pulmonary or peripheral edema
- Weight loss
- Decrease in blood pressure
- Increase in urine output
- Decrease in calcium level

Thiazide diuretics

SELECT PROTOTYPE MEDICATION: Hydrochlorothiazide

OTHER MEDICATIONS
- Chlorothiazide
- Methyclothiazide
- Thiazide-type diuretics
  - Indapamide
  - Chlorthalidone
  - Metolazone

PURPOSE

EXPECTED PHARMACOLOGICAL ACTION

- Thiazide diuretics work in the early distal convoluted tubule.
- Blocks the reabsorption of sodium and chloride, and prevents the reabsorption of water at this site
- Promotes diuresis when renal function is not impaired

THERAPEUTIC USES

- Thiazide diuretics are often the medication of first choice for essential hypertension.
- These medications are used for edema of mild to moderate heart failure and liver and kidney disease.
- Thiazide diuretics often are used in combination with antihypertensive agents for blood pressure control.
- These medications are used to reduce urine production in clients who have diabetes insipidus.
- These medications promote reabsorption of calcium and can reduce the risk for postmenopausal osteoporosis.

COMPLICATIONS

Dehydration and hyponatremia

NURSING CONSIDERATIONS
- Assess/monitor clients for manifestations of dehydration (dry mouth, increased thirst, minimal urine output, weight loss).
- Monitor electrolytes and weight.
- Report urine output less than 30 mL/hr. Stop medication and notify the provider.

Hypokalemia and hypochloremia

NURSING CONSIDERATIONS
- Monitor cardiac status and K+ levels, especially if taking digoxin.
- Report a decrease in K+ level (less than 3.5 mEq/L).
- Teach clients to consume foods high in potassium.
- Teach clients to recognize manifestations of hypokalemia (nausea/vomiting, general weakness, fatigue, leg cramps).

Hyperglycemia

NURSING CONSIDERATIONS: Monitor for an increase in blood glucose levels.

Hyperuricemia, hypomagnesemia, increased LDL cholesterol

NURSING CONSIDERATIONS
- Monitor uric acid, magnesium, LDL cholesterol, and HDL cholesterol levels.
- Instruct clients to observe for manifestations of low magnesium levels (e.g., weakness, muscle twitching, and tremors).

CONTRAINDICATIONS/PRECAUTIONS

- Avoid administering thiazide diuretics during pregnancy because the medication decreases maternal blood volume and decreases placental perfusion, causing a compromise in the nutrients supplied to the fetus.
- If a thiazide diuretic is indicated during lactation, advise clients not to breastfeed because the diuretic enters the milk and is harmful to the infant.
- Contraindicated in clients who have renal impairment.
- Use cautiously in clients who have cardiovascular disease, diabetes mellitus, hypokalemia, hyperlipidemia, hypomagnesemia, and gout. Use cautiously in clients taking digoxin, lithium, or antihypertensives.

INTERACTIONS

- Medication and food interactions are the same as for loop diuretic medication.
- Thiazide diuretics cause no risk of hearing loss and can be combined with ototoxic medications.

NURSING ADMINISTRATIONS

- Chlorothiazide is administered orally and IV; all others can are given orally.
- Obtain baseline data, including orthostatic blood pressure, weight, electrolytes, and location and extent of edema.
- Monitor potassium levels.
- Instruct clients to take the medication first thing in the morning; if twice-a-day dosing is prescribed, be sure the second dose is taken by 1400 to prevent nocturia.
- Encourage clients to consume foods high in potassium and maintain adequate fluid intake (1,500 mL/day, unless contraindicated).
- If GI upset occurs, clients should take the medication with or after meals.
- Alternate-day dosing can decrease electrolyte imbalances.
- Weigh clients at the same time each day with same amount of clothing and bed linen (if using a bed scale), usually upon awakening.
- Monitor blood pressure and I&O.
- If potassium level drops below 3.5 mEq/L, monitor the ECG, and notify the provider because the client might require a potassium supplement.
- If the medication is used for hypertension, teach clients to self-monitor blood pressure and weight by keeping a log.
- Advise clients to get up slowly to minimize postural hypotension, monitor blood pressure, and assess for hypovolemia. If faintness or dizziness occurs, instruct clients to sit or lie down.
- Teach clients to report significant weight loss, lightheadedness, dizziness, GI distress, or general weakness to the provider. These can indicate hypokalemia or hypovolemia.
- Instruct clients who have diabetes to monitor for elevated blood glucose levels.
- Instruct clients to observe for manifestations of low magnesium levels (e.g., weakness, muscle twitching, and tremors).

NURSING EVALUATION OF MEDICATION EFFECTIVENESS

Depending on therapeutic intent, effectiveness is evidenced by the following.
- Decrease in blood pressure
- Decrease in edema
- Increase in urine output
- Reduced urine output in diabetes insipidus
- Preserved bone integrity in postmenopausal women.

Potassium-sparing diuretics

SELECT PROTOTYPE MEDICATION: Spironolactone

OTHER MEDICATIONS
- Triamterene
- Amiloride

PURPOSE

EXPECTED PHARMACOLOGICAL ACTION

Potassium-sparing diuretics block the action of aldosterone (sodium and water retention), which results in potassium retention and the excretion of sodium and water.

THERAPEUTIC USES

- Potassium-sparing diuretics are combined with other diuretics (loop and thiazide diuretics) for potassium-sparing effects to treat hypertension and edema.
- Administered for heart failure.
- Potassium-sparing diuretics block actions of aldosterone in primary hyperaldosteronism by retaining potassium and increasing sodium excretion, causing an opposite effect of the action of aldosterone in the distal nephrons.
- Therapeutic effects can take 12 to 48 hr.

ROUTE OF ADMINISTRATION: Oral

COMPLICATIONS

Hyperkalemia

NURSING CONSIDERATIONS
- Monitor potassium level. Initiate cardiac monitoring for serum potassium greater than 5 mEq/L.
- Monitor electrolytes and for manifestations of hyperkalemia, such as weakness, fatigue, dyspnea, and dysrhythmias.
- Treat hyperkalemia by discontinuing medication, restricting potassium in the diet. If needed,, administer a potassium-excreting diuretic, or administer glucose and insulin IV to drive potassium back into the cell.
- Do not administer potassium supplements or other potassium-sparing diuretics in conjunction with spironolactone.
- Caution is recommended when administered with angiotensin-converting enzyme (ACE) inhibitors, angiotensin receptor blockers, and direct renin inhibitors because these can cause elevated potassium levels.

Endocrine effects

Male clients: Deepened voice, impotence

Female clients: Irregularities of menstrual cycle

NURSING CONSIDERATIONS
- Advise clients to observe for adverse effects.
- Clients should notify the provider if these responses occur.

Drowsiness, metabolic acidosis

NURSING CONSIDERATIONS
- Instruct client to avoid activities that require alertness until effects of medication are known.
- Monitor for metabolic acidosis, such as drowsiness, and restlessness.

CONTRAINDICATIONS/PRECAUTIONS

- Do not administer to clients who have hyperkalemia, are taking potassium supplements, or another potassium sparing diuretic.
- Do not administer to clients who have severe kidney failure and anuria.
- Use with caution in clients who have kidney or liver disease, electrolyte imbalances, or metabolic acidosis.

INTERACTIONS

Concurrent use of ACE inhibitors, angiotensin receptor blockers, and direct renin inhibitors increases the risk of hyperkalemia.
NURSING CONSIDERATIONS: Monitor the client's K+ levels. Notify the provider if K+ is greater than 5.0 mEq/L. Avoid concurrent use.

Concurrent use of potassium supplements, salt substitutes, and another potassium sparing diuretic increases the risk of hyperkalemia.
NURSING CONSIDERATIONS: Avoid concurrent use.

NURSING ADMINISTRATION

- Obtain baseline data.
- Weigh clients at the same time each day with same amount of clothing and bed linen (if using a bed scale), usually upon awakening.
- Monitor blood pressure and I&O.
- Monitor ECG periodically.
- Monitor potassium levels.
- Teach clients to avoid salt substitutes that contain potassium and reduce intake of potassium-rich foods, such as oranges, bananas, and dates.
- Teach clients to self-monitor blood pressure.
- Instruct clients to keep a log of blood pressure and weight.
- Warn clients that triamterene can turn urine a bluish color.
- Instruct client to report cramps, diarrhea, thirst, altered menstruation, or deepened voice.
- Instruct client to avoid activities that require alertness until effects of medication are known.

NURSING EVALUATION OF MEDICATION EFFECTIVENESS

Depending on therapeutic intent, effectiveness is evidenced by the following.
- Maintenance of normal potassium levels: 3.5 to 5.0 mEq/L
- Weight loss
- Decrease in blood pressure and edema

Osmotic diuretics

SELECT PROTOTYPE MEDICATION: Mannitol

PURPOSE

EXPECTED PHARMACOLOGICAL ACTION

Osmotic diuretics reduce intracranial pressure and intraocular pressure by raising serum osmolality and drawing fluid back into the vascular and extravascular space.

THERAPEUTIC USES

- Prevents kidney failure in specific situations, such as hypovolemic shock and severe hypotension, because mannitol is not reabsorbed and remains in the nephron, drawing off water, thus preserving urine flow and preventing kidney failure.
- Decreases intracranial pressure (ICP) caused by cerebral edema by drawing off fluid from the brain into the bloodstream.
- Decreases intraocular pressure by drawing ocular fluid into the bloodstream.
- Promotes sodium retention and water excretion in clients who have hyponatremia and fluid volume excess.
- Administered for the oliguria phase of acute kidney injury.

COMPLICATIONS

Heart failure, pulmonary edema
NURSING CONSIDERATIONS: If manifestations of heart failure develop (dyspnea, weakness, fatigue, distended neck veins, and/or weight gain), stop the medication immediately, and notify the provider.

Rebound increased intracranial pressure
NURSING CONSIDERATIONS: Monitor for increased ICP, such as change in level of consciousness, change in pupils, headache, nausea, and vomiting.

Fluid and electrolyte imbalances, metabolic acidosis
NURSING CONSIDERATIONS: Monitor laboratory values. Monitor for manifestations of metabolic acidosis, such as drowsiness and restlessness.

CONTRAINDICATIONS/PRECAUTIONS

This medication is contraindicated in clients who have active intracranial bleed, anuria, severe pulmonary edema, severe dehydration, and renal failure. Use extreme caution in clients who have heart failure, are pregnant or breast feeding, renal insufficiency, and electrolyte imbalances.

INTERACTIONS

Lithium excretion through the kidneys is increased.
NURSING CONSIDERATIONS: Monitor lithium levels.

Increase risk for hypokalemia with cardiac glycosides.
NURSING CONSIDERATIONS: Monitor potassium and ECG.

NURSING ADMINISTRATION

- Administer mannitol by continuous IV infusion.
- To prevent administering microscopic crystals, use a filter needle when drawing from the vial and a filter in the IV tubing.
- Monitor daily weight, I&O, and serum electrolytes.
- Monitor for manifestations of dehydration, and increased edema.
- Obtain baseline data, including orthostatic blood pressure, weight, electrolytes, and location and extent of edema.
- Weigh clients at the same time each day with same amount of clothing and bed linen (if using a bed scale), usually upon awakening.
- Monitor blood pressure
- If potassium level drops below 3.5 mEq/L, monitor the ECG, and notify the provider because the client might require a potassium supplement.
- Advise clients to get up slowly to minimize postural hypotension, monitor blood pressure, and assess for hypovolemia. If faintness or dizziness occurs, instruct clients to sit or lie down.
- Teach clients to report significant weight loss, lightheadedness, dizziness, GI distress, or general weakness to the provider. These can indicate hypokalemia or hypovolemia.
- Monitor for increased ICP, such as change in level of consciousness, change in pupils, headache, nausea, and vomiting.
- Monitor for metabolic acidosis, such as drowsiness and restlessness.

NURSING EVALUATION OF MEDICATION EFFECTIVENESS

Depending on therapeutic intent, effectiveness is evidenced by the following.
- Normal kidney function as demonstrated by
  - Urine output of at least 30 mL/hr
  - Serum creatinine 0.6 to 1.3 mg/dL for men and 0.5 to 1.1 mg/dL for women
  - BUN levels 10 to 20 mg/dL
- Decrease in intracranial pressure
- Decrease in intraocular pressure

Application Exercises

1. A nursing is planning care for a client who is receiving furosemide IV for peripheral edema. Which of the following interventions should the nurse include in the plan of care? (Select all that apply.)

   A. Assess for tinnitus.

   B. Report urine output 50 mL/hr.

   C. Monitor serum potassium levels.

   D. Elevate the head of bed slowly before ambulation.

   E. Recommend eating a banana daily.

2. A nurse is providing information to a client who has a new prescription for hydrochlorothiazide. Which of the following information should the nurse include?

   A. Take the medication with food.

   B. Plan to take the medication at bedtime.

   C. Expect increased swelling of the ankles.

   D. Fluid intake should be limited in the morning.

3. A nurse is monitoring a client who is receiving spironolactone. Which of the following findings should the nurse report to the provider?

   A. Serum sodium 144 mEq/L

   B. Urine output 120 mL in 4 hr

   C. Serum potassium 5.2 mEq/L

   D. Blood pressure 140/90 mm Hg

4. A nurse is caring for a client who has increased intracranial pressure and is receiving mannitol. Which of the following findings should the nurse report to the provider?

   A. Blood glucose 150 mg/dL

   B. Urine output 40 mL/hr

   C. Dyspnea

   D. Bilateral equal pupil size

5. A nurse is planning caring for a client who is has a new prescription for torsemide. The nurse should plan to monitor for which of the following adverse reactions of this medications? (Select all that apply.)

   A. Respiratory acidosis

   B. Hypokalemia

   C. Hypotension

   D. Ototoxicity

   E. Ventricular dysrhythmias

PRACTICE Active Learning Scenario

A charge nurse is reviewing the use of loop diuretics with a group of nurses. Use the ATI Active Learning Template: Medication to complete this item.

THERAPEUTIC USES: Identify two.

COMPLICATIONS: Describe three adverse effects.

NURSING INTERVENTIONS: Describe two interventions for each of the three adverse effects.

Application Exercises Key

1. A. **CORRECT:** An adverse effect of furosemide is ototoxicity. Manifestations of tinnitus should be reported to the provider.

   B. A urine output of 50 mL/hr is within the expected reference range. A urine output less than 30 mL/hr is a manifestation of dehydration and the nurse should notify the provider.

   C. **CORRECT:** A decrease in serum potassium levels is an adverse effect of furosemide, and the nurse should notify the provider.

   D. **CORRECT:** Slowly elevating the head of the bed will prevent the client from developing orthostatic hypotension, which is a manifestation of hypovolemia.

   E. **CORRECT:** A banana is high in potassium. The nurse should encourage the client to eat foods high in potassium to prevent hypokalemia.

   Ⓝ *NCLEX® Connection: Pharmacological and Parenteral Therapies, Parenteral/Intravenous Therapies*

2. A. **CORRECT:** The client should take hydrochlorothiazide with or after meals to prevent gastrointestinal upset.

   B. The client should take hydrochlorothiazide in the morning or no later than 1400, and not at bedtime, to prevent nocturia.

   C. The client should expect decreased swelling of the ankles.

   D. The client should maintain an adequate fluid intake (1,500 mL) throughout the day unless contraindicated.

   Ⓝ *NCLEX® Connection: Pharmacological and Parenteral Therapies, Medication Administration*

3. A. Serum sodium of 144 mEq/L is within the expected reference range.

   B. Urine output of 30 mL/hr or 120 mL in 4 hr is within the expected reference range.

   C. **CORRECT:** Serum potassium of 5.2 mEq/L indicates hyperkalemia. Because spironolactone causes potassium retention, the nurse should withhold the medication and notify the provider.

   D. A blood pressure of 140/90 mm Hg is within the expected reference range.

   Ⓝ *NCLEX® Connection: Pharmacological and Parenteral Therapies, Adverse Effects/Contraindications/Side Effects/Interactions*

4. A. This blood glucose is within the expected reference range.

   B. Urine output of 40 mL/hr is within the expected reference range.

   C. **CORRECT:** Dyspnea is a manifestation of heart failure, an adverse effect of mannitol. The nurse should stop the medication and notify the provider.

   D. Bilateral equal pupil size is an expected finding and can indicate reduction in intracranial pressure.

   Ⓝ *NCLEX® Connection: Pharmacological and Parenteral Therapies, Adverse Effects/Contraindications/Side Effects/Interactions*

5. A. The nurse should plan to monitor for metabolic alkalosis.

   B. **CORRECT:** The nurse should plan to monitor for hypokalemia, which is an adverse effect of a loop diuretic.

   C. **CORRECT:** The nurse should plan to monitor for hypotension.

   D. **CORRECT:** The nurse should plan to monitor the client for ototoxicity.

   E. **CORRECT:** The nurse should plan to monitor for ventricular dysrhythmias, which is a manifestation of hypokalemia, an adverse effect of torsemide.

   Ⓝ *NCLEX® Connection: Pharmacological and Parenteral Therapies, Adverse Effects/Contraindications/Side Effects/Interactions*

PRACTICE Answer

Using the ATI Active Learning Template: Medication

THERAPEUTIC USES
- Used when there is an emergent need for rapid mobilization of fluid
- Pulmonary edema caused by heart failure
- Liver, cardiac, or kidney disease
- Hypertension
- Unlabeled use: Hypercalcemia

COMPLICATIONS
- Dehydration
- Hypotension
- Ototoxicity
- Hypokalemia

NURSING INTERVENTIONS
- Dehydration: Assess for dry mouth, increased thirst, low urine output, weight loss.
- Hypotension: Monitor orthostatic blood pressure and pulse; monitor for manifestations of postural hypotension.
- Ototoxicity: Assess for tinnitus; avoid administering ototoxic medications.
- Hypokalemia: Monitor laboratory values; offer potassium-rich foods; assess for general weakness, nausea, and vomiting.

Ⓝ *NCLEX® Connection: Pharmacological and Parenteral Therapies, Medication Administration*

CHAPTER 20

CHAPTER 20 *Medications Affecting Blood Pressure*

Blood pressure is controlled in a variety of ways with many medications that are used alone or in combination. Guidelines for pharmacological management of hypertension are found in The Eighth Report of the Joint National Committee on Prevention, Detection, Evaluation, and Treatment of High Blood Pressure released in 2013 by the U.S. Department of Health and Human Services.

Angiotensin-converting enzyme inhibitors

SELECT PROTOTYPE MEDICATION: Captopril

OTHER MEDICATIONS
- Enalapril
- Enalaprilat
- Fosinopril
- Lisinopril
- Ramipril
- Moexipril
- Benazepril

PURPOSE

EXPECTED PHARMACOLOGICAL ACTION: Angiotensin-converting enzyme (ACE) inhibitors reduce production of angiotensin II by blocking the conversion of angiotensin I to angiotensin II and increasing levels of bradykinin, leading to the following.
- Vasodilation (mostly arteriole)
- Excretion of sodium and water, and retention of potassium by actions in the kidneys
- Reduction in pathological changes in the blood vessels and heart that result from the presence of angiotensin II and aldosterone

THERAPEUTIC USES
- Hypertension
- Heart failure
- Myocardial infarction (to decrease mortality and to decrease risk of heart failure and left ventricular dysfunction)
- Diabetic and nondiabetic nephropathy
- For clients at high risk for a cardiovascular event, ramipril is used to prevent MI, stroke, or death.

COMPLICATIONS

First-dose orthostatic hypotension

NURSING CONSIDERATIONS
- If the client is already taking a diuretic, stop the medication temporarily for 2 to 3 days prior to the start of an ACE inhibitor.
- Taking another type of antihypertensive medication increases the hypotensive effects of an ACE inhibitor.
- Start treatment with a low dosage of the medication.
- Monitor blood pressure for 2 hr after initiation of treatment. Qs
- Instruct clients to change positions slowly and to lie down if feeling dizzy, lightheaded, or faint.

Cough

Related to inhibition of kinase II (alternative name for ACE), which results in increase in bradykinin

CLIENT EDUCATION: Inform clients of the possibility of experiencing a dry cough and to notify the provider. Discontinue the medication.

Hyperkalemia

NURSING CONSIDERATIONS
- Monitor potassium levels to maintain a level within the expected reference range of 3.5 to 5 mEq/L.
- Advise clients to avoid the use of salt substitutes containing potassium.
- Monitor for manifestations of hyperkalemia, such as numbness and tingling and paresthesia in hands and feet.

Rash and dysgeusia (altered taste)

Primarily with captopril

NURSING CONSIDERATIONS
- Clients should inform the provider if these effects occur.
- Adverse effects will stop with discontinuation of the medication.

Angioedema

Swelling of the tongue and oral pharynx

NURSING CONSIDERATIONS
- Treat severe effects with subcutaneous injection of epinephrine.
- Discontinue medication.

Neutropenia

Rare but serious complication of captopril

NURSING CONSIDERATIONS
- Monitor WBC counts every 2 weeks for 3 months, then periodically.
- This condition is reversible when detected early.
- Inform clients to notify the provider at the first indications of infection (fever, sore throat). Discontinue medication.

CONTRAINDICATIONS/PRECAUTIONS

- Pregnancy Risk Category D during the second and third trimester, related to fetal injury. Qs
- Contraindicated in clients who have history of allergy/angioedema to ACE inhibitors, in bilateral renal artery stenosis, or in clients who have a single kidney.
- Use cautiously in clients who have kidney impairment and collagen vascular disease because they are at greater risk for developing neutropenia. Closely monitor these clients for manifestations of infection.

INTERACTIONS

Diuretics can contribute to first-dose hypotension.
NURSING CONSIDERATIONS: Advise clients to temporarily stop taking diuretics 2 to 3 days before the start of therapy with an ACE inhibitor.

Antihypertensive medications can have an additive hypotensive effect.
NURSING CONSIDERATIONS: Advise clients that dosage of medication might need to be adjusted if ACE inhibitors are added to the treatment regimen.

Potassium supplements and potassium-sparing diuretics increase the risk of hyperkalemia.
NURSING CONSIDERATIONS: Clients should only take potassium supplements if prescribed. Clients should avoid salt substitutes that contain potassium.

ACE inhibitors can increase levels of lithium.
NURSING CONSIDERATIONS: Monitor lithium levels to avoid toxicity.

Use of NSAIDs can decrease the antihypertensive effect of ACE inhibitors.
NURSING CONSIDERATIONS: Avoid concurrent use.

NURSING ADMINISTRATION

- Administer ACE inhibitors orally except enalaprilat, which is the only ACE inhibitor for IV use. QEBP
- Advise clients that the medication is prescribed as a single formulation or in combination with hydrochlorothiazide (a thiazide diuretic).
- Advise clients that blood pressure is monitored after the first dose for at least 2 hr to detect hypotension.
- Instruct clients to take captopril and moexipril at least 1 hr before meals. Other ACE inhibitors are taken with or without food.
- Advise clients to notify the provider if cough, rash, dysgeusia (altered taste), or indications of infection occur.
- Advise client to rise slowly from sitting.
- Advise client to avoid activities that require alertness until effects are known.
- Advise clients to report if pregnancy is suspected.

Angiotensin II receptor blockers

SELECT PROTOTYPE MEDICATION: Losartan

OTHER MEDICATIONS
- Valsartan
- Irbesartan
- Candesartan
- Olmesartan
- Telmisartan

PURPOSE

EXPECTED PHARMACOLOGICAL ACTION: These medications block the action of angiotensin II in the body. This results in the following.
- Vasodilation (arterioles and veins)
- Excretion of sodium and water (by decreasing release of aldosterone)

THERAPEUTIC USES
- Hypertension
- Heart failure (valsartan and candesartan)
- Stroke prevention (losartan)
- Delay progression of diabetic nephropathy (irbesartan and losartan)
- Protect against MI, stroke, and death from cardiac causes in individuals unable to tolerate ACE inhibitors (telmisartan)
- Reduce mortality following an acute myocardial infarction (valsartan)
- Slow the development of diabetic retinopathy (losartan)

COMPLICATIONS

The major difference between angiotensin II receptor blockers (ARBs) and ACE inhibitors is that ARBs block the actions of angiotensin II and ACE inhibitors block the formation of angiotensin II.

Angioedema

NURSING CONSIDERATIONS
- Advise clients to observe for manifestations (skin wheals, swelling of tongue and pharynx) and to notify provider immediately.
- Treat severe effects with subcutaneous injection of epinephrine.
- Discontinue medication.

Fetal injury

CLIENT EDUCATION
- Advise women of risk during the second and third trimester of pregnancy.
- Advise women of childbearing age to use contraception while on this medication.

Hypotension

NURSING CONSIDERATIONS: Monitor blood pressure. Advise clients to rise slowly from a sitting position.

Dizziness, lightheadedness

CLIENT EDUCATION: Instruct clients to avoid activities that require alertness until effects are known.

CONTRAINDICATIONS/PRECAUTIONS

- Pregnancy Risk Category D. ARBs cause fetal damage in the second and third trimesters. Discontinue as early in pregnancy as possible. Qs
- These medications are contraindicated in clients who have renal stenosis when present bilaterally or in a single remaining kidney because of the risk for kidney injury.
- Use cautiously in clients who experienced angioedema with ACE inhibitor.

INTERACTIONS

Antihypertensive medications can have an additive effect when used with ARBs.
NURSING CONSIDERATIONS: Adjust dosage of medication if ACE inhibitors are added to the treatment regimen.

Increased risk for lithium toxicity
NURSING CONSIDERATIONS: Monitor lithium levels and adjust dosage.

NURSING ADMINISTRATION

- Administer medications by oral route. QEBP
- Advise clients that medication is prescribed as a single formulation or in combination with hydrochlorothiazide.
- Take ARBs with or without food.
- Advise clients who have heart failure to monitor weight and edema.

Aldosterone antagonists

SELECT PROTOTYPE MEDICATION: Eplerenone

OTHER MEDICATION: Spironolactone

PURPOSE

EXPECTED PHARMACOLOGICAL ACTION: Aldosterone antagonists reduce blood volume by blocking aldosterone receptors in the kidney, thus promoting excretion of sodium and water and retention of potassium.

THERAPEUTIC USES
- Hypertension
- Heart failure

COMPLICATIONS

Hyperkalemia, hyponatremia

NURSING CONSIDERATIONS
- Monitor serum potassium and sodium levels periodically.
- Advise client not to use potassium supplements or salt substitutes containing potassium.
- Advise client to monitor and report manifestations of hyperkalemia, such as paresthesia and tingling of hands and feet.

Flu-like manifestations

Fatigue, headache, diarrhea, abdominal pain, cough

CLIENT EDUCATION: Advise client to report severe manifestations to provider.

Gynecomastia

Enlargement and tenderness of male breast tissue

CLIENT EDUCATION: Advise the client to report severe manifestations to the provider.

Dizziness, fatigue

CLIENT EDUCATION: Avoid activities that require alertness until reaction is known.

CONTRAINDICATIONS/PRECAUTIONS

- Contraindicated in clients who have high potassium levels, kidney impairment, hepatic disease, and type 2 diabetes mellitus with microalbuminuria. Qs
- Use cautiously in clients who have liver impairment.

INTERACTIONS

Verapamil, ACE inhibitors, ARBs, erythromycin, potassium-sparing diuretics, NSAIDs, and ketoconazole can increase risk of hyperkalemia.
NURSING CONSIDERATIONS
- Monitor serum potassium more frequently if client must take these medication concurrently.
- Teach client the manifestations of hyperkalemia.

Lithium toxicity can occur if it is taken concurrently.
NURSING CONSIDERATIONS: Monitor clients on lithium more frequently for lithium toxicity.

Grapefruit and grapefruit juice inhibit metabolism of eplerenone.
NURSING CONSIDERATIONS: Advise client to avoid grapefruit.

Concurrent use with diuretics increase risk for orthostatic hypotension.
NURSING CONSIDERATIONS
- Advise clients to rise slowly from sitting.
- Monitor blood pressure.

NURSING ADMINISTRATION

- Administer orally with or without food. QEBP
- Do not administer with potassium supplements.

Direct renin inhibitors

SELECT PROTOTYPE MEDICATION: Aliskiren

PURPOSE

EXPECTED PHARMACOLOGICAL ACTION: Binds with renin to inhibit production of angiotensin I, thus decreasing production of both angiotensin II and aldosterone.

THERAPEUTIC USE: Relieves hypertension when used alone or with another antihypertensive medication.

COMPLICATIONS

Angioedema, rash, and cough

Angioedema is swelling of the pharynx, tongue, glottis

CLIENT EDUCATION: Teach client to monitor for rash and angioedema. Stop medication and notify provider, or call 911 for severe manifestations.

Hyperkalemia

NURSING CONSIDERATIONS
- Monitor serum potassium periodically during treatment.
- Advise client not to use potassium supplements or salt substitutes containing potassium.
- Advise client to monitor and report manifestations of hyperkalemia, such as paresthesia and tingling of hands and feet.

Diarrhea

- Dose-related
- Seen most often in females and older adult clients

NURSING CONSIDERATIONS
- Teach client to notify provider for severe diarrhea.
- Monitor for dehydration, especially in older adults. ©

Hypotension

NURSING CONSIDERATIONS
- Monitor blood pressure. Advise clients to rise slowly from sitting.
- Advise clients to avoid activities that require alertness until effects are known.

CONTRAINDICATIONS/PRECAUTIONS

- Pregnancy Risk Category D. Qs
- Advise women of childbearing age to use contraception and discontinue medication if pregnancy occurs.
- Contraindicated in clients who have hyperkalemia
- Use cautiously in older adults and clients who have asthma, other respiratory disorders, history of angioedema, diabetes mellitus, renal stenosis, hypotension, or kidney or hepatic disease.

INTERACTIONS

Decreases serum levels of furosemide.
NURSING CONSIDERATIONS: Possible need to increase furosemide dosage.

Increases effect of other antihypertensive medications.
NURSING CONSIDERATIONS: Monitor blood pressure for hypotension when combinations are used.

Atorvastatin and ketoconazole increase levels of aliskiren.
NURSING CONSIDERATIONS: Monitor for hypotension if used concurrently.

High-fat foods reduce absorption.
NURSING CONSIDERATIONS: Advise client to not take medication with foods high in fat.

Increased hyperkalemia with ACE inhibitors, potassium supplements, and potassium-sparing diuretics.
NURSING CONSIDERATIONS: Monitor potassium levels and for manifestations of hyperkalemia. Avoid concurrent use.

NURSING ADMINISTRATION

- High-fat meals interfere with absorption. Instruct clients to take at the same time daily away from foods high in fat. QEBP
- Available alone or in combination tablets with a variety of other antihypertensives (e.g., hydrochlorothiazide, a diuretic; valsartan, an ARB).

Calcium channel blockers

SELECT PROTOTYPE MEDICATIONS
- Nifedipine
- Verapamil
- Diltiazem

OTHER MEDICATIONS
- Amlodipine
- Felodipine
- Nicardipine

PURPOSE

EXPECTED PHARMACOLOGICAL ACTION

Nifedipine

- Blocking of calcium channels in blood vessels leads to vasodilation of vascular smooth muscle (peripheral arterioles) and arteries/arterioles of the heart.
- Nifedipine acts primarily on arterioles. Veins are not significantly affected.

Verapamil, diltiazem

- Blocking of calcium channels in blood vessels leads to vasodilation of peripheral arterioles and arteries/arterioles of the heart.
- Blocking of calcium channels in the myocardium, SA node, and AV node leads to a decreased force of contraction, decreased heart rate, and slowing of the rate of conduction through the AV node.
- These medications act on arterioles and the heart at therapeutic doses.
- Veins are not significantly affected.

THERAPEUTIC USES

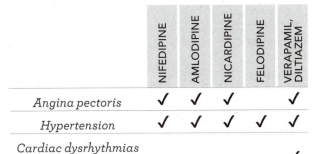

	NIFEDIPINE	AMLODIPINE	NICARDIPINE	FELODIPINE	VERAPAMIL, DILTIAZEM
Angina pectoris	✓	✓	✓		✓
Hypertension	✓	✓	✓	✓	✓
Cardiac dysrhythmias (atrial fibrillation, atrial flutter, SVT)					✓

COMPLICATIONS

NIFEDIPINE

Reflex tachycardia

NURSING CONSIDERATIONS
- Monitor clients for an increased heart rate.
- Administer a beta-blocker (metoprolol) to counteract tachycardia.

Acute toxicity

NURSING CONSIDERATIONS
- With excessive doses, the heart, in addition to blood vessels, is affected.
- Monitor vital signs and ECG. Provide gastric lavage and cathartic if indicated.
- Administer medications (norepinephrine, calcium, isoproterenol, lidocaine, and IV fluids).
- Have equipment for cardioversion and cardiac pacer available.

Orthostatic hypotension and peripheral edema

NURSING CONSIDERATIONS
- Monitor blood pressure, edema, and daily weight.
- Instruct clients to observe for swelling in the lower extremities, and notify the provider if it occurs.
- A diuretic can be prescribed to control edema.
- Instruct clients about the manifestations of postural hypotension (lightheadedness, dizziness). If these occur, advise clients to sit or lie down. Can be minimized by getting up slowly.

VERAPAMIL, DILTIAZEM

Orthostatic hypotension and peripheral edema

NURSING CONSIDERATIONS
- Monitor blood pressure, edema, and daily weight.
- Instruct clients to observe for swelling in the lower extremities, and notify the provider if it occurs.
- A diuretic can be prescribed to control edema.
- Instruct clients about the manifestations of postural hypotension (lightheadedness, dizziness). If these occur, advise clients to sit or lie down. Can be minimized by getting up slowly.

Constipation (primarily verapamil)

CLIENT EDUCATION: Advise clients to increase intake of high fiber food and oral fluids, if not restricted.

Suppression of cardiac function

Bradycardia, heart failure

NURSING CONSIDERATIONS
- Monitor ECG, pulse rate, and rhythm.
- Advise clients to observe for suppression of cardiac function (slow pulse, activity intolerance), and to notify provider if these occur. Discontinue medication if needed.

Dysrhythmias

QRS complex is widened and QT interval is prolonged.

NURSING CONSIDERATIONS: Monitor vital signs and ECG.

Acute toxicity

Resulting in hypotension, bradycardia, AV block, and ventricular tachydysrhythmias

NURSING CONSIDERATIONS
- Monitor vital signs and ECG. Gastric lavage and cathartic can be indicated.
- Administer medications (norepinephrine, calcium, isoproterenol, lidocaine, and IV fluids).
- Have equipment for cardioversion and cardiac pacer available.

CONTRAINDICATIONS/PRECAUTIONS

- Pregnancy Risk Category C. **Qs**
- Nifedipine is contraindicated in clients who are in cardiogenic shock.
- Use nifedipine with caution in clients who have acute MI, unstable angina, aortic stenosis, hypotension, sick sinus syndrome, and second- or third-degree AV block.
- Verapamil is contraindicated in clients who have hypotension, heart block, digoxin toxicity, severe heart failure, and during lactation.
- Use cautiously in older adults and clients who have kidney or liver disorders, mild to moderate heart failure, or GERD. **G**

INTERACTIONS

NIFEDIPINE

Beta-blockers, such as metoprolol, are used to decrease reflex tachycardia.
NURSING CONSIDERATIONS: Monitor for excessive slowing of heart rate.

Cimetidine, ranitidine, and grapefruit juice can lead to toxicity.
NURSING CONSIDERATIONS
- Monitor for indications of toxicity (decrease in blood pressure, increase in heart rate, and flushing).
- Advise clients to avoid drinking grapefruit juice.
- Avoid concurrent use with cimetidine and ranitidine.

VERAPAMIL, DILTIAZEM

Verapamil can increase digoxin levels, increasing the risk of digoxin toxicity. Digoxin can cause an additive effect and intensify AV conduction suppression.
NURSING CONSIDERATIONS
- Monitor digoxin levels to maintain therapeutic range.
- Monitor vital signs for bradycardia and for manifestations of AV block, such as a reduced ventricular rate.

Concurrent use of beta-blockers can lead to heart failure, AV block, and bradycardia.
NURSING CONSIDERATIONS
- Allow several hours between administration of IV verapamil and beta-blockers.
- Monitor ECG and heart rate.

Consuming grapefruit juice and verapamil or diltiazem can lead to toxicity.
NURSING CONSIDERATIONS
- Monitor for indications of toxicity, such as decrease in blood pressure, decrease in heart rate, and AV block.
- Advise clients to avoid drinking grapefruit juice.

NURSING ADMINISTRATION

- Advise clients not to chew or crush sustained-release tablets.
- For IV administration of verapamil, administer injections slowly over a period of 2 to 3 min. Q EBP
- Advise clients who have angina to record pain frequency, intensity, duration, and location. Notify the provider if attacks increase in frequency, intensity, and/or duration.
- Teach clients to monitor blood pressure and heart rate, as well as keep a blood pressure record. Withhold medication and notify provider for pulse less than 50/min and systolic blood pressure less than 90 mm Hg.
- Advise client to change positions slowly and to avoid activities that require alertness until effects are known.

Alpha adrenergic blockers (sympatholytics)

SELECT PROTOTYPE MEDICATION: Prazosin

OTHER MEDICATIONS
- Doxazosin
- Terazosin

PURPOSE

EXPECTED PHARMACOLOGICAL ACTION

Selective alpha$_1$ blockade results in the following.
- Venous and arterial dilation
- Smooth muscle relaxation of the prostatic capsule and bladder neck

THERAPEUTIC USES

- Primary hypertension.
- Doxazosin and terazosin are used to decrease manifestations of benign prostatic hyperplasia (BPH), which include urgency, frequency, and dysuria.

COMPLICATIONS

First-dose orthostatic hypotension

NURSING CONSIDERATIONS
- Start treatment with low dosage of medication.
- First dose often is given at night.
- Monitor blood pressure for 2 to 6 hr after initiation of treatment.
- Instruct clients to avoid activities requiring mental alertness for the first 12 to 24 hr.
- Instruct clients to change positions slowly and to lie down if feeling dizzy, lightheaded, or faint.

CONTRAINDICATIONS/PRECAUTIONS

- Pregnancy Risk Category C. Qs
- Contraindicated in clients who have hypotension.
- Use cautiously clients who have angina pectoris or renal insufficiency, and in older adults. G

INTERACTIONS

Antihypertensive medications can have an additive hypotensive effect.
NURSING CONSIDERATIONS
- Instruct clients to observe for indications of hypotension (dizziness, lightheadedness, faintness).
- Instruct clients to lie down if these manifestations occur, and to change positions slowly.

NURSING ADMINISTRATION

- Instruct clients that the medication can be taken with food.
- Recommend that clients take the initial dose at bedtime to decrease "first-dose" hypotensive effect.
- Advise client about safety measures to minimize effects of orthostatic hypotension/dizziness.

Centrally acting alpha₂ agonists

SELECT PROTOTYPE MEDICATION: Clonidine

OTHER MEDICATIONS
- Guanfacine
- Methyldopa

PURPOSE

EXPECTED PHARMACOLOGICAL ACTION

These medications act within the CNS to decrease sympathetic outflow resulting in decreased stimulation of the adrenergic receptors (both alpha and beta receptors) of the heart and peripheral vascular system.
- Decrease in sympathetic outflow to the myocardium results in bradycardia and decreased cardiac output (CO).
- Decrease in sympathetic outflow to the peripheral vasculature results in vasodilation, which leads to decreased blood pressure.

THERAPEUTIC USES

- Primary hypertension (administered alone, with a diuretic, or with another antihypertensive agent)
- Severe cancer pain (administered parenterally by epidural infusion)

INVESTIGATIONAL USE
- Migraine headache
- Flushing from menopause
- Management of ADHD and Tourette syndrome
- Management of withdrawal from alcohol, tobacco, and opioids

COMPLICATIONS

Drowsiness and sedation

NURSING CONSIDERATIONS
- Drowsiness will diminish as use of medication continues.
- Advise clients to avoid activities that require mental alertness until manifestations subside.

Dry mouth

CLIENT EDUCATION
- Advise clients to be compliant with medication regimen.
- Reassure clients that dry mouth usually resolves in 2 to 4 weeks.
- Encourage clients to chew gum or suck on hard candy, and to take small amounts of water or ice chips.

Rebound hypertension if abruptly discontinued

NURSING CONSIDERATIONS
- Advise clients not to discontinue treatment without consulting the provider.
- Discontinue clonidine gradually over 2 to 4 days.

CONTRAINDICATIONS/PRECAUTIONS

- Clonidine is Pregnancy Risk Category C. Methyldopa and guanfacine are Pregnancy Risk Category B.
- Avoid use during lactation. Qs
- Avoid use of transdermal patch on affected skin in scleroderma and systemic lupus erythematosus.
- Contraindicated in clients who have a bleeding disorder or are on anticoagulants.
- Use cautiously in clients who have had a stroke, asthma, COPD, recent MI, diabetes mellitus, major depressive disorder, or chronic kidney disease.

INTERACTIONS

Antihypertensive medications can have an additive hypotensive effect.
NURSING CONSIDERATIONS
- Instruct clients to observe for manifestations of hypotension (dizziness, lightheadedness, faintness).
- Instruct clients to lie down if feeling dizzy, lightheaded, or faint, and change positions slowly.

Concurrent use of prazosin, MAOIs, and tricyclic antidepressants can counteract the antihypertensive effect of clonidine.
NURSING CONSIDERATIONS: Monitor clients for therapeutic effect. Monitor blood pressure. Do not use concurrently.

Additive CNS depression can occur with concurrent use of other CNS depressants, such as alcohol.
NURSING CONSIDERATIONS: Advise clients of additive CNS depression with alcohol, and encourage clients to avoid use.

NURSING ADMINISTRATION

- Administer medication by oral, epidural, and transdermal routes.
- Medication is usually administered twice a day in divided doses. Take larger dose at bedtime to decrease the occurrence of daytime sleepiness. QEBP
- Transdermal patches are applied every seven days. Advise clients to apply patch on hairless, intact skin on torso or upper arm.

Beta adrenergic blockers (sympatholytics)

SELECT PROTOTYPE MEDICATIONS

Cardioselective: Beta$_1$ (affects only the heart)
- Metoprolol
- Atenolol
- Esmolol

Nonselective: Beta$_1$ and beta$_2$ (affecting both the heart and lungs)
- Propranolol
- Nadolol

Alpha and beta blockers
- Carvedilol
- Labetalol

PURPOSE

EXPECTED PHARMACOLOGICAL ACTION

- In cardiac conditions, the primary effects of beta-adrenergic blockers are a result of beta$_1$-adrenergic blockade in the myocardium and in the electrical conduction system of the heart.
- Decreased heart rate (negative chronotropic [rate] action).
- Decreased myocardial contractility (negative inotropic [force] action); decreases cardiac output.
- Decreased rate of conduction through the AV node (negative dromotropic action).
- Alpha blockade adds vasodilation in medications such as carvedilol and labetalol.
- Reduces release of renin which decreases angiotensin II and causes vasodilation and promotes excretion of sodium and water.

THERAPEUTIC USES

- Primary hypertension (exact mechanism unknown: long-term use causes reduction in peripheral vascular resistance).
- Angina, tachydysrhythmias, heart failure, and myocardial infarction.
- Suppresses reflex tachycardia due to vasodilators. Other uses can include treatment of hyperthyroidism, migraine headache, pheochromocytoma, and glaucoma.

COMPLICATIONS

BETA$_1$ BLOCKADE: METOPROLOL, PROPRANOLOL

Bradycardia

NURSING CONSIDERATIONS
- Monitor pulse. If below 50/min, hold medication and notify the provider.
- Use cautiously in clients who have diabetes mellitus. This medication can mask tachycardia, an early manifestation of low blood glucose. Advise clients to monitor blood glucose to detect hypoglycemia.

Decreased cardiac output

NURSING CONSIDERATIONS
- Use cautiously with clients who have heart failure. Doses are started very low and titrated to the desired level.
- Advise clients to observe for manifestations of worsening heart failure (shortness of breath, edema, weight gain, fatigue).
- Notify the provider if manifestations occur.

AV block

NURSING CONSIDERATIONS: Obtain a baseline ECG and monitor.

Orthostatic hypotension

CLIENT EDUCATION
- Advise clients to sit or lie down if experiencing dizziness or faintness.
- Advise clients to avoid sudden changes of position and rise slowly.

Rebound myocardium excitation

NURSING CONSIDERATIONS
- The myocardium becomes sensitized to catecholamines with long-term use of beta-blockers.
- Advise clients not to stop taking beta-blockers abruptly, but to follow the provider's instructions.
- Discontinue use of beta-blockers over 1 to 2 weeks.

BETA$_2$ BLOCKADE: PROPRANOLOL

Bronchoconstriction

NURSING CONSIDERATIONS
- Avoid in clients who have asthma.
- Clients who have asthma should receive a beta$_1$ selective agent.

Glycogenolysis is inhibited

NURSING CONSIDERATIONS
- Clients who have diabetes mellitus rely on the breakdown of glycogen into glucose to manage low blood glucose (can happen with insulin overdose).
- In addition, a decreased heart rate can further mask manifestations of impending low blood glucose level. Clients who have diabetes mellitus receive a beta$_1$ selective agent.

CONTRAINDICATIONS/PRECAUTIONS
- Contraindicated in clients who have AV block and sinus bradycardia. **Qs**
- Nonselective beta-adrenergic blockers are contraindicated in clients who have asthma, bronchospasm, and heart failure.
- Use cardioselective beta-adrenergic blockers cautiously in clients who have asthma.
- In general, use beta-adrenergic blockers cautiously in clients who have myasthenia gravis, hypotension, peripheral vascular disease, diabetes mellitus, depression, and in older adults and those who have a history of severe allergies. **Ⓒ**

INTERACTIONS

BETA$_1$ BLOCKADE: METOPROLOL, PROPRANOLOL

Calcium channel blockers (CCB) verapamil and diltiazem intensify the effects of beta-blockers
- Decreased heart rate
- Decreased myocardial contractility
- Decreased rate of conduction through the AV node
- NURSING CONSIDERATIONS
  - Monitor ECG and blood pressure.
  - Monitor clients closely if taking a CCB and beta-blocker concurrently. Reduce dose if needed.

Concurrent use of antihypertensive medications with beta-blockers can intensify the hypotensive effect of both medications.
NURSING CONSIDERATIONS: Monitor for a drop in blood pressure.

BETA$_2$ BLOCKADE: PROPRANOLOL

Propranolol use can mask the hypoglycemic effect of insulin and prevent the breakdown of fat in response to hypoglycemia.
NURSING CONSIDERATIONS: Monitor blood glucose levels.

NURSING ADMINISTRATION
- Administer medications orally, usually once or twice a day.
- Atenolol, metoprolol, labetalol, and propranolol can be administered by the IV route.
- Advise clients not to discontinue medication without consulting the provider.
- Advise clients to avoid sudden changes in position to prevent occurrence of orthostatic hypotension.
- Instruct clients not to crush or chew extended-release tablets.
- Teach clients to self-monitor heart rate and blood pressure at home on a daily basis.
- Take with food to increase absorption.

NURSING EVALUATION OF MEDICATION EFFECTIVENESS

Depending on therapeutic intent, effectiveness is evidenced by the following.
- Absence of chest pain
- Absence of cardiac dysrhythmias
- Normotensive blood pressure readings
- Control of heart failure manifestations

Medications for hypertensive crisis

SELECT PROTOTYPE MEDICATION: Nitroprusside (centrally-acting vasodilator)

OTHER MEDICATIONS
- Nitroglycerin (vasodilator)
- Nicardipine (calcium channel blocker)
- Clevidipine (calcium channel blocker)
- Enalaprilat (ACE inhibitor)
- Esmolol (beta blocker)

PURPOSE

EXPECTED PHARMACOLOGICAL ACTION: Direct vasodilation of arteries and veins resulting in rapid reduction of blood pressure (decreased preload and afterload)

THERAPEUTIC USES: Hypertensive crisis

COMPLICATIONS

Excessive hypotension

NURSING CONSIDERATIONS
- Administer medication slowly because rapid administration will cause blood pressure to go down rapidly.
- Monitor blood pressure and ECG continuously.
- Keep client supine during administration. Q EBP

Cyanide poisoning/thiocyanate toxicity

- Headache and drowsiness, and can lead to cardiac arrest
- Nitroprusside only

NURSING CONSIDERATIONS
- Clients who have liver dysfunction are at increased risk.
- Risk of cyanide poisoning is reduced by administering medication for no longer than 3 days, and at a rate of 5 mcg/kg/min or less. Avoid prolonged use of nitroprusside.
- Manifestations include weakness, disorientation and delirium. Administer thiosulfate to reverse effects.
- Monitor plasma levels if used for more than 3 days. Level should be maintained at less than 10 mg/dL.
- Discontinue medication if cyanide toxicity occurs.

Bradycardia, tachycardia, ECG changes

NURSING CONSIDERATIONS: Monitor ECG for changes.

CONTRAINDICATIONS/PRECAUTIONS

- Pregnancy Risk Category C.
- Contraindicated in clients who have heart failure with reduced peripheral vascular resistance, and AV shunt. ©
- Use cautiously in clients who have liver and kidney disease, hypothyroidism, hypovolemia, or fluid and electrolyte imbalances, and in older adults.

INTERACTIONS

Do not administer nitroprusside in the same infusion as any other medication.

NURSING ADMINISTRATION

- Prepare medication by adding to diluent for IV infusion.
- Note color of solution. Solution can be light brown in color. Discard solution of any other color. Q EBP
- Protect IV container and tubing from light.
- Discard medication after 24 hr.
- Monitor vital signs and ECG continuously.

NURSING EVALUATION OF MEDICATION EFFECTIVENESS

Depending on therapeutic intent, effectiveness is evidenced by the following.
- Decrease in blood pressure and maintenance of normotensive blood pressure.
- Improvement of heart failure such as ability to perform activities of daily living, improved breath sounds, and absence of edema.

Application Exercises

1. A nurse is reviewing the health record of a client who asks about using propranolol to treat hypertension. The nurse should recognize which of the following conditions is a contraindication for taking propranolol?

   A. Asthma

   B. Glaucoma

   C. Hypertension

   D. Tachycardia

2. A nurse is teaching a client who has a new prescription for verapamil to control hypertension. Which of the following instructions should the nurse include?

   A. Increase the amount of dietary fiber in the diet.

   B. Drink grapefruit juice daily to increase vitamin C intake.

   C. Decrease the amount of calcium in the diet.

   D. Withhold food for 1 hr after the medication is taken.

3. A nurse is caring for a client who has a new prescription for captopril for hypertension. The nurse should monitor the client for which of the following adverse effects of this medication?

   A. Hypokalemia

   B. Hypernatremia

   C. Neutropenia

   D. Bradycardia

4. A nurse in an acute care facility is caring for a client who is receiving IV nitroprusside for hypertensive crisis. The nurse should monitor the client for which of the following adverse reactions to this medication?

   A. Intestinal ileus

   B. Neutropenia

   C. Delirium

   D. Hyperthermia

5. A nurse is planning to administer a first dose of captopril to a client who has hypertension. Which of the following medications can intensify first dose hypotension? (Select all that apply.)

   A. Simvastatin

   B. Hydrochlorothiazide

   C. Phenytoin

   D. Clonidine

   E. Aliskiren

PRACTICE Active Learning Scenario

A nurse in an outpatient facility is teaching a client who has a new prescription for aliskiren to treat hypertension. What should the nurse teach the client about this medication? Use the ATI Active Learning Template: Medication to complete this item.

THERAPEUTIC USES: Identify the therapeutic use for aliskiren.

COMPLICATIONS: List two adverse effects of this medication.

NURSING INTERVENTIONS: Describe one test to monitor.

CLIENT EDUCATION: Identify two teaching points.

Application Exercises Key

1. A. **CORRECT:** Propranolol is a nonselective beta-adrenergic blocker that blocks both beta$_1$ and beta$_2$ receptors. Blockade of beta$_2$ receptors in the lungs causes bronchoconstriction, so it is contraindicated in clients who have asthma.

   B. Propranolol is not contraindicated in clients who have glaucoma.

   C. Propranolol is prescribed to treat hypertension. It is not contraindicated for clients who have this disorder.

   D. Propranolol is prescribed to treat tachydysrhythmias, such as tachycardia. It is contraindicated in clients who have bradycardia and heart block.

   Ⓝ *NCLEX® Connection: Pharmacological and Parenteral Therapies, Adverse Effects/Contraindications/Side Effects/Interactions*

2. A. **CORRECT:** Increasing dietary fiber intake can help prevent constipation, an adverse effect of verapamil.

   B. Clients should be taught to avoid drinking grapefruit juice when taking verapamil because concurrent use can lead to toxicity. In addition, it is not necessary to take extra vitamin C when taking verapamil.

   C. There is no restriction on dietary calcium intake for clients taking verapamil.

   D. There is no restriction regarding food when taking verapamil. Clients can take verapamil with food to prevent GI upset.

   Ⓝ *NCLEX® Connection: Pharmacological and Parenteral Therapies, Medication Administration*

3. A. Hyperkalemia, rather than hypokalemia, is a risk for clients taking ACE inhibitors.

   B. ACE inhibitors cause excretion of sodium and water. Hypernatremia is not a risk for the client taking an ACE inhibitor.

   C. **CORRECT:** Neutropenia is a serious adverse effect that can occur in clients taking an ACE inhibitor. The nurse should monitor the client's CBC and teach the client to report indications of infection to the provider.

   D. Tachycardia is an adverse effect of ACE inhibitors.

   Ⓝ *NCLEX® Connection: Pharmacological and Parenteral Therapies, Adverse Effects/Contraindications/Side Effects/Interactions*

4. A. Headache is an adverse effect of nitroprusside, not intestinal ileus.

   B. Bradycardia is an adverse effect of nitroprusside, not neutropenia.

   C. **CORRECT:** Delirium and other mental status changes can occur in thiocyanate toxicity when IV nitroprusside is infused at a high dosage. Monitor thiocyanate level during therapy to remain below 10 mg/dL.

   D. Hypotension is an adverse effect of nitroprusside, not hyperthermia.

   Ⓝ *NCLEX® Connection: Pharmacological and Parenteral Therapies, Parenteral/Intravenous Therapies*

5. A. Simvastatin, an antilipemic medication that lowers cholesterol, does not interact with captopril and does not intensify first-dose hypotension.

   B. **CORRECT:** Hydrochlorothiazide, a thiazide diuretic, is often used to treat hypertension. Diuretics can intensify first-dose orthostatic hypotension caused by captopril and can continue to interact with antihypertensive medications to cause hypotension. The nurse should monitor clients carefully for hypotension, especially after the first dose of captopril and keep the client safe from injury.

   C. Phenytoin, an antiseizure medication, does not interact with captopril and does not intensify first dose hypotension.

   D. **CORRECT:** Clonidine, a centrally acting alpha$_2$ agonist, is an antihypertensive medication that can interact with captopril to intensify first-dose orthostatic hypotension. The nurse should monitor clients carefully for hypotension, especially after the first dose of captopril, and keep the client safe from injury.

   E. **CORRECT:** Aliskiren, a direct renin inhibitor, is an antihypertensive medication that can interact with captopril to intensify its first-dose orthostatic hypotension. The nurse should monitor clients carefully for hypotension, especially after the first dose of captopril, and keep the client safe from injury.

   Ⓝ *NCLEX® Connection: Pharmacological and Parenteral Therapies, Adverse Effects/Contraindications/Side Effects/Interactions*

PRACTICE Answer

Using the ATI Active Learning Template: Medication

THERAPEUTIC USES: Aliskiren binds with renin to inhibit production of angiotensin I, thus decreasing production of both angiotensin II and aldosterone. Aliskiren is used solely for treating hypertension alone or in combination with other antihypertensives.

COMPLICATIONS
- Diarrhea: dose-related, occurs most frequently in females and older adult clients
- Risk for angioedema and rash caused by allergy to the medication
- Hyperkalemia
- Hypotension

NURSING INTERVENTIONS: The nurse should monitor serum electrolytes, paying close attention to potassium levels, because the client is at risk for hyperkalemia. This is especially important when the client takes ACE inhibitors concurrently, because these medications also raise potassium levels.

CLIENT EDUCATION
- Advise clients not to take aliskiren with foods high in fat, which decreases absorption of the medication.
- Advise clients not to take potassium supplements or salt substitutes containing potassium.
- Female clients should be instructed not to take aliskiren during pregnancy.
- Teach the client that if a rash or angioedema occurs, discontinue aliskiren and notify the provider.
- The client should call 911 if severe manifestations of allergy are present.

   Ⓝ *NCLEX® Connection: Pharmacological and Parenteral Therapies, Medication Administration*

CHAPTER 21   *Cardiac Glycosides
and Heart Failure*

Heart failure results from inadequate pumping of the heart muscle with manifestations caused by the heart's inability to meet the circulation needs of the whole body. Decreased tissue perfusion results in fatigue, shortness of breath, weakness, and activity intolerance.

Heart failure causes a reduction in cardiac output (CO) and affects heart rate, stroke volume (SV), preload, and afterload. There are two types of heart failure: left-sided (with pulmonary manifestations such as dyspnea, cough, and oliguria) and right-sided (systemic congestion with peripheral edema, jugular vein distention, weight gain).

Diuretics, ACE inhibitors, angiotensin II receptor blockers (ARBs), and beta adrenergic blockers are the medications of choice for treatment of heart failure. Cardiac glycosides are indicated if these medications are unable to control manifestations.

Cardiac glycosides

SELECT PROTOTYPE MEDICATION: Digoxin

PURPOSE

EXPECTED PHARMACOLOGICAL ACTION

Positive inotropic effect: increased force of myocardial contraction
- Increased force and efficiency of myocardial contraction improves the heart's effectiveness as a pump, improving stroke volume and cardiac output.

Negative chronotropic effect: decreased heart rate
- At therapeutic levels, digoxin slows the rate of sinoatrial (SA) node depolarization and the rate of impulses through the conduction system of the heart.
- A decreased heart rate gives the ventricles more time to fill with blood coming from the atria, which leads to increased SV and increased CO.

THERAPEUTIC USES

As a second-line medication
- Treatment of heart failure
- Dysrhythmias (atrial fibrillation)
- Can reduce manifestations, but does not prolong life

COMPLICATIONS

Dysrhythmias, cardiotoxicity

- Dysrhythmias caused by interfering with the electrical conduction in the myocardium)
- Cardiotoxicity leading to bradycardia

NURSING CONSIDERATIONS
- Conditions that increase the risk of developing digoxin-induced dysrhythmias include hypokalemia, increased serum digoxin levels, and heart disease. Older adult clients are particularly at risk. Ⓖ
- Monitor serum levels of K+ to maintain a level between 3.5 to 5.0 mEq/L.
- Instruct clients to report manifestations of hypokalemia (nausea/vomiting, general weakness). Potassium supplements are prescribed if clients are concurrently taking a diuretic.
- Teach clients to consume high-potassium foods (green leafy vegetables, bananas, potatoes).
- Monitor digoxin level.
- Therapeutic serum levels can vary, but usually range from 0.5 to 0.8 ng/mL.
- Dosages should be based on serum levels and client response to medication.
- Teach clients to monitor pulse rate, and recognize and report changes, such as irregular rate with early or extra beats.

GI effects

Include anorexia (usually the first manifestation of toxicity), nausea, vomiting, and abdominal pain

CLIENT EDUCATION: Teach clients to monitor for these effects and report to the provider if they occur.

CNS effects

Include fatigue, weakness, vision changes (diplopia, blurred vision, yellow-green or white halos around objects)

CLIENT EDUCATION: Teach clients to monitor for these effects and report to the provider if they occur.

CONTRAINDICATIONS/PRECAUTIONS

- Pregnancy Risk Category C. Ⓠs
- Contraindicated in clients who have disturbances in ventricular rhythm, including ventricular fibrillation, ventricular tachycardia, and second- and third-degree heart block.
- Use cautiously in clients who have hypokalemia, partial AV block, advanced heart failure, and impaired kidney function.

INTERACTIONS

Thiazide diuretics, such as hydrochlorothiazide, and loop diuretics, such as furosemide, can lead to hypokalemia, which increases the risk of developing dysrhythmias.
NURSING CONSIDERATIONS
- Monitor and maintain K+ level between 3.5 and 5.0 mEq/L.
- Treat hypokalemia with potassium supplements or a potassium-sparing diuretic.

ACE inhibitors and ARBs increase the risk of hyperkalemia, which can lead to decreased therapeutic effects of digoxin.
NURSING CONSIDERATIONS
- Use cautiously if these medications are used with potassium supplements or a potassium-sparing diuretic.
- Maintain K+ level between 3.5 to 5.0 mEq/L.

Sympathomimetic medications such as dopamine complement the inotropic action of digoxin and increase the rate and force of heart muscle contraction. These medications can increase the risk of tachydysrhythmias.
NURSING CONSIDERATIONS: Monitor ECG. Instruct clients to measure pulse rate and report palpitations.

Quinidine increases the risk of digoxin toxicity when used concurrently by displacing digoxin from its binding site and reducing kidney excretion.
NURSING CONSIDERATIONS: Avoid concurrent use.

Verapamil increases plasma levels of digoxin.
NURSING CONSIDERATIONS: If used concurrently, decrease digoxin dose. Concurrent use is usually avoided because of verapamil cardiosuppression action counteracting the action of digoxin.

Antacids decrease absorption of digoxin and can decrease its effectiveness.
NURSING CONSIDERATIONS: Advise clients to talk to the provider before taking any antacids.

NURSING ADMINISTRATION

- Advise clients to take the medication as prescribed. If a dose is missed, the next dose should not be doubled. Q_EBP
- Check pulse rate and rhythm before administration of digoxin and record. Notify the provider if heart rate is less than 60/min in an adult, less than 70/min in children, and less than 90/min in infants.
- Administer digoxin at the same time daily.
- Monitor digoxin levels periodically during treatment and maintain therapeutic levels between 0.5 and 0.8 ng/mL to prevent digoxin toxicity.
- Avoid taking OTC medications to prevent adverse effects and medication interactions.
- Instruct clients to observe for manifestations of hypokalemia, such as muscle weakness, and to notify the provider if they occur.
- Instruct clients to observe for indications of digoxin toxicity (fatigue, weakness, vision changes, GI effects), and to notify the provider if they occur.
- If administering IV digoxin, infuse over at least 5 min, (10 to 15 min in clients who have pulmonary edema) and monitor client for dysrhythmias. Q_EBP

MANAGEMENT OF DIGOXIN TOXICITY
- Stop digoxin and potassium-sparing medication immediately.
- Monitor K+ levels. For levels less than 3.5 mEq/L, administer potassium IV or by mouth. Do not give any further K+ if the level is greater than 5.0 mEq/L.
- Treat dysrhythmias with phenytoin or lidocaine.
- Treat bradycardia with atropine.
- For excessive overdose, activated charcoal, cholestyramine, or digoxin immune Fab can be used to bind digoxin and prevent absorption.

NURSING EVALUATION OF MEDICATION EFFECTIVENESS

Depending on therapeutic intent, effectiveness is evidenced by the following.
- Control of heart failure
- Absence of cardiac dysrhythmias

Adrenergic agonists

SELECT PROTOTYPE MEDICATION: Catecholamines
- Epinephrine
- Dopamine
- Dobutamine
- Isoproterenol
- Norepinephrine

OTHER MEDICATIONS
- Albuterol
- Ephedrine

PURPOSE

SITE/RESPONSE

Alpha₁ receptors

- Activation of receptors in arterioles of skin, viscera and mucous membranes, and veins leads to vasoconstriction.
- Mydriasis (dilation of pupil)

Beta₁ receptors

- Heart stimulation leads to increased heart rate, increased myocardial contractility, and increased rate of conduction through the AV node.
- Activation of receptors in the kidney lead to the release of renin.

Beta₂ receptors

- Activation of receptors in the arterioles of the heart, lungs, and skeletal muscles leads to vasodilation.
- Bronchial stimulation leads to bronchodilation.
- Activation of receptors in uterine smooth muscle causes relaxation.
- Activation of receptors in the liver cause glycogenolysis.
- Skeletal muscle receptor activation leads to muscle contraction.

Dopamine receptors

Activation of receptors in the kidney cause the renal blood vessels to dilate.

MEDICATIONS

Epinephrine

Alpha$_1$ receptors
- PHARMACOLOGICAL ACTION: Vasoconstriction
- THERAPEUTIC USE
  - Slows absorption of local anesthetics
  - Manages superficial bleeding
  - Decreased congestion of nasal mucosa
  - Increased blood pressure

Beta$_1$ receptors
- PHARMACOLOGICAL ACTION
  - Increased heart rate
  - Increased myocardial contractility
  - Increased rate of conduction through the AV node
  - Increased cardiac output
  - Improved tissue perfusion
- THERAPEUTIC USE: Treatment of AV block, heart failure, shock, and cardiac arrest

Beta$_2$ receptors
- PHARMACOLOGICAL ACTION: Bronchodilation
- THERAPEUTIC USE: Asthma

Dopamine

Low dose: Beta$_1$
- PHARMACOLOGICAL ACTION: Renal blood vessel dilation
- THERAPEUTIC USE
  - Shock
  - Heart failure
  - Acute kidney injury

Moderate dose: Beta$_1$
- PHARMACOLOGICAL ACTION
  - Renal blood vessel dilation
  - Increased heart rate
  - Increased myocardial contractility
  - Increased rate of conduction through the AV node
- THERAPEUTIC USE
  - Shock
  - Heart failure

High dose: Beta$_1$, alpha$_1$
- PHARMACOLOGICAL ACTION
  - Renal blood vessel constriction
  - Increased heart rate
  - Increased myocardial contractility
  - Increased rate of conduction through the AV node
  - Vasoconstriction
- THERAPEUTIC USE
  - Shock
  - Heart failure

Dobutamine

Beta$_1$
- PHARMACOLOGICAL ACTION
  - Increased heart rate
  - Increased myocardial contractility and cardiac output
  - Increased rate of conduction through the AV node
- THERAPEUTIC USE: Heart failure

COMPLICATIONS

EPINEPHRINE

Vasoconstriction

Hypertensive crisis due to activation of alpha$_1$ receptors in the heart.

NURSING CONSIDERATIONS
- Provide for continuous cardiac and blood pressure monitoring.
- Report changes in vital signs to the provider.

Cardiac complications

Dysrhythmias due to activation of beta$_1$ receptors in the heart. Beta$_1$ receptor activation also increases the workload of the heart and increases oxygen demand, leading to the development of angina.

NURSING CONSIDERATIONS
- Provide for continuous cardiac monitoring.
- Monitor clients closely for dysrhythmias, change in heart rate, and chest pain.
- Notify the provider of dysrhythmias, increased heart rate, and chest pain. Treat per protocol.

DOPAMINE

Cardiac complications

Beta$_1$ receptor activation in the heart can cause dysrhythmias. Beta$_1$ receptor activation also increases the workload of the heart and increases oxygen demand, leading to development of angina.

NURSING CONSIDERATIONS
- Provide for continuous cardiac monitoring.
- Monitor clients closely for dysrhythmias, change in heart rate, and chest pain.
- Notify the provider of dysrhythmias, increased heart rate, and chest pain. Treat per protocol.

Necrosis

Can occur from extravasation of high doses of dopamine

NURSING CONSIDERATIONS
- Monitor IV site carefully. Infuse through central IV line if possible. Qs
- Discontinue infusion at first indication of irritation.
- If extravasation occurs, administer phentolamine, an alpha blocker to counteract alpha mediated vasoconstriction.

DOBUTAMINE

Increased heart rate

NURSING CONSIDERATIONS
- Provide continuous cardiac monitoring.
- Report changes in vital signs to the provider.

CONTRAINDICATIONS/PRECAUTIONS

- Epinephrine and dopamine are Pregnancy Risk Category C. Qs
- Dobutamine is Pregnancy Risk Category B.
- Dopamine is contraindicated in clients who have tachydysrhythmias, and ventricular fibrillation.
- Use dopamine and dobutamine cautiously in clients who have hyperthyroidism, angina, history of myocardial infarction, hypertension, and diabetes.
- Epinephrine should be used with caution in clients who have hyperthyroidism, angina, cardiac dysrhythmias, and hypertension.

INTERACTIONS

MAOIs prevent inactivation of epinephrine and therefore prolong the effects of epinephrine. MAOIs used with dobutamine and dopamine can cause cardiotoxicity.
NURSING CONSIDERATIONS: Avoid use of MAOIs in clients receiving epinephrine, dopamine, and dobutamine.

Tricyclic antidepressants block uptake of epinephrine, dopamine, and dobutamine, which will prolong and intensify effects of epinephrine.
NURSING CONSIDERATIONS: Clients taking these medications concurrently might need a lowered dosage of epinephrine, dopamine, and dobutamine.

General anesthetics can cause the heart to become hypersensitive to the effects of epinephrine, dopamine, and dobutamine, leading to dysrhythmias.
NURSING CONSIDERATIONS
- Perform continuous ECG monitoring.
- Notify the provider of evidence of chest pain, dysrhythmias, and increased heart rate.

Alpha-adrenergic blocking agents, such as phentolamine, block action at alpha receptors.
NURSING CONSIDERATIONS: Phentolamine can be used to treat epinephrine toxicity and extravasation of epinephrine, and dopamine. QEBP

Beta-adrenergic blocking agents, such as propranolol, block action at beta receptors.
NURSING CONSIDERATIONS: Use propranolol to treat chest pain and dysrhythmias.

Diuretics promote beneficial effects of dopamine.
NURSING CONSIDERATIONS: Monitor for therapeutic effects.

NURSING ADMINISTRATION

- These medications must be administered IV by continuous infusion. QEBP
- Use an IV pump to control infusion.
- Dosage is titrated based on blood pressure response.
- Stop the infusion of dopamine at first evidence of infiltration. Extravasation can be treated with local injection of an alpha-adrenergic blocking agent, such as phentolamine.
- Assess/monitor for chest pain. Notify the provider if chest pain occurs.
- Monitor urine output frequently for indications of decreased kidney perfusion.
- Monitor ECG continuously, and notify provider of indications of tachycardia or dysrhythmias.
- Monitor perfusion to extremities.
- Monitor cardiac output, pulmonary capillary wedge pressure, central venous pressure.

NURSING EVALUATION OF MEDICATION EFFECTIVENESS

Depending on therapeutic intent, effectiveness is evidenced by improved perfusion as evidenced by urine output of greater than or equal to 30 mL/hr (with adequate kidney function), improved mental status, and systolic blood pressure maintained at greater than or equal to 90 mm Hg.

Application Exercises

1. A nurse in a provider's office is monitoring serum electrolytes for four older adult clients who take digoxin. Which of the following electrolyte values increases a client's risk for digoxin toxicity?

    A. Calcium 9.2 mg/dL

    B. Calcium 10.3 mg/dL

    C. Potassium 3.4 mEq/L

    D. Potassium 4.8 mEq/L

2. A nurse is caring for an older adult client who has a new prescription for digoxin and takes multiple other medications. The nurse should recognize that concurrent use of which of the following medications places the client at risk for digoxin toxicity?

    A. Phenytoin

    B. Verapamil

    C. Warfarin

    D. Aluminum hydroxide

3. A nurse is administering a dopamine infusion at a low dose to a client who has severe heart failure. Which of the following findings is an expected effect of this medication?

    A. Lowered heart rate

    B. Increased myocardial contractility

    C. Decreased conduction through the AV node

    D. Vasoconstriction of renal blood vessels

4. A nurse is providing teaching to a client who has a new prescription for digoxin. The nurse should instruct the client to monitor and report which of the following adverse effects that is a manifestation digoxin toxicity? (Select all that apply.)

    A. Fatigue

    B. Constipation

    C. Anorexia

    D. Rash

    E. Diplopia

5. A nurse is teaching a client who has a new prescription for digoxin to treat heart failure. Which of the following instructions should the nurse include in the teaching?

    A. Contact provider if heart rate is less than 60/min.

    B. Check pulse rate for 30 seconds and multiply result by 2.

    C. Increase intake of sodium.

    D. Take with food if nausea occurs.

PRACTICE Active Learning Scenario

A nurse is caring for a client who has heart failure and a new prescription for digoxin 0.125 mg PO daily. What should the nurse teach the client about this medication? Use the ATI Active Learning Template: Medication to complete this item.

THERAPEUTIC USES

COMPLICATIONS: Identify two adverse effects.

NURSING INTERVENTIONS: Describe two diagnostic tests to monitor.

CLIENT EDUCATION: Include three teaching points.

Application Exercises Key

1. A. Calcium 9.2 mg/dL is within the expected reference range and does not put a client at risk for digoxin toxicity.

   B. Calcium 10.3 mg/dL is within the expected reference range and does not put a client at risk for digoxin toxicity.

   C. **CORRECT:** Potassium 3.4 mEq/L is below the expected reference range and puts a client at risk for digoxin toxicity. Low potassium can cause fatal dysrhythmias, especially in older clients who take digoxin. The nurse should notify the provider, who might prescribe a potassium supplement or a potassium-sparing diuretic for the client.

   D. A potassium level of 4.8 mEq/L is within the expected reference range and does not put a client at risk for digoxin toxicity.

   Ⓝ *NCLEX® Connection: Pharmacological and Parenteral Therapies, Adverse Effects/Contraindications/Side Effects/Interactions*

2. A. Phenytoin, an antiseizure and antidysrhythmic medication, does not increase a client's risk for digoxin toxicity. When given as an antidysrhythmic, phenytoin can treat dysrhythmias caused by digoxin toxicity.

   B. **CORRECT:** Verapamil, a calcium-channel blocker, can increase digoxin levels. If these medications are given concurrently, the digoxin dosage might be decreased and the nurse should monitor digoxin levels carefully.

   C. Warfarin does not interact with digoxin to increase digoxin levels.

   D. Antacids, such as aluminum hydroxide, decrease absorption of digoxin and can decrease digoxin levels and effectiveness.

   Ⓝ *NCLEX® Connection: Pharmacological and Parenteral Therapies, Adverse Effects/Contraindications/Side Effects/Interactions*

3. A. At a low dose, dopamine stimulates beta$_1$ receptors, which increases heart rate. At high doses, dopamine stimulates alpha$_1$ receptors, which can decrease heart rate.

   B. **CORRECT:** The nurse should expect dopamine to cause increased myocardial contractility, which also increases cardiac output. This occurs with the stimulation of beta$_1$ receptors and is a positive inotropic effect of dopamine when it is administered at a low dose.

   C. At a low dose, dopamine stimulates beta$_1$ receptors, which increases conduction through the AV node.

   D. At a low dose, dopamine stimulates beta$_1$ receptors, which dilates renal blood vessels. In high doses, dopamine stimulates alpha$_1$ receptors, which can constrict renal blood vessels.

   Ⓝ *NCLEX® Connection: Pharmacological and Parenteral Therapies, Parenteral/Intravenous Therapies*

4. A. **CORRECT:** Fatigue and weakness are early CNS findings that can indicate digoxin toxicity.

   B. Nausea, vomiting, and diarrhea, rather than constipation, are GI manifestations of digoxin toxicity.

   C. **CORRECT:** GI disturbances, such as anorexia, are manifestations of digoxin toxicity.

   D. Rash is not a manifestation of digoxin toxicity.

   E. **CORRECT:** Visual changes, such as diplopia and yellow-tinged vision, are manifestations of digoxin toxicity.

   Ⓝ *NCLEX® Connection: Pharmacological and Parenteral Therapies, Adverse Effects/Contraindications/Side Effects/Interactions*

5. A. **CORRECT:** The client should contact the provider for a heart rate less than 60/min.

   B. The client should check her pulse rate for 1 full minute before each dose.

   C. The client should reduce intake of sodium and avoid excess fluids.

   D. The client should report nausea to the provider because it is a manifestation of digoxin toxicity.

   Ⓝ *NCLEX® Connection: Pharmacological and Parenteral Therapies, Adverse Effects/Contraindications/Side Effects/Interactions*

PRACTICE Answer

Using the ATI Active Learning Template: Medication

THERAPEUTIC USES: Digoxin improves the heart's pumping effectiveness, and increases cardiac output and stroke volume. It decreases heart rate by slowing depolarization through the SA node, thus allowing more time for the ventricles to fill with blood. Due to these effects, digoxin is used to treat heart failure, atrial fibrillation, and some other tachydysrhythmias.

COMPLICATIONS: The client should monitor for manifestations of digoxin toxicity, which include GI effects (nausea, vomiting, diarrhea), CNS effects (fatigue, weakness), visual effects (yellow-tinged vision, halos around lights, diplopia), heart rate less than 60/min in adults, or skipped beats when checking the pulse.

NURSING INTERVENTIONS
- Monitor digoxin serum levels periodically during treatment. The expected reference range is 0.5 to 0.8 ng/mL.
- Monitor serum potassium levels because hypokalemia can cause cardiac dysrhythmias, especially in older adult clients. Monitoring ECG is also important to check for dysrhythmias.

CLIENT EDUCATION
- Teach the client to take oral digoxin at the same time each day. The client should not skip a dose or take more than the prescribed dose each day.
- Teach the client to monitor for manifestations of toxicity.
- Advise the client to report any new prescriptions and to contact provider before taking OTC medications, because digoxin interacts with many other substances.

Ⓝ *NCLEX® Connection: Pharmacological and Parenteral Therapies, Medication Administration*

UNIT 4   MEDICATIONS AFFECTING THE
          CARDIOVASCULAR SYSTEM

CHAPTER 22 *Angina*

Anginal pain often manifests as a sudden pain beneath the sternum radiating to the left shoulder, arm, and jaw. It is a result of inadequate supply of oxygen to meet the myocardial demand. Pharmacological management is aimed at prevention of myocardial ischemia, pain, myocardial infarction, and death.

Anginal pain is managed with organic nitrates, beta-adrenergic blocking agents, calcium channel blockers, and ranolazine. Clients who have chronic stable angina should concurrently take an antiplatelet agent such as aspirin or clopidogrel, a cholesterol-lowering agent, and an ACE inhibitor to prevent myocardial infarction and death.

Organic nitrates

SELECT PROTOTYPE MEDICATION: Nitroglycerin (NTG)
- Oral extended-release capsules
- Sublingual tablet
- Translingual spray
- Topical ointment
- Transdermal patch
- Intravenous

OTHER MEDICATIONS
- Isosorbide dinitrate (sublingual)
- Isosorbide mononitrate (oral)

PURPOSE

EXPECTED PHARMACOLOGICAL ACTION

- In chronic stable exertional angina, nitroglycerin dilates veins and decreases venous return (preload), which decreases cardiac oxygen demand.
- In variant (Prinzmetal's or vasospastic) angina, nitroglycerin prevents or reduces coronary artery spasm, thus increasing oxygen supply.

THERAPEUTIC USES

- Treatment of acute angina attack
- Prophylaxis of chronic stable angina or variant angina

COMPLICATIONS

Headache

CLIENT EDUCATION
- Instruct clients to use aspirin or acetaminophen to relieve pain.
- Clients should notify the provider if headache does not resolve in a few weeks. Dosage can be reduced.

Orthostatic hypotension

CLIENT EDUCATION
- Advise clients to sit or lie down if experiencing dizziness or faintness.
- Clients should avoid sudden changes of position and rise slowly.

Reflex tachycardia

NURSING CONSIDERATIONS
- Monitor vital signs.
- Administer a beta-blocker such as metoprolol if needed.

Tolerance

NURSING CONSIDERATIONS
- Use lowest dose needed to achieve effect.
- Take all long-acting forms of nitroglycerin with a medication-free period each day. This action reduces the risk of tolerance.

CONTRAINDICATIONS/PRECAUTIONS

- Pregnancy Risk Category C.
- This medication is contraindicated in clients who have hypersensitivity to nitrates.
- Nitroglycerin is contraindicated in clients who have severe anemia, closed-angle glaucoma, and traumatic head injury because the medication can increase intracranial pressure.
- Use cautiously in clients taking antihypertensive medications, and clients who have hyperthyroidism or kidney or liver dysfunction.

INTERACTIONS

Use of alcohol can contribute to the hypotensive effect of nitroglycerin.
NURSING CONSIDERATIONS: Advise clients to avoid use of alcohol.

Antihypertensive medications, such as beta-blockers, calcium channel blockers, and diuretics can contribute to hypotensive effect.
NURSING CONSIDERATIONS: Use nitroglycerin cautiously in clients receiving these medications.

Use of PDE5 inhibitors (sildenafil, tadalafil, vardenafil) and nitroglycerin can result in life-threatening hypotension.
NURSING CONSIDERATIONS: Instruct clients not to take these medications if prescribed nitroglycerin.

NURSING ADMINISTRATION

Sublingual tablet and translingual spray

TYPES
- Rapid onset
- Short duration

USE
- Treat acute attack
- Prophylaxis of acute attack

NURSING CONSIDERATIONS
- Use this rapid-acting nitrate at the first indication of chest pain. Do not wait until pain is severe. Qs
- Use prior to activity that is known to cause chest pain, such as climbing a flight of stairs.

For sublingual tablet
- Place the tablet under the tongue and allow it to dissolve.
- Store tablets in original bottles, and in a cool, dark place.
- Spray translingual spray against oral mucosa and do not inhale.

Sustained-release oral capsules

TYPES
- Slow onset
- Long duration

USE: Long-term prophylaxis against anginal attacks

NURSING CONSIDERATIONS
- Swallow capsules without crushing or chewing.
- Take capsules on an empty stomach with at least 8 oz of water.

Transdermal

TYPES
- Slow onset
- Long duration

USE: Long-term prophylaxis against anginal attacks

NURSING CONSIDERATIONS
- To ensure appropriate dose, patches should not be cut.
- Place the patch on a hairless area of skin (chest, back, or abdomen) and rotate sites to prevent skin irritation.
- Remove old patch, wash skin with soap and water, and dry thoroughly before applying new patch.
- Remove the patch at night to reduce the risk of developing tolerance to nitroglycerin. Be medication-free between 10 and 12 hr/day. QEBP

Topical ointment

TYPES
- Slow onset
- Long duration

USE: Long-term prophylaxis against anginal attacks

NURSING CONSIDERATIONS
- Remove the prior dose before a new dose is applied. Measure specific dose with applicator paper and spread over 2.5 to 3.5 inches of the paper.
- Apply to a clean, hairless area of the body, and cover with clear plastic wrap.
- Follow same guidelines for site selection as for transdermal patch.
- Avoid touching ointment with the hands.

Intravenous

USE
- Control of angina not responding to other medications
- Control of blood pressure or induced hypotension during surgery
- Heart failure resulting from acute MI

NURSING CONSIDERATIONS
- Administer with IV tubing supplied by manufacturer using a glass IV bottle.
- Administer continuously due to short duration of action.
- Start at a slow rate, usually 5 mcg/min, and titrate gradually until desired response is achieved.
- Provide continuous cardiac and blood pressure monitoring during administration.

TREATMENT OF ANGINAL ATTACK USING SUBLINGUAL TABLETS OR TRANSLINGUAL SPRAY

- Stop activity. Sit or lie down. QEBP
- Immediately put one sublingual tablet under the tongue and let it dissolve. Rest for 5 min.
- If pain not relieved by first tablet, call 911, then take a second tablet.
- After another 5 min, take a third tablet if pain is still not relieved. Do not take more than three sublingual tablets.
- If using nitroglycerin translingual spray, one spray substitutes for one sublingual tablet when treating an anginal attack.

CLIENT EDUCATION
- Advise clients not to stop taking long-acting nitroglycerin abruptly and follow the provider's instructions.
- Advise clients who have angina to record pain frequency, intensity, duration, and location. Notify the provider if attacks increase in frequency, intensity, and/or duration.
- Do not crush or chew oral nitroglycerin or isosorbide tablets.

NURSING EVALUATION OF MEDICATION EFFECTIVENESS

Depending on therapeutic intent, effectiveness is evidenced by the following.
- Prevention and termination of acute anginal attacks
- Long-term management of stable angina
- Control of perioperative blood pressure
- Control of heart failure following acute MI

Antianginal agent

SELECT PROTOTYPE MEDICATION: Ranolazine

PURPOSE

EXPECTED PHARMACOLOGICAL ACTION: Lowers cardiac oxygen demand and thereby improves exercise tolerance and decreases pain

THERAPEUTIC USES: Chronic stable angina in combination with amlodipine, a beta adrenergic blocker, or an organic≈nitrate

COMPLICATIONS

QT prolongation

Can increase the risk for torsades de pointes

NURSING CONSIDERATIONS
- Monitor ECG. Do not use in clients who have a prolonged QT or are taking other medications that prolong QT.
- Advise client to report palpitations, chest pain or dyspnea.

Elevated blood pressure

NURSING CONSIDERATIONS: Monitor blood pressure.

CONTRAINDICATIONS/PRECAUTIONS

- Pregnancy Risk Category C. Qs
- Ranolazine is contraindicated in clients who have QT prolongation or in clients taking other medications that can result in QT prolongation, and clients who have hepatic impairment, ventricular tachycardia, ventricular dysrhythmias, and hypokalemia.
- Use cautiously in older adult clients, and in clients who have hypotension or kidney impairment. Ⓖ

INTERACTIONS

Inhibitors of CYP3A4 can increase levels of ranolazine and lead to torsades de pointes.
- Agents include grapefruit juice, HIV protease inhibitors, macrolide antibiotics, azole antifungals, and verapamil.
- NURSING CONSIDERATIONS: Avoid concurrent use.

Quinidine and sotalol can further prolong QT interval.
NURSING CONSIDERATIONS: Avoid concurrent use.

Concurrent use of digoxin and simvastatin increases serum levels of digoxin and simvastatin.
NURSING CONSIDERATIONS
- Monitor digoxin level.
- Instruct client to report muscle weakness.

NURSING ADMINISTRATION

- Administer as an extended release oral tablet, twice daily with or without food. Do not crush or chew tablet. Qᴇʙᴾ
- Obtain baseline and monitor ECG for QT prolongation.
- Obtain baseline and monitor digoxin level with concurrent use.
- Can take concurrently with other antianginal medications, such as nitroglycerin.
- Monitor blood pressure and pulse periodically.
- Instruct clients that ranolazine is not indicated for the treatment of an acute anginal attack.

NURSING EVALUATION OF MEDICATION EFFECTIVENESS

Depending on therapeutic intent, effectiveness can be evidenced by the following.
- Prevention of acute anginal attacks
- Long-term management of stable angina

Application Exercises

1. A nurse is teaching a client who has angina pectoris and is learning how to treat acute anginal attacks. The clients asks, "What is my next step if I take one tablet, wait 5 minutes, but still have anginal pain?" Which of the following responses should the nurse make?

   A. "Take two more sublingual tablets at the same time."

   B. "Call the emergency response team."

   C. "Take a sustained-release nitroglycerin capsule."

   D. "Wait another 5 minutes then take a second sublingual tablet."

2. A nurse is teaching a client who has a new prescription for nitroglycerin transdermal patch for angina pectoris. Which of the following instructions should the nurse include?

   A. Remove the patch each evening.

   B. Cut each patch in half if angina attacks are under control.

   C. Take off the nitroglycerin patch for 30 min if a headache occurs.

   D. Apply a new patch every 48 hr.

3. A nurse is taking a medication history from a client who has angina and is to begin taking ranolazine. The nurse should report which of the following medications in the client's history that can interact with ranolazine? (Select all that apply.)

   A. Digoxin

   B. Simvastatin

   C. Verapamil

   D. Amlodipine

   E. Nitroglycerin transdermal patch

4. A nurse is caring for a client who is prescribed isosorbide mononitrate for chronic stable angina and develops reflex tachycardia. Which of the following medications should the nurse expect to administer?

   A. Furosemide

   B. Captopril

   C. Ranolazine

   D. Metoprolol

5. A nurse is teaching a client who has angina how to use nitroglycerin transdermal ointment. The nurse should include which of the following instructions?

   A. "Remove the prior dose before applying a new dose."

   B. "Rub the ointment directly into your skin until it is no longer visible."

   C. "Cover the applied ointment with a clean gauze pad."

   D. "Apply the ointment to the same skin area each time."

PRACTICE Active Learning Scenario

A nurse is caring for a client who has angina pectoris and a new prescription for oral nitroglycerin capsules. What should the nurse teach the client about this medication? Use the ATI Active Learning Template: Medication to complete this item.

THERAPEUTIC USES: Identify similarities and differences for the forms of nitroglycerin: oral, sublingual, and transdermal.

COMPLICATIONS: Identify two adverse effects of the medication.

NURSING INTERVENTIONS: Describe three nursing actions for clients taking nitroglycerin oral capsules.

Application Exercises Key

1. A. The client should not take two sublingual doses at once.

   B. **CORRECT:** The next step is to call 911 and then take a second sublingual tablet. If the first tablet does not work, the client might be having a myocardial infarction. The client can take a third tablet if the second one has not relieved the pain after waiting an additional 5 minutes.

   C. Taking an oral sustained-release capsule is not indicated to treat an acute anginal attack.

   D. The client should not wait an additional 5 minutes before taking a second tablet. The client should call 911 because he might be having a myocardial infarction.

   Ⓝ *NCLEX® Connection: Pharmacological and Parenteral Therapies, Medication Administration*

2. A. **CORRECT:** In order to prevent tolerance to nitroglycerin, the client should remove the patch for 10 to 12 hr during each 24-hr period.

   B. The client should always apply a whole patch to ensure he receives the prescribed dosage. The patches are available in many dosages.

   C. The nurse should not instruct the client to remove patches for a 30-min period if a headache occurs. The client should notify the provider if headaches do not resolve because the dose of nitroglycerin might need to be decreased.

   D. The client should apply a new patch every 24 hr.

   Ⓝ *NCLEX® Connection: Pharmacological and Parenteral Therapies, Medication Administration*

3. A. **CORRECT:** Concurrent use with ranolazine increases serum levels of digoxin, so digoxin toxicity can result.

   B. **CORRECT:** Concurrent use with ranolazine increases serum levels of simvastatin, so liver toxicity can result.

   C. **CORRECT:** Verapamil is an inhibitor of CYP3A4, which can increase levels of ranolazine and lead to the dysrhythmia torsades de pointes.

   D. Amlodipine, a calcium channel blocker, is used for hypertension and stable angina. It is prescribed along with ranolazine to treat angina.

   E. Nitroglycerin transdermal patches are prescribed along with ranolazine to treat angina.

   Ⓝ *NCLEX® Connection: Pharmacological and Parenteral Therapies, Adverse Effects/Contraindications/Side Effects/Interactions*

4. A. Furosemide, a loop diuretic, treats hypertension and edema associated with heart failure. It is not used to treat tachycardia.

   B. Captopril, an ACE inhibitor, treats hypertension or heart failure. It is not used to treat tachycardia.

   C. Ranolazine, an antianginal medication, treats stable angina pectoris. It is not used to treat tachycardia.

   D. **CORRECT:** Metoprolol, a beta adrenergic blocker, is used to treat hypertension and stable angina pectoris, and is often prescribed to decrease heart rate in clients who have tachycardia.

   Ⓝ *NCLEX® Connection: Pharmacological and Parenteral Therapies, Expected Actions/Outcomes*

5. A. **CORRECT:** The client should remove the prior dose before applying a new dose to prevent toxicity.

   B. The ointment should not be rubbed directly onto the skin. It is also important to tell the client not to touch the ointment with the fingers. The client should use the applicator that comes with the ointment to measure the correct dose and then spread the ointment onto the pre-marked paper, before applying the ointment-covered paper to the skin.

   C. The client should cover the applied ointment with a transparent dressing and tape securely to the skin. Do not cover the medication with gauze.

   D. The client should rotate application sites each time the ointment is applied. The client should select a clean, hairless area of the body.

   Ⓝ *NCLEX® Connection: Pharmacological and Parenteral Therapies, Medication Administration*

PRACTICE Answer

Using the ATI Active Learning Template: Medication

THERAPEUTIC USES: Sublingual tablets or spray are used to treat an angina attack after it begins, while the oral tablets, transdermal patch, and transdermal ointment are used for prevention of angina. The capsules and transdermal forms have a slower onset and longer duration of action than the sublingual forms. Sublingual nitroglycerin begins working within 2 min, but the duration of action is only 30 min. Oral forms are taken several times daily, but duration of action is several hours.

COMPLICATIONS: Major adverse effects include headache, dizziness caused by hypotension, and rebound tachycardia.

NURSING INTERVENTIONS
- The nurse should teach the client that the oral sustained-release form of nitroglycerin should not be used to abort an angina attack. In addition, it should be taken on an empty stomach with at least 8 oz of water and must be swallowed whole.
- The nurse should teach the client not to perform activities that require alertness if dizziness is experienced while taking oral nitroglycerin.
- The client should inform the provider if headaches are persistent because the dose of nitroglycerin might need to be decreased.
- The client should inform the provider if tachycardia occurs, because a beta-adrenergic blocker or other medication can be prescribed to slow the pulse rate.

Ⓝ *NCLEX® Connection: Pharmacological and Parenteral Therapies, Medication Administration*

UNIT 4   MEDICATIONS AFFECTING THE
CARDIOVASCULAR SYSTEM

CHAPTER 23 *Medications Affecting Cardiac Rhythm*

Medications affecting cardiac rhythm act by altering cardiac electrophysiologic function in order to treat or prevent dysrhythmias.

Electrophysiological changes can include prolonging the AV node; increasing or reducing conduction speed; altering ectopic pacemakers and SA node; reducing myocardial excitability; lengthening effective refractory period; and stimulating the autonomic nervous system.

There are four main classification groups of antidysrhythmics: sodium channel blockers, beta-adrenergic blockers, potassium channel blockers, and calcium channel blockers.

Toxicity is major concern for antidysrhythmic medications. Medication toxicity can lead to increased cardiac dysrhythmias.

Antidysrhythmic medications

CLASS I MEDICATIONS

Sodium channel blockers slow cardiac conduction velocity They are divided into three groups: IA, IB, and IC.

Class IA

SELECT PROTOTYPE MEDICATION: Procainamide (oral, IV)

OTHER MEDICATIONS
- Quinidine
- Disopyramide

Class IB

SELECT PROTOTYPE MEDICATION: Lidocaine (IV)

OTHER MEDICATIONS
- Mexiletine
- Phenytoin

Class IC

SELECT PROTOTYPE MEDICATION: Propafenone (oral)

OTHER MEDICATIONS: Flecainide

CLASS II MEDICATIONS

Beta-adrenergic blockers prevent sympathetic nervous system stimulation of the heart.

SELECT PROTOTYPE MEDICATION: Propranolol (oral, IV)

OTHER MEDICATIONS
- Esmolol
- Acebutolol

CLASS III MEDICATIONS

Potassium channel blockers prolong the action potential and refractory period of the cardiac cycle.

SELECT PROTOTYPE MEDICATION: Amiodarone (oral, IV)

OTHER MEDICATIONS
- Sotalol
- Ibutilide
- Dofetilide

CLASS IV MEDICATIONS

Calcium channel blockers prolongs cardiac conduction, depresses depolarization and decreases oxygen demand of the heart.

SELECT PROTOTYPE MEDICATION: Verapamil (oral, IV)

OTHER MEDICATIONS: Diltiazem

OTHER MEDICATIONS

- Adenosine (IV)
- Digoxin (oral, IV)

PURPOSE

Class IA

EXPECTED PHARMACOLOGICAL ACTION
- Slow impulse conductions in the atria, ventricles, and His-Purkinje system
- Delay repolarization

THERAPEUTIC USES
- Supraventricular tachycardia (SVT)
- Ventricular tachycardia
- Atrial flutter
- Atrial fibrillation

Class IB

EXPECTED PHARMACOLOGICAL ACTION
- Decrease electrical conduction
- Decrease automaticity
- Increase rate of repolarization

THERAPEUTIC USE: Short-term use only for ventricular dysrhythmias

Class IC

EXPECTED PHARMACOLOGICAL ACTION
- Decrease conduction velocity in atria, ventricles, and His-Purkinje system
- Delay ventricular repolarization

THERAPEUTIC USE: SVT

Class II

EXPECTED PHARMACOLOGICAL ACTION
- Decrease heart rate
- Decrease automaticity through the SA node, decrease velocity of conduction through the AV node, decrease myocardial contractility
- Decrease atrial ectopic stimulation

THERAPEUTIC USES: Atrial fibrillation, atrial flutter, paroxysmal SVT, hypertension, angina, PVCs

Class III

EXPECTED PHARMACOLOGICAL ACTION
- Delays repolarization
- Prolongs action potential
- Reduced automaticity in the SA node
- Reduced contractility and conduction in the AV node, ventricles, and His-Purkinje system
- Dilates coronary blood vessels

THERAPEUTIC USES
- Conversion of atrial fibrillation: oral route
- Recurrent ventricular fibrillation
- Recurrent ventricular tachycardia
- Atrial flutter

Class IV calcium channel blockers, verapamil, diltiazem

EXPECTED PHARMACOLOGICAL ACTION
- Decrease force of contraction
- Decrease heart rate
- Slow rate of conduction through the SA and AV nodes

THERAPEUTIC USES
- Atrial fibrillation and flutter
- SVT
- Hypertension
- Angina pectoris

Adenosine

EXPECTED PHARMACOLOGICAL ACTION: Decrease electrical conduction through AV node

THERAPEUTIC USES
- Paroxysmal SVT
- Wolff-Parkinson-White syndrome

Digoxin

EXPECTED PHARMACOLOGICAL ACTION
- Decrease electrical conduction through AV node
- Increase myocardial contraction

THERAPEUTIC USES: Heart failure, atrial fibrillation and flutter, paroxysmal SVT

COMPLICATIONS

PROCAINAMIDE

Systemic lupus syndrome

Fever, painful and swollen joints, butterfly-shaped rash on face

NURSING CONSIDERATIONS
- Manifestations resolve with discontinuation of medication.
- Control effects with NSAIDs.
- Monitor for nuclear antibody titers (ANA). If ANA titer is present and increases, discontinue medication.

Neutropenia and thrombocytopenia

NURSING CONSIDERATIONS
- Monitor weekly complete blood counts for the first 12 weeks, then periodically. Qs
- Monitor for indications of infection and bleeding. Stop medication if there is evidence of bone marrow suppression.

Cardiotoxicity

Widening of the QRS by more than 50%, increasing of the QT interval, and prolonging of the PR interval are indications of procainamide cardiotoxicity.

NURSING CONSIDERATIONS
- Monitor medication levels (therapeutic procainamide level is 4 to 10 mcg/mL).
- Monitor for other manifestations of toxicity, such as confusion, drowsiness, and vomiting.
- Monitor vital signs and ECG.
- If dysrhythmias occur, hold medication and contact the provider.

Hypotension

NURSING CONSIDERATIONS: Monitor blood pressure. Might need to withhold medication for hypotension.

LIDOCAINE

CNS effects

Drowsiness, altered mental status, paresthesias, seizures

NURSING CONSIDERATIONS
- Carefully monitor clients and notify the provider if manifestations occur.
- Administer phenytoin to control seizure activity.

Respiratory arrest

NURSING CONSIDERATIONS
- Monitor vital signs and ECG.
- Ensure resuscitation equipment ready at bedside. Qs

PROPAFENONE

Bradycardia, heart failure, dizziness, weakness, hypotension, bronchospasm

NURSING CONSIDERATIONS: Monitor heart rate, blood pressure. Monitor for chest pain, dyspnea, crackles, weight gain, or edema.

PROPRANOLOL

Hypotension, bradycardia, heart failure, AV block, fatigue, bronchospasm in clients who have asthma

NURSING CONSIDERATIONS
- Monitor blood pressure and heart rate. Monitor for chest pain, dyspnea, crackles, weight gain, or edema. Check apical pulse prior to dosage.
- Notify provider for pulse rate less than 50/min, or other prescribed rate.

AMIODARONE

Pulmonary toxicity

NURSING CONSIDERATIONS
- Obtain baseline chest x-ray and pulmonary function tests.
- Continue to monitor pulmonary function through course of therapy.
- Advise clients to observe for dyspnea, cough, and chest pain.
- Notify the provider if effects occur.

Sinus bradycardia and AV block

Can lead to heart failure

NURSING CONSIDERATIONS
- Monitor blood pressure and ECG.
- Monitor for indications of heart failure (dyspnea, cough, chest pain, neck vein distention, crackles) and notify the provider if they occur.
- If AV block occurs, medication should be discontinued. Insert a pacemaker if indicated.
- Discontinue medication if indicated.

Visual disturbances

Photophobia, blurred vision, can lead to blindness

NURSING CONSIDERATIONS: Advise clients to report visual disturbances.

Other effects

Can include liver and thyroid dysfunction, GI disturbances, CNS effects, photosensitivity, and blue-gray discoloration to skin

NURSING CONSIDERATIONS
- Obtain baseline liver and thyroid function and monitor periodically.
- Advise clients to avoid sun lamps, and wear sunscreen and protective clothing.
- Advise clients to observe for manifestations, and report to the provider if they occur.

Phlebitis with IV administration

NURSING CONSIDERATIONS: Use of central venous catheter is indicated. Qs

Hypotension, bradycardia, AV block

NURSING CONSIDERATIONS: Monitor cardiac status and blood pressure.

VERAPAMIL

Bradycardia, hypotension, heart failure, constipation, peripheral edema

NURSING CONSIDERATIONS
- Monitor ECG and blood pressure. Treat severe hypotension with IV fluid therapy, modified Trendelenburg position, or IV calcium gluconate.
- Reduce dose in clients who have a history of heart failure. Increase fiber and fluids as prescribed. Monitor for chest pain, dyspnea, crackles, weight gain, or edema. Check apical pulse prior to dosage.
- Notify provider for pulse rate less than 50/min, or other prescribed rate.

ADENOSINE

Sinus bradycardia, hypotension, dyspnea, vasodilation

Sinus bradycardia (decreased conduction through AV node), hypotension, dyspnea (bronchoconstriction), flushing of face (vasodilation)

NURSING CONSIDERATIONS
- Monitor ECG. Effects usually last 1 min or less.
- Monitor for manifestations, and notify the provider if they occur.

DIGOXIN

Bradycardia, hypotension, toxicity

NURSING CONSIDERATIONS
- Monitor apical heart rate. Hold dose for heart rate less than 60/min.
- Monitor digoxin level. Optimal therapeutic level is 0.5 to 0.8 ng/mL.
- Monitor for indications of digoxin toxicity: anorexia, nausea, vomiting, visual disturbances, dysrhythmias
- Monitor potassium level. Hypokalemia increases risk for toxicity; keep potassium level between 3.5 and 5.0 mEq/L.

CONTRAINDICATIONS/PRECAUTIONS

Procainamide

- Pregnancy Risk Category C.
- Contraindicated in clients who have hypersensitivity to procaine or quinidine, complete heart block, atypical ventricular tachycardia, and systemic lupus erythematosus.
- Use cautiously in clients who have partial AV block, myasthenia gravis, liver or kidney disorders, heart failure, and digoxin toxicity.

Lidocaine

- Pregnancy Risk Category B.
- Contraindicated in clients who have Stokes-Adams syndrome, Wolff-Parkinson-White syndrome, and severe heart block.
- Use cautiously in clients who have liver and kidney dysfunction, second-degree heart block, sinus bradycardia, and heart failure.

Propafenone

- Pregnancy Risk Category C.
- Contraindicated in clients who have AV block, severe heart failure, severe hypotension, and cardiogenic shock.
- Use cautiously in older adult clients and clients who have heart failure, liver or kidney dysfunction, and chronic respiratory disorders.

Propranolol

- Pregnancy Risk Category C.
- Contraindicated in clients who have greater than first-degree AV block, heart failure, and bradycardia.
- Use cautiously in clients who have Wolff-Parkinson-White syndrome; diabetes mellitus; or liver, thyroid, or respiratory dysfunction.

Amiodarone

- Pregnancy Risk Category D.
- Contraindicated in newborns, infants, and clients who have AV block and bradycardia.
- Use cautiously in clients who have liver, thyroid, or respiratory dysfunction; heart failure; and fluid and electrolyte imbalances.

Verapamil

- Pregnancy Risk Category C.
- Contraindicated in clients who have greater than first-degree AV block (unless they have a working pacemaker), atrial fib/flutter, severe heart failure, and severe hypotension.
- IV form is contraindicated in ventricular tachycardia and for clients taking beta blockers.
- Use cautiously in clients who have liver or kidney dysfunction, heart failure, hypotension, or are taking digoxin or beta blockers.

Adenosine

- Pregnancy Risk Category C.
- Contraindicated in clients who have second- and third-degree heart block, AV block, atrial flutter, and atrial fibrillation.
- Use cautiously in older adults and clients who have asthma.

Digoxin

- Pregnancy Risk Category C.
- Contraindicated in clients who have ventricular tachycardia or ventricular fibrillation not caused by heart failure.
- Use cautiously in clients who have AV block, bradycardia, kidney disease, hypothyroidism, and cardiomyopathy.

INTERACTIONS

Procainamide

Antidysrhythmics have additive effects and can increase the risk for toxicity.
NURSING CONSIDERATIONS
- Monitor heart rate and rhythm.
- Notify the provider of change or start of new dysrhythmia.

Beta blockers, cimetidine, and ranitidine can increase procainamide effects.
NURSING CONSIDERATIONS: Avoid concurrent use. Monitor ECG and blood pressure. Reduce dose if needed.

Antihypertensives have an additive hypotensive effect.
NURSING CONSIDERATIONS: Monitor blood pressure and notify the provider if there is a significant decrease.

Lidocaine

Cimetidine, beta blockers, and phenytoin can decrease metabolism of lidocaine, increasing risk of toxicity.
NURSING CONSIDERATIONS
- Monitor client for CNS depression (sedation, irritability, seizures).
- Monitor lidocaine level. Reduce dosage.

Propafenone

Propafenone can slow medication metabolism and cause an increase in the levels of digoxin, oral anticoagulants, and propranolol.
NURSING CONSIDERATIONS
- Monitor for medication toxicity.
- Monitor coagulation.

Quinidine and amiodarone increase risk of propafenone toxicity.
NURSING CONSIDERATIONS: Do not use concurrently.

Grapefruit juice can reduce propafenone metabolism and cause toxicity.
NURSING CONSIDERATIONS: Advise clients to avoid grapefruit juice.

Propranolol

Verapamil and diltiazem have additive cardiosuppression effects.
NURSING CONSIDERATIONS: Monitor ECG, heart rate, and blood pressure.

Propranolol use can mask the hypoglycemic effect of insulin and prevent the breakdown of fat in response to hypoglycemia.
NURSING CONSIDERATIONS: Use with caution. Monitor blood glucose levels.

Amiodarone

Amiodarone can increase plasma levels of quinidine, procainamide, digoxin, diltiazem, and warfarin.
NURSING CONSIDERATIONS: Lower dosages of these medications. Monitor ECG.

Cholestyramine decreases levels of amiodarone.
NURSING CONSIDERATIONS: Monitor for therapeutic effects.

Diuretics, other antidysrhythmics, and antibiotics (erythromycin, azithromycin) can increase the risk of dysrhythmias
NURSING CONSIDERATIONS: Use cautiously with clients taking these medications.

Concurrent use of beta blockers, verapamil, and diltiazem can lead to bradycardia.
NURSING CONSIDERATIONS: Monitor clients closely.

Propranolol can increase digoxin level.
NURSING CONSIDERATIONS: Monitor digoxin level. Monitor heart rate.

Consuming grapefruit juice can lead to toxicity.
NURSING CONSIDERATIONS: Advise clients to avoid drinking grapefruit juice. Qs

Verapamil

Concurrent use of atenolol, esmolol, or propranolol can cause additive effects of both medications.
NURSING CONSIDERATIONS: Monitor ECG. Reduce dosages if needed.

Verapamil can potentiate carbamazepine and digoxin. Increased risk for heart block with concurrent use with digoxin.
NURSING CONSIDERATIONS: Monitor medication levels, heart rate, and ECG.

Beta blockers can cause heart failure, AV block, and bradycardia.
NURSING CONSIDERATIONS: Monitor heart rate and ECG; monitor for heart failure. Use caution.

Grapefruit juice can reduce verapamil metabolism and cause toxicity.
NURSING CONSIDERATIONS: Advise clients to avoid grapefruit juice.

Adenosine

Methylxanthines, such as theophylline and caffeine, block receptors for adenosine and therefore prevent therapeutic effect.
NURSING CONSIDERATIONS: Avoid concurrent use.

Cellular uptake of dipyridamole is blocked, leading to intensification of effects of adenosine.
NURSING CONSIDERATIONS: Monitor for indications of excessive dosage, and notify the provider if these occur.

Digoxin

Amiodarone, quinidine, verapamil, diltiazem, propafenone, and flecainide are antidysrhythmics, which increase digoxin levels.
NURSING CONSIDERATIONS: Monitor for medication level and for toxicity. Reduce medication dosage if needed.

Corticosteroids, diuretics, thiazides, and amphotericin B can cause decreased potassium level.
NURSING CONSIDERATIONS: Monitor potassium and monitor medication levels for toxicity.

Antacids and metoclopramide can decrease digoxin absorption.
NURSING CONSIDERATIONS
- Monitor blood levels and effective response.
- Give dosages at wide intervals.

NURSING ADMINISTRATION

Procainamide

CLIENT EDUCATION
- Advise clients to take medications as prescribed.
- Advise clients not crush or chew sustained-released preparations.

Lidocaine

NURSING CONSIDERATIONS
- IV administration is usually started with a loading dose, which is weight-based, followed by a maintenance dose of 1 to 4 mg/min.
- Adjust the rate according to cardiac response.
- Usually used for no more than 24 hr.
- Never administer lidocaine preparation that contains epinephrine (usually in lidocaine used for local anesthesia). Severe hypertension or dysrhythmias can occur. Qs

Propafenone

NURSING CONSIDERATIONS
- Monitor ECG during treatment.
- Monitor for bradycardia and hypotension. Monitor for dizziness or weakness.
- Instruct clients to take the medication with food.

Propranolol

NURSING CONSIDERATIONS

- Instruct clients to check pulse daily and notify the provider for pulse rate less than 50/min, or other prescribed rate.
- Administer IV propranolol no faster than 1 mg/min.

Amiodarone

NURSING CONSIDERATIONS

- Amiodarone is highly toxic. Monitor closely for adverse effects.
- Inform clients that adverse effects can continue for an extended period of time after the medication is discontinued.
- Provide clients with written information regarding potential toxicities.

Verapamil

NURSING CONSIDERATIONS

- Monitor heart rate before doses and notify provider for HR less than 50/min. Verapamil can cause orthostatic hypotension. Advise clients to change positions slowly. Client might need to lie flat until dizziness subsides.
- Avoid activities that require alertness until effects are known.
- Advise clients to notify the provider for peripheral edema, chest pain, or shortness of breath.

Adenosine

NURSING CONSIDERATIONS

- Adenosine has a very short half-life, so adverse reactions are mild and last for less than 1 min.
- Administration should be by IV bolus, flushed with saline following administration. Q EBP

Digoxin

CLIENT EDUCATION

- Instruct clients to take apical pulse for 1 min before taking a dose. If the heart rate is less than 60/min, the client should hold the dose and notify the provider.
- Advise clients to eat a high-potassium diet.

NURSING EVALUATION OF MEDICATION EFFECTIVENESS

Depending on therapeutic intent, effectiveness is evidenced by the following.
- Improvement of manifestations (chest pain, shortness of breath, bradycardia, or tachycardia)
- Absence of dysrhythmias
- Return to baseline ECG, heart rate, and regular rhythm

Application Exercises

1. A nurse is assessing a client who is taking amiodarone to treat atrial fibrillation. Which of the following findings is a manifestation of amiodarone toxicity?

   A. Light yellow urine

   B. Report of tinnitus

   C. Productive cough

   D. Blue-gray skin discoloration

2. A nurse is caring for a client who received IV verapamil to treat supraventricular tachycardia (SVT). The client's pulse rate is now 98/min and his blood pressure is 74/44 mg Hg. The nurse should anticipate a prescription for which of the following IV medications?

   A. Calcium gluconate

   B. Sodium bicarbonate

   C. Potassium chloride

   D. Magnesium sulfate

3. A nurse is assessing a client who is taking digoxin to treat heart failure. Which of the following findings is a manifestation of digoxin toxicity?

   A. Bruising

   B. Report of metallic taste

   C. Muscle pain

   D. Report of anorexia

4. A nurse is assessing a client who has taken procainamide to treat dysrhythmias for the last 12 months. The nurse should assess the client for which of the following adverse effects of this medication? (Select all that apply.)

   A. Hypertension

   B. Widened QRS complex

   C. Narrowed QT interval

   D. Easy bruising

   E. Swollen joints

5. A nurse is preparing to administer propranolol to a client who has a dysrhythmia. Which of the following actions should the nurse plan to take?

   A. Hold propranolol for an apical pulse greater than 100/min.

   B. Administer propranolol to increase the client's blood pressure.

   C. Assist the client when she sits up or stands after taking this medication.

   D. Check for hypokalemia frequently due to the risk for propranolol toxicity.

PRACTICE Active Learning Scenario

A nurse is preparing to provide teaching to a client who has a new prescription for verapamil for recurrent supraventricular tachycardia. What should the nurse teach the client about this medication? Use the ATI Active Learning Template: Medication to complete this item.

THERAPEUTIC USES

COMPLICATIONS: Identify three adverse effects.

NURSING INTERVENTIONS: Describe three, including diagnostic tests the nurse should monitor.

Application Exercises Key

1. A. Light yellow urine is an expected finding and does not indicate toxicity.

   B. Ototoxicity can occur with aminoglycoside antibiotics, but does not indicate amiodarone toxicity.

   C. **CORRECT:** Productive cough can indicate pulmonary toxicity or heart failure. The nurse should assess for cough, chest pain, and shortness of breath.

   D. A blue-gray skin discoloration can occur in clients who are taking amiodarone with sun exposure and should resolve.

   Ⓝ *NCLEX® Connection: Pharmacological and Parenteral Therapies, Adverse Effects/Contraindications/Side Effects/Interactions*

2. A. **CORRECT:** Reverse severe hypotension caused by verapamil with calcium gluconate, given slowly IV. The calcium counteracts vasodilation caused by verapamil. Other measures to increase blood pressure can include IV fluid therapy and placing the client in a modified Trendelenburg position.

   B. IV sodium bicarbonate is used to treat metabolic acidosis. It is not used to increase blood pressure in clients who have received verapamil.

   C. IV potassium chloride is used to treat hypokalemia. It is not used to increase blood pressure in clients who have received verapamil.

   D. IV magnesium sulfate is used to treat ventricular dysrhythmias, such as torsades de pointe. It is not used to increase blood pressure in clients who have received verapamil.

   Ⓝ *NCLEX® Connection: Pharmacological and Parenteral Therapies, Expected Actions/Outcomes*

3. A. Bruising is an adverse effect of anticoagulants and antiplatelet medications.

   B. Metallic taste is an adverse effect of captopril and certain antibiotics.

   C. Weakness is a manifestation of digoxin toxicity, not muscle pain.

   D. **CORRECT:** Anorexia, blurred vision, stomach pain, and diarrhea are manifestations of digoxin toxicity.

   Ⓝ *NCLEX® Connection: Pharmacological and Parenteral Therapies, Adverse Effects/Contraindications/Side Effects/Interactions*

4. A. Hypotension, rather than hypertension, is an adverse effect of procainamide.

   B. **CORRECT:** On the ECG, procainamide can cause a widened QRS complex, which is a manifestation of cardiotoxicity if the QRS complex becomes widened by more than 50% of the expected reference range.

   C. On the ECG, procainamide can cause a prolonged QT interval, a manifestation of cardiotoxicity.

   D. **CORRECT:** Procainamide can cause bone marrow depression, with neutropenia (infection) and thrombocytopenia (easy bruising, bleeding).

   E. **CORRECT:** Systemic lupus erythematosus-like syndrome can occur as an adverse effect of procainamide. Manifestations include swollen, painful joints. Clients who take procainamide in large doses or for more than 1 year are at risk.

   Ⓝ *NCLEX® Connection: Pharmacological and Parenteral Therapies, Adverse Effects/Contraindications/Side Effects/Interactions*

5. A. Propranolol is a beta-adrenergic blocker that is used to slow tachydysrhythmias. The nurse should not hold the medication for a pulse greater than 100/min, but should hold it for a very low pulse rate, such as less than 50/min.

   B. Propranolol is used to treat hypertension and is not administered to increase the client's blood pressure.

   C. **CORRECT:** Propranolol can cause orthostatic hypotension, so it is important assess for dizziness during ambulation or when moving to a sitting position.

   D. Propranolol can increase potassium level. The client is at risk for toxicity with digoxin, rather than propranolol, when the serum potassium is low.

   Ⓝ *NCLEX® Connection: Pharmacological and Parenteral Therapies, Medication Administration*

PRACTICE Answer

Using the ATI Active Learning Template: Medication

THERAPEUTIC USES: Verapamil is a calcium channel blocker and a class IV antidysrhythmic medication that decreases heart rate, slows conduction through both the SA and AV nodes, and decreases force of contraction of the heart. It is used to treat supraventricular tachycardia (SVT).

COMPLICATIONS
- Bradycardia
- Hypotension
- Heart failure
- Constipation

NURSING INTERVENTIONS
- Monitor both kidney and liver function because the medication dosage might need to be lowered if either kidney or liver impairment are present.
- Monitor blood pressure and pulse.
- Monitor periodic ECG testing for dysrhythmias and for improvement of SVT.
- Assess for manifestations of heart failure, such as dyspnea and crackles in the lungs.
- Question the client about dizziness, which can occur due to hypotension.
- Teach the client to move slowly from lying to sitting or standing and to avoid driving or operating heavy machinery until effects of verapamil are known.

Ⓝ *NCLEX® Connection: Pharmacological and Parenteral Therapies, Medication Administration*

UNIT 4   MEDICATIONS AFFECTING THE
CARDIOVASCULAR SYSTEM

CHAPTER 24 *Antilipemic Agents*

Antilipemic agents work in different ways to help lower low-density lipoprotein (LDL) cholesterol levels, raise high-density lipoprotein (HDL) cholesterol levels, and possibly decrease very low-density lipoprotein (VLDL) levels. These medications should be used along with lifestyle modifications such as regular activity, diet, and weight control.

Prior to starting these medications, the client should have lab work including baseline levels of total cholesterol, LDL cholesterol, HDL cholesterol, and triglycerides. These blood values should be monitored periodically throughout the course of therapy. In addition, baseline liver and kidney function tests should be obtained and monitored periodically.

Medications are not considered first-line therapy for coronary artery disease and should only be used if lifestyle changes do not reduce the LDL cholesterol to an acceptable level.

Medication classifications include HMG-CoA reductase inhibitors (statins), cholesterol absorption inhibitors, bile-acid sequestrants, nicotinic acid, fibrates, and antisense oligonucleotide.

HMG-CoA reductase inhibitors (statins)

SELECT PROTOTYPE MEDICATION: Atorvastatin

OTHER MEDICATIONS
- Simvastatin
- Lovastatin
- Pravastatin
- Rosuvastatin
- Fluvastatin
- Pitavastatin

COMBINATION MEDICATIONS
- Simvastatin and ezetimibe
- Simvastatin and niacin
- Lovastatin and niacin

PURPOSE

EXPECTED PHARMACOLOGICAL ACTIONS
- Decrease manufacture of LDL and VLDL cholesterol.
- Increase manufacture of HDL.
- Other beneficial effects include promotion of vasodilation, and decrease in plaque site inflammation, thromboembolism, and risk of atrial fibrillation.

THERAPEUTIC USES
- Primary hypercholesterolemia
- Prevention of coronary events (primary and secondary)
- Protection against myocardial infarction (MI) and stroke for clients who have diabetes mellitus
- Increasing levels of HDL in clients who have primary hypercholesterolemia
- Primary prevention in clients who have normal LDL

COMPLICATIONS

Hepatotoxicity

Evidenced by increase in aspartate transaminase (AST)

NURSING CONSIDERATIONS
- Obtain baseline liver function.
- Monitor liver function tests after 12 weeks and then every 6 months.
- Advise clients to observe for indications of liver dysfunction (anorexia, vomiting, nausea, jaundice), and to notify the provider if manifestations occur.
- Advise clients to avoid alcohol.
- Medication might be discontinued if liver function tests are above the expected reference range.

Myopathy

- Evidenced by muscle aches, pain, and tenderness
- Can progress to myositis or rhabdomyolysis

NURSING CONSIDERATIONS
- Obtain baseline creatine kinase (CK) level.
- Monitor CK levels periodically while on treatment.
- Advise clients to report muscle aches, pain, and tenderness.
- Medication might be discontinued if CK levels are elevated.

CONTRAINDICATIONS/PRECAUTIONS
- Pregnancy Risk Category X. Qs
- Contraindicated in clients who have a liver disorder or are breastfeeding.
- For clients of Asian descent, rosuvastatin should be avoided or prescribed in a smaller dose than for other clients.
- Use cautiously in clients who have previously had liver disease, acute infections, electrolyte imbalance, or severe metabolic disorders. Dosage of several statins (lovastatin, pitavastatin, pravastatin, rosuvastatin, and simvastatin) should be reduced for clients who have severe kidney impairment.

INTERACTIONS

Fibrates (gemfibrozil, fenofibrate) and ezetimibe increase the risk of myopathy.
NURSING CONSIDERATIONS
- Obtain baseline CK level.
- Monitor CK levels periodically during treatment.
- Advise clients to report muscle aches and pain.
- Medication might be discontinued if CK levels are elevated.

Medications that suppress CYP3A4, such as erythromycin and ketoconazole, along with HIV protease inhibitors, amiodarone, and cyclosporine can increase levels of some statins when taken concurrently.
NURSING CONSIDERATIONS
- Avoid atorvastatin, lovastatin, and simvastatin.
- Dosage of statin might need to be decreased.
- Advise clients to inform the provider of all medications currently taken.

Grapefruit juice suppresses CYP3A4 and can increase levels of statins.
NURSING CONSIDERATIONS: Clients taking statins should avoid grapefruit and grapefruit juice.

NURSING ADMINISTRATION

- Administer statins via oral route.
- Administer lovastatin with evening meal. Other statins can be taken without food, but evening dosing is best because most cholesterol is synthesized during the night. Q**EBP**
- Atorvastatin or fluvastatin should be used in clients who have impaired kidney function. For other statins, dosages will be reduced.
- Advise clients about the importance of obtaining baseline cholesterol, HDL, LDL, and triglyceride levels, as well as liver and kidney function tests, and monitoring periodically during treatment.

Cholesterol absorption inhibitor

SELECT PROTOTYPE MEDICATION: Ezetimibe

PURPOSE

EXPECTED PHARMACOLOGICAL ACTION

Ezetimibe inhibits absorption of cholesterol secreted in the bile and from food.

THERAPEUTIC USES

- Clients who have modified diets can use this medication as an adjunct to help lower LDL cholesterol.
- Medication can be used alone or in combination with a statin medication.

COMPLICATIONS

Hepatitis

NURSING CONSIDERATIONS
- Obtain baseline liver function.
- Advise clients to observe for liver dysfunction (anorexia, vomiting, nausea, jaundice) and to notify the provider if effects occur.
- Advise clients to avoid alcohol.
- Medication might be discontinued if liver function tests are abnormal.

Myopathy

NURSING CONSIDERATIONS
- Obtain baseline CK level.
- Monitor CK levels periodically while on treatment.
- Advise clients to notify the provider if manifestations such as muscle aches and pains occur.
- Medication might be discontinued if CK levels are elevated.

CONTRAINDICATIONS/PRECAUTIONS

- Pregnancy Risk Category X. Q**s**
- Contraindicated in clients who have active moderate-to-severe liver disorders, especially those taking a statin concurrently.
- Use caution in older adults and in clients who have mild liver disorders. Ⓖ

INTERACTIONS

Bile acid sequestrants, such as cholestyramine, interfere with absorption.
NURSING CONSIDERATIONS: Advise clients to take ezetimibe 1 hr before or 4 hr after taking bile sequestrants.

Statins, such as atorvastatin, can increase the risk of liver dysfunction and myopathy.
NURSING CONSIDERATIONS
- Obtain baseline liver function tests and monitor periodically. Advise clients to observe for indications of liver damage (anorexia, vomiting, nausea). The provider should be notified, and the medication will most likely be discontinued.
- Advise clients to notify the provider of manifestations such as muscle aches and pains.
- Medication might be discontinued if CK levels are elevated.

Concurrent use with fibrates, such as gemfibrozil, increases the risk of cholelithiasis and myopathy.
NURSING CONSIDERATIONS: Ezetimibe is not recommended for use with fibrates.

Levels of ezetimibe can be increased with concurrent use of cyclosporine.
NURSING CONSIDERATIONS: Monitor for adverse effects (liver damage, myopathy).

NURSING ADMINISTRATION

- Advise the client to report muscle aches and pain.
- Medication might be discontinued if CK levels are elevated.
- Advise clients about the importance of obtaining baseline cholesterol, HDL, LDL, and triglyceride levels, as well as liver and kidney function tests, and monitor periodically during treatment.
- Advise clients to follow a low-fat, low-cholesterol diet and to get involved in a regular exercise regimen. Qᴘᴄᴄ
- Clients can take this medication in a fixed-dose combination with simvastatin.

Bile-acid sequestrants

SELECT PROTOTYPE MEDICATION: Colesevelam

OTHER MEDICATION: Colestipol

PURPOSE

EXPECTED PHARMACOLOGICAL ACTION: Decrease in LDL cholesterol

THERAPEUTIC USE: May be used alone or as an adjunct with a HMG-CoA reductase inhibitor, such as atorvastatin, and with dietary measures to lower cholesterol levels.

COMPLICATIONS

Constipation

NURSING CONSIDERATIONS: Advise clients to increase the intake of high-fiber food and oral fluids, if not restricted.

CONTRAINDICATIONS/PRECAUTIONS

- Colesevelam is Pregnancy Risk Category B. Colestipol is Pregnancy Risk Category C. Qs
- Colesevelam is contraindicated in clients who have bowel obstruction or pancreatitis caused by high triglycerides.
- Use cautiously in clients who have biliary disorders and diabetes mellitus, and in older adults. Ⓖ

INTERACTIONS

Bile-acid sequestrants interfere with absorption of many medications, including levothyroxine; second-generation sulfonylureas, such as glipizide; phenytoin; fat-soluble vitamins (A, D, E, K); and oral contraceptives. They also form insoluble complexes with thiazide diuretics, digoxin, and warfarin.

CLIENT EDUCATION
- Advise clients to take other medications 4 hr before taking bile sequestrants.
- Advise clients to inform the provider of all medications currently taken.

NURSING ADMINISTRATION

- Colesevelam is taken orally in tablet form. It should be taken with food and 8 oz of water, and not concurrently with other medications. Qᴇʙᴘ
- Colestipol is supplied as oral tablet that should not be crushed or chewed. Give 30 min before a meal.
- Colestipol is also supplied in a powder formulation. Advise clients to use an adequate amount of fluid (4 to 8 oz) to dissolve the medication. This will prevent irritation or impaction of the esophagus.

Nicotinic acid, niacin

PURPOSE

EXPECTED PHARMACOLOGICAL ACTION

Decrease in LDL cholesterol and triglyceride levels

THERAPEUTIC USES

- For clients at risk for pancreatitis and elevated triglyceride levels
- Lower elevated LDL cholesterol and triglycerides, and raise HDL levels

COMPLICATIONS

GI distress

Usually self-limiting

CLIENT EDUCATION: Advise client to take with food.

Facial flushing and feeling of warmth, tingling of hands and feet (temporary)

CLIENT EDUCATION: Advise client to take aspirin 30 min before each dose.

Hyperglycemia

NURSING CONSIDERATIONS: Monitor blood glucose levels.

Hepatotoxicity

NURSING CONSIDERATIONS
- Obtain baseline liver function tests and monitor periodically.
- Advise clients to observe for indications of liver dysfunction (anorexia, vomiting, nausea, jaundice), and to notify the provider if these occur.
- Medication might be discontinued if liver function tests are abnormal.

Hyperuricemia

NURSING CONSIDERATIONS
- Monitor kidney function, BUN, and creatinine, I&O.
- Encourage adequate fluid intake of 2 to 3 L of water each day from food and beverage sources unless contraindicated.
- Administer allopurinol if uric acid level is elevated.

CONTRAINDICATIONS/PRECAUTIONS

- Pregnancy Risk Category C. Qs
- Contraindicated in clients who have liver disease and gout.
- Use cautiously in clients who have diabetes mellitus, asymptomatic hyperuricemia, and peptic ulcer disease.

NURSING ADMINISTRATION

- Administer by oral route, either in tablet or liquid form. Tablet can be standard form or time-released.
  - Administer standard form three times a day with or after meals. QEBP
  - Administer time-released formulations once in the evening.
- Advise clients that dosage is much larger than dosage when taken as vitamin supplement.

Fibrates

SELECT PROTOTYPE MEDICATION: Gemfibrozil

OTHER MEDICATIONS: Fenofibrate

PURPOSE

EXPECTED PHARMACOLOGICAL ACTION

- Decrease in triglyceride levels (increase in VLDL excretion for clients unable to lower triglyceride levels with lifestyle modification or other antilipemic medications)
- Increase in HDL levels by promoting production of precursors to HDLs

THERAPEUTIC USES

- Reduction of plasma triglycerides (VLDL)
- Increased levels of HDL

COMPLICATIONS

GI distress

Usually mild and self-limiting

Gallstones

CLIENT EDUCATION
- Advise clients to observe for indications of gallbladder disease (right upper quadrant pain, fat intolerance, bloating).
- Advise clients to notify the provider if manifestations occur.

Myopathy (muscle tenderness, pain)

- Obtain baseline CK level.
- Monitor CK levels periodically during treatment.
- Monitor for muscle aches, pain, and tenderness, and notify the provider if adverse effects occur.
- Stop medication if CK levels are elevated.

Hepatotoxicity

NURSING CONSIDERATIONS
- Obtain baseline liver function tests, and monitor periodically.
- Advise clients to observe for indications of liver dysfunction (anorexia, vomiting, nausea, jaundice), and to notify the provider if manifestations occur.
- Stop medication if liver function tests are abnormal.

CONTRAINDICATIONS/PRECAUTIONS

- Pregnancy Risk Category C Qs
- Contraindicated in clients who have liver disorders, severe kidney dysfunction, and gallbladder disease

INTERACTIONS

With concurrent use, warfarin increases the risk of bleeding.
NURSING CONSIDERATIONS
- Obtain baseline prothrombin time (PT) and INR, and perform periodic monitoring.
- Advise clients to report indications of bleeding (bruising, bleeding gums), and notify the provider if these occur.

Statins increase the risk of myopathy.
NURSING CONSIDERATIONS: Avoid using concurrently.

NURSING ADMINISTRATION

- Administer via oral route.
- Advise clients to take medication 30 min prior to breakfast and dinner. QEBP

Antisense oligonucleotide

SELECT PROTOTYPE MEDICATION: Mipomersen

PURPOSE

EXPECTED PHARMACOLOGICAL ACTION: Inhibits synthesis of apolipoprotein B-100 and thus decreases LDL, non-HDL, total cholesterol, and apolipoprotein B.

THERAPEUTIC USES: Reduces cholesterol levels in clients who have homozygous familial hypercholesterolemia

COMPLICATIONS

Liver toxicity

NURSING CONSIDERATIONS: Baseline ALT, AST, alkaline phosphatase, and total bilirubin should be checked before beginning medication and regularly during therapy.

CLIENT EDUCATION: Advise the client to avoid alcohol consumption while taking this medication.

Flu-like manifestations, nausea, headache

CLIENT EDUCATION: Instruct the client to report manifestations to provider.

Hypertension

NURSING CONSIDERATIONS: Monitor blood pressure regularly while taking this medication.

Musculoskeletal pain

CLIENT EDUCATION: Instruct the client to report pain to the provider.

CONTRAINDICATIONS/PRECAUTIONS

- Pregnancy Risk Category B
- Use caution in older adults (increased risk for hypertension, hepatic injury). Ⓒ
- Use caution in clients who are breastfeeding or have kidney disease. Qs

INTERACTIONS

Acetaminophen, methotrexate, tetracyclines, and tamoxifen increase levels of mipomersen and can increase risk for liver damage.
NURSING CONSIDERATIONS
- Review client medications with the provider.
- Teach the client to use an alternative to acetaminophen for mild pain relief.

NURSING ADMINISTRATION

- Administered subcutaneously into the abdomen, thigh, or outer arm once weekly on the same day of the week. Q EBP
- For missed doses, give the missed dose at least 3 days before the next dose is due.

Application Exercises

1. A nurse is providing teaching to a client who is starting simvastatin. Which of the following information should the nurse include in the teaching?
   - A. Take this medication in the evening.
   - B. Change position slowly when rising from a chair.
   - C. Maintain a steady intake of green leafy vegetables.
   - D. Consume no more than 1 L/day of fluid.

2. A nurse is collecting data from a client who is taking gemfibrozil. Which of the following assessment findings should the nurse identify as an adverse reaction to the medication?
   - A. Mental status changes
   - B. Tremor
   - C. Jaundice
   - D. Pneumonia

3. A nurse is teaching a client who is taking digoxin and has a new prescription for colesevelam. Which of the following instructions should the nurse include in the teaching?
   - A. "Take digoxin with your morning dose of colesevelam."
   - B. "Your sodium and potassium levels will be monitored periodically while taking colesevelam."
   - C. "Watch for bleeding or bruising while taking colesevelam."
   - D. "Take colesevelam with food and at least one glass of water."

4. A nurse is completing a nursing history for a client who takes simvastatin. The nurse should identify which of the following disorders as a contraindication to adding ezetimibe to the client's medications?
   - A. History of severe constipation
   - B. History of hypertension
   - C. Active hepatitis C
   - D. Type 2 diabetes mellitus

5. A nurse is caring for a client who has a new prescription for niacin to reduce cholesterol. The nurse should monitor for which of the following findings as an adverse effect of niacin? (Select all that apply.)
   - A. Muscle aches
   - B. Hyperglycemia
   - C. Hearing loss
   - D. Flushing of the skin
   - E. Jaundice

PRACTICE Active Learning Scenario

A nurse is providing care for a client who has elevated total cholesterol, LDL, and triglycerides, and has a new prescription for atorvastatin once daily. The client has type 2 diabetes mellitus and hypertension. What should the nurse teach the client about atorvastatin? Use the ATI Active Learning Template: Medication to complete this item.

THERAPEUTIC USES: Identify for atorvastatin.

COMPLICATIONS: Identify two adverse effects.

NURSING INTERVENTIONS: Describe three two tests to monitor.

CLIENT EDUCATION: Include two teaching points.

Application Exercises Key

1. A. **CORRECT:** The client should take simvastatin in the evening because nighttime is when the most cholesterol is synthesized in the body. Taking statin medications in the evening increases medication effectiveness.

   B. Changing position slowly might be necessary when taking an antihypertensive medication, but it is not necessary after taking simvastatin.

   C. Consuming a steady intake of green vegetables is important for clients taking warfarin, but does not help lower cholesterol when taking simvastatin.

   D. There is no indication for taking less than 1 L/day of fluid when taking simvastatin.

   Ⓝ *NCLEX® Connection: Pharmacological and Parenteral Therapies, Medication Administration*

2. A. Mental status changes do not occur as adverse effects of gemfibrozil.

   B. Tremor does not occur as an adverse effect of gemfibrozil.

   C. **CORRECT:** Jaundice, anorexia, and upper abdominal discomfort can be findings in liver impairment, which can occur in clients taking gemfibrozil.

   D. Pneumonia is not an adverse effect of gemfibrozil.

   Ⓝ *NCLEX® Connection: Pharmacological and Parenteral Therapies, Adverse Effects/Contraindications/Side Effects/Interactions*

3. A. Many medications, including digoxin, should be taken 4 hr before colesevelam to prevent decreased absorption of the other medications.

   B. Serum electrolytes are not checked periodically while taking colesevelam. However, total cholesterol, LDL, HDL, and triglycerides are checked, as well as blood glucose and HbA1C levels for clients who have diabetes mellitus.

   C. Bleeding and bruising are not expected effects caused by colesevelam.

   D. **CORRECT:** Colesevelam should be taken with food and at least 8 oz of water.

   Ⓝ *NCLEX® Connection: Pharmacological and Parenteral Therapies, Medication Administration*

4. A. Unlike the bile-acid sequestrants, ezetimibe does not cause constipation and is not contraindicated in clients who have a history of constipation.

   B. A history of hypertension is not a contraindication to taking ezetimibe along with simvastatin.

   C. **CORRECT:** Ezetimibe is contraindicated in clients who have an active moderate-to-severe liver disorder, especially if the client is already taking a statin, such as simvastatin.

   D. Type 2 diabetes mellitus is not a contraindication to taking ezetimibe along with simvastatin.

   Ⓝ *NCLEX® Connection: Pharmacological and Parenteral Therapies, Adverse Effects/Contraindications/Side Effects/Interactions*

5. A. Myopathy (muscles aches) can occur with statins and other antilipemic medications, but this is not an adverse effect of niacin.

   B. **CORRECT:** Hyperglycemia can occur as an adverse effect of niacin. The nurse should plan to monitor blood glucose periodically.

   C. Hearing loss is not an adverse effect of taking niacin.

   D. **CORRECT:** Flushing of the skin, along with tingling of the extremities, occurs soon after taking niacin. The effect should decrease in a few weeks, and can be minimized by taking an aspirin tablet 30 min before the niacin.

   E. **CORRECT:** Niacin can cause liver disorders, so the nurse should monitor for jaundice, abdominal pain, and anorexia.

   Ⓝ *NCLEX® Connection: Pharmacological and Parenteral Therapies, Adverse Effects/Contraindications/Side Effects/Interactions*

PRACTICE Answer

Using the ATI Active Learning Template: Medication

THERAPEUTIC USES: Atorvastatin decreases LDL and triglycerides, and elevates HDL. It reduces the risk for cardiovascular events, such as myocardial infarction, and also provides secondary prevention in clients who have had a cardiovascular event. In clients who have diabetes mellitus and hypertension, atorvastatin can reduce mortality by controlling cholesterol levels.

COMPLICATIONS
- Muscle pain/tenderness (myopathy)
- Liver toxicity with findings such as jaundice, upper abdominal pain, anorexia, and nausea

NURSING INTERVENTIONS: Monitor baseline and periodic cholesterol levels (including LDL, HDL, and triglycerides), creatine kinase levels for myopathy, and liver function tests for liver toxicity.

CLIENT EDUCATION
- Instruct the client about additional ways to help decrease cholesterol and improve health, such as exercise, low-fat diet, weight control, and smoking cessation.
- Instruct the client to take atorvastatin in the evening without regard to meals. (Antilipemic agents are given in the evening because cholesterol is mostly synthesized during the night.)

Ⓝ *NCLEX® Connection: Pharmacological and Parenteral Therapies, Medication Administration*

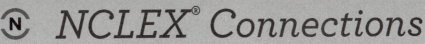
When reviewing the following chapters, keep in mind the relevant topics and tasks of the NCLEX outline, in particular:

Client Needs: Pharmacological and Parenteral Therapies

ADVERSE EFFECTS/CONTRAINDICATIONS/SIDE EFFECTS/ INTERACTIONS: Evaluate and document the client's response to actions taken to counteract side effects and adverse effects of medications and parenteral therapy.

DOSAGE CALCULATION: Perform calculations needed for medication administration.

CHAPTER 25 *Medications Affecting Coagulation*

Pharmaceutical agents that modify coagulation are used to prevent clot formation or break apart an existing clot. These medications work in the blood to alter the clotting cascade, prevent platelet aggregation, or dissolve a clot. All carry a significant risk of bleeding.

The goal of medications that alter coagulation is to increase circulation and perfusion, decrease pain, and prevent further tissue damage.

The groups of medications used include oral and parenteral anticoagulants, direct thrombin inhibitors, direct inhibitors of factor Xa, antiplatelet medications, and thrombolytic agents.

Parenteral anticoagulants

SELECT PROTOTYPE MEDICATION: Heparin

Low molecular weight heparins

SELECT PROTOTYPE MEDICATION: Enoxaparin

OTHER MEDICATIONS: Dalteparin

Activated factor Xa inhibitor

SELECT PROTOTYPE MEDICATION: Fondaparinux

PURPOSE

EXPECTED PHARMACOLOGICAL ACTION

These parenteral anticoagulants prevent clotting by activating antithrombin, thus indirectly inactivating both thrombin and factor Xa. This inhibits fibrin formation.

THERAPEUTIC USES

Heparin
- Conditions necessitating prompt anticoagulant activity (evolving stroke, pulmonary embolism, massive deep-vein thrombosis)
- An adjunct for clients having open heart surgery or renal dialysis
- Low-dose therapy for prophylaxis against postoperative venous thrombosis (for example, hip/knee or abdominal surgery)
- Treatment of disseminated intravascular coagulation

Low molecular weight heparins
- Prevent deep-vein thrombosis (DVT) in clients who are postoperative.
- Treat DVT and pulmonary embolism.
- Prevent complications in angina, non-Q wave MI, and ST elevation MI.

Activated factor Xa inhibitor (fondaparinux)
- Prevent DVT and pulmonary embolism in postoperative clients.
- Treat acute DVT or pulmonary embolism in conjunction with warfarin.

COMPLICATIONS

Heparin

Hemorrhage secondary to heparin overdose
NURSING CONSIDERATIONS
- Monitor vital signs.
- Advise clients to observe for bleeding: increased heart rate, decreased blood pressure, bruising, petechiae, hematomas, black tarry stools.
- In the case of overdose, stop heparin, administer protamine, and avoid aspirin.
- Monitor activated partial thromboplastin time (aPTT). Keep value at 1.5 to 2 times the baseline. Q EBP

Heparin-induced thrombocytopenia
- Evidenced by low platelet count and increased development of thrombi: mediated by antibody development (white clot syndrome)
- NURSING CONSIDERATIONS
  ○ Monitor platelet count periodically throughout treatment, especially in the first month.
  ○ Stop heparin if platelet count is less than 100,000/mm³. Nonheparin anticoagulants, such as lepirudin or argatroban, can be used as a substitute if anticoagulation is still needed.

Hypersensitivity reactions (chills, fever, urticaria)
NURSING CONSIDERATIONS: Administer a small test dose prior to the administration of heparin.

Toxicity/overdose
NURSING CONSIDERATIONS
- Administer protamine, which binds with heparin and forms a heparin-protamine complex that has no anticoagulant properties.
- Protamine should be administered slowly IV, no faster than 20 mg/min or 50 mg in 10 min.
- Do not exceed 100 mg in a 2-hr period. Administer carefully to prevent protamine overdose (excessive anticoagulation).

Enoxaparin

Hemorrhage
NURSING CONSIDERATIONS
- Monitor vital signs.
- Advise clients to observe for bleeding: increased heart rate, decreased blood pressure, bruising, petechiae, hematomas, black tarry stools.
- Monitor platelet count. Instruct client to avoid aspirin.

Neurologic damage from hematoma formed during spinal or epidural anesthesia
NURSING CONSIDERATIONS: In clients who have spinal or epidural anesthesia: Assess insertion site for indications of hematoma formation, such as redness or swelling. Monitor sensation and movement of lower extremities. Notify provider of abnormal findings.

Thrombocytopenia evidenced by low platelet count
NURSING CONSIDERATIONS
- Monitor platelets. Discontinue medication for platelet count less than 100,000/mm^3.

Toxicity/overdose
NURSING CONSIDERATIONS
- Administer protamine (heparin antagonist)
- Protamine should be administered slowly IV, no faster than 20 mg/min or 50 mg in 10 min.

Fondaparinux

Hemorrhage
NURSING CONSIDERATIONS
- Monitor vital signs.
- Advise clients to observe for bleeding: increased heart rate, decreased blood pressure, bruising, petechiae, hematomas, black tarry stools.
- Monitor platelet count. Instruct clients to avoid aspirin.

Neurologic damage from hematoma formed during spinal or epidural anesthesia
NURSING CONSIDERATIONS: In clients who have spinal or epidural anesthesia: Assess insertion site for indications of hematoma formation such as redness or swelling. Monitor sensation and movement of lower extremities. Notify provider of abnormal findings.

Thrombocytopenia evidenced by low platelet count
NURSING CONSIDERATIONS: Monitor platelets. Discontinue medication for platelet count less than 100,000/mm^3.

CONTRAINDICATIONS/PRECAUTIONS

- Parenteral anticoagulants are contraindicated in clients who have low platelet counts (thrombocytopenia) or uncontrollable bleeding. Qs
- These medications should not be used during or following surgeries of the eye(s), brain, or spinal cord; lumbar puncture; or regional anesthesia.
- Use cautiously in clients who have hemophilia, increased capillary permeability, dissecting aneurysm, peptic ulcer disease, severe hypertension, hepatic or kidney disease, or threatened abortion.

INTERACTIONS

Antiplatelet agents such as aspirin, NSAIDs, and other anticoagulants can increase risk for bleeding.
NURSING CONSIDERATIONS
- Avoid concurrent use when possible.
- Monitor carefully for evidence of bleeding.
- Take precautionary measures to avoid injury (limit venipunctures and injections).

NURSING ADMINISTRATION

These medications cannot be absorbed by the intestinal tract and must be given via subcutaneous injection or IV infusion.

Heparin QEBP

- Obtain baseline vital signs.
- Obtain baseline and monitor complete blood count (CBC), platelet count, and hematocrit levels.
- Read label carefully. Heparin is dispensed in units and in a variety of concentrations.
- Check dosages with another nurse before administration.
- Use an infusion pump for continuous IV administration. Monitor rate of infusion every 30 to 60 min. Qs
- Monitor aPTT every 4 to 6 hr until appropriate dose is determined, then monitor daily.
- For subcutaneous injections, use a 20- to 22-gauge needle to withdraw medication from the vial. Then, change the needle to a smaller needle (25- or 26-gauge, 1/2 to 5/8 inches long).
- Administer deep subcutaneous injections in the abdomen, ensuring a distance of 2 inches from the umbilicus. Do not aspirate.
- Apply gentle pressure for 1 to 2 min after the injection. Rotate and record injection sites.
- Instruct clients to monitor for indications of bleeding: bruising, gums bleeding, abdominal pain, nose bleeds, coffee-ground emesis, and tarry stools.
- Instruct clients to avoid the use of over-the-counter (OTC) NSAIDs, aspirin, or medications containing salicylates.
- Advise clients to use an electric razor for shaving and to brush with a soft toothbrush.

Enoxaparin/fondaparinux

- Monitoring is not required. These medications are acceptable for home use.
- Provide instruction regarding self-administration. Medications can be available in prefilled syringes.
- For subcutaneous injections when a prefilled syringe is not available, use a 20- to 22-gauge needle to withdraw medication from the vial. Then, change to a small needle (25- or 26-gauge, 1/2 to 5/8 inches long). Deep subcutaneous injections should be administered in the abdomen, ensuring a distance of 2 inches from the umbilicus. Do not aspirate.
- Prefilled syringes are available in various dosages for subcutaneous injection. Rotate sites between right and left anterolateral and posterolateral abdominal walls at least 2 inches from umbilicus. Do not expel the air bubble in the syringe unless adjustments must be made to the dose. Pinch up an area of skin, inject at a 90° angle, and insert needle completely. Do not aspirate. Inject entire contents of syringe. Ⓠ EBP
- Do not rub the site for 1 to 2 min after the injection. Rotate and record injection sites.
- Instruct clients to monitor for indications of bleeding, such as bruising, gums bleeding, abdominal pain, nose bleeds, coffee-ground emesis, and tarry stools.
- Instruct clients to avoid the use of OTC NSAIDs, aspirin, or medications containing salicylates.
- Advise client to use an electric razor for shaving and to brush with a soft toothbrush.

NURSING EVALUATION OF MEDICATION EFFECTIVENESS

Depending on therapeutic intent, effectiveness can be evidenced by the following.

Heparin: aPTT levels of 60 to 80 seconds

Heparin, enoxaparin, and fondaparinux: No development or no further development of venous thrombi or emboli

Oral anticoagulant

SELECT PROTOTYPE MEDICATION: Warfarin

PURPOSE

EXPECTED PHARMACOLOGICAL ACTION:
Oral anticoagulants antagonize vitamin K, thereby preventing the synthesis of four coagulation factors: factor VII, IX, X, and prothrombin.

THERAPEUTIC USES
- Treatment of venous thrombosis
- Treatment of thrombus formation in clients who have atrial fibrillation or prosthetic heart valves
- Prevention of recurrent myocardial infarction, transient ischemic attacks, pulmonary embolus, and DVT

COMPLICATIONS

Hemorrhage

NURSING CONSIDERATIONS
- Monitor vital signs.
- Advise clients to observe for bleeding (increased heart rate, decreased blood pressure, bruising, petechiae, hematomas, black tarry stools).
- Obtain baseline prothrombin time (PT), and monitor levels of PT and international normalized ratio (INR) periodically.
- In the case of a warfarin overdose, discontinue administration of warfarin, and administer vitamin K_1.

Hepatitis

NURSING CONSIDERATIONS: Monitor liver enzymes. Assess for jaundice.

Toxicity/overdose

NURSING CONSIDERATIONS
- Administer vitamin K_1 to promote synthesis of coagulation factors VII, IX, X, and prothrombin.
- Administer IV vitamin K_1 slowly and in a diluted solution to prevent anaphylactoid-type reaction. Ⓠ s
- Administer small doses of vitamin K_1 (2.5 mg PO, 0.5 to 1 mg IV) to prevent development of resistance to warfarin.
- If vitamin K_1 cannot control bleeding, administer fresh frozen plasma or whole blood.

CONTRAINDICATIONS/PRECAUTIONS

- Classified as Pregnancy Risk Category X due to high risk of fetal hemorrhage, fetal death, and CNS defects. Advise clients to notify the provider if they become pregnant during warfarin therapy. If anticoagulation is needed during pregnancy, heparin can be safely used. Qs
- Contraindicated in clients who have low platelet counts (thrombocytopenia) or uncontrollable bleeding.
- Contraindicated during or following surgeries of the eye(s), brain, or spinal cord; lumbar puncture; or regional anesthesia.
- Contraindicated in clients who have vitamin K deficiencies, liver disorders, and alcohol use disorder due to the additive risk of bleeding.
- Use cautiously in clients who have hemophilia, dissecting aneurysm, peptic ulcer disease, severe hypertension, or threatened abortion.

INTERACTIONS

Concurrent use of heparin, aspirin, acetaminophen, glucocorticoids, sulfonamides, and parenteral cephalosporins increases effects of warfarin, which increases the risk for bleeding.

NURSING CONSIDERATIONS
- Avoid concurrent use if possible.
- Instruct clients to observe for inclusion of aspirin in OTC medications.
- If used concurrently, monitor carefully for indications of bleeding and increased PT, INR, and aPTT levels.
- Medication dosage should be adjusted accordingly.

Concurrent use of phenobarbital, carbamazepine, phenytoin, oral contraceptives, and vitamin K decreases anticoagulant effects.

NURSING CONSIDERATIONS
- Avoid concurrent use if possible.
- If used concurrently, monitor carefully for reduced PT and INR levels.
- Medication dosage should be adjusted accordingly.

Foods high in vitamin K, such as dark green leafy vegetables (lettuce, cooked spinach), cabbage, broccoli, Brussels sprouts, mayonnaise, and canola and soybean oil, can decrease anticoagulant effects with excessive intake.

NURSING CONSIDERATIONS
- Provide clients with a list of foods high in vitamin K.
- Instruct clients to maintain a consistent intake of vitamin K to avoid sudden fluctuations that could affect the action of warfarin. Qs

Multiple other medications interact with warfarin.

NURSING CONSIDERATIONS: Take a complete medication history for clients taking warfarin, and advise clients to inform the provider if any new medication is started.

NURSING ADMINISTRATION

- Administration is usually oral, once daily, and at the same time each day.
- Obtain baseline vital signs.
- Monitor PT levels (therapeutic level 18 to 24 seconds) and INR levels (therapeutic levels 2 to 3). INR levels are the most accurate. Hold dose and notify the provider if these levels exceed therapeutic ranges. QEBP
- Obtain baseline and monitor CBC, platelet count, and Hct levels.
- Instruct clients that anticoagulant effects can take 8 to 12 hr, and full therapeutic effect is not achieved for 3 to 5 days. For clients in the hospital setting, explain the need for continued heparin infusion when starting oral warfarin.
- Advise clients that anticoagulation effects can persist for up to 5 days following discontinuation of medication due to a long half-life.
- Advise clients to avoid alcohol and OTC and nonprescription medications to prevent adverse effects and medication interactions, such as risk of bleeding.
- Advise clients to employ nonpharmacological measures to avoid development of thrombi, including avoiding sitting for prolonged periods of time, not wearing constricting clothing, and elevating and moving legs when sitting.
- Advise clients to wear a medical alert bracelet indicating warfarin use.
- Be prepared to administer vitamin K_1 for warfarin overdose.
- Teach clients to self-monitor PT and INR at home as appropriate. QPCC
- Plan for frequent PT monitoring for clients who are prescribed medications that interact with warfarin. The client is at greatest risk for harm when the interacting medication is being deleted or added. Frequent PT monitoring allows for dosage adjustments as necessary.
- Advise clients to record dosage, route, and time of warfarin administration on a daily basis.
- Advise clients to notify the provider regarding warfarin use.
- Advise clients to use a soft-bristle toothbrush to prevent gum bleeding and an electric razor for shaving.

NURSING EVALUATION OF MEDICATION EFFECTIVENESS

Depending on therapeutic intent, effectiveness can be evidenced by the following.
- PT 1.5 to 2 times control
- INR of 2 to 3 for treatment of acute myocardial infarction, atrial fibrillation, pulmonary embolism, venous thrombosis, or tissue heart valves
- INR of 3 to 4.5 for mechanical heart valve or recurrent systemic embolism
- No development or no further development of venous thrombi

Direct thrombin inhibitors

SELECT PROTOTYPE MEDICATION: Dabigatran

OTHER MEDICATIONS
- **Hirudin analogs:** Bivalirudin, desirudin, lepirudin
- Argatroban

PURPOSE

EXPECTED PHARMACOLOGICAL ACTION: These medications work by directly inhibiting thrombin, thus preventing a thrombus from developing.

THERAPEUTIC USES
- **Dabigatran** prevents stroke or embolism in clients who have atrial fibrillation not caused by valvular heart disease. It is also used to treat DVT and to prevent pulmonary embolism.
- **Bivalirudin** is given concurrently with aspirin for clients who undergo coronary angioplasty.
- **Argatroban** is used to prevent or treat thrombosis in clients who cannot take heparin due to heparin-induced thrombocytopenia.
- **Desirudin** is administered to clients having hip replacement surgery to prevent DVT.

COMPLICATIONS

Bleeding (GI, GU, cranial, and other sites)

NURSING CONSIDERATIONS
- Teach clients to report manifestations of bleeding to the provider.
- For severe bleeding, no antidote to dabigatran is available. Dialysis or injections of recombinant factor VIIa can be used.
- Clients undergoing elective surgery should stop taking dabigatran before surgery.

GI effects

GI discomfort, nausea, vomiting, esophageal reflux, ulcer formation

NURSING CONSIDERATIONS
- Take dabigatran with food.
- The client might need a proton pump inhibitor, such as omeprazole, or an H_2 receptor antagonist, such as ranitidine, for these manifestations.

Other effects

Bivalirudin can also cause back pain, nausea, hypotension, and headache.

NURSING CONSIDERATIONS: Monitor vital signs and assess for headache when taking this medication.

CONTRAINDICATIONS/PRECAUTIONS

- Dabigatran and argatroban are Pregnancy Risk Category C. Bivalirudin and lepirudin are Pregnancy Risk Category B.
- Contraindicated in clients who have active bleeding or allergy to the medication. Qs
- Use cautiously in clients who have liver impairment or who are at risk for bleeding.
- Use dabigatran, bivalirudin, desirudin, and lepirudin cautiously in clients who have kidney impairment.

INTERACTIONS

Rifampin decreases levels of dabigatran.
NURSING CONSIDERATIONS: Use cautiously together, and watch for therapeutic effect.

Other thrombolytics and anticoagulants can increase risk for bleeding with argatroban, desirudin, bivalirudin, or dabigatran.
NURSING CONSIDERATIONS: Monitor coagulation studies carefully with concurrent use.

NURSING ADMINISTRATION

- Dabigatran is available in oral capsules that should be swallowed whole and can be taken with or without food. The container should be used within 30 days of opening. Discontinue other anticoagulants when starting dabigatran.
- Bivalirudin and lepirudin are administered IV by direct bolus or continuous infusion.
- Argatroban is administrated IV by continuous infusion to prevent or treat thrombus formation, or as a bolus during percutaneous coronary intervention. Before starting, discontinue heparin and check aPTT.
- Desirudin is administered by deep subcutaneous injection into the abdomen or thigh.

Direct inhibitor of factor Xa

SELECT PROTOTYPE MEDICATION: Rivaroxaban

PURPOSE

EXPECTED PHARMACOLOGICAL ACTION: Provides anticoagulation selectively and directly by inhibiting factor Xa.

THERAPEUTIC USES: Used in clients who have atrial fibrillation and in the prevention of DVT and pulmonary embolism in clients who are undergoing total hip or knee arthroplasty. Also used for prophylaxis for stroke and embolism in clients who have nonvalvular atrial fibrillation.

COMPLICATIONS

Bleeding

GI, GU, cranial, retinal, or epidural bleeding following removal of epidural catheter

NURSING CONSIDERATIONS
- Teach the client to report bleeding, bruising, headache, or eye pain.
- Monitor hemoglobin and hematocrit.
- Wait at least 18 hr following last dose to remove an epidural catheter, and wait 6 hr after removal before starting rivaroxaban again. Qs
- No antidote is available for severe bleeding, and dialysis is ineffective in removing the medication from the bloodstream. Activated charcoal can be given to prevent further absorption.

Elevated liver enzymes and bilirubin

Liver enzymes: ALT, AST, and GGT

NURSING CONSIDERATIONS
- Monitor baseline and periodic liver function.
- Report elevated values to provider.

CONTRAINDICATIONS/PRECAUTIONS

- Pregnancy Risk Category C. Increased risk of hemorrhage in pregnancy. Qs
- Contraindicated clients who have previous allergy to rivaroxaban, or who have active bleeding, severe kidney impairment, or moderate to severe liver impairment.
- Use cautiously in clients taking anticoagulants, antiplatelet medications, or fibrinolytics, and clients who have mild liver or moderate kidney impairment.

INTERACTIONS

Bleeding risk is increased when taking erythromycin, diltiazem, verapamil, quinidine, or amiodarone.
NURSING CONSIDERATIONS: Monitor carefully for bleeding if these medications are taken concurrently.

Rifampin, carbamazepine, phenytoin, and St. John's wort can decrease rivaroxaban levels.
NURSING CONSIDERATIONS: Monitor for therapeutic effect in clients who take medications concurrently.

NURSING ADMINISTRATION

- Administer tablets orally, once daily, with or without food, and at the same time each day. QEBP
- For stroke and systemic embolism prevention, administer orally once daily with the evening meal.
- Monitor hemoglobin, hematocrit, and liver and kidney function periodically during treatment.

Antiplatelets

Antiplatelet/salicylic

SELECT PROTOTYPE MEDICATION: Aspirin

Antiplatelet/glycoprotein inhibitors

SELECT PROTOTYPE MEDICATION: Abciximab

OTHER MEDICATIONS: Eptifibatide, tirofiban

Antiplatelet/ADP inhibitors

SELECT PROTOTYPE MEDICATIONS: Clopidogrel

OTHER MEDICATIONS: Ticlopidine

Antiplatelet/arterial vasodilator

SELECT PROTOTYPE MEDICATION: Pentoxifylline

OTHER MEDICATIONS: Dipyridamole, cilostazol

PURPOSE

EXPECTED PHARMACOLOGICAL ACTIONS
- Antiplatelets prevent platelets from clumping together by inhibiting enzymes and factors that normally lead to arterial clotting.
- Antiplatelet medications inhibit platelet aggregation at the onset of the clotting process. These medications alter bleeding time.

THERAPEUTIC USES
- Primary prevention of acute myocardial infarction
- Prevention of reinfarction in clients following an acute myocardial infarction
- Prevention of ischemic stroke or transient ischemic attack
- Acute coronary syndromes (abciximab, tirofiban, eptifibatide, clopidogrel)
- Intermittent claudication (cilostazol, pentoxifylline, dipyridamole)

ROUTES OF ADMINISTRATION
- Aspirin: Oral
- Abciximab: IV
- Clopidogrel: Oral
- Pentoxifylline: Oral

COMPLICATIONS

Aspirin

GI effects (nausea, vomiting, dyspepsia)
NURSING CONSIDERATIONS
- Advise clients to use enteric-coated tablets and to take aspirin with food. Ⓠ EBP
- Concurrent use of a proton pump inhibitor, such as omeprazole, might decrease GI effects.

Hemorrhagic stroke
CLIENT EDUCATION: Advise clients to observe for weakness, dizziness, and headache, and to notify the provider if effects occur.

Prolonged bleeding time, gastric bleed, thrombocytopenia
NURSING CONSIDERATIONS: Monitor bleeding time. Monitor for gastric bleed, such as coffee-ground emesis or bloody, tarry stools. Monitor for bruising, petechiae, and bleeding gums.

Tinnitus, hearing loss
NURSING CONSIDERATIONS
- Monitor for hearing loss.
- If manifestations occur, withhold the dose and notify the provider.

Abciximab

Hypotension and bradycardia
NURSING CONSIDERATIONS: Monitor heart rate and blood pressure.

Prolonged bleeding time, gastric bleed, thrombocytopenia, bleed from cardiac catheterization site
NURSING CONSIDERATIONS
- Monitor bleeding time.
- Monitor for gastric bleed (coffee-ground emesis or bloody, tarry stools).
- Monitor for bruising, petechiae, and bleeding gums.
- Apply pressure to the cardiac catheter access site.

Clopidogrel

Bleeding
Prolonged bleeding time, gastric bleed, thrombocytopenia
NURSING CONSIDERATIONS
- Monitor bleeding time.
- Monitor for gastric bleed (coffee-ground emesis or bloody, tarry stools).
- Monitor for bruising, petechiae, and bleeding gums.
- Apply pressure to cardiac catheter access.

GI effects (diarrhea, dyspepsia, pain)
CLIENT EDUCATION: Teach the client to monitor for effects and notify the provider.

Pentoxifylline

Dyspepsia, nausea, vomiting
NURSING CONSIDERATIONS
- Take with food.
- Do not crush or chew medication.
- Monitor hydration if GI upset occurs.

CONTRAINDICATIONS/PRECAUTIONS

Aspirin

- Pregnancy Risk Category D in the third trimester.
- Contraindicated in clients who have bleeding disorders and thrombocytopenia.
- Use cautiously in clients who have peptic ulcer disease and severe kidney or hepatic disorders. Do not give to children or adolescents who have fever or recent chickenpox.
- Use with caution in older adults. Ⓖ

Abciximab

- Pregnancy Risk Category C.
- Contraindications include clients who have bleeding disorders, thrombocytopenia, recent stroke, AV malformation, aneurysm, uncontrolled hypertension, and recent major surgery.
- Use cautiously in clients who have peptic ulcer disease and severe kidney or hepatic disorders.

Clopidogrel

- Pregnancy Risk Category B
- Contraindications include clients who have bleeding disorders, thrombocytopenia, peptic ulcer disease, and intracranial bleed.
- Use cautiously in clients who have peptic ulcer disease and severe kidney or hepatic disorders. Clients who are breastfeeding should not take this medication.

Pentoxifylline

- Pregnancy Risk Category C.
- Contraindicated for clients who have bleeding disorders or retinal or cerebral bleeds.

INTERACTIONS

Aspirin

Concurrent use of other medications that enhance bleeding (NSAIDs, heparin, warfarin, thrombolytics, antiplatelets) increases risk for bleeding.
NURSING CONSIDERATIONS
- Advise clients to avoid concurrent use.
- If used concurrently, monitor carefully for indications of bleeding.

Urine acidifiers (ammonium chloride) can increase aspirin levels.
NURSING CONSIDERATIONS: Monitor for aspirin toxicity (hearing loss, tinnitus).

Concurrent use of aspirin can reduce hypertensive action of beta blockers.
NURSING CONSIDERATIONS: Monitor blood pressure.

Corticosteroids can increase aspirin excretion and decrease aspirin effects. These medications can increase risk for GI bleed.

NURSING CONSIDERATIONS
- Monitor for decreased aspirin effectiveness.
- Monitor for gastric bleed (coffee-ground emesis and tarry or bloody stools).

Caffeine can increase aspirin absorption.

NURSING CONSIDERATIONS: Monitor for toxicity.

Abciximab

Concurrent use of other medications that enhance bleeding (NSAIDs, heparin, warfarin, thrombolytics, antiplatelets) increases risk for bleeding.

NURSING CONSIDERATIONS
- Advise clients to avoid concurrent use.
- If used concurrently, monitor carefully for indications of bleeding.

Clopidogrel

Concurrent use of other medications that enhance bleeding (NSAIDs, heparin, warfarin, thrombolytics, antiplatelets) increases risk for bleeding.

NURSING CONSIDERATIONS
- Advise clients to avoid concurrent use.
- If used concurrently, monitor carefully for indications of bleeding.

Proton pump inhibitors decrease effectiveness.

NURSING CONSIDERATIONS: If needed for GI effects, pantoprazole interferes the least with platelet inhibition.

Pentoxifylline

Concurrent use of anticoagulants increases risk for bleeding.

NURSING CONSIDERATIONS: Monitor PT and INR. Clients can require reduced dosage.

Pentoxifylline can increase levels of theophylline.

NURSING CONSIDERATIONS: Monitor theophylline level. Clients can require reduced dosage.

NURSING ADMINISTRATION

- Advise clients that prevention of strokes, myocardial infarctions, and reinfarction can be accomplished with low-dose aspirin (81 mg).
- Aspirin 325 mg should be taken during initial acute episode of myocardial infarction.
- Advise clients to notify the provider regarding aspirin use. Qs
- Clopidogrel is sometimes prescribed concurrently with aspirin, which increases the risk for bleeding. Clopidogrel should be discontinued 7 days before an elective surgery.

NURSING EVALUATION OF MEDICATION EFFECTIVENESS

Depending on therapeutic intent, effectiveness can be evidenced by absence of arterial thrombosis, adequate tissue perfusion, and blood flow without occurrence of abnormal bleeding.

Thrombolytic medications

SELECT PROTOTYPE MEDICATION: Alteplase, often called tPA (tissue plasminogen activator)

OTHER MEDICATIONS
- Tenecteplase
- Reteplase

PURPOSE

EXPECTED PHARMACOLOGICAL ACTION: Thrombolytic medications dissolve clots that have already formed. Clots are dissolved by conversion of plasminogen to plasmin, which destroys fibrinogen and other clotting factors.

THERAPEUTIC USES
- Treat acute myocardial infarction (all three medications).
- Treat massive pulmonary emboli (alteplase only).
- Treat acute ischemic stroke (alteplase only).
- Restore patency to central IV catheters (alteplase only).

ROUTE OF ADMINISTRATION: IV only

COMPLICATIONS

ALTEPLASE

Bleeding

Serious risk of bleeding from different sites
- Internal bleeding: GI or GU tracts and cerebral bleeding
- Superficial bleeding: wounds, IV catheter sites

NURSING CONSIDERATIONS
- Limit venipunctures and injections.
- Apply pressure dressings to recent wounds.
- Monitor for changes in vital signs, alterations in level of consciousness, weakness, and indications of intracranial bleeding.
- Notify the provider if manifestations occur.
- Monitor aPTT and PT, Hgb, and Hct.

CONTRAINDICATIONS/PRECAUTIONS

- Pregnancy Risk Category C.
- Because of the additive risk for serious bleeding, use is contraindicated in clients who have the following. Qs
  - Any prior intracranial hemorrhage (hemorrhagic stroke)
  - Known structural cerebral vascular lesion (arteriovenous malformation)
  - Active internal bleeding
  - History of significant closed head or spinal trauma within past 2 months
  - Acute pericarditis or bacterial endocarditis
  - Brain tumors
  - Severe hepatic or kidney disorders
- Use cautiously in clients who have severe hypertension, cerebral vascular disorders, recent GU or GI bleeding, or major surgery within past 10 days, and in older adult clients.

INTERACTIONS

Concurrent use of other medications that enhance bleeding (NSAIDs, heparin, warfarin, thrombolytics, antiplatelets) increases risk for bleeding.

NURSING CONSIDERATIONS: If used concurrently, monitor the client carefully for indications of bleeding.

NURSING ADMINISTRATION

- Use of thrombolytic agents should take place as soon as possible after onset of manifestations (within 3 hr is best). Qᴇʙᴘ
- Clients receiving a thrombolytic agent should be monitored in a setting that provides for close supervision and continuous monitoring during and after administration of the medication.
- Obtain baseline platelet counts, hemoglobin (Hgb), hematocrit (Hct), aPTT, PT, INR, and fibrinogen levels. Monitor periodically.
- Obtain baseline vital signs (heart rate, blood pressure), and monitor frequently per protocol.
- Nursing care includes continuous monitoring of hemodynamic status to assess for therapeutic and adverse effects of thrombolytic (relief of chest pain, indications of bleeding). Follow facility protocol.
- Provide for client safety per facility protocol.
- Ensure adequate IV access for administration of emergency medications and availability of emergency equipment.

- Do not mix any medications in an IV with thrombolytic agents.
- Minimize bruising or bleeding by limiting venipunctures and subcutaneous/IM injections. Hold direct pressure to injection site or ABG site for up to 30 min until oozing stops. Qs
- Discontinue thrombolytic therapy if life-threatening bleeding occurs. Treat blood loss with whole blood, packed red blood cells, and/or fresh frozen plasma. Ensure that IV aminocaproic acid is available for administration in the event of excessive fibrinolysis.
- Following thrombolytic therapy, administer heparin or aspirin as prescribed to decrease the risk of rethrombosis.
- Following thrombolytic therapy, administer beta blockers as prescribed to decrease myocardial oxygen consumption and to reduce the incidence and severity of reperfusion arrhythmias.
- Administer H_2 antagonists, such as ranitidine, or proton pump inhibitors, such as omeprazole, as prescribed to prevent GI bleeding.

NURSING EVALUATION OF MEDICATION EFFECTIVENESS

Depending on therapeutic intent, effectiveness can be evidenced by evidence of thrombus lysis and restoration of circulation (relief of chest pain, reduction of initial ST segment injury pattern as shown on ECG 60 to 90 min after start of therapy).

Application Exercises

1. A nurse is planning to administer subcutaneous enoxaparin 40 mg using a prefilled syringe of enoxaparin 40 mg/0.4 mL to an adult client following hip arthroplasty. Which of the following actions should the nurse plan to take?
   - A. Expel the air bubble from the prefilled syringe before injecting.
   - B. Insert the needle completely into the client's tissue.
   - C. Administer the injection in the client's thigh.
   - D. Aspirate carefully after inserting the needle into the client's skin.

2. A nurse is caring for a hospitalized client who is receiving IV heparin for a deep-vein thrombosis. The client begins vomiting blood. After the heparin has been stopped, which of the following medications should the nurse prepare to administer?
   - A. Vitamin K₁
   - B. Atropine
   - C. Protamine
   - D. Calcium gluconate

3. A nurse is planning to administer IV alteplase to a client who is demonstrating manifestations of a massive pulmonary embolism. Which of the following interventions should the nurse plan to take?
   - A. Administer IM enoxaparin along with the alteplase dose.
   - B. Hold direct pressure on puncture sites for up to 30 min.
   - C. Administer aminocaproic acid IV prior to alteplase infusion.
   - D. Prepare to administer alteplase within 8 hr of manifestation onset.

4. A nurse is monitoring a client who takes aspirin 81 mg PO daily. The nurse should identify which of the following manifestations as adverse effects of daily aspirin therapy? (Select all that apply.)
   - A. Hypertension
   - B. Coffee-ground emesis
   - C. Tinnitus
   - D. Paresthesias of the extremities
   - E. Nausea

5. A nurse is caring for a client who has atrial fibrillation and a new prescription for dabigatran to prevent development of thrombosis. Which of the following medications is prescribed concurrently to treat an adverse effect of dabigatran?
   - A. Vitamin K₁
   - B. Protamine
   - C. Omeprazole
   - D. Probenecid

Application Exercises Key

1. A. The nurse should not expel the air bubble in the prefilled syringe prior to injection because the medication has been premeasured, and expelling the air could cause medication to be lost. An exception would be if the dosage needed to be adjusted prior to the injection.

   B. **CORRECT:** The nurse should inject the needle on the prefilled syringe completely when administering enoxaparin in order to administer the medication by deep subcutaneous injection.

   C. A deep subcutaneous injection should be administered into the subcutaneous tissue of the abdomen, at least 2 inches away from the umbilicus.

   D. The nurse should not aspirate when administering enoxaparin or other heparin products subcutaneously.

   (N) *NCLEX® Connection: Pharmacological and Parenteral Therapies, Medication Administration*

2. A. Vitamin K₁ is used to reverse the effects of warfarin.

   B. Atropine is used to reverse bradycardia caused by beta adrenergic blockers.

   C. **CORRECT:** Protamine reverses the anticoagulant effect of heparin.

   D. Calcium gluconate is used to treat magnesium sulfate toxicity.

   (N) *NCLEX® Connection: Pharmacological and Parenteral Therapies, Parenteral/Intravenous Therapies*

3. A. Enoxaparin is only available in a subcutaneous form. Subcutaneous and IM injections and other punctures should be avoided due to bleeding risk when alteplase is administered.

   B. **CORRECT:** The nurse should plan to hold direct pressure on puncture sites for 10 to 30 min or until oozing of blood stops.

   C. Aminocaproic acid is an antidote to alteplase and should only be administered in the event of serious bleeding that does not stop after blood products are administered or other remedies are tried. It would not be given prior to alteplase administration.

   D. Alteplase must be administered as soon as possible after manifestations of myocardial infarction, pulmonary embolism, or cerebral vascular accident begin. Three hours is often the limit; client outcomes would be decreased if 8 hr elapsed before beginning alteplase.

   (N) *NCLEX® Connection: Pharmacological and Parenteral Therapies, Medication Administration*

4. A. Hypotension and shock can result if severe aspirin allergy occurs, but hypertension is not an adverse effect of aspirin therapy.

   B. **CORRECT:** GI bleeding with dark stools or coffee-ground emesis can be an adverse effect of aspirin therapy.

   C. **CORRECT:** Tinnitus and hearing loss can occur as an adverse effect of aspirin therapy

   D. Paresthesias of the extremities are not adverse effects of aspirin therapy.

   E. **CORRECT:** Nausea, vomiting, and abdominal pain can occur as a result of aspirin therapy.

   (N) *NCLEX® Connection: Pharmacological and Parenteral Therapies, Adverse Effects/Contraindications/Side Effects/Interactions*

5. A. Vitamin K₁ is used to treat hemorrhage or overdose of warfarin, but it is not an antidote for dabigatran.

   B. Protamine is used to treat severe hemorrhage or overdose of heparin, but is not an antidote for dabigatran.

   C. **CORRECT:** Omeprazole or another proton pump inhibitor is prescribed for a client who is taking dabigatran and has abdominal pain and other GI findings that can occur as adverse effects of dabigatran. The nurse should advise the client who has GI effects to take dabigatran with food.

   D. Probenecid is used to treat gout and gouty arthritis, and is not indicated to treat an adverse effect of dabigatran.

   (N) *NCLEX® Connection: Pharmacological and Parenteral Therapies, Medication Administration*

PRACTICE Active Learning Scenario

A nurse is teaching a client who has a new prescription for clopidogrel following a myocardial infarction. What should the nurse teach the client about this medication? Use the ATI Active Learning Template: Medication to complete this item.

THERAPEUTIC USES: Identify for clopidogrel in this client.

COMPLICATIONS: Identify two adverse effects for this medication.

NURSING INTERVENTIONS: Describe three, including one test the nurse should monitor periodically.

PRACTICE Answer

Using the ATI Active Learning Template: Medication

THERAPEUTIC USES: Clopidogrel inhibits platelet aggregation and prolongs bleeding time. It is used to prevent myocardial infarction (MI) or stroke in clients who have already had an MI or stroke.

COMPLICATIONS: Like other platelet inhibitors, clopidogrel can cause bleeding due to thrombocytopenia. It can also cause GI effects, such as abdominal pain, nausea, and diarrhea.

NURSING INTERVENTIONS

- The nurse should plan to monitor the platelet count periodically while the client takes clopidogrel.
- Teach the client to monitor for bleeding. The client should watch for black stools, coffee-ground emesis, blood in the urine, nose bleeds, unusual bruising, or petechiae. The client should inform the provider if these occur and about GI effects.
- The nurse should be aware of all medications the client is taking, because risk for bleeding increases if the medication is taken with anticoagulants or antiplatelet medications. Clopidogrel is sometimes administered concurrently with aspirin, and that increases the risk for bleeding. The medication should be discontinued 7 days before any elective surgery.

(N) *NCLEX® Connection: Pharmacological and Parenteral Therapies, Medication Administration*

UNIT 5   MEDICATIONS AFFECTING THE
          HEMATOLOGIC SYSTEM

CHAPTER 26 *Growth Factors*

Blood cells and platelets are produced in the body by the biological process hematopoiesis. In the body, this process is naturally controlled by hormones, also known as hematopoietic growth factors.

THERAPEUTIC PURPOSES

Genetically engineered products are available for therapeutic purposes.
- Replacement of neutrophils and platelets after chemotherapy
- Hastening of bone marrow function after a bone marrow transplant
- Increase in red blood cell production for clients who have chronic kidney disease

HEMATOPOIETIC GROWTH FACTORS

There are three groups of hematopoietic growth factors.

ERYTHROPOIETIC GROWTH FACTORS: also known as erythropoiesis stimulating agents (ESAs)
- Biological name: erythropoietin

LEUKOPOIETIC GROWTH FACTORS
- Biological names
  ○ Granulocyte colony stimulating factor
  ○ Granulocyte-macrophage colony-stimulating factor

THROMBOPOIETIC GROWTH FACTOR: Interleukin-11

Erythropoietic growth factors

SELECT PROTOTYPE MEDICATION: Epoetin alfa: erythropoietin

OTHER MEDICATIONS: Darbepoetin alfa: long-acting erythropoietin

PURPOSE

EXPECTED PHARMACOLOGICAL ACTION

Hematopoietic growth factors act on the bone marrow to increase production of red blood cells.

THERAPEUTIC USES

Epoetin alfa
- Anemia related to chronic kidney disease
- For clients who have anemia caused by chemotherapy (nonmyeloid cancers)
- To increase erythrocyte counts in clients who will undergo elective surgery
- For clients who have anemia caused by taking zidovudine for HIV/AIDS

Darbepoetin alfa: For clients who have chronic kidney disease and clients who have anemia caused by chemotherapy (nonmyeloid cancer)

COMPLICATIONS

Hypertension

Secondary to elevations in hematocrit level

NURSING CONSIDERATIONS: Monitor Hgb levels and blood pressure. If elevated, administer antihypertensive medications.

Risk for a thrombotic event

- Such as myocardial infarction or stroke if the client has a Hgb of 11 g/dL or higher, or an increase of more than 1 g/dL in 2 weeks.
- Seizures can also occur with a too-rapid rise in the blood counts.

NURSING CONSIDERATIONS
- Decrease dosage when these limits are reached. Therapy can be resumed when Hgb drops to acceptable level, but dosage should be reduced.
- Consider placing client on seizure precautions if rapid increase in Hgb or blood pressure occurs.

Deep-vein thrombosis

Increased risk in preoperative clients

NURSING CONSIDERATIONS: Prophylactic use of an anticoagulant might be needed for preoperative clients.

Headache and body aches

NURSING CONSIDERATIONS: Report headaches that are frequent or severe to the provider. Hypertension can be the cause.

CONTRAINDICATIONS/PRECAUTIONS

- Pregnancy Risk Category C. Qs
- Contraindicated in clients who have uncontrolled hypertension.
- Contraindicated in clients who have some cancers due to possible increase in tumor growth.

NURSING ADMINISTRATION

- Obtain baseline blood pressure. In clients who have chronic kidney disease, control hypertension before the start of treatment. QEBP
- Monitor blood pressure frequently, because adjustments in antihypertensive medication can also be required as treatment progresses.
- Administer by subcutaneous or IV bolus injection. Dosage is based on the client's weight.
- Do not agitate the vial of medication. Use each vial for one dose, and do not put the needle back into the vial when withdrawing the medication.
- Do not mix the medication with any other medication in the syringe.
- Dosing is usually three times/week, but can be once per week with some types of chemotherapy.
- Monitor iron levels, and implement measures to ensure an iron level that is within the expected reference range. RBC growth depends on adequate quantities of iron, folic acid, and vitamin B_{12}. Without adequate levels of these, erythropoietin is significantly less effective.
- Monitor Hgb and Hct twice per week until the target range is reached.
- Assure that clients receive the FDA's Risk Evaluation and Mitigation Strategy medication guide that explains risks and benefits of ESAs. The medication guide also discusses ways clients can help minimize risks of the medication. QPCC
- The longer-acting forms are administered less frequently.

NURSING EVALUATION OF MEDICATION EFFECTIVENESS

Depending on therapeutic intent, effectiveness can be evidenced by Hgb level of 10 to 11 g/dL and maximum Hct of 33%.

Leukopoietic growth factors

SELECT PROTOTYPE MEDICATION: Filgrastim

OTHER MEDICATION: Pegfilgrastim

PURPOSE

EXPECTED PHARMACOLOGICAL ACTION: Leukopoietic growth factors stimulate the bone marrow to increase production of neutrophils.

THERAPEUTIC USES
- Decreases the risk of infection in clients who have neutropenia, from cancer and other conditions
- To build up numbers of hematopoietic stem cells prior to harvesting for autologous transplant

COMPLICATIONS

Bone pain

NURSING CONSIDERATIONS
- Monitor for bone pain, and notify the provider.
- Administer acetaminophen, or opioid analgesic if acetaminophen is not effective.

Leukocytosis

NURSING CONSIDERATIONS
- Monitor CBC two times per week during treatment.
- Decrease dose or interrupt treatment if WBC is greater than 100,000/mm³ or absolute neutrophil count exceeds 10,000/mm³.

Splenomegaly and risk of splenic rupture

With long-term use

NURSING CONSIDERATIONS: Evaluate reports of left upper quadrant abdominal pain or shoulder tip pain carefully, and report to provider.

CONTRAINDICATIONS/PRECAUTIONS

- Pregnancy Risk Category C. Qs
- Contraindicated in clients who are sensitive to *Escherichia coli* protein.
- Use cautiously in clients who have cancer of the bone marrow, sickle cell disease, or respiratory disease, and in women who are breastfeeding and in children.

NURSING ADMINISTRATION

- Administer filgrastim via intermittent IV bolus, continuous IV, subcutaneous infusion, or subcutaneous injection.
- Do not agitate the vial of medication. Use each vial for one dose, and do not combine with other medications. Do not put the needle back into the vial when withdrawing the medication. Q EBP
- Monitor CBC two times per week.
- If the client will be administering subcutaneous filgrastim at home, provide thorough instruction on self-administration procedures.
- Administer pegfilgrastim by subcutaneous injection 24 hr after each round of chemotherapy. The client must then wait at least 14 days before starting the next round of chemotherapy.

NURSING EVALUATION OF MEDICATION EFFECTIVENESS

Depending on therapeutic intent, effectiveness can be evidenced by the following.
- Absence of infection
- WBC count and differential within expected reference ranges

Granulocyte-macrophage colony-stimulating factor

SELECT PROTOTYPE MEDICATION: Sargramostim

PURPOSE

EXPECTED PHARMACOLOGICAL ACTION: This medication acts on the bone marrow to increase production of white blood cells (neutrophils, monocytes, macrophages, eosinophils).

THERAPEUTIC USES
- Hastens bone marrow function after bone marrow transplant
- Used in the treatment of failed bone marrow transplant
- Given to older adult clients who have acute myelogenous leukemia after induction of chemotherapy to accelerate neutrophil recovery and decrease incidence of life-threatening infections

COMPLICATIONS

Diarrhea, weakness, rash, malaise, and bone pain

NURSING CONSIDERATIONS
- Monitor for adverse effects, and notify the provider if they occur.
- Administer acetaminophen.

Leukocytosis, thrombocytosis

NURSING CONSIDERATIONS
- Monitor CBC two times per week during treatment.
- Reduce dose or interrupt treatment for absolute neutrophil count 20,000/mm^3 or greater, WBC 50,000/mm3 or greater, or platelets 500,000/mm^3 or greater.

First IV dose effect

Tachycardia, hypotension, chills, fever, diaphoresis, dyspnea

NURSING CONSIDERATIONS: Assess carefully for these effects, and notify the provider if they occur.

CONTRAINDICATIONS/PRECAUTIONS

- Pregnancy Risk Category C.
- Contraindicated in clients allergic to yeast and certain other products.
- Use cautiously in clients who have lung, cardiac, kidney, or hepatic disease; hypoxia; peripheral edema; or pleural or pericardial effusion.
- Use cautiously in clients who have cancer of the bone marrow.

NURSING ADMINISTRATION

- Obtain baseline CBC, differential, and platelet count. Monitor periodically during treatment. Q EBP
- When administered subcutaneously, reconstitute with sterile water. Mix contents gently, but do not shake vial.
- Administer by IV infusion, diluted and without an in-line membrane filter. Slow or discontinue infusion if client who has pre-existing heart failure or respiratory disorders experiences increase in dyspnea.

NURSING EVALUATION OF MEDICATION EFFECTIVENESS

Depending on therapeutic intent, effectiveness can be evidenced by the following.
- Absence of infection
- WBC and differential within expected reference ranges

Thrombopoietic growth factors

SELECT PROTOTYPE MEDICATION: Oprelvekin

PURPOSE

EXPECTED PHARMACOLOGICAL ACTION: Increases the production of platelets

THERAPEUTIC USES: Decreases thrombocytopenia and the need for platelet transfusions in clients receiving chemotherapy

COMPLICATIONS

Fluid retention

Peripheral edema, dyspnea on exertion

NURSING CONSIDERATIONS
- Monitor I&O.
- Use cautiously in clients who have a history of heart failure or pleural effusion. If adverse effects occur, stop the medication and notify the provider.

Cardiac dysrhythmias

Tachycardia, atrial fibrillation, atrial flutter

NURSING CONSIDERATIONS
- Use cautiously in clients who have a history of cardiac dysrhythmias.
- Monitor vital signs, heart rate, and heart rhythm.
- If adverse effects occur, stop the medication and notify the provider.

Eye effects

Conjunctival injection, transient blurring of vision, papilledema (inflammation of the eye and eyelid)

NURSING CONSIDERATIONS: Advise the client to observe for adverse effects. The medication should be withheld until notification of the provider.

Allergic reactions, possible anaphylaxis

NURSING CONSIDERATIONS: Observe carefully for allergic reactions. Stop the medication and notify the provider if adverse effects occur.

CONTRAINDICATIONS/PRECAUTIONS

- Generally contraindicated in clients who have cancer of the bone marrow, because they can stimulate tumor growth. Qs
- Use cautiously in clients who have heart failure and pleural effusion.

NURSING ADMINISTRATION

- Obtain baseline CBC, platelet count, and electrolytes. QEBP
- Oprelvekin should not be agitated or combined with other medications.
- Administer oprelvekin once daily by subcutaneous injection until platelet count reaches the prescribed level.

NURSING EVALUATION OF MEDICATION EFFECTIVENESS

Depending on therapeutic intent, effectiveness can be evidenced by platelet count greater than 50,000/mm³.

Application Exercises

1. A nurse is caring for a client who is receiving daily doses of oprelvekin. Which of the following laboratory values should the nurse monitor to determine effectiveness of this medication?

   A. Hemoglobin

   B. Absolute neutrophil count

   C. Platelet count

   D. Total white blood count

2. A nurse is preparing to administer filgrastim for the first time to a client who has just undergone a bone marrow transplant. Which of the following interventions is appropriate?

   A. Administer IM in a large muscle mass to prevent injury.

   B. Ensure that the medication is refrigerated until just prior to administration.

   C. Shake vial gently to mix well before withdrawing dose.

   D. Discard vial after removing one dose of the medication.

3. A nurse is monitoring a client who is receiving epoetin alfa for adverse effects. The nurse should identify which of the following findings as an adverse effect of this medication? (Select all that apply)

   A. Leukocytosis

   B. Hypertension

   C. Edema

   D. Blurred vision

   E. Headache

4. A nurse is assessing a client who has chronic neutropenia and who has been receiving filgrastim. Which of the following actions should the nurse take to assess for an adverse effect of filgrastim?

   A. Assess for bone pain.

   B. Assess for right lower quadrant pain.

   C. Auscultate for crackles in the bases of the lungs.

   D. Auscultate the chest to listen for a heart murmur.

PRACTICE Active Learning Scenario

A nurse is teaching a client who has chronic kidney disease and a new prescription for subcutaneous epoetin alfa three times weekly. What should the nurse teach the client about this medication? Use the ATI Active Learning Template: Medication to complete this item.

THERAPEUTIC USES: Identify for epoetin alfa in this client.

COMPLICATIONS: Identify two adverse effects the client should watch for.

NURSING INTERVENTIONS: Describe four, including two tests the nurse should monitor periodically.

Application Exercises Key

1. A. Hemoglobin levels should be monitored for a client receiving epoetin alfa.

   B. Absolute neutrophil count should be monitored for a client receiving filgrastim.

   C. **CORRECT:** The expected outcome for oprelvekin is a platelet count greater than 50,000/mm³.

   D. A total WBC should be monitored for a client receiving sargramostim.

   Ⓝ *NCLEX® Connection: Pharmacological and Parenteral Therapies, Expected Actions/Outcomes*

2. A. Filgrastim is not administered by the IM route.

   B. The nurse should allow the medication to reach room temperature prior to administration.

   C. Before withdrawing a dose of filgrastim, the nurse should take care not to shake the medication vial.

   D. **CORRECT:** Only one dose of filgrastim should be withdrawn from the vial and the vial should then be discarded.

   Ⓝ *NCLEX® Connection: Pharmacological and Parenteral Therapies, Medication Administration*

3. A. Leukocytosis is an adverse effect of filgrastim, rather than for epoetin alfa.

   B. **CORRECT:** Hypertension is an adverse effect of epoetin alfa that the nurse should monitor for throughout treatment.

   C. Edema is an adverse effect of oprelvekin caused by fluid retention, rather than of epoetin alfa.

   D. Blurred vision is an adverse effect of oprelvekin, rather than of epoetin alfa.

   E. **CORRECT:** Headache is an adverse effect of epoetin alfa.

   Ⓝ *NCLEX® Connection: Pharmacological and Parenteral Therapies, Adverse Effects/Contraindications/Side Effects/Interactions*

4. A. **CORRECT:** Bone pain is a dose-related adverse effect of filgrastim. It can be treated with acetaminophen and, if necessary, an opioid analgesic.

   B. Palpating gently for right lower quadrant pain can be a necessary part of the nurse's assessment, but will not assess for an adverse effect of filgrastim.

   C. Auscultating for crackles in the bases of the lungs can be a necessary part of the nurse's assessment, but will not assess for an adverse effect of filgrastim.

   D. Auscultating the chest to listen for a heart murmur can be a necessary part of the nurse's assessment, but will not assess for an adverse effect of filgrastim.

   Ⓝ *NCLEX® Connection: Pharmacological and Parenteral Therapies, Adverse Effects/Contraindications/Side Effects/Interactions*

PRACTICE Answer

Using the ATI Active Learning Template: Medication

THERAPEUTIC USES: Erythropoietin, a substance that stimulates bone marrow to produce red blood cells, is produced by the kidney. In clients who have chronic kidney disease, erythropoietin is no longer present and anemia results. Epoetin alfa stimulates production of red blood cells in these clients.

COMPLICATIONS
- Headaches and myalgia (body aches)
- Thrombotic events, such as myocardial infarction and stroke
- Hypertension (common, sometimes serious)
- A too-rapid increase (Hgb greater than 1 g/dL over 2 weeks, or Hgb greater than 10 g/dL) can worsen hypertension, increase risk of thrombosis, and cause seizures.

NURSING INTERVENTIONS
- Monitor baseline iron levels, CBC with differential, and platelet count.
- Monitor Hgb and Hct twice weekly until blood counts stabilize.
- Calculate dosages carefully. Both subcutaneous and IV epoetin alfa have dosages based on the client's weight. Do not shake the epoetin alfa vial, and discard vial after one dose is removed.
- Monitor blood pressure carefully, and report increases to the provider. Question the client about frequency and severity of headaches, which could be an indication of increasing blood pressure or a simple adverse effect.

Ⓝ *NCLEX® Connection: Pharmacological and Parenteral Therapies, Medication Administration*

UNIT 5   MEDICATIONS AFFECTING THE
HEMATOLOGIC SYSTEM

CHAPTER 27   *Blood and*
Blood Products

Blood and blood products are used to increase intravascular volume, replace clotting factors and components of blood, replace blood loss, and improve oxygen carrying capacity. Blood products include whole blood and components of blood, such as packed red blood cells, platelets, plasma, white blood cells, and albumin.

PURPOSE

Whole blood

EXPECTED PHARMACOLOGICAL ACTION: Increases circulating blood volume

THERAPEUTIC USES
- Replacement therapy for acute blood loss secondary to traumatic injuries or surgical procedures
- Volume expansion in clients who have extensive burn injury, dehydration, shock

TYPE OF REACTION
- Acute hemolytic reaction
- Febrile nonhemolytic reaction
- Anaphylactic reactions
- Mild allergic reactions
- Circulatory overload
- Hyperkalemia
- Transfusion-associated graft-versus-host disease
- Sepsis

Packed red blood cells (PRBCs)

EXPECTED PHARMACOLOGICAL ACTION: Increases the number of RBCs

THERAPEUTIC USES
- PRBCs indicated in severe symptomatic anemia (Hgb 6 to 10 g/dL)
- Hemoglobinopathies
- Medication-induced hemolytic anemia
- Erythroblastosis fetalis

TYPE OF REACTION
- Acute hemolytic reaction
- Febrile nonhemolytic reaction
- Anaphylactic reactions
- Mild allergic reactions
- Hyperkalemia
- Transfusion-associated graft-versus-host disease
- Sepsis

Platelet concentrate

EXPECTED PHARMACOLOGICAL ACTION:
Increases platelet counts

THERAPEUTIC USES
- Platelets indicated in thrombocytopenia for a platelet count less than 20,000/mm³ (aplastic anemia, chemotherapy-induced bone marrow suppression)
- Platelets indicated in active bleeding for a platelet count less than 50,000/mm³

TYPE OF REACTION
- Febrile nonhemolytic reaction
- Mild allergic reactions
- Sepsis

Fresh frozen plasma (FFP)

EXPECTED PHARMACOLOGICAL ACTION: Replaces coagulation factors

THERAPEUTIC USES
- Active bleeding or massive hemorrhage
- Extensive burns
- Shock
- Disseminated intravascular coagulation
- Antithrombin III deficiency
- Thrombotic thrombocytopenic purpura
- Reversal of anticoagulation effects of warfarin
- Replacement therapy for coagulation factors II, V, VII, IX, X, and XI

TYPE OF REACTION
- Acute hemolytic reaction
- Febrile nonhemolytic reaction
- Anaphylactic reactions
- Mild allergic reactions
- Circulatory overload
- Sepsis

Pheresed granulocytes

EXPECTED PHARMACOLOGICAL ACTION:
Replaces neutrophils/granulocytes

THERAPEUTIC USES
- Severe neutropenia (absolute neutrophil count less than 500/mm³)
- Life-threatening bacterial/fungal infection not responding to antibiotic therapy
- Neonatal sepsis
- Neutrophil dysfunction

TYPE OF REACTION
- Acute hemolytic reaction
- Febrile nonhemolytic reaction
- Anaphylactic reactions
- Mild allergic reactions
- Circulatory overload
- Sepsis (infusion of contaminated products)

Albumin

EXPECTED PHARMACOLOGICAL ACTION: Expands circulating blood volume by exerting oncotic pressure

THERAPEUTIC USES
- Hypovolemia
- Hypoalbuminemia
- Burns
- Adult respiratory distress
- Cardiopulmonary bypass surgery
- Hemolytic disease of the newborn

TYPE OF REACTION: Risk for fluid volume excess, such as pulmonary edema

COMPLICATIONS

Acute hemolytic reaction

Chills, fever, low back pain, tachycardia, tachypnea, hypotension

NURSING CONSIDERATIONS
- Prevent by performing all safety checks, following facility protocol carefully. Ensure client identity (using two nurses) and that Rh and ABO types are compatible.
- Assess vital signs at baseline and by facility protocol during the first 15 to 30 min. Stay with the client during that time. Continue to take vital signs at least hourly or by facility policy.
- Acute hemolytic reaction usually occurs during first 50 mL of infusion, but onset can be delayed.
- If manifestations occur, stop infusion immediately, keeping IV line open with 0.9% sodium chloride and new IV tubing. Notify the provider.

Febrile nonhemolytic reaction, fever, headache

- Febrile nonhemolytic reaction: most common (sudden chills)
- Fever: increase in temperature greater than 1° C from baseline

NURSING CONSIDERATIONS
- Observe for manifestations of a reaction and stop the transfusion if they occur, keeping the IV line open with 0.9% sodium chloride.
- Notify the provider immediately.
- Administer acetaminophen for fever.

Anaphylactic reactions

Anxiety, urticaria, wheezing, shock, cardiac arrest

NURSING CONSIDERATIONS
- If manifestations occur, stop the transfusion and notify the provider immediately, keeping the IV line open with 0.9% sodium chloride.
- Initiate CPR if necessary.
- Have epinephrine ready for IM or IV injection.

Mild allergic reactions (flushing, itching, urticaria)

NURSING CONSIDERATIONS
- Note that a client who has a history of allergic reaction to blood transfusion or has undergone a stem cell transplant might receive a prescription for washed (leukocyte-poor) red blood cells to prevent allergic reaction.
- If manifestations occur, stop the transfusion and notify the provider immediately, keeping the IV line open with 0.9% sodium chloride.
- If manifestations are very mild and there is no respiratory compromise, antihistamines may be prescribed and the transfusion restarted slowly.

Circulatory overload

Cough, shortness of breath, crackles, hypertension, tachycardia, distended neck veins

NURSING CONSIDERATIONS
- Observe for manifestations of fluid volume excess.
- In older adults or clients at risk for overload, transfuse 1 unit of PRBCs over 2 to 4 hr, avoiding any concurrent fluid infusion into another IV site. Monitor vital signs every 15 min throughout transfusion. If possible, wait 2 hr between units of blood when multiple units have been prescribed.
- If manifestations occur, stop the transfusion, place the client in a sitting position with the legs down, and notify the provider.
- Administer diuretics and oxygen as appropriate.
- Monitor I&O.
- Prior to any transfusion, assess kidney, respiratory, and cardiovascular function for risk of overload.

Sepsis

Rapid onset of chills and fever, vomiting, diarrhea, hypotension, shock

NURSING CONSIDERATIONS
- Ensure IV access, and have equipment prepared prior to removing blood product from refrigeration.
- Inspect blood product for gas bubbles, discoloration, or cloudiness (which can indicate bacterial contamination) and return to blood bank if abnormalities are seen.
- Transfuse unit of blood within 4 hr after removal from refrigeration.
- Observe for sepsis during and following transfusion.
- Stop the transfusion, and keep the line open with 0.9% sodium chloride.
- Notify the provider immediately if manifestations of sepsis occur.
- Obtain blood culture, send transfusion bag for analysis for possible contaminants, and treat sepsis with antibiotics, IV fluids, vasopressors, and steroids.

Hyperkalemia due to lysis of blood cells

Bradycardia, hypotension, irregular heartbeat, paresthesias of extremities, muscle twitching, potassium level 5.0 mEq/L or greater

NURSING CONSIDERATIONS

- Be aware that lysis of blood cells is more likely in products that were previously frozen or older than 1 week.
- Check potassium level before transfusion to obtain baseline.
- Notify the provider immediately for manifestations of hyperkalemia.

Transfusion-associated graft-versus-host disease

Rare, and occurring 1 to 2 weeks following transfusion

MANIFESTATIONS: Nausea, vomiting, weight loss, hepatitis, thrombocytopenia

NURSING CONSIDERATIONS

- Can be prevented by using irradiated blood products that contain decreased T-cells and cytokines.
- Teach clients to report manifestations to the provider.

CONTRAINDICATIONS/PRECAUTIONS

- Contraindicated in clients who have hypersensitivity reactions.
- Observe culturally sensitive or religious issues regarding blood transfusion, such as for clients who are Jehovah's Witnesses. Infusing colloids and other plasma expanders can be acceptable. QPCC

NURSING ADMINISTRATION

- Obtain baseline laboratory values: Hgb, Hct, platelet count, total protein, albumin levels, PT, PTT, fibrinogen, potassium, pH, and serum calcium.
- Prior to start of transfusion, assess laboratory values and blood transfusion history, verify the prescription, and ensure that client has signed consent for transfusion. Assess for risk of fluid overload. A diuretic may be prescribed between units for clients at risk for fluid overload. Qs
- Obtain baseline vital signs before beginning transfusion. Stay with the client, and monitor vital signs per facility policy for 15 to 30 min and then at least hourly until completed.
- Assess existing infusion site for patency or infection. Ensure that a 20-gauge or larger IV catheter is used to avoid hemolysis of blood cells.
- Obtain the blood product from the blood bank just before beginning transfusion (no more than 30 min between taking unit of PRBCs from blood bank refrigeration and beginning of transfusion). Ensure transfusion is complete at least 4 hr after product is taken from the blood bank refrigerator.
- Carefully perform all safety checks to ensure correct product is administered to the correct client. Qs

- Use only 0.9% sodium chloride solution to administer with blood products; prime IV and blood tubing with this solution. Use a blood filter for most blood products and either a Y-type or straight tubing set depending on facility policy. Change tubing after every 2 units to prevent bacterial sepsis.
- For platelet transfusion, use a specialized platelet filter with shorter tubing. Platelets stick onto the standard blood administration filter and to the longer tubing so it is important to use a platelet filter.
- Document blood product type, blood bank number of product, total volume infused, time of start and completion of transfusion, vital signs, and any adverse effects, as well as actions taken.
- Observe universal precautions during handling and administration of blood products.
- Do not administer blood products with any other medications.

COMPLETE TRANSFUSION WITHIN SPECIFIED TIME. QEBP
- **Whole blood, PRBCs:** about 250 mL/unit; infuse within 2 to 4 hr.
- **Platelet concentrate:** about 300 mL/unit; infuse within 15 to 30 min/unit.
- **FFP:** about 200 mL/unit; infuse over 30 to 60 min/unit.
- **White blood cells:** about 400 mL/unit; infuse over 45 min to 1 hr.
- **Albumin**
  - 5%: 250 to 500 mL bottle; infuse 1 to 10 mL/min.
  - 25%: 50 to 100 mL bottle; infuse 4 mL/min.

IF A BLOOD TRANSFUSION REACTION IS NOTED
- Stop the transfusion and notify the provider immediately. Qs
- Do not turn on IV fluids that are connected to the Y tubing because the remaining blood in the Y tubing will be infused and aggravate the client's reaction. Administer 0.9% sodium chloride through new tubing.
- Document start and completion times of transfusion, total volume of transfusion, and client response to the transfusion.
- Stay with the client, and monitor vital signs and urinary output.
- Notify the blood bank, recheck the identification tag and numbers on the blood bag, and send the blood bag and IV tubing to the blood bank for analysis.
- Obtain a urine specimen, and send to the laboratory to determine RBC hemolysis. Insert an indwelling catheter if hemolytic reaction is suspected to monitor urine output.
- Repeat type and cross match. Obtain CBC and bilirubin to determine hemolysis.
- Complete a transfusion log sheet, which includes complete record of baseline vital signs, ongoing monitoring, and client response to transfusion. Incorporate this in the medical record.

CONSIDERATIONS FOR OLDER ADULT CLIENTS ©

- Use caution to prevent overload of fluid. Transfuse whole blood or PRBCs slowly, over 2 to 4 hr. If possible, wait 2 hr between transfusion of multiple units.
- Take vital signs every 15 min throughout the procedure. Monitor for findings of fluid overload frequently during and after the transfusion.

FOR MASSIVE TRANSFUSION

Greater than or equal to replacement of total blood volume in 24 hr, about 10 units for an adult or 5 units in 4 hr

- Monitor platelets, PT, and aPTT every 5 units and replace as needed.
- Monitor potassium and calcium levels.
- Monitor ECG for changes associated with hypokalemia, hyperkalemia, or hypocalcemia.
- Warm blood using blood warmer to prevent hypothermia.

AUTOLOGOUS BLOOD TRANSFUSION

- Several weeks prior to elective surgery the client donates blood which can be used for that client after surgery.
- Weekly blood collection can be done if client has normal laboratory values. Iron supplements are prescribed.
- Fresh blood can be saved for up to 40 days, or blood can be frozen for up to 10 years before use for a client who has a rare blood type.
- Autologous transfusion prevents some blood reactions (e.g., acute hemolytic), but client is still at risk for circulatory overload and sepsis.

Application Exercises

1. A nurse is preparing to administer a transfusion of 300 mL of pooled platelets for a client who has severe thrombocytopenia. The nurse should plan to administer the transfusion over which of the following time frames?

   A. Within 30 min/unit

   B. Within 60 min/unit

   C. Within 2 hr/unit

   D. Within 4 hr/unit

2. A nurse is transfusing a unit of packed red blood cells (PRBCs) for a client who has anemia due to chemotherapy. The client reports a sudden headache and chills. The client's temperature is 2° F higher than her baseline. In addition to notifying the provider, which of the following actions should the nurse take? (Select all that apply.)

   A. Stop the transfusion.

   B. Place the client in an upright position with feet down.

   C. Remove the blood bag and tubing from the IV catheter.

   D. Obtain a urine specimen.

   E. Infuse dextrose 5% in water through the IV.

3. A nurse is preparing to transfuse a unit of packed red blood cells (PRBCs) for a client who has severe anemia. Which of the following interventions will prevent an acute hemolytic reaction?

   A. Ensure that the client has a patent IV line before obtaining blood product from the refrigerator.

   B. Obtain help from another nurse to confirm the correct client and blood product.

   C. Take a complete set of vital signs before beginning transfusion and periodically during the transfusion.

   D. Stay with the client for the first 15 to 30 min of the transfusion.

4. A nurse is caring for a hospitalized client who has an activated partial thromboplastin time (aPTT) greater than 1.5 times the expected reference range. Which of the following blood products should the nurse prepare to transfuse?

   A. Whole blood

   B. Platelets

   C. Fresh frozen plasma

   D. Packed red blood cells

5. A nurse is assessing a client during transfusion of a unit of whole blood. The client develops a cough, shortness of breath, elevated blood pressure, and distended neck veins. The nurse should anticipate a prescription for which of the following medications?

   A. Epinephrine

   B. Lorazepam

   C. Furosemide

   D. Diphenhydramine

PRACTICE Active Learning Scenario

A nurse is preparing to transfuse a unit of packed red blood cells (PRBCs) for an older adult client who has who has a GI bleed and Hgb 6.0 g/dL. Use the ATI Active Learning Template: Therapeutic Procedure to complete this item.

OUTCOMES/EVALUATION: What assessment data would indicate to the nurse that transfusion of PRBCs is indicated in this client?

1. A. **CORRECT:** Platelets are fragile and should be administered quickly to reduce the risk of clumping. The nurse should administer the platelets within 15 to 30 min/unit.

   B. The nurse should administer fresh frozen plasma within 30 to 60 min/unit.

   C. The nurse should administer a unit of whole blood or PRBCs within 2 to 4 hr.

   D. The nurse should administer a unit of whole blood or PRBCs within 2 to 4 hr.

   Ⓝ *NCLEX® Connection: Pharmacological and Parenteral Therapies, Parenteral/Intravenous Therapies*

2. A. **CORRECT:** The nurse should stop the transfusion for a rise in temperature of 2° F and reports of chills and fever. The client can be having a hemolytic reaction to the blood or a febrile reaction.

   B. The nurse should place a client who has circulatory overload in the upright position with the feet down. This client's manifestations do not indicate circulatory overload.

   C. **CORRECT:** The nurse should avoid infusing more PRBCs into the client's vein, and should remove the blood bag and tubing from the client's IV catheter.

   D. **CORRECT:** Obtaining a urine specimen to check for hemolysis is standard procedure when the client has a reaction to a blood transfusion.

   E. The nurse should only infuse 0.9% sodium chloride into the client's IV along with a transfusion of PRBCs. The nurse should infuse 0.9% sodium chloride until a new prescription is received.

   Ⓝ *NCLEX® Connection: Pharmacological and Parenteral Therapies, Adverse Effects/Contraindications/Side Effects/Interactions*

3. A. Ensuring that the client has a patent IV line before obtaining the blood product is important but will not prevent an acute hemolytic reaction.

   B. **CORRECT:** Identifying and matching the correct blood product with the correct client will prevent an acute hemolytic reaction from occurring because this reaction is caused by ABO or Rh incompatibility.

   C. Taking vital signs before and during the transfusion can ensure prompt identification and treatment of an acute hemolytic reaction, but will not prevent it from occurring.

   D. Staying with the client for the first 15 to 30 min of the transfusion can ensure prompt identification and treatment of an acute hemolytic reaction but will not prevent it from occurring.

   Ⓝ *NCLEX® Connection: Pharmacological and Parenteral Therapies, Expected Actions/Outcomes*

4. A. Whole blood is transfused in clients who have experienced acute blood loss or who require volume expansion in addition to replacement of red blood cells. It is not indicated for clients who have an elevated aPTT.

   B. Platelets are transfused for clients who have severe thrombocytopenia and are not indicated for clients who have an elevated aPTT.

   C. **CORRECT:** Fresh frozen plasma is indicated for a client who has an elevated aPTT because it replaces coagulation factors and can help prevent bleeding.

   D. PRBCs are transfused for clients who are severely anemic but who do not require the extra plasma found in a unit of whole blood. PRBCs are not indicated for clients who have an elevated aPTT.

   Ⓝ *NCLEX® Connection: Pharmacological and Parenteral Therapies, Expected Actions/Outcomes*

5. A. Epinephrine may be prescribed for a client who has anaphylactic shock caused by a severe allergic reaction, but is not indicated for the manifestations assessed in this client.

   B. Lorazepam, a benzodiazepine, may be prescribed for a client who has severe anxiety, but it is not indicated for the manifestations assessed in this client.

   C. **CORRECT:** Furosemide, a loop diuretic, may be prescribed to relieve manifestations of circulatory overload.

   D. Diphenhydramine, a histamine blocker, may be prescribed to treat mild allergic reactions, but it is not indicated for the manifestations assessed in this client.

   Ⓝ *NCLEX® Connection: Pharmacological and Parenteral Therapies, Medication Administration*

PRACTICE Answer

Using the ATI Active Learning Template: Therapeutic Procedure

OUTCOMES/EVALUATION: A client who lost blood from a GI bleed can need a unit of PRBCs if his Hgb is below 10 g/dL and he is demonstrating manifestations of hypovolemia (increase in pulse and respiration rate; decrease in blood pressure; low oxygen saturation; cool and pale or cyanotic; decreased capillary refill time; decreased urinary output). If hypoxic, the client will exhibit decreased level of consciousness and confusion. PRBCs restore red blood cells and improve oxygenation. If the client has lost a large amount of fluid volume, whole blood, rather than PRBCs, can be indicated.

Ⓝ *NCLEX® Connection: Pharmacological and Parenteral Therapies, Expected Actions/Outcomes*

When reviewing the following chapters, keep in mind the relevant topics and tasks of the NCLEX outline, in particular:

Client Needs: Pharmacological and Parenteral Therapies

ADVERSE EFFECTS/CONTRAINDICATIONS/SIDE EFFECTS/ INTERACTIONS: Document side effects and adverse effects of medications and parenteral therapy.

EXPECTED ACTIONS/OUTCOMES: Evaluate client response to medication.

PARENTERAL/INTRAVENOUS THERAPIES: Evaluate the client's response to intermittent parenteral fluid therapy.

CHAPTER 28 *Peptic Ulcer Disease*

Pharmacological management of peptic ulcer disease addresses the imbalance between gastric mucosal defenses, including mucus and bicarbonate, and antagonistic factors such as *H. pylori* infection, gastric acid, pepsin, smoking, and use of NSAIDs.

For clients who have *H. pylori*, antibiotics are used to eradicate the disease process. All of the other medications prescribed are used to promote healing of the GI tract.

Therapeutic management outcomes include reduction of manifestations, promotion of healing, prevention of complications, and prevention of recurrence.

Antibiotics

SELECT PROTOTYPE MEDICATIONS
- Amoxicillin
- Bismuth
- Clarithromycin
- Metronidazole
- Tetracycline
- Tinidazole

PURPOSE

EXPECTED PHARMACOLOGICAL ACTION: Eradication of *H. pylori* bacteria

THERAPEUTIC USES: Therapy should include combination of two or three antibiotics for 14 days to increase effectiveness and to minimize the development of medication resistance. Qpcc

NURSING ADMINISTRATION

- Advise client to take amoxicillin, clarithromycin, and metronidazole with food to decrease gastric disturbances.
- Advise clients that adverse effects of nausea and diarrhea are common.
- Remind clients to take the full course of prescribed medications.

Histamine$_2$-receptor antagonists

SELECT PROTOTYPE MEDICATION: Ranitidine

OTHER MEDICATIONS
- Cimetidine
- Famotidine
- Nizatidine: PO use only

PURPOSE

EXPECTED PHARMACOLOGICAL ACTION: Block H_2 receptors, which reduces the volume of gastric acid and lowers the concentration of hydrogen ions in the stomach

THERAPEUTIC USES
- Prescribed for gastric and duodenal ulcers, GERD, hypersecretory conditions (Zollinger–Ellison syndrome), aspiration pneumonitis, heartburn, and acid indigestion
- Used in conjunction with antibiotics to treat ulcers caused by *H. pylori*

COMPLICATIONS

CIMETIDINE

Blocked androgen receptors

Resulting in decreased libido, gynecomastia, and impotence.

CLIENT EDUCATION: Inform clients of these possible effects.

CNS effects (lethargy, depression, confusion)

NURSING CONSIDERATIONS
- These effects are seen more often in older adults who have kidney or liver dysfunction.
- Cimetidine should be avoided in older adults.

RANITIDINE

Constipation, diarrhea, nausea

NURSING CONSIDERATIONS: Report these effects to the provider.

FAMOTIDINE

Dizziness, drowsiness and constipation.

CLIENT EDUCATION: Avoid tasks that require alertness, and take medication at bedtime.

CONTRAINDICATIONS/PRECAUTIONS

- These medications are Pregnancy Risk Category B.
- Use in older adults can cause antiadrenergic effects (impotence) and CNS effects (confusion). Ⓖ
- H₂-receptor antagonists decrease gastric acidity, which promotes bacterial colonization of the stomach and the respiratory tract. Use cautiously in clients who are at a high risk for pneumonia, including clients who have chronic obstructive pulmonary disease (COPD).

INTERACTIONS

Cimetidine can inhibit medication-metabolizing enzymes and thus increase the levels of warfarin, phenytoin, theophylline, and lidocaine.

NURSING CONSIDERATIONS

- In clients taking warfarin, monitor for indications of bleeding.
- Monitor INR and PT levels, and adjust warfarin dosages accordingly. Ⓠ EBP
- In clients taking phenytoin, theophylline, and lidocaine, monitor serum levels and adjust dosages accordingly.

Concurrent use of antacids can decrease absorption of histamine₂-receptor antagonists.

NURSING CONSIDERATIONS: Advise clients not to take an antacid 1 hr before or after taking a histamine₂-receptor antagonist.

NURSING ADMINISTRATION

- Cimetidine, ranitidine, and famotidine can be administered IV for acute situations.
- Advise clients to eat meals on a regular schedule in a relaxed setting, and to not overeat.
- Instruct clients to avoid foods that promote gastric acid secretion, such as caffeine beverages and decaffeinated ad caffeinated coffee.
- Inform clients that adequate rest and reduction of stress can promote healing.
- Clients should avoid smoking, which can delay healing.
- Encourage clients to avoid aspirin and other NSAIDs unless taking low-dose aspirin therapy for prevention of cardiovascular disease.
- Alcohol can exacerbate peptic ulcer disease. Advise clients to avoid drinking alcohol.
- Availability of these medications OTC can discourage clients from seeking appropriate health care. Encourage clients to see a provider if manifestations persist.
- The medication regimen can be complex, often requiring clients to take two or three different medications for an extended period of time. Encourage clients to adhere to the medication regimen, and provide support.
- Ranitidine can be taken with or without food.
- Treatment of peptic ulcer disease is usually started as an oral dose twice a day until the ulcer is healed, followed by a maintenance dose, which usually is taken once a day at bedtime.
- Teach clients to notify the provider for any indication of obvious or occult GI bleeding, such as coffee-ground emesis.

Proton pump inhibitor

SELECT PROTOTYPE MEDICATION: Omeprazole

OTHER MEDICATIONS
- Pantoprazole
- Lansoprazole
- Dexlansoprazole
- Rabeprazole
- Esomeprazole

PURPOSE

EXPECTED PHARMACOLOGICAL ACTION: Block basal and stimulated acid production, and reduce gastric acid secretion by irreversibly inhibiting the enzyme that produces gastric acid

THERAPEUTIC USE: Prescribed for gastric and duodenal ulcers, erosive esophagitis, GERD, and hypersecretory conditions, such as Zollinger-Ellison syndrome

COMPLICATIONS

Minor adverse effects with short-term treatment include headache, diarrhea, nausea, and vomiting.

LONG-TERM TREATMENT

Pneumonia

CLIENT EDUCATION: Inform clients of these possible effects and to monitor and report manifestations of a respiratory infection.

Osteoporosis and fractures

CLIENT EDUCATION: Advise clients to increase vitamin D and calcium intake.

Rebound acid hypersecretion

CLIENT EDUCATION: Advise clients to take a low dose if possible and to taper slowly to discontinue.

Hypomagnesemia

CLIENT EDUCATION: Advise clients to monitor and report manifestations of hypomagnesemia, such as tremors, muscle cramps, and seizures.

CONTRAINDICATIONS/PRECAUTIONS

- These medications are Pregnancy Risk Category C.
- Contraindicated for clients hypersensitive to medication and during lactation.
- Use cautiously in children and with clients who have dysphagia or liver disease.
- These medications increase the risk for pneumonia. Use cautiously in clients at high risk for pneumonia, including clients who have COPD.

INTERACTIONS

Digoxin and phenytoin levels can increase when used concurrently with omeprazole.
NURSING CONSIDERATIONS: Monitor digoxin and phenytoin levels carefully if prescribed concurrently.

Absorption of ketoconazole, itraconazole, and atazanavir is decreased when taken concurrently with proton pump inhibitors.
NURSING CONSIDERATIONS: Avoid concurrent use. If necessary to administer concurrently, separate medication administration by 2 to 12 hr.

The beneficial effects of clopidogrel can decrease with concurrent use.
NURSING CONSIDERATIONS: Monitor for thrombotic events.

NURSING ADMINISTRATION

- Do not crush, chew, or break sustained-release capsules.
- Do not open capsule and sprinkle contents over food to facilitate swallowing.
- Clients should take omeprazole once per day prior to eating in the morning.
- Encourage clients to avoid alcohol and irritating medications, such as NSAIDs.
- Active ulcers should be treated for 4 to 6 weeks.
- Pantoprazole can be administered to clients intravenously. In addition to low incidence of headache and diarrhea, there can be irritation at the injection site leading to thrombophlebitis. Monitor the IV site for indications of inflammation (redness, swelling, local pain), and change the IV site if indicated.
- Teach clients to notify the provider for any indication of obvious or occult GI bleeding, such as coffee-ground emesis.

Mucosal protectant

SELECT PROTOTYPE MEDICATION: Sucralfate

PURPOSE

EXPECTED PHARMACOLOGICAL ACTION
- The acidic environment of the stomach and duodenum changes sucralfate into a protective barrier that adheres to an ulcer. This protects the ulcer from further injury from acid and pepsin.
- This viscous substance can stick to the ulcer for up to 6 hr.

THERAPEUTIC USES
- Sucralfate is used for clients who have acute duodenal ulcers and those requiring maintenance therapy.
- Sucralfate is not absorbed. Therefore, it has no systemic effects.
- Investigational use of sucralfate includes gastric ulcers and GERD.

COMPLICATIONS

Constipation

CLIENT EDUCATION: To prevent constipation, encourage clients to increase dietary fiber and drink at least 1,500 mL/day if fluids are not restricted.

CONTRAINDICATIONS/PRECAUTIONS

- Pregnancy Risk Category B.
- Contraindicated in clients who are hypersensitive to the medication.
- Use cautiously in clients who have chronic kidney disease.

INTERACTIONS

Sucralfate can interfere with the absorption of phenytoin, digoxin, warfarin, and ciprofloxacin.
NURSING CONSIDERATIONS: Maintain a 2-hr interval between these medications and sucralfate to minimize this interaction.

Antacids interfere with the absorption of sucralfate.
NURSING CONSIDERATIONS: Take sucralfate 30 min before or after antacids.

NURSING ADMINISTRATION

- Assist clients with the medication regimen.
- Instruct clients that sucralfate should be taken four times a day, 1 hr before meals, and again at bedtime.
- Clients can break or dissolve the medication in water, but should not crush or chew the tablet.
- Encourage clients to complete the course of treatment.

Antacids

SELECT PROTOTYPE MEDICATION: Aluminum hydroxide

OTHER MEDICATIONS
- Magnesium hydroxide
- Calcium carbonate

PURPOSE

EXPECTED PHARMACOLOGICAL ACTION
- Antacids neutralize gastric acid by producing neutral salts, and inactivating pepsin.
- Mucosal protection can occur from stimulation of the production of prostaglandins.

THERAPEUTIC USES: Antacids are used in clients to treat peptic ulcer disease and GERD by promoting healing and relieving pain.

COMPLICATIONS

Constipation, diarrhea

Aluminum and calcium compounds: Constipation

Magnesium compounds: Diarrhea

CLIENT EDUCATION
- Advise clients that use of these compounds can be alternated to offset intestinal effects and normalize bowel function. Q EBP
- If a client has difficulty managing bowel function, recommend a combination product that contains aluminum hydroxide and magnesium hydroxide.

Fluid retention

Antacids containing sodium can result in fluid retention.

CLIENT EDUCATION: Teach clients who have hypertension or heart failure to avoid antacids that contain sodium.

Hypophosphatemia, hypomagnesemia

Possible effects of aluminum hydroxide

NURSING CONSIDERATIONS: Monitor electrolyte levels.

Toxicity, hypermagnesemia

Magnesium compounds can lead to toxicity and hypermagnesemia in clients who have impaired kidney function.

CLIENT EDUCATION
- Teach clients who have impaired kidney function to avoid antacids that contain magnesium.
- Monitor for CNS depression.

CONTRAINDICATIONS/PRECAUTIONS

- Aluminum hydroxide is Pregnancy Risk Category C.
- Antacids should be used with caution in clients who have GI perforation or obstruction.
- Use cautiously in clients who have abdominal pain.

INTERACTIONS

Aluminum compounds bind to phenytoin, and tetracycline interferes with absorption.
CLIENT EDUCATION: Teach clients to take these medications 4 to 6 hr apart.

NURSING ADMINISTRATION

- Clients taking tablets should be instructed to chew the tablets thoroughly and then drink at least 8 oz of water or milk.
- Teach clients to shake liquid formulations to ensure even dispersion of the medication.
- Compliance is difficult for clients due to the frequency of administration. Medication can be administered seven times a day: 1 hr and 3 hr after meals, and again at bedtime. Encourage compliance by reinforcing the intended effect of the antacid (such as relief of pain, healing of ulcer). Q PCC
- Teach clients to take all medications at least 1 hr before or after taking an antacid.

Prostaglandin E analog

SELECT PROTOTYPE MEDICATION: Misoprostol

PURPOSE

EXPECTED PHARMACOLOGICAL ACTION

Acts as an endogenous prostaglandin in the GI tract that decreases acid secretion, increases the secretion of bicarbonate and protective mucus, and promotes vasodilation to maintain submucosal blood flow. These actions serve to prevent gastric ulcers.

THERAPEUTIC USES

- Used in clients taking long-term NSAIDs to prevent gastric ulcers.
- Unlabeled use: Used in clients who are pregnant only to induce labor by causing cervical ripening.

COMPLICATIONS

Diarrhea

With concurrent use of magnesium antacids

NURSING CONSIDERATIONS
- Instruct clients to notify the provider of diarrhea or abdominal pain.
- Reduce dosage if needed.

Dysmenorrhea, spotting

NURSING CONSIDERATIONS
- Instruct clients to notify the provider if dysmenorrhea and spotting occur.
- The provider might discontinue the medication.

CONTRAINDICATIONS/PRECAUTIONS

- Pregnancy Risk Category X
- If women of childbearing years use misoprostol, they must be able to comply with birth-control measures, be given oral and written warnings about the adverse effects, have a negative serum pregnancy test 2 weeks prior to initiating therapy, and begin therapy only on the second or third day of the menstrual cycle. Qs

NURSING ADMINISTRATION

Teach clients to take misoprostol with meals and at bedtime.

NURSING EVALUATION OF MEDICATION EFFECTIVENESS

Depending on therapeutic intent, effectiveness can be evidenced by the following.
- Reduced frequency or absence of GERD manifestations (heartburn, bloating, belching)
- Absence of GI bleeding
- Healing of gastric and duodenal ulcers
- No reoccurrence of ulcer

Application Exercises

1. A nurse is providing instructions to a client who has a prescription for amoxicillin and clarithromycin to treat a peptic ulcer. Which of the following information should the nurse include in the teaching?

- A. "Take these medications with food."
- B. "These medications can turn your stool black"
- C. "These medications can cause photosensitivity."
- D. "The purpose of these medications is to decrease the pH of gastric juices in the stomach."

2. A nurse is teaching a client who has a new prescription for omeprazole for management of heartburn. Which of the following information should the nurse include in the teaching?

- A. Take this medication at bedtime.
- B. This medication decreases the production of gastric acid.
- C. Take this medication 2 hr after eating.
- D. This medication can cause hyperkalemia.

3. A nurse is teaching a client who is taking sucralfate PO for peptic ulcer disease has a new prescription for phenytoin to control seizures. Which of the following instructions should the nurse include?

- A. Take an antacid with the sucralfate.
- B. Take sucralfate with a glass of milk.
- C. Allow a 2-hr interval between these medications.
- D. Chew the sucralfate thoroughly before swallowing.

4. A nurse is caring for four clients who have peptic ulcer disease. The nurse should recognize misoprostol is contraindicated for which of the following clients?

- A. A client who is pregnant
- B. A client who has osteoarthritis
- C. A client who has a kidney stone
- D. A client who has a urinary tract infection

5. A nurse is providing a client who has peptic ulcer disease with instructions about managing his condition. Which of the following instructions should the nurse include? (Select all that apply.)

- A. "Eat a bedtime snack."
- B. "Drink decaffeinated coffee"
- C. "Low-dose aspirin therapy should be avoided."
- D. "Seek measures to reduce stress."
- E. "Avoid smoking."

PRACTICE Active Learning Scenario

A nurse is caring for a female client who has a prescription for aluminum hydroxide suspension to treat peptic ulcer disease . Use the ATI Active Learning Template: Medication to complete this item.

THERAPEUTIC USES: Identify the therapeutic use of aluminum hydroxide.

CLIENT EDUCATION: Identify three instructions the nurse should include regarding taking this medication.

1. A. **CORRECT:** The nurse should instruct the client to take these medications with food to reduce GI disturbances.

    B. Bismuth can cause stool to turn black. Black stool can be a manifestation of gastric bleeding.

    C. Tetracycline can cause photosensitivity.

    D. Antacids neutralize the pH of the gastric juices in the stomach.

    Ⓝ NCLEX® Connection: Pharmacological and Parenteral Therapies, Medication Administration

2. A. Omeprazole is administered in the morning for treatment of heartburn.

    B. **CORRECT:** Omeprazole reduces gastric acid secretion by inhibiting the enzyme that produces gastric acid.

    C. Omeprazole is administered before meals with a glass of water.

    D. Omeprazole can cause hypomagnesemia.

    Ⓝ NCLEX® Connection: Pharmacological and Parenteral Therapies, Medication Administration

3. A. Antacids can interfere with the effects of sucralfate, so the client should allow a 30 min interval between the sucralfate and the antacid.

    B. Sucralfate should be taken on an empty stomach, 1 hr before meals.

    C. **CORRECT:** Sucralfate can interfere with the absorption of phenytoin, so the client should allow a 2-hr interval between the sucralfate and phenytoin.

    D. The client should swallow the sucralfate whole.

    Ⓝ NCLEX® Connection: Pharmacological and Parenteral Therapies, Medication Administration

4. A. **CORRECT:** Misoprostol can induce labor and is contraindicated in pregnancy.

    B. There are no contraindications for use in clients who have osteoarthritis.

    C. There are no contraindications for use in clients who have kidney stones.

    D. There are no contraindications for use in clients who have urinary tract infections.

    Ⓝ NCLEX® Connection: Pharmacological and Parenteral Therapies, Adverse Effects/Contraindications/Side Effects/Interactions

5. A. The client should avoid a bedtime snack to reduce gastric acid secretion.

    B. The client should avoid caffeinated and decaffeinated coffee to reduce gastrin release.

    C. Although frequent use of NSAIDs can decrease prostaglandin production resulting in injury to gastric tissue, low-dose aspirin therapy is permitted.

    D. **CORRECT:** Reducing stress is beneficial for healing of the ulcer and prevention of complications.

    E. **CORRECT:** Smoking inhibits healing of the ulcer.

    Ⓝ NCLEX® Connection: Pharmacological and Parenteral Therapies, Medication Administration

PRACTICE Answer

Using the ATI Active Learning Template: Medication

THERAPEUTIC USES: Aluminum hydroxide raises the pH of gastric contents, which reduces irritation of stomach mucosa, resulting in relief of pain.

CLIENT EDUCATION

- Aluminum hydroxide is rated Pregnancy Risk Category C. Discontinue use and notify provider if you become pregnant.
- Shake the medication prior to taking each dose in order to disperse the medication.
- Take other medications at least 1 hr before or after taking aluminum hydroxide.
- Aluminum hydroxide can cause constipation. Notify the provider if it persists. You might need to alternate this antacid with one that is a magnesium compound and has diarrhea as an adverse effect.
- Continue to take the medication even after you no longer have manifestations so that the ulcer will continue to heal.
- The medication is prescribed at frequent dosing intervals to promote healing of the ulcer. Seven times a day, 1 hr before, 3 hr after meals, and at bedtime is a common dosing schedule.

Ⓝ NCLEX® Connection: Pharmacological and Parenteral Therapies, Medication Administration

UNIT 6 MEDICATIONS AFFECTING THE
GASTROINTESTINAL SYSTEM AND NUTRITION

CHAPTER 29 *Gastrointestinal Disorders*

The medications in this section affect some aspect of the gastrointestinal tract to treat or prevent nausea, vomiting, motion sickness, diarrhea, or constipation; treat hiatal hernia by controlling reflux; and treat gastroesophageal reflux disease (GERD) by increasing gastric motility, protecting stomach lining, and inhibiting secretion of gastric acid.

Medications include antiemetics, laxatives, antidiarrheals, prokinetic agents, medications for irritable bowel syndrome (IBS), 5-aminosalicylates, probiotics, and medications for hiatal hernia.

Antiemetics

SELECT PROTOTYPE MEDICATIONS
- **Glucocorticoids:** Dexamethasone
- **Substance P/neurokinin₁ antagonists:** Aprepitant
- **Serotonin antagonists:** Ondansetron, granisetron
- **Dopamine antagonists:** Prochlorperazine, metoclopramide, promethazine
- **Cannabinoids:** Dronabinol
- **Anticholinergics:** Scopolamine
- **Antihistamines:** Dimenhydrinate, hydroxyzine
- **Benzodiazepines:** Lorazepam

PURPOSE

Glucocorticoids: dexamethasone

EXPECTED PHARMACOLOGICAL ACTION: The antiemetic mechanism is unknown.

THERAPEUTIC USES
- Usually used in combination with other antiemetics to treat chemotherapy-induced nausea and vomiting (CINV).
- Administer PO or IV.

Substance P/neurokinin₁ antagonists: aprepitant

EXPECTED PHARMACOLOGICAL ACTION: Inhibits substance P/neurokinin₁ in the brain.

THERAPEUTIC USES
- For best results, it should be used in combination with a glucocorticoid or serotonin antagonist to prevent postoperative nausea, vomiting, and CINV.
- Extended duration of action makes it effective for immediate use and delayed response.
- Administer PO or IV.

Serotonin antagonist: ondansetron

EXPECTED PHARMACOLOGICAL ACTION: Prevents emesis by blocking the serotonin receptors in the chemoreceptor trigger zone (CTZ), and antagonizing the serotonin receptors on the afferent vagal neurons that travel from the upper GI tract to the CTZ.

THERAPEUTIC USES
- Prevents emesis related to chemotherapy, radiation therapy, and postoperative recovery.
- Administer PO, IM, or IV.

Dopamine antagonists: prochlorperazine (a subset of phenothiazine)

EXPECTED PHARMACOLOGICAL ACTION: Antiemetic effects result from blockade of dopamine receptors in the CTZ.

THERAPEUTIC USES
- Prevents emesis related to chemotherapy, opioids, and postoperative recovery.
- Administer PO, IM, or IV.

Cannabinoids: dronabinol

EXPECTED PHARMACOLOGICAL ACTION: Antiemetic mechanism is unknown.

THERAPEUTIC USES
- To control CINV and to increase appetite in clients who have AIDS.
- Administer PO.

Anticholinergic: scopolamine

EXPECTED PHARMACOLOGICAL ACTION: Interferes with the transmission of nerve impulses traveling from the vestibular apparatus of the inner ear to the vomiting center (VC) in the brain.

THERAPEUTIC USES
- Treats motion sickness.
- Administer transdermally, PO, IV, or subcutaneously.

Antihistamines: dimenhydrinate

EXPECTED PHARMACOLOGICAL ACTION: Muscarinic and histaminergic receptors in nerve pathways that connect the inner ear and VC are blocked.

THERAPEUTIC USES
- Treats motion sickness.
- Administer PO, IM, or IV.

Benzodiazepines: lorazepam

EXPECTED PHARMACOLOGICAL ACTION: Depresses nerve function at multiple CNS sites.

THERAPEUTIC USES
- Used in combination with other medications to suppress CINV.
- Administer PO, IM, or IV

COMPLICATIONS

Substance P/neurokinin₁ antagonist: aprepitant

Fatigue, diarrhea, dizziness, possible liver damage
NURSING CONSIDERATIONS
- Treat headache with nonopioid analgesics.
- Monitor stool pattern.
- Monitor liver function tests periodically

Serotonin antagonist: ondansetron

Headache, diarrhea, dizziness
NURSING CONSIDERATIONS
- Treat headache with nonopioid analgesics.
- Monitor stool pattern.

Prolonged QT interval can lead to a serious dysrhythmia (torsades de pointes).
NURSING CONSIDERATIONS: Monitor ECG in clients who have cardiac disorders.

Dopamine antagonists: prochlorperazine

Extrapyramidal symptoms (EPSs)
NURSING CONSIDERATIONS
- Inform clients of possible adverse effects (restlessness, anxiety, spasms of face and neck).
- Advise clients to stop the medication and inform the provider if EPSs occur.
- Administer an anticholinergic medication, such as diphenhydramine or benztropine, to treat EPSs.

Hypotension
NURSING CONSIDERATIONS
- Monitor clients receiving antihypertensive medications for low blood pressure.
- Instruct clients to rise slowly from lying to standing to prevent dizziness and falls. **Qs**

Sedation
NURSING CONSIDERATIONS
- Inform clients of the potential for sedation.
- Advise clients to avoid activities that require alertness, such as driving.

Anticholinergic effects
- Dry mouth, urinary retention, constipation
- NURSING CONSIDERATIONS
  ○ Instruct clients to increase fluid intake.
  ○ Instruct clients to increase physical activity by engaging in regular exercise.
  ○ Tell clients to suck on hard candy or chew gum to help relieve dry mouth.
  ○ Administer a stimulant laxative such as senna to counteract a decrease in bowel motility, or stool softeners such as docusate sodium to prevent constipation.
  ○ Advise clients to void every 4 hr. Monitor I&O, and palpate the lower abdomen area every 4 to 6 hr to assess the bladder.

Cannabinoids: dronabinol

Potential for dissociation, dysphoria
NURSING CONSIDERATIONS: Avoid using in clients who have mental health disorders.

Hypotension, tachycardia
NURSING CONSIDERATIONS: Use cautiously in clients who have cardiovascular disorders. **Qs**

Anticholinergics (scopolamine) and antihistamines (dimenhydrinate)

Sedation
CLIENT EDUCATION
- Inform clients of the potential for sedation.
- Advise clients to avoid activities that require alertness, such as driving.

Anticholinergic effects
- Dry mouth, urinary retention, constipation
- NURSING CONSIDERATIONS
  ○ Instruct clients to increase fluid intake.
  ○ Instruct clients to increase physical activity by engaging in regular exercise.
  ○ Tell clients to suck on hard candy or chew gum to help relieve dry mouth.
  ○ Administer a stimulant laxative such as senna to counteract a decrease in bowel motility, or stool softeners such as docusate sodium to prevent constipation.
  ○ Advise clients to void every 4 hr. Monitor I&O, and palpate the lower abdomen area every 4 to 6 hr to assess the bladder.

CONTRAINDICATIONS/PRECAUTIONS

- Ondansetron should not be given to clients who have long QT syndrome. Qs
- Use dopamine antagonists cautiously, if at all, with children and older adults due to the increased risk of extrapyramidal side effects.
- Dopamine antagonists, antihistamines, and anticholinergic antiemetics should be used cautiously in clients who have urinary retention or obstruction, asthma, and narrow angle glaucoma.
- Aprepitant should be used cautiously in children and in clients who have severe liver and kidney disease.
- Promethazine is contraindicated in children younger than 2 years old and should be used with extreme caution in older children.

INTERACTIONS

CNS depressants, such as opioids and alcohol, can intensify CNS depression of antiemetics.
NURSING CONSIDERATIONS: Advise clients that CNS depression is more likely and to avoid activities that require mental alertness.

Concurrent use of antihypertensives can intensify hypotensive effects of antiemetics.
NURSING CONSIDERATIONS:
- Advise clients to sit or lie down if lightheadedness or dizziness occur. Clients should avoid sudden changes in position by moving slowly from a lying to a sitting or standing position.
- Provide assistance with ambulation as needed.

Concurrent use of anticholinergic medications (antihistamines) can intensify anticholinergic effects of antiemetics.
NURSING CONSIDERATIONS: Provide teaching to reduce anticholinergic effects (sipping on fluids, use of laxatives, voiding on a regular basis).

NURSING ADMINISTRATION

- Antiemetics prevent or treat nausea and vomiting from various causes. Nursing assessment can identify the underlying related factors and verify that the appropriate medication is used.
- When a client is receiving a chemotherapy agent, the client can experience CINV. To prevent CINV, antiemetics are administered prior to chemotherapy as this is more effective than treating nausea that is already occurring. Combining three antiemetics is more effective than the use of a single antiemetic. QEBP
- Transdermal scopolamine is applied as a patch behind the ear several hours prior to surgery or 4 hr before travel when motion sickness is anticipated. Change every 3 days.

NURSING EVALUATION OF MEDICATION EFFECTIVENESS

Depending on therapeutic intent, effectiveness can be evidenced by absence of nausea and vomiting.

Laxatives

SELECT PROTOTYPE MEDICATIONS
- Psyllium
- Docusate sodium
- Bisacodyl
- Magnesium hydroxide

OTHER MEDICATIONS
- Senna
- Lactulose

PURPOSE

Bulk-forming laxatives: psyllium

EXPECTED PHARMACOLOGICAL ACTION: Bulk-forming laxatives soften fecal mass and increase bulk, which is identical to the action of dietary fiber.

THERAPEUTIC USES
- Decrease diarrhea in clients who have diverticulosis and IBS.
- Control stool for clients who have an ileostomy or colostomy.
- Promote defecation in older adults who have a decrease in peristalsis due to age-related changes in the GI tract. Ⓖ

Surfactant laxatives: docusate sodium

EXPECTED PHARMACOLOGICAL ACTION: Surfactant laxatives lower surface tension of the stool to allow penetration of water.

THERAPEUTIC USES
- Relieve constipation related to pregnancy or opioid use.
- Prevent painful elimination in clients who have conditions such as hemorrhoids or following a procedure such as episiotomy.
- Prevent straining in clients who have conditions such as cerebral aneurysm or following myocardial infarction.
- Decrease the risk of fecal impaction in immobile clients and promote defecation in older adults who have decreased peristalsis due to age-related changes in the GI tract.

Stimulant laxatives: bisacodyl

EXPECTED PHARMACOLOGICAL ACTION: Stimulant laxatives result in stimulation of intestinal peristalsis.

THERAPEUTIC USES
- Prepare client prior to surgery or diagnostic tests, such as a colonoscopy.
- Short-term treatment of constipation caused by high-dose opioid use.

Osmotic laxatives: magnesium hydroxide

EXPECTED PHARMACOLOGICAL ACTION: Osmotic laxatives draw water into the intestine to increase the mass of stool, stretching musculature, which results in peristalsis.

THERAPEUTIC USES
- **Low dose:** Prevent painful elimination (clients who have episiotomy or hemorrhoids).
- **High dose:** Client preparation prior to surgery or diagnostic tests, such as a colonoscopy.
- Rapid evacuation of the bowel after ingestion of poisons or following anthelmintic therapy to rid the body of dead parasites.

COMPLICATIONS

GI irritation

CLIENT EDUCATION: Instruct clients not to crush or chew enteric-coated tablets.

Rectal burning sensation, leading to proctitis

CLIENT EDUCATION: Discourage clients from using bisacodyl suppositories on a regular basis.

Toxic magnesium levels

Laxatives with magnesium salts, such as magnesium hydroxide, can lead to accumulation of toxic levels of magnesium.

CLIENT EDUCATION: Advise clients who have impaired kidney function to read labels carefully and to avoid laxatives that contain magnesium.

Sodium absorption and fluid retention

Laxatives with sodium salts, such as sodium phosphate, place clients at risk for sodium absorption and fluid retention.

CLIENT EDUCATION
- Advise clients who have heart disease to read labels carefully and to avoid laxatives that contain sodium.
- Advise clients who have kidney disease and who are taking medications that alter kidney function to avoid laxatives that contain sodium. Qs

Dehydration

Osmotic diuretics can cause dehydration.

NURSING CONSIDERATIONS
- Monitor I&O.
- Monitor/assess for manifestations of dehydration, such as poor skin turgor.
- Encourage clients to increase water intake to at least 8 to 10 glasses of water per day.

CONTRAINDICATIONS/PRECAUTIONS

- Laxatives are contraindicated in clients who have fecal impaction, bowel obstruction, and acute surgical abdomen to prevent perforation. Qs
- Laxatives are contraindicated in clients who have nausea, cramping, and abdominal pain.
- Laxatives, with the exception of bulk-forming laxatives, are contraindicated in clients who have ulcerative colitis and diverticulitis.
- Use cautiously during pregnancy and lactation. Bisacodyl and docusate are Pregnancy Risk Category C.

INTERACTIONS

Milk and antacids can destroy enteric coating of bisacodyl.
CLIENT EDUCATION: Instruct clients to take bisacodyl at least 1 hr apart from ingesting these substances.

NURSING ADMINISTRATION

- Obtain a complete history of laxative use, and provide teaching as appropriate. Qpcc
- Teach clients that chronic laxative use can lead to fluid and electrolyte imbalances.
- To promote defecation and resumption of normal bowel function, instruct clients to increase high-fiber foods (e.g., bran, fresh fruits and vegetables) in the daily diet and to increase amounts of fluids. Recommend at least 2 to 3 L/day from beverages and food sources.
- Encourage clients to maintain a regular exercise regimen to improve bowel function.
- Instruct clients to take bulk-forming and surfactant laxatives with 8 oz water.

NURSING EVALUATION OF MEDICATION EFFECTIVENESS

Depending on therapeutic intent, effectiveness can be evidenced by the following.
- Return to regular bowel function
- Evacuation of bowel in preparation for surgery or diagnostic tests

Antidiarrheals

SELECT PROTOTYPE MEDICATION: Diphenoxylate plus atropine

OTHER MEDICATIONS
- Loperamide
- Paregoric

PURPOSE

EXPECTED PHARMACOLOGICAL ACTION: Antidiarrheals activate opioid receptors in the GI tract to decrease intestinal motility and to increase the absorption of fluid and sodium in the intestine.

THERAPEUTIC USES
- **Specific antidiarrheal agents** can be used to treat the underlying cause of diarrhea. For example, antibiotics can be used to treat diarrhea caused by a bacterial infection.
- **Nonspecific antidiarrheal agents** provide symptomatic treatment of diarrhea (decrease in frequency and fluid content of stool).

COMPLICATIONS

- At recommended doses for diarrhea, diphenoxylate does not affect the CNS system.
- At high doses, clients can experience typical opioid effects, such as euphoria or CNS depression. However, the addition of atropine, which has unpleasant adverse effects (blurred vision, dry mouth, urinary retention, constipation, tachycardia) in diphenoxylate discourages ingestion of doses higher than those prescribed.

CONTRAINDICATIONS/PRECAUTIONS

- There is an increased risk of megacolon in clients who have inflammatory bowel disorders. This could lead to a serious complication, such as perforation of the bowel.
- Diphenoxylate is contraindicated in clients who have severe electrolyte imbalance or dehydration. It is Controlled Substance Category V. Qs
- Paregoric is contraindicated in clients who have COPD.
- Antidiarrheals are Pregnancy Risk Category C.

INTERACTIONS

Alcohol and other CNS depressants can enhance CNS depression.

NURSING ADMINISTRATION

- Administer initial dose of diphenoxylate plus atropine 5 mg. Titrate to the client's response. The maximum dose 8 tabs/day.
- Loperamide is an analog of the opioid meperidine. This medication is not a controlled substance, and at high doses does not mimic morphine-like effects.
- Advise clients who have diarrhea to drink small amounts of clear liquids or a commercial oral electrolyte solution to maintain electrolyte balance for the first 24 hr. Qᴘᴄᴄ
- Advise clients to avoid drinking plain water because it does not contain necessary electrolytes that have been lost in the stool.
- Advise clients to avoid caffeine. Caffeine exacerbates diarrhea by increasing GI motility.
- Clients who have severe cases of diarrhea can be hospitalized for management of dehydration.
- Management of dehydration should include monitoring of weight, I&O, and vital signs. A hypotonic solution such as 0.45% sodium chloride might be prescribed.

NURSING EVALUATION OF MEDICATION EFFECTIVENESS

Depending on therapeutic intent, effectiveness can be evidenced by return of normal bowel pattern as evidenced by decrease in frequency and fluid volume of stool.

Prokinetic agents

SELECT PROTOTYPE MEDICATION: Metoclopramide

PURPOSE

EXPECTED PHARMACOLOGICAL ACTION
- If the CTZ is activated (e.g., by chemotherapy) the CTZ in turn activates the vomiting center to expel gastric contents. Metoclopramide controls nausea and vomiting by blocking dopamine and serotonin receptors in the CTZ.
- Metoclopramide augments action of acetylcholine, which causes an increase in upper GI motility, increasing peristalsis.

THERAPEUTIC USES
- Control of postoperative and chemotherapy-induced nausea and vomiting, as well as facilitation of intubation and examination of the GI tract.
- The oral form is used for diabetic gastroparesis (delayed stomach emptying with gas and bloating) and management of GERD through its ability to increase gastric motility.

COMPLICATIONS

Extrapyramidal symptoms

NURSING CONSIDERATIONS
- Inform clients of the possible adverse effects, such as restlessness, anxiety, and spasms of the face and neck.
- Administer an antihistamine, such as diphenhydramine, to minimize EPSs.

Sedation

CLIENT EDUCATION
- Inform clients of the potential for sedation.
- Advise clients to avoid activities that require alertness, such as driving.

Diarrhea

NURSING CONSIDERATIONS: Monitor bowel function and for indications of dehydration.

CONTRAINDICATIONS/PRECAUTIONS

- Contraindicated in clients who have GI perforation, GI bleeding, bowel obstruction, and hemorrhage.
- Contraindicated in clients who have a seizure disorder due to an increased risk of seizures.
- Use cautiously in children and older adults due to the increased risk for EPS.

INTERACTIONS

Concurrent use of alcohol and other CNS depressants increases the risk of seizures and sedation.
NURSING CONSIDERATIONS
- Advise clients to avoid the use of alcohol.
- Use cautiously with other CNS depressants.

Opioids and anticholinergics decrease the effects of metoclopramide.
NURSING CONSIDERATIONS: Advise clients to avoid using opioids and medications with anticholinergic effects.

NURSING ADMINISTRATION

- Monitor for CNS depression and EPSs.
- The medication can be given orally or IV. If the IV dose 10 mg or less, it may be administered IVP undiluted over 2 min. If the dose is greater than 10 mg, it should be diluted and infused over 15 min. Dilute the medication in at least 50 mL dextrose 5% in water, sodium chloride, or lactated Ringer's. Q**EBP**

NURSING EVALUATION OF MEDICATION EFFECTIVENESS

Depending on therapeutic intent, effectiveness can be evidenced by absence of nausea and vomiting.

Medications for irritable bowel syndrome with diarrhea (IBS-D)

SELECT PROTOTYPE MEDICATION: Alosetron

PURPOSE

EXPECTED PHARMACOLOGICAL ACTION: Selective blockade of 5-HT3 receptors, which innervate the viscera and result in increased firmness in stool and decrease in urgency and frequency of defecation.

THERAPEUTIC USES: Approved only for female clients who have severe IBS-D that has lasted more than 6 months and has been resistant to conventional management.

COMPLICATIONS

Constipation

Can result in GI toxicity, such as ischemic colitis, bowel obstruction, impaction, or perforation

NURSING CONSIDERATIONS
- Because of the potentially fatal outcome of GI toxicity, only clients who meet specific criteria and are willing to sign a treatment agreement may receive prescriptions for the medication. Q**s**
- Instruct clients to watch for rectal bleeding, bloody diarrhea, or abdominal pain and report to the provider. Medication should be discontinued.

CONTRAINDICATIONS/PRECAUTIONS

Contraindicated for clients who have chronic constipation, history of bowel obstruction, Crohn's disease, ulcerative colitis, impaired intestinal circulation, diverticulitis, or thrombophlebitis.

INTERACTIONS

Medications that induce cytochrome P450 enzymes, such as phenobarbital, can decrease levels of alosetron.
NURSING CONSIDERATIONS: Monitor the effectiveness of medication.

NURSING ADMINISTRATION

- Instruct clients that manifestations should resolve within 1 to 4 weeks but will return 1 week after medication is discontinued.
- Dosage will start as once a day and may be increased to BID.

NURSING EVALUATION OF MEDICATION EFFECTIVENESS

Depending on therapeutic intent, effectiveness can be evidenced by relief of diarrhea, and decrease in urgency and frequency of defecation.

Medications for irritable bowel syndrome with constipation (IBS-C)

SELECT PROTOTYPE MEDICATION: Lubiprostone

PURPOSE

EXPECTED PHARMACOLOGICAL ACTION

Increases fluid secretion in the intestine to promote intestinal motility

THERAPEUTIC USES

- Irritable bowel syndrome with constipation in women
- Chronic constipation

COMPLICATIONS

Diarrhea

NURSING CONSIDERATIONS: Monitor frequency of stools. Notify the provider if severe diarrhea occurs.

Nausea

CLIENT EDUCATION: Instruct clients to take the medication with food.

CONTRAINDICATIONS/PRECAUTIONS

- Pregnancy Risk Category C
- Contraindicated for clients who have bowel obstruction

INTERACTIONS

No significant interactions

NURSING ADMINISTRATION

- Instruct clients to take the medication with food to decrease nausea.
- Oral dosage should be taken BID.

NURSING EVALUATION OF MEDICATION EFFECTIVENESS

Depending on therapeutic intent, effectiveness can be evidenced by relief of constipation.

5-Aminosalicylates

SELECT PROTOTYPE MEDICATION: Sulfasalazine

OTHER MEDICATIONS FOR IBD
- **5-aminosalicylates:** Mesalamine, olsalazine
- **Glucocorticoids:** Hydrocortisone
- **Immunosuppressants:** Azathioprine
- **Immunomodulator:** Infliximab
- **Antibiotics:** Metronidazole

PURPOSE

EXPECTED PHARMACOLOGICAL ACTION: Decrease inflammation by inhibiting prostaglandin synthesis

THERAPEUTIC USES
- IBS, Crohn's disease, ulcerative colitis
- IBD is controlled, rather than cured, by these medications, which often are used in combination therapy.

COMPLICATIONS

Blood disorders

Include agranulocytosis, hemolytic and macrocytic anemia

NURSING CONSIDERATIONS: Monitor complete blood count.

Nausea, cramps, rash, arthralgia

NURSING CONSIDERATIONS: Notify the provider if adverse effects persist.

CONTRAINDICATIONS/PRECAUTIONS

- Women who are pregnant, plan to become pregnant, or who are breastfeeding should consult the provider about continued use of sulfasalazine.
- 5-aminosalicylates are contraindicated in clients who have sensitivity to sulfonamides, salicylates, or thiazide diuretics.
- Use cautiously in older adults. Ⓒ
- Use cautiously in clients who have liver or kidney disease or blood dyscrasias.

INTERACTIONS

- Iron and antibiotics can alter the absorption of sulfasalazine.
- Mesalamine can decrease the absorption of digoxin.

NURSING ADMINISTRATION

Ensure that controlled-release and enteric-coated forms of the medications are not crushed or chewed.

NURSING EVALUATION OF MEDICATION EFFECTIVENESS

Depending on therapeutic intent, effectiveness can be evidenced by the following.
- Decreased bowel inflammation and relief of GI distress
- Return to normal bowel function

Probiotics: Dietary supplements

PURPOSE

EXPECTED PHARMACOLOGICAL ACTION: Various preparations of bacteria and yeast, which are normal flora of the intestine and colon, help to metabolize foods, promote nutrient absorption, and reduce colonization by pathogenic bacteria. They also can increase nonspecific cellular and humoral immunity.

THERAPEUTIC USE: Probiotics are used to treat the manifestations of IBS, ulcerative colitis, and *Clostridium difficile*-associated diarrhea and rotavirus diarrhea in children.

COMPLICATIONS

Flatulence and bloating

INTERACTIONS

If antibiotics or antifungals are used concurrently, they should be administered at least 2 hr apart from probiotics. ⓆEBP

Medications for hiatal hernia

For complications and other information about these medications, refer to **CHAPTER 28: PEPTIC ULCER DISEASE**.

PROTON PUMP INHIBITORS
- Omeprazole
- Esomeprazole
- Lansoprazole

ANTACIDS
- Aluminum hydroxide
- Sodium bicarbonate
- Calcium carbonate

PURPOSE

EXPECTED PHARMACOLOGICAL ACTION

Proton pump inhibitors block the final step of gastric acid production to prevent reflux in sliding hiatal hernia.

Antacids neutralize gastric acid to provide relief of manifestations such as heartburn, belching, dysphagia.

NURSING EVALUATION OF MEDICATION EFFECTIVENESS

Reduced frequency of manifestations of hiatal hernia such as heartburn, belching, and dysphagia.

Application Exercises

1. A nurse is caring for a client who received prochlorperazine 4 hr ago. The client reports spasms of his face. The nurse should anticipate a prescription for which of the following medications?

   A. Fomepizole

   B. Naloxone

   C. Phytonadione

   D. Diphenhydramine

2. A nurse is planning to administer ondansetron IV for an older adult client who has a history of diabetes mellitus and cardiac myopathy and is receiving chemotherapy for cancer. For which of the following adverse effects of ondansetron should the nurse monitor? (Select all that apply.)

   A. Headache

   B. Diarrhea

   C. Shortened PR interval

   D. Hyperglycemia

   E. Prolonged QT interval

3. A nurse is providing instructions about the use of laxatives to a client who has heart failure. The nurse should tell the client he should avoid which of the following laxatives?

   A. Sodium phosphate

   B. Psyllium

   C. Bisacodyl

   D. Polyethylene glycol

4. A nurse is caring for a client who has diabetes and is experiencing nausea due to gastroparesis. The nurse should anticipate a prescription for which of the following medications?

   A. Lubiprostone

   B. Metoclopramide

   C. Bisacodyl

   D. Loperamide

5. A nurse is providing information about probiotic supplements to a male client. Which of the following information should the nurse include? (Select all that apply.)

   A. "Probiotics are micro-organisms that are normally found in the GI tract."

   B. "Probiotics are used to treat *Clostridium difficile*."

   C. "Probiotics are used to treat benign prostatic hyperplasia."

   D. "You can experience bloating while taking probiotic supplements."

   E. "If you are prescribed an antibiotic, you should take it at the same time you take your probiotic supplement."

PRACTICE Active Learning Scenario

A nurse is caring for a client who has a prescription for sulfasalazine. Use the ATI Active Learning Template: Medication to complete this item to include the following sections.

THERAPEUTIC USES: Identify two therapeutic uses for sulfasalazine.

COMPLICATIONS: Identify two blood disorders that occur as a complication with the use of sulfasalazine.

MEDICATION ADMINISTRATION: Identify how frequently the client should take the medication.

Application Exercises Key

1. A. Fomepizole is an antidote used to treat ethylene glycol poisoning.

   B. Naloxone is used to treat opioid overdose.

   C. Vitamin K₁ is used to treat warfarin overdose.

   D. **CORRECT:** An adverse effect of prochlorperazine is acute dystonia, which is evidenced by spasms of the muscles in the face, neck, and tongue. Diphenhydramine is used to suppress extrapyramidal effects of prochlorperazine.

   (N) *NCLEX® Connection: Pharmacological and Parenteral Therapies, Expected Actions/Outcomes*

2. A. **CORRECT:** Headache is a common adverse effect of ondansetron.

   B. **CORRECT:** Diarrhea or constipation are both adverse effects of ondansetron.

   C. A shortened PR interval is not an adverse effect of ondansetron.

   D. Ondansetron does not affect blood glucose.

   E. **CORRECT:** A prolonged QT interval is a possible adverse effect of ondansetron that can lead to torsades de pointes, a serious dysrhythmia.

   (N) *NCLEX® Connection: Pharmacological and Parenteral Therapies, Adverse Effects/Contraindications/Side Effects/Interactions*

3. A. **CORRECT:** Typically, clients who have heart failure are on a sodium-restricted diet. Absorption of sodium from sodium phosphate causes fluid retention and is contraindicated for clients who have heart failure.

   B. Psyllium is not absorbed by the intestine and is not contraindicated for clients who have heart failure.

   C. Bisacodyl does not appear to have systemic effects and is not contraindicated for clients who have heart failure.

   D. Polyethylene glycol is contraindicated in a number of GI conditions, but it is not contraindicated for clients who have heart failure.

   (N) *NCLEX® Connection: Pharmacological and Parenteral Therapies, Adverse Effects/Contraindications/Side Effects/Interactions*

4. A. Lubiprostone is a medication used to treat irritable bowel syndrome with constipation in women.

   B. **CORRECT:** Metoclopramide is a dopamine antagonist that is used to treat nausea and also increases gastric motility. It can relieve the bloating and nausea of diabetic gastroparesis.

   C. Bisacodyl is a stimulant laxative that is used for short-term treatment of constipation.

   D. Loperamide is an antidiarrheal agent that decreases gastrointestinal peristalsis.

   (N) *NCLEX® Connection: Pharmacological and Parenteral Therapies, Adverse Effects/Contraindications/Side Effects/Interactions*

5. A. **CORRECT:** Probiotics consist of lactobacilli, bifidobacteria, and *Saccharomyces boulardii*, which normally are found in the digestive tract.

   B. **CORRECT:** Probiotics are used to treat a number of GI conditions, including irritable bowel syndrome, diarrhea associated with *Clostridium difficile*, and ulcerative colitis.

   C. Saw palmetto is a supplement that clients might use to treat benign prostatic hyperplasia.

   D. **CORRECT:** Flatulence and bloating are adverse effects of probiotic supplements.

   E. The client should take the probiotic supplement at least 2 hr after taking an antibiotic or antifungal medication. Antibiotics and antifungal medications destroy bacteria and yeast found in probiotic supplements.

   (N) *NCLEX® Connection: Pharmacological and Parenteral Therapies, Medication Administration*

PRACTICE Answer

Using the ATI Active Learning Template: Medication

THERAPEUTIC USES: Crohn's disease and ulcerative colitis

COMPLICATIONS: Complications that occur with the use of sulfasalazine include agranulocytosis, and hemolytic and macrocytic anemia.

MEDICATION ADMINISTRATION: The client should take sulfasalazine four times per day in divided doses.

(N) *NCLEX® Connection: Pharmacological and Parenteral Therapies, Medication Administration*

CHAPTER 30

Vitamins, Minerals, and Supplements

Vitamins and minerals have important roles in the body, including the production of red blood cells, building bones, making hormones, regulating body fluid volume, and supporting nerve cell function. Vitamin and mineral deficiencies can increase the risk for health problems, such as anemias, heart disease, cancers, and osteoporosis. Supplements of vitamins and minerals can help prevent multiple health conditions.

Iron preparations

SELECT PROTOTYPE MEDICATIONS
- Oral: Ferrous sulfate
- Parenteral: Iron dextran

OTHER MEDICATIONS
- Oral: Ferrous gluconate, ferrous fumarate
- Parenteral: Ferumoxytol, iron sucrose, sodium-ferric gluconate complex (SFGC)

PURPOSE

EXPECTED PHARMACOLOGICAL ACTION: Iron preparations provide iron needed for RBC development and oxygen transport to cells. During times of increased growth (in growing children or during pregnancy) or when RBCs are in high demand (after blood loss), the need for iron can be greatly increased. Iron is poorly absorbed by the body, so relatively large amounts must be ingested orally to increase Hgb and Hct levels.

THERAPEUTIC USES
- Iron preparations are used to treat and prevent iron-deficiency anemia.
  - **Ferumoxytol** is limited to clients who have chronic kidney disease, regardless if on dialysis or receiving erythropoietin. Ferumoxytol requires only two doses over 3 to 8 days compared with SFGC and iron sucrose, which require 3 to 10 doses over several weeks.
  - **SFGC** is used for clients who are undergoing long-term hemodialysis and are deficient in iron.
  - **Iron sucrose** is used for clients who have chronic kidney disease, are receiving erythropoietin, and are hemodialysis- or peritoneal dialysis-dependent; and clients who have chronic kidney disease, are not receiving erythropoietin, and are not dialysis-dependent.

- Iron preparations are used to prevent iron deficiency anemia for clients who are at an increased risk, such as infants, children, and pregnant women.
- Parenteral forms should only be used in clients who are unable to take oral medications, in which case the IV route is preferred.

COMPLICATIONS

GI distress (nausea, constipation, heartburn)

NURSING CONSIDERATIONS
- If intolerable, administer medication with food, but this greatly reduces absorption.
- Can need to reduce dosage
- Monitor the client's bowel pattern and intervene as appropriate. This side effect usually resolves with continued use.

Teeth staining (liquid form)

NURSING CONSIDERATIONS: Teach clients to dilute liquid iron with water or juice, drink with a straw, and rinse mouth after swallowing.

Staining of skin and other tissues (IM injections)

NURSING CONSIDERATIONS
- Give IM doses deep IM using Z-track technique.
- Avoid this route if possible.

Anaphylaxis

- Risk with parenteral administration of iron dextran.
- Anaphylaxis is triggered by the dextran in iron dextran, not by the iron.
- Anaphylaxis is minimal with SFGC, iron sucrose, and ferumoxytol.

NURSING CONSIDERATIONS
- IV route is safer than IM.
- Administer a test dose and observe the client closely. No test dose is needed before administering ferumoxytol and iron sucrose.
- Administer slowly, and use manufacturer's recommendation for specific product.
- Be prepared with life-support equipment and epinephrine.

Hypotension

Can progress to circulatory collapse with parenteral administration

NURSING CONSIDERATIONS: Monitor vital signs when administering parenteral iron.

Fatal iron toxicity in children

Can occur when an overdose of iron (2 to 10 g) is ingested

NURSING CONSIDERATIONS
- Manifestations of toxicity include severe GI symptoms, shock, acidosis, and liver and heart failure. The chelating agent deferoxamine, given parenterally, is used to treat toxicity.
- Avoid using oral and parenteral iron concurrently.

CONTRAINDICATIONS/PRECAUTIONS

- Contraindicated for clients who have previous hypersensitivity to iron, anemias other than iron-deficiency anemia.
- Oral preparations should be used with caution in clients who have peptic ulcer disease, regional enteritis, ulcerative colitis, and severe liver disease.

Concurrent administration of antacids or tetracyclines reduces absorption of iron.
NURSING CONSIDERATIONS
- Separate use by at least 2 hr.
- Vitamin C increases absorption, but also increases incidence of GI complications.

Caffeine and dairy products can interfere with absorption.
NURSING CONSIDERATIONS: Avoid caffeine and dairy intake when taking medication.

Food reduces absorption but reduces gastric distress.
NURSING CONSIDERATIONS: Take with food at the start of therapy if gastric distress occurs.

NURSING ADMINISTRATION

NURSING CARE
- Instruct clients to take iron on an empty stomach, such as 1 hr before meals, as stomach acid increases absorption.
- Instruct clients to take with food if GI adverse effects occur. This might increase adherence to therapy even though absorption is also decreased.
- Instruct clients to space doses at approximately equal intervals throughout day to most efficiently increase red blood cell production.
- Inform clients to anticipate a harmless dark green or black color of stool.
- Teach clients to dilute liquid iron with water or juice, drink with a straw, and rinse the mouth after swallowing.
- Instruct clients to increase water and fiber intake (unless contraindicated) and to maintain an exercise program to counter the constipation effects.
- Advise clients that therapy can last 1 to 2 months. Usually, dietary intake will be sufficient after Hgb has returned to a therapeutic level.
- Encourage concurrent intake of appropriate quantities of foods high in iron (liver, egg yolks, muscle meats, yeast, grains, green leafy vegetables).

NURSING EVALUATION OF MEDICATION EFFECTIVENESS

Depending on therapeutic intent, effectiveness is evidenced by the following.
- Increased reticulocyte count is expected at least 1 week after beginning iron therapy.
- Increase in hemoglobin of 2 g/dL is expected 1 month after beginning therapy.
- Fatigue and pallor (skin, mucous membranes) should subside, and the client reports increased energy level.

Vitamin B$_{12}$/Cyanocobalamin

SELECT PROTOTYPE MEDICATION: Vitamin B$_{12}$

OTHER MEDICATIONS: Intranasal cyanocobalamin

PURPOSE

EXPECTED PHARMACOLOGICAL ACTION
- Vitamin B$_{12}$ is necessary to convert folic acid from its inactive form to its active form. All cells rely on folic acid for DNA production.
- Vitamin B$_{12}$ deficiency can result in megaloblastic (macrocytic) anemia and cause dysrhythmias and heart failure if not corrected. Vitamin B$_{12}$ is administered to prevent or correct deficiency. Damage to rapidly multiplying cells can affect the skin and mucous membranes, causing GI disturbances. Neurologic damage, which includes numbness and tingling of extremities and CNS damage caused by demyelination of neurons, can result from deficiency of this vitamin.
- Vitamin B$_{12}$ deficiency affects all blood cells produced in the bone marrow.
  - Loss of erythrocytes leads to heart failure, cerebral vascular insufficiency, and hypoxia.
  - Loss of leukocytes leads to infections.
  - Loss of thrombocytes leads to bleeding and hemorrhage.
- Loss of intrinsic factor within the cells of the stomach causes an inability to absorb vitamin B$_{12}$, making it necessary to administer parenteral or intranasal vitamin B$_{12}$ or high doses of oral B$_{12}$ for the rest of the client's life.

THERAPEUTIC USES
- Treatment of vitamin B$_{12}$ deficiency
- Megaloblastic (macrocytic) anemia related to vitamin B$_{12}$ deficiency

COMPLICATIONS

Hypokalemia

Secondary to the increased RBC production effects of vitamin B$_{12}$

NURSING CONSIDERATIONS
- Monitor potassium levels during the start of treatment.
- Observe clients for manifestations of potassium deficiency (muscle weakness, irregular cardiac rhythm).
- Clients might require potassium supplements.

CONTRAINDICATIONS/PRECAUTIONS

- Vitamin B$_{12}$ deficiency should not be treated only with folic acid. Treatment with folic acid alone can reverse the hematologic effects of the deficiency but can allow neurologic damage to progress. If folic acid is used for a client who has vitamin B$_{12}$ deficiency, ensure that dosage of vitamin B$_{12}$ is adequate.
- Oral and intranasal cyanocobalamin are Pregnancy Risk Category A.
- Parenteral cyanocobalamin is Pregnancy Risk Category C.

INTERACTIONS

Masks manifestations of vitamin B$_{12}$ deficiency with concurrent administration of folic acid
NURSING CONSIDERATIONS: Make sure that clients receive adequate doses of vitamin B$_{12}$ when using folic acid.

NURSING ADMINISTRATION

NURSING CARE

- Obtain baseline vitamin B$_{12}$, Hgb, Hct, RBC, reticulocyte counts, and folate levels. Monitor periodically.
- Monitor for manifestations of vitamin B$_{12}$ deficiency, such as beefy red tongue, pallor, and neuropathy.
- Cyanocobalamin is administered intranasally, orally, IM, or subcutaneously. Injections are painful and usually reserved for clients who have significant reduced ability to absorb vitamin B$_{12}$, such as lack of intrinsic factor (pernicious anemia), enteritis, and partial removal of the stomach.
- Clients who have malabsorption syndrome can use intranasal or parenteral preparations.
- Intranasal cyanocobalamin should be administered 1 hr before or after eating hot foods, which can cause the medication to be removed from nasal passages without being absorbed, because of increased nasal secretions.
- Clients who have irreversible malabsorption syndrome (parietal cell atrophy or total gastrectomy) will need lifelong treatment, usually parenterally. If oral therapy is used, doses must be very high.
  ○ Encourage concurrent intake of quantities of foods high in vitamin B$_{12}$, such as dairy products.
  ○ Perform a Schilling test to determine vitamin B$_{12}$ absorption in the gastrointestinal tract.
  ○ Measurement of plasma B$_{12}$ levels helps determine the need for therapy.
  ○ Advise clients to adhere to prescribed laboratory tests. Monitor blood counts and vitamin B$_{12}$ levels every 3 to 6 months.

NURSING EVALUATION OF MEDICATION EFFECTIVENESS

Depending on therapeutic intent, effectiveness can be evidenced by the following.
- Disappearance of megaloblasts (in 2 to 3 weeks)
- Increased reticulocyte count
- Increase in hematocrit
- Improvement of neurologic injury, such as absence of tingling sensation of hands and feet and numbness of extremities. Improvement can take months, and some clients never attain full recovery.

Folic acid

SELECT PROTOTYPE MEDICATION: Folic acid

PURPOSE

EXPECTED PHARMACOLOGICAL ACTION: Folic acid is essential in the production of DNA and erythropoiesis (RBC, WBC, and platelets).

THERAPEUTIC USES
- Treatment of megaloblastic (macrocytic) anemia secondary to folic acid deficiency
- Prevention of neural tube defects that can occur early during pregnancy (thus needed for all women of child-bearing age who might become pregnant)
- Treatment of malabsorption syndrome, such as sprue
- Supplement for alcohol use disorder (due to poor dietary intake of folic acid and injury to the liver)

CONTRAINDICATIONS/PRECAUTIONS

Avoid indiscriminate use of folic acid to reduce the risk of masking manifestations of vitamin B$_{12}$ deficiency.

INTERACTIONS

Folic acid levels are decreased by methotrexate and sulfonamides.
NURSING CONSIDERATIONS: Avoid concurrent use of these medications.

Folic acid can decrease phenytoin serum levels because of increased metabolism.
NURSING CONSIDERATIONS: Monitor serum phenytoin levels.

NURSING ADMINISTRATION

NURSING CARE

- Assess for manifestations of megaloblastic anemia (pallor, easy fatigability, palpitations, paresthesias of hands or feet).
- Obtain baseline folic acid, Hgb and Hct levels, and RBC and reticulocyte counts. Monitor periodically.
- Advise clients who have folic acid deficiency to concurrently increase intake of food sources of folic acid, such as liver, green leafy vegetables, citrus fruits, and dried peas and beans. Monitor for risk factors indicating that folic acid therapy is needed, such as heavy alcohol use and child-bearing age.

NURSING EVALUATION OF MEDICATION EFFECTIVENESS

Depending on therapeutic intent, effectiveness is evidenced by the following.
- Folate level within expected reference range
- Return of RBC, reticulocyte count, and Hgb and Hct to levels within expected reference range
- Improvement of anemia findings such as absence of pallor, dyspnea, easy fatigability
- Absence of neural tube defects in newborns

Potassium supplements

SELECT PROTOTYPE MEDICATION: Potassium chloride

OTHER MEDICATIONS
- Potassium gluconate
- Potassium phosphate
- Potassium bicarbonate

PURPOSE

EXPECTED PHARMACOLOGICAL ACTION
Potassium is essential for conducting nerve impulses, maintaining electrical excitability of muscle, and regulation of acid/base balance.

THERAPEUTIC USES
- Treating hypokalemia (potassium less than 3.5 mEq/L).
- For clients receiving diuretics resulting in potassium loss, such as furosemide
- For clients who have potassium loss due to excessive or prolonged vomiting, diarrhea, excessive use of laxatives, intestinal drainage, and GI fistula

COMPLICATIONS

Local GI ulceration and GI distress

Nausea, vomiting, diarrhea, abdominal discomfort, and esophagitis with oral administration

CLIENT EDUCATION
- Instruct clients to take the medication with meals or at least 8 oz of water to minimize GI discomfort and prevent ulceration.
- Teach clients not to dissolve the tablet in the mouth because oral ulceration will develop.

Hyperkalemia (potassium more than 5.0 mEq/L)

NURSING CONSIDERATIONS
- Hyperkalemia rarely occurs with oral administration.
- Monitor clients receiving IV potassium for manifestations of hyperkalemia, such as bradycardia, ECG changes, vomiting, confusion, anxiety, dyspnea, weakness, numbness, and tingling.
- Severe hyperkalemia can require treatment, such as calcium salt, glucose and insulin, sodium bicarbonate, sodium polystyrene sulfonate, peritoneal dialysis, or hemodialysis.

CONTRAINDICATIONS/PRECAUTIONS

Contraindicated for clients who have severe kidney disease or hypoaldosteronism

INTERACTIONS

Concurrent use of potassium-sparing diuretics, such as spironolactone, or ACE inhibitors (lisinopril) increases the risk of hyperkalemia.
NURSING CONSIDERATIONS: Avoid concurrent use.

NURSING ADMINISTRATION

ORAL FORMULATIONS
- Mix powdered formulations in at least 120 mL (4 oz) of liquid.
- Advise clients to take potassium chloride with a meal or at least 8 oz of water to reduce the risk of adverse GI effects.
- Instruct clients not to crush extended-release tablets.
- Instruct clients to notify the provider if they have difficulty swallowing the pills. Medication is supplied as a powder or a sustained-release tablet that is easier to tolerate.

IV ADMINISTRATION
- Never administer IV bolus. Rapid IV infusion can result in fatal hyperkalemia. Qs
- Use an IV infusion pump to control the infusion rate.
- Dilute potassium and give no more than 40 mEq/L of IV solution to prevent vein irritation.
- Infuse slowly, generally no faster than 10 mEq/hr.
- Cardiac monitoring is indicated for serum potassium levels outside of expected reference ranges. ECG changes, such as prolonged PR interval and peaked T-waves, can indicate potassium toxicity.
- Infuse potassium through a large bore needle. Assess the IV site for local irritation, phlebitis, and infiltration. Discontinue the IV immediately if infiltration occurs.
- Monitor I&O to ensure an adequate urine output of at least 30 mL/hr.

NURSING EVALUATION OF MEDICATION EFFECTIVENESS

Depending on therapeutic intent, effectiveness is evidenced by serum potassium level within the expected reference range (3.5 to 5.0 mEq/L).

Magnesium sulfate

SELECT PROTOTYPE MEDICATION
- Parenteral: Magnesium sulfate
- Oral: Magnesium hydroxide, magnesium oxide, magnesium citrate

> Magnesium hydroxide and magnesium oxide act as antacids when administered in a low dose, and all three act as laxatives.

PURPOSE

EXPECTED PHARMACOLOGICAL ACTION: Magnesium activates many intracellular enzymes, binds the messenger RNA to ribosomes, and plays a role in regulating skeletal muscle contractility and blood coagulation.

THERAPEUTIC USES
- Magnesium supplements are used for clients who have hypomagnesemia (magnesium level less than 1.3 mEq/L).
- Oral preparations of magnesium sulfate are used to prevent or treat low magnesium levels and as laxatives.
- Parenteral magnesium is used for clients who have severe hypomagnesemia.
- IV magnesium sulfate is used to stop preterm labor and as an anticonvulsant during labor and delivery.

COMPLICATIONS

Muscle weakness, flaccid paralysis, painful muscle contractions, suppression of AV conduction through the heart, respiratory depression

NURSING CONSIDERATIONS
- IV administration requires careful monitoring of cardiac and neuromuscular status.
- Monitor serum magnesium levels.
- Avoid administering with neuromuscular blocking agents, which can potentiate respiratory depression and apnea.
- Have IV calcium available to reverse the effects of magnesium. Qs

Diarrhea

NURSING CONSIDERATIONS
- Monitor electrolyte levels for electrolyte loss from diarrhea.
- Monitor I&O, and observe for manifestations of dehydration.

CONTRAINDICATIONS/PRECAUTIONS
- Magnesium is Pregnancy Risk Category A.
- Contraindicated in clients who have AV block, rectal bleeding, nausea, vomiting, and abdominal pain.
- Use cautiously with clients who have renal and/or cardiac disease.

INTERACTIONS
- Magnesium sulfate can decrease the absorption of tetracyclines and digoxin.
- Monitor the therapeutic effect to determine if absorption has been affected.

NURSING ADMINISTRATION

NURSING CARE
- Monitor serum magnesium, calcium, and phosphorus.
- Monitor blood pressure, heart rate, and respiratory rate when given intravenously.
- Assess for depressed or absent deep tendon reflexes as a manifestation of toxicity.
- Calcium gluconate is given for magnesium sulfate toxicity. Always have an injectable form of calcium gluconate available when administering magnesium sulfate by IV. Qs
- Teach clients about dietary sources of magnesium (whole-grain cereals, nuts, legumes, green leafy vegetables, bananas).

NURSING EVALUATION OF MEDICATION EFFECTIVENESS

Depending on therapeutic intent, effectiveness is evidenced by serum magnesium levels within expected reference range (1.3 to 2.1 mEq/L).

Herbal supplements

- Herbal supplements are widely used but less tested and regulated than conventional medications. Dosages are less precise than for more regulated medications. Because different formulations are not standardized, it can be difficult to know which preparations can provide therapeutic effects.
- Supplements are regulated by the FDA for manufacturing devoid of impurities, and for accurate labeling.

Aloe, aloe vera

- Acts as a topical anti-inflammatory, analgesic, and cathartic
- Soothes pain
- Heals burns
- Softens skin
- Laxative

ADVERSE EFFECTS AND PRECAUTIONS
- Skin preparations: Possible hypersensitivity
- Laxative: Possible fluid and electrolyte imbalances
- Increases menstrual flow when taken during menses
- Avoid in clients who have kidney disorders.

INTERACTIONS: Interacts with digoxin, diuretics, corticosteroids and antidysrhythmics

NURSING ADMINISTRATION: Teach clients to recognize manifestations of fluid and electrolyte imbalance if using as a laxative.

Black cohosh

- Acts as an estrogen substitute
- Mechanism of action is unknown
- Treats manifestations of menopause

ADVERSE EFFECTS AND PRECAUTIONS
- GI distress, lightheadedness, headache, rash, weight gain
- Avoid taking during pregnancy, especially the first two trimesters of pregnancy.
- Limit use to no longer than 6 months due to lack of information regarding long-term effects.

INTERACTIONS
- Increases effects of antihypertensive medications
- Can increase effect of estrogen medications
- Increases hypoglycemia in clients taking insulin or other medications for diabetes

NURSING ADMINISTRATION: Question clients who take antihypertensives, insulin, or hypoglycemic agents, or clients who might be pregnant about possible use of black cohosh.

Echinacea

- Stimulates the immune system
- Decreases inflammation
- Topically heals skin disorders, wounds, and burns
- Possibly treats viruses (common cold, herpes simplex)
- Used to increase T-lymphocyte, tumor necrosis factor, and interferon production

ADVERSE EFFECTS
- Bitter taste
- Mild GI symptoms or fever can occur.
- Allergic reactions, especially in clients who are allergic to plants such as ragweed or others in the daisy family

INTERACTIONS: With chronic use (more than 6 months), echinacea can decrease positive effects of medications for tuberculosis, HIV, or cancer.

NURSING ADMINISTRATION
- Echinacea is available in many forms, including dried roots, plants, extracts, and teas.
- Question clients who have tuberculosis, cancer, HIV, lupus erythematosus, and rheumatoid arthritis about concurrent use. Advise these clients to talk to the provider.

Feverfew

- Can block platelet aggregation
- Can block a factor that causes migraines
- Can decrease the number and severity of migraine headaches (does not treat an existing migraine)

ADVERSE EFFECTS AND PRECAUTIONS
- Mild GI symptoms
- Post-feverfew syndrome can occur, causing agitation, tiredness, inability to sleep, headache, and joint discomfort.
- Can cause allergic reactions in clients allergic to ragweed or echinacea

INTERACTIONS
- Can cause increased risk of bleeding in clients taking NSAIDs, heparin, and warfarin
- Discontinue 2 weeks before elective surgery.

NURSING ADMINISTRATION: Question clients about concurrent use of NSAIDs, heparin, and warfarin.

Garlic

- When crushed, forms the enzyme allicin
- Blocks LDL cholesterol and raises HDL cholesterol; lowers triglycerides
- Suppresses platelet aggregation and disrupts coagulation
- Acts as a vasodilator (can lower blood pressure)

ADVERSE EFFECTS: GI symptoms

INTERACTIONS
- Due to antiplatelet qualities, can increase risk of bleeding in clients taking NSAIDs, warfarin, and heparin
- Decreases levels of saquinavir (a medication for HIV treatment) and cyclosporine

NURSING ADMINISTRATION
- Question clients about concurrent use of NSAIDs, heparin, and warfarin.
- Have clients who are taking antiplatelet or anticoagulant medication, cyclosporine, or saquinavir contact their provider.

Ginger root

- Relieves vertigo and nausea
- Increases intestinal motility
- Increases gastric mucous production
- Decreases GI spasms
- Produces an anti-inflammatory effect
- Suppresses platelet aggregation
- Used to treat morning sickness, motion sickness, nausea from surgery
- Can decrease pain and stiffness of rheumatoid arthritis

ADVERSE EFFECTS AND PRECAUTIONS
- Use cautiously in clients who are pregnant because high doses can cause uterine contractions.
- Adverse effects are unknown, with potential CNS depression and cardiac dysrhythmias with very large overdose.

INTERACTIONS
- Interacts with medications that interfere with coagulation (NSAIDS, warfarin, and heparin).
- Can increase hypoglycemic effects of diabetes medications

NURSING ADMINISTRATION
- Question clients about concurrent use with NSAIDs, heparin, and warfarin.
- Monitor for hypoglycemia if the client takes insulin or other medication for diabetes.

Ginkgo biloba

- Promotes vasodilation: Decreases leg pain caused from occlusive arterial disorders
- Decreases platelet aggregation: Can decrease risk of thrombosis
- Decreases bronchospasm
- Increases blood flow to the brain: Thought to improve memory (dementia, Alzheimer's disease), but studies do not indicate effectiveness

ADVERSE EFFECTS AND PRECAUTIONS
- Mild GI upset, headache, lightheadedness, which can be decreased by reducing dose
- Should be taken with caution in clients at risk for seizures

INTERACTIONS
- Can interact with medications that lower the seizure threshold, such as antihistamines, antidepressants, and antipsychotics
- Can interfere with coagulation

NURSING ADMINISTRATION
- Question clients regarding history of antidepressant use (imipramine), which causes a decrease in seizure threshold.
- Question clients about concurrent use with NSAIDs, heparin, and warfarin.

Glucosamine

- Stimulates cells to make cartilage and synovial fluid
- Suppresses inflammation of the joints and cartilage degradation
- Treats osteoarthritis of the knee, hip, and wrist

ADVERSE EFFECTS AND PRECAUTIONS
- Mild GI upset (nausea, heartburn)
- Use with caution with shellfish allergy.

INTERACTIONS: Use caution if taking antiplatelet or anticoagulant medication.

NURSING ADMINISTRATION: Question clients about concurrent use with NSAIDs, heparin, and warfarin.

Kava

> ❗ Causes liver injury Qs

- Possibly acts on gamma-aminobutyric acid (GABA) receptors in the CNS
- Promotes sleep
- Decreases anxiety
- Promotes muscle relaxation without affecting concentration

ADVERSE EFFECTS AND PRECAUTIONS
- Chronic use causes dry, flaky skin and jaundice.
- Chronic use and large doses can cause liver damage, including severe liver failure.

INTERACTIONS: Can cause sedation when taken concurrently with CNS depressants.

NURSING ADMINISTRATION
- Question clients taking any CNS depressant, including alcohol, about use of kava.
- Ask clients who have any liver condition about concurrent use.

Ma huang

> ❗ Can cause hypertension, tachycardia, stroke, myocardial infarction. Qs

- Stimulates the CNS
- Suppresses the appetite
- Used for weight loss
- Constricts arterioles: Increases heart rate and blood pressure
- Bronchodilator: Treats colds, influenza, and allergies

ADVERSE EFFECTS AND PRECAUTIONS
- Because it contains ephedrine, ma huang can stimulate the cardiovascular system. At high doses, it can cause death from hypertension and dysrhythmias.
- Stimulation of CNS can cause euphoria. In high doses, it can cause psychosis.

INTERACTIONS
- Interacts with CNS stimulants to potentiate their effect
- Can cause severe hypertension when taken with monoamine oxidase inhibitor antidepressants
- Interacts with antihypertensive medications, decreasing effects

NURSING ADMINISTRATION
- Question clients carefully about other medications.
- Products that include more than 10 mg/dose are forbidden to be sold in the U.S.

St. John's wort

- Affects serotonin, producing antidepressant effects: Used for mild depression
- Used orally as an analgesic to relieve pain and inflammation
- Applied topically for infection

ADVERSE EFFECTS
- Mild adverse effects, including dry mouth, lightheadedness, constipation, GI symptoms
- Skin rash when exposed to sunlight

INTERACTIONS
- Can cause serotonin syndrome when combined with other antidepressants, amphetamine, and cocaine
- Decreases effectiveness of oral contraceptives, cyclosporine, warfarin, digoxin, calcium-channel blockers, steroids, HIV protease inhibitors, and some anticancer medications

NURSING ADMINISTRATION
- Question clients taking any of the medications with which this substance interacts about concurrent use.
- Encourage clients using St. John's wort to prevent prolonged sun exposure and use sunscreen.

Saw palmetto

Can decrease prostate symptoms of hyperplasia

ADVERSE EFFECTS AND PRECAUTIONS: Few adverse effects; can cause mild GI effects

INTERACTIONS
- Possible additive effects with finasteride
- Can interact with antiplatelet and anticoagulant medications
- Pregnancy Risk Category X **Qs**

NURSING ADMINISTRATION
- Question clients about use before prostate-specific antigen tests.
- Question clients about concurrent use with aspirin, heparin, and warfarin.

Valerian

- Increases GABA to prevent insomnia (similar to benzodiazepines)
- Reduces anxiety-related restlessness
- Drowsiness effect increases over time

ADVERSE EFFECTS AND PRECAUTIONS
- Can cause drowsiness, lightheadedness, depression
- Risk of physical dependence

PRECAUTION
- Clients who have mental health disorders should use with caution.
- Should be avoided by women who are pregnant or lactating.

INTERACTIONS: It is not known if valerian potentiates effects of CNS depressants

NURSING ADMINISTRATION: Clients taking valerian should be warned about the possibility of drowsiness when operating motor vehicles and other equipment.

1. A nurse is teaching a client who has anemia and a new prescription for a liquid iron supplement. Which of the following information should the nurse include in the teaching? (Select all that apply.)

   A. "Add foods that are high in fiber to your diet."

   B. "Rinse your mouth after taking the medication."

   C. "Expect stools to be green or black in color."

   D. "Take the medication with a glass of milk."

   E. "Add red meat to your diet."

2. A nurse is caring for a client who has increased liver enzymes and is taking herbal supplements. Which of the following herbal supplements should the nurse report to the provider?

   A. Glucosamine

   B. Saw palmetto

   C. Kava

   D. St. John's wort

3. A nurse is evaluating a group of clients at a health fair to identify the need for folic acid therapy. Which of the following clients require folic acid therapy? (Select all that apply.)

   A. 12-year-old child who has iron deficiency anemia

   B. 24-year-old female who has no health problems

   C. 44-year-old male who has hypertension

   D. 55–year-old female who has alcohol use disorder

   E. 35-year-old male who has type 2 diabetes mellitus

4. A nurse is preparing to administer potassium chloride IV to a client who has hypokalemia. Which of the following actions should the nurse take? (Select all that apply.)

   A. Infuse medication through a large-bore needle.

   B. Monitor urine output to ensure at least 20 mL/hr.

   C. Administer medication via direct IV bolus.

   D. Implement cardiac monitoring.

   E. Administer the infusion using an IV pump.

5. A nurse is caring for a client who requests information on the use of feverfew. Which of the following responses should the nurse make?

   A. "It is used to treat skin infections."

   B. "It can decrease the frequency of migraine headaches."

   C. "It can lessen the nasal congestion in the common cold."

   D. "It can relieve nausea of morning sickness during pregnancy."

6. A nurse is completing an assessment of a client's current medications. The client states she also takes gingko biloba. Which of the following medications is contraindicated for a client taking gingko biloba?

   A. Acetaminophen

   B. Warfarin

   C. Digoxin

   D. Lisinopril

PRACTICE Active Learning Scenario

A nurse is educating a client about a new prescription for cyanocobalamin. What should the nurse include in the teaching? Use the ATI Active Learning Template: Medication to complete this item.

EXPECTED PHARMACOLOGICAL ACTION

CLIENT EDUCATION: Describe four teaching points for the client.

EVALUATION OF MEDICATION EFFECTIVENESS: Describe two nursing interventions.

1. A. **CORRECT:** Foods high in fiber can prevent constipation, which can occur when taking iron supplements.

   B. **CORRECT:** Iron supplements can stain teeth when taken in a liquid form. The client should rinse orally after taking the medication.

   C. **CORRECT:** Dark green or black stools can occur when taking iron supplements. The client should anticipate this effect.

   D. Dairy products and caffeine can decrease the absorption of iron supplements. Iron supplements are maximally absorbed when taken on an empty stomach or 1 hr before meals.

   E. **CORRECT:** Red meats are high in iron and recommended for a client to improve anemia when taken concurrently with iron supplements.

   (N) *NCLEX® Connection: Pharmacological and Parenteral Therapies, Medication Administration*

2. A. Glucosamine can increase bleeding and should be used with caution in clients who are taking antiplatelet medications or anticoagulants.

   B. Saw palmetto can cause mild GI effects, and should be used with caution in clients who are taking antiplatelet medications or anticoagulants.

   C. **CORRECT:** Chronic use or high doses of kava can cause liver damage, including severe liver failure.

   D. Garlic can cause GI symptoms and should be used with caution in clients who are taking antiplatelet medications or anticoagulants.

   (N) *NCLEX® Connection: Pharmacological and Parenteral Therapies, Adverse Effects/Contraindications/Side Effects/Interactions*

3. A. The client who has iron deficiency anemia requires treatment with iron supplements,.

   B. **CORRECT:** The female client of childbearing age should take folic acid to prevent neural tube defects in the fetus.

   C. The client who has hypertension requires treatment with diet, exercise, and antihypertensive medication.

   D. **CORRECT:** The client who has alcohol use disorder can require folic acid therapy. Excess alcohol consumption leads to poor dietary intake of folic acid and injury to the liver.

   E. The client who has type 2 diabetes mellitus requires treatment with diet, exercise, and hyperglycemic medication.

   (N) *NCLEX® Connection: Pharmacological and Parenteral Therapies, Expected Actions/Outcomes*

4. A. **CORRECT:** Infuse potassium through a large-bore needle to prevent vein irritation, phlebitis, and infiltration.

   B. The nurse monitors urine output to ensure at least 30 mL/hr for adequate kidney function.

   C. Administer IV potassium slowly, no faster than 10 mEq/hr. Rapid administration can result in fatal hyperkalemia.

   D. **CORRECT:** Implement cardiac monitoring to detect cardiac dysrhythmias in a client receiving IV potassium.

   E. **CORRECT:** Administer IV potassium using an infusion pump to prevent fatal hyperkalemia due to a rapid infusion rate.

   (N) *NCLEX® Connection: Pharmacological and Parenteral Therapies, Parenteral/Intravenous Therapies*

5. A. Aloe is used to treat tissue injury.

   B. **CORRECT:** Feverfew is used to decrease the frequency of migraine headaches, but it has not been proven to relieve an existing migraine headache.

   C. Echinacea is used to can relieve manifestations of the common cold.

   D. Ginger root is used to relieve nausea caused from morning sickness during pregnancy.

   (N) *NCLEX® Connection: Pharmacological and Parenteral Therapies, Medication Administration*

6. A. Aspirin should be used with caution in clients taking ginkgo biloba because ginkgo biloba can suppress coagulation.

   B. **CORRECT:** Warfarin is contraindicated for a client taking gingko biloba because ginkgo biloba can suppress coagulation and increase the risk of bleeding or hemorrhage.

   C. Decongestants are contraindicated for a client taking gingko biloba. Digoxin is not contraindicated for a client taking gingko biloba.

   D. Antipsychotic medications are contraindicated for a client taking gingko biloba. Lisinopril is not contraindicated for a client taking gingko biloba.

   (N) *NCLEX® Connection: Pharmacological and Parenteral Therapies, Adverse Effects/Contraindications/Side Effects/Interactions*

PRACTICE Answer

Using the ATI Active Learning Template: Medication

EXPECTED PHARMACOLOGICAL ACTION: Cyanocobalamin converts folic acid from an inactive form to an active form. It corrects megaloblastic anemia related to a deficiency of vitamin B_{12}.

CLIENT EDUCATION
- Review manifestations of hypokalemia.
- Discuss the use of potassium supplements, if prescribed.
- Discuss dietary sources of potassium.
- Encourage foods high in vitamin B_{12}.
- Administer intranasal cyanocobalamin 1 hr before or after eating hot foods when nasal secretions are decreased.
- Periodic laboratory testing of Hgb, Hct, RBC, reticulocyte count, and folate levels is advised.

EVALUATION OF MEDICATION EFFECTIVENESS
- Review laboratory values for increased reticulocyte count and macrocytes and Hgb and Hct levels within the expected reference range.
- Assess for improvement of neurologic manifestations (numbness, tingling of hands and feet).

(N) *NCLEX® Connection: Pharmacological and Parenteral Therapies, Medication Administration*

When reviewing the following chapters, keep in mind the relevant topics and tasks of the NCLEX outline, in particular:

Client Needs: Pharmacological and Parenteral Therapies

ADVERSE EFFECTS/CONTRAINDICATIONS/SIDE EFFECTS/ INTERACTIONS: Document side effects and adverse effects of medications and parenteral therapy.

MEDICATION ADMINISTRATION: Review pertinent data prior to medication administration.

CHAPTER 31

Medications Affecting the Reproductive Tract

Medications that affect the reproductive system include hormones that stimulate puberty (such as estrogen and progesterone in females, and testosterone in males), replace a hormonal deficiency (male or female), or prevent pregnancy in women (oral contraceptives).

Medications that are used to treat benign prostatic hyperplasia (BPH) include 5-alpha reductase inhibitors and alpha$_1$-adrenergic antagonists. Phosphodiesterase type 5 (PDE5) inhibitors are used to treat erectile dysfunction.

Estrogens

SELECT PROTOTYPE MEDICATIONS:
Conjugated equine estrogens

OTHER MEDICATIONS
- Estradiol
- Estradiol hemihydrate

ROUTE OF ADMINISTRATION
- **Oral, transdermal, intravaginal, IM, and IV:**
  Transdermal therapy reduces incidents of nausea and vomiting. A smaller dose is prescribed, and there is a reduction of fluctuation of blood estrogen levels and a reduced risk of complications.
- **IV and IM:** Rare

PURPOSE

EXPECTED PHARMACOLOGICAL ACTION
Estrogens are hormones needed for growth and maturation of the female reproductive tract, development of secondary sex characteristics, and are active in the follicular phase of the menstrual cycle. Estrogens block bone resorption and reduce low-density lipoprotein (LDL) levels. At high levels, estrogens suppress the release of a follicle-stimulating hormone (FSH) needed for conception. Estrogens also can promote or suppress blood coagulation.

THERAPEUTIC USES
- Contraception
- Acne in women and girls older than 15 years who want contraception
- Relief of moderate to severe postmenopausal manifestations, such as hot flashes, mood changes
- Prevention of postmenopausal osteoporosis
- Treatment of dysfunctional uterine bleeding
- Treatment of prostate cancer, and hypogonadism
- Treatment of moderate to severe symptoms of vulvar atrophy

COMPLICATIONS

Endometrial and ovarian cancers

When estrogen is used alone for postmenopausal therapy

NURSING CONSIDERATIONS
- Administer progestins along with estrogen.
- Instruct clients to report persistent vaginal bleeding if they have an intact uterus.
- Advise clients to have an endometrial biopsy every 2 years and pelvic exam yearly.

Potential risk for estrogen-dependent breast cancer

More often in postmenopausal women who use estrogen with progestin

NURSING CONSIDERATIONS
- Rule out estrogen-dependent breast cancer prior to starting therapy.
- Encourage clients to examine their breasts regularly. Obtain yearly breast exams by a provider, and periodic mammograms.

Embolic events

- Such as MI, pulmonary embolism, DVT, stroke
- Women older than 60 have increased risk of myocardial infarction and coronary heart disease.

NURSING CONSIDERATIONS
- Encourage clients to avoid all nicotine products.
- Monitor for pain, swelling, warmth, or erythema of lower legs.
- Teach clients how to reduce risk of cardiovascular disease.

CONTRAINDICATIONS/PRECAUTIONS

- Pregnancy Risk Category X
- Contraindicated for clients who have the following. Qs
  - Client or family history of heart disease
  - Atypical vaginal bleeding that is undiagnosed
  - Breast or estrogen-dependent cancer
  - History or risk of thromboembolic disease
- Use cautiously during breastfeeding because estrogens decrease quantity and quality of milk and are excreted in breast milk.
- Use cautiously in prepubescent girls. If administered, monitor bone growth and check periodically for early epiphyseal plate closure.

INTERACTIONS

Estrogens can reduce the effectiveness of warfarin.
NURSING CONSIDERATIONS
- If used concurrently, monitor international normalized ratio (INR) and prothrombin time (PT).
- Warfarin doses might need to be adjusted.

Concurrent use of phenytoin can decrease the effectiveness of estrogens.
NURSING CONSIDERATIONS: Monitor for decreased estrogen effects. An alternative form of birth control might be indicated.

Concurrent use of corticosteroids can increase effects of the corticosteroid.
NURSING CONSIDERATIONS: Monitor for increased corticosteroid effects.

Smoking increases risk for thrombophlebitis.
NURSING CONSIDERATIONS: Advise clients not to smoke. Use alternative treatment if smoking persists.

Concurrent use of anticoagulants, oral hypoglycemics, and thyroid medications can cause a decrease in the action of these medications.
NURSING CONSIDERATIONS: Monitor for decreased effects, and adjust dosages as needed. Monitor glucose and thyroid levels.

NURSING ADMINISTRATION

- Instruct clients to take the medication at the same time each day (e.g., at bedtime).
- Apply estrogen patches to the skin of the trunk. Avoid the breasts and waistline.
- Instruct clients to report menstrual changes, such as dysmenorrhea, amenorrhea, breakthrough bleeding, or breast changes.
- Encourage clients to perform monthly breast self-examinations and schedule annual gynecologic and breast examinations with the provider.
- Advise clients to notify the provider of any swelling or redness in legs, shortness of breath, or chest pain.
- Discontinue prior to knee or hip surgery or any surgical procedures that can cause extensive immobilization.

NURSING EVALUATION OF MEDICATION EFFECTIVENESS

Depending on therapeutic intent, effectiveness is evidenced by the following.
- No evidence of conception
- Relief of severe postmenopausal manifestations (hot flashes, mood changes)
- Reduction in dysfunctional uterine bleeding
- Decrease in spread of prostate cancer

Progesterones

SELECT PROTOTYPE MEDICATION: Medroxyprogesterone

OTHER MEDICATIONS
- Norethindrone
- Megestrol acetate

ROUTES OF ADMINISTRATION: Oral, IM, subcutaneous, transdermal, and intravaginal

PURPOSE

EXPECTED PHARMACOLOGICAL ACTION
Progesterones induce favorable conditions for fetal growth and development and maintain pregnancy. A drop in progesterone levels results in menstruation.

THERAPEUTIC USES
- Use progestins alone or with estrogens for contraception.
- Progestins counter adverse effects of estrogen in menopausal hormone therapy.
- Progestins are used to treat the following.
  - Dysfunctional uterine bleeding due to hormonal imbalance
  - Amenorrhea due to hormonal imbalance
  - Endometriosis
  - Advanced cancer of the endometrium, breast, and kidney
- Can be used in women who are undergoing in vitro fertilization, and in some clients to prevent preterm birth.

COMPLICATIONS

Breast cancer

In postmenopausal women in combination with estrogens

CLIENT EDUCATION: Encourage clients to perform regular breast self-examinations and get mammograms.

Thromboembolic events

MI, pulmonary embolism, thrombophlebitis, stroke

NURSING CONSIDERATIONS
- Discourage clients from smoking.
- Monitor for pain, swelling, warmth, or erythema of lower legs.
- Advise clients to notify the provider of chest pain or shortness of breath.

Breakthrough bleeding, amenorrhea, breast tenderness

NURSING CONSIDERATIONS
- Obtain baseline breast exam and Pap smear.
- Instruct clients to report abnormal vaginal bleeding.

Edema

NURSING CONSIDERATIONS: Monitor blood pressure, I&O, and weight gain.

Jaundice

NURSING CONSIDERATIONS: Monitor for indications of jaundice, such as yellowing of the skin and sclera of the eyes. Monitor liver enzymes.

Migraine headaches

NURSING CONSIDERATIONS: Notify the provider of severe headache.

Birth defects/spontaneous abortion

NURSING CONSIDERATIONS: Notify the provider if pregnancy is planned or suspected.

CONTRAINDICATIONS/PRECAUTIONS

- Pregnancy Risk Category B
- Contraindicated in clients who have the following. Qs
  - Undiagnosed vaginal bleeding
  - History of thromboembolic disease, cardiovascular, or cerebrovascular disease
  - History of breast or genital cancers
- Use cautiously in clients who have diabetes mellitus, seizures disorders, and migraine headaches.

INTERACTIONS

Use of carbamazepine, phenobarbital, phenytoin, and rifampin can decrease contraceptive effectiveness.
NURSING CONSIDERATIONS: Additional contraceptive measures might be needed with concurrent use of these medications.

Concurrent use with corticosteroids and anticoagulants can cause decreased bone density.
CLIENT EDUCATION: Instruct clients to increase calcium and vitamin D intake. Avoid concurrent use.

Smoking increases risk for thrombophlebitis.
CLIENT EDUCATION: Advise clients not to smoke. Use alternative treatment if smoking persists.

NURSING ADMINISTRATION

- Instruct clients to anticipate withdrawal bleeding 3 to 7 days after stopping the medication. Qpcc
- Notify the provider if pregnancy is planned or suspected.

NURSING EVALUATION OF MEDICATION EFFECTIVENESS

Depending on therapeutic intent, effectiveness is evidenced by the following.
- Restoration of hormonal balance with control of uterine bleeding
- Restoration of menses
- Decrease in endometrial hyperplasia in postmenopausal women receiving concurrent estrogen
- Control of the spread of endometrial cancer

Hormonal contraceptives

SELECT PROTOTYPE MEDICATIONS

- Estrogen-progestin combinations contain estrogen and progestin and are referred to as combination oral contraceptives (OCs). OCs that contain progestin only are often referred to as minipills.
- Combination oral contraceptives with estrogen plus a progestin
  - Ethinyl estradiol and norethindrone
  - Ethinyl estradiol and drospirenone
  - Combination oral contraceptives are classified as monophasic, biphasic, triphasic, or quadriphasic. With monophasic OCs, the dosage of estrogen to progestin remains the same throughout the cycle. With the other classifications, the estrogen/progestin changes to duplicate a typical menstrual cycle.
- Progestin-only oral contraceptives: Norethindrone

OTHER MEDICATIONS

- Transdermal patch: Ethinyl estradiol and norelgestromin
- Vaginal contraceptive ring: Ethinyl estradiol and etonogestrel
- Parenteral: Depot medroxyprogesterone acetate available for IM use and for subcutaneous use
- Etonogestrel implants

ROUTE OF ADMINISTRATION

- Oral, transdermal, intravaginal, intrauterine, IM, subcutaneous, subdermal
- Combination OCs are given in a cyclic pattern, usually in a 28-day regimen. They can also be given in extended-cycle schedules.

PURPOSE

EXPECTED PHARMACOLOGICAL ACTION: Oral contraceptives stop conception by preventing ovulation. They also thicken the cervical mucus and alter the endometrial lining to reduce the chance of fertilization.

THERAPEUTIC USES: Hormonal contraceptives are used to prevent pregnancy.

COMPLICATIONS

Thromboembolic events

- MI, pulmonary embolism, thrombophlebitis, stroke
- Unlikely with progestin-only OCs

CLIENT EDUCATION
- Discourage clients from smoking.
- Instruct clients to report warmth, edema, tenderness, or pain in lower legs.

Hypertension

NURSING CONSIDERATIONS: Monitor and take actions to maintain blood pressure.

Breakthrough or irregular uterine bleeding

NURSING CONSIDERATIONS
- Instruct clients to record duration and frequency of breakthrough bleeding.
- Evaluate for possible pregnancy if two or more menstrual periods are missed.

Breast cancer

NURSING CONSIDERATIONS: Oral contraceptives can increase growth of a pre-existing breast cancer. Do not give to women who have breast cancer.

Hyperglycemia

NURSING CONSIDERATIONS: Monitor glucose in clients who have diabetes mellitus. Adjust antihyperglycemics as needed.

Hyperkalemia

With combination OC that contains drospirenone

NURSING CONSIDERATIONS: Do not use combination OC with drospirenone in clients at risk for hyperkalemia, such as renal insufficiency or adrenal insufficiency.

CONTRAINDICATIONS/PRECAUTIONS

- Pregnancy Risk Category X
- Contraindicated for clients who Qs
  - Are smokers and over the age of 35.
  - Have a history of thrombophlebitis and cardiovascular events.
  - Have a family history or risk factors for breast cancer.
  - Are experiencing abnormal vaginal bleeding.
- Use cautiously in clients who have hypertension, diabetes mellitus, gallbladder disease, uterine leiomyoma, seizures, and migraine headaches.

INTERACTIONS

Oral contraceptive effectiveness decreases with use of carbamazepine, phenobarbital; antibiotics, especially penicillins and cephalosporins; phenytoin, and rifampin.
NURSING CONSIDERATIONS: Additional contraceptive measures might be needed with concurrent use of these medications.

Oral contraceptives decrease the effects of warfarin and oral hypoglycemics.
NURSING CONSIDERATIONS: Monitor INR, PT, and glucose levels, and adjust dosages accordingly.

Oral contraceptives can increase the effects of theophylline and imipramine.
NURSING CONSIDERATIONS: Monitor for signs of toxicity.

NURSING ADMINISTRATION

- Check for pregnancy prior to start of therapy. Qpcc
- Instruct clients to take pills at the same time each day.
- Instruct clients to take medication for 21 days followed by 7 days of no medication (or inert pill). For the traditional 28-day cycle OCs, begin the sequence on the first day or first Sunday after the onset of menses.
- If one or more pills are missed in the first week, take one pill as soon as possible and continue on with the pack. Use an additional form of contraception for 7 days.
- If one or two pills are missed in the second or third week, take one as soon as possible and continue on with the active pills in the pack but skip the placebos and go straight to the new pack once all of the active pills have been taken.
- If three or more pills are missed during the second or third week, follow the same instructions for missing two pills. Use an additional form of contraception for 7 days.
- Extended-cycle OCs are taken for longer than the typical 28-day cycle. Eighty-four days is common, but some preparations are taken continuously.

> For example, for extended-cycle OC taken for 84 days, the client has withdrawal bleeding four times per year. Some extended-cycle OC are taken continuously, and the client does not have withdrawal bleeding.

- Encourage clients who smoke to quit.
- Advise client to report swelling or redness in legs, shortness of breath, or severe headache.

NURSING EVALUATION OF MEDICATION EFFECTIVENESS

Depending on therapeutic intent, effectiveness is confirmed by no evidence of conception.

Androgens

SELECT PROTOTYPE MEDICATION: Testosterone

OTHER MEDICATIONS: Methyltestosterone

ROUTE OF ADMINISTRATION: IM, transdermal, implantable pellets, buccal tablets

PURPOSE

EXPECTED PHARMACOLOGICAL ACTION
The hormone-receptor complex acts on cellular DNA to promote specific mRNA molecules and production of proteins, resulting in the following.
- Development of sex traits in men and the production and maturation of sperm
- Increase in skeletal muscle
- Increase in synthesis of erythropoietin

THERAPEUTIC USES
- Hypogonadism in males
- Delayed puberty in boys
- Androgen replacement in testicular failure
- Anemia not responsive to traditional therapy
- Postmenopausal breast cancer
- Muscle wasting in male clients who have AIDS

COMPLICATIONS

Androgenic (virilization) effects

- In women, these medications can cause irregularity or cessation of menses, hirsutism, weight gain, acne, lowering of voice, growth of clitoris, vaginitis, and baldness.
- In boys and men, these medications can cause acne, priapism, increased facial and body hair, and penile enlargement.

NURSING CONSIDERATIONS
- Advise clients of possible medication effects.
- Advise women to report occurrence of these effects.
- Medication might be discontinued to prevent permanent changes.

Epiphyseal closure

Premature closure of epiphysis in boys can reduce mature height.

NURSING CONSIDERATIONS: Monitor epiphysis with serial X-rays.

Cholestatic hepatitis, jaundice

NURSING CONSIDERATIONS
- Monitor for indications of jaundice, such as yellowing of the skin and sclera of the eyes.
- Monitor liver enzymes.

Hypercholesterolemia

These medications can decrease high-density lipoproteins (HDL) and increase LDL.

NURSING CONSIDERATIONS
- Monitor cholesterol levels.
- Advise clients to adjust diet to reduce cholesterol levels.

Increase in growth of prostate cancer

NURSING CONSIDERATIONS
- Do not give to clients who have prostate cancer.
- Monitor for prostate cancer.

Polycythemia

NURSING CONSIDERATIONS: Monitor hemoglobin and hematocrit.

Edema from salt and water retention

NURSING CONSIDERATIONS
- Instruct clients to monitor for weight gain and swelling of extremities, and report these to the provider.
- Medication can be discontinued.

High abuse potential

NURSING CONSIDERATIONS: Identify high-risk groups, and educate regarding abuse potential and possible health risks.

Hypercalcemia

NURSING CONSIDERATIONS: Monitor electrolytes and for manifestations of hypercalcemia, such as lethargy, nausea, vomiting, and constipation.

Hypoglycemia in clients who have diabetes mellitus

NURSING CONSIDERATIONS: Monitor glucose and adjust antihyperglycemic medications.

CONTRAINDICATIONS/PRECAUTIONS

- Pregnancy Risk Category X
- Contraindicated in older adult clients and men who have prostate or breast cancer, severe cardiac, renal, or liver disease. ⓒ
- Use cautiously in clients who have heart failure, hypercalcemia, or hypertension.

INTERACTIONS

Androgens can alter effects of oral anticoagulants.
NURSING CONSIDERATIONS: Monitor PT and INR.

Androgens can alter effects of insulins and antidiabetic agents.
NURSING CONSIDERATIONS: Monitor glucose level, and adjust dosages.

Concurrent use of androgens and hepatotoxic medications can increase risk for hepatotoxicity.
NURSING CONSIDERATIONS: Monitor liver enzymes. Assess for jaundice.

NURSING ADMINISTRATION

- Instruct clients using gel formulations to wash their hands after every application due to the possibility of skin-to-skin transfer to others. Cover application with clothing after gel has dried and wash off before skin to skin contact with another person.
- Inject IM formulations into a large muscle and rotate injection sites. Qpcc
- Monitor women for acne and manifestations of masculinization (facial hair, baldness, deepened voice).
- Advise clients to use a barrier method of birth control.
- Advise clients to reduce cholesterol in the diet.
- Advise clients at risk about abuse potential.
- Obtain daily weights.

NURSING EVALUATION OF MEDICATION EFFECTIVENESS

Depending on therapeutic intent, effectiveness is evidenced by the following.
- Puberty is induced in boys.
- Testosterone is increased in men.
- There is a decrease in the progression of breast cancer in women. Medication produces expected results with minimal adverse effects.

5-Alpha reductase inhibitors

SELECT PROTOTYPE MEDICATIONS: Finasteride

OTHER MEDICATIONS: Dutasteride

ROUTE OF ADMINISTRATION: Oral

PURPOSE

EXPECTED PHARMACOLOGICAL ACTION: Decreases usable testosterone by inhibiting the converting enzyme, causing a reduction of the prostate size and increased hair growth

THERAPEUTIC USES
- Benign prostatic hyperplasia
- Male pattern baldness

COMPLICATIONS

Decreased libido, ejaculate volume

CLIENT EDUCATION: Advise clients to notify the provider if adverse effects occur.

Gynecomastia

CLIENT EDUCATION: Advise clients to notify the provider if adverse effects occur.

CONTRAINDICATIONS/PRECAUTIONS

- Pregnancy Risk Category X
- Contraindicated in clients who have medication hypersensitivity.
- Use with caution in clients who have liver disease.

INTERACTIONS

None significant

NURSING ADMINISTRATION

- Advise clients that therapeutic effects can take 6 months or longer.
- Pregnant women should not handle crushed or broken medication. Qs
- Advise clients not to donate blood unless medication has been discontinued for at least 1 month.

NURSING EVALUATION OF MEDICATION EFFECTIVENESS

Depending on therapeutic intent, effectiveness is evidenced by the following.
- Prostate size is decreased, and the client is able to urinate effectively.
- Prostate-specific antigen (PSA) levels have decreased from baseline.
- Client has increased hair growth.

Alpha$_1$-adrenergic antagonists

SELECT PROTOTYPE MEDICATION
Selective alpha$_1$ receptor antagonist: Tamsulosin

OTHER MEDICATIONS
- Selective alpha$_1$ receptor antagonist: Silodosin
- Nonselective alpha$_1$ receptor antagonists
  - Alfuzosin
  - Terazosin
  - Doxazosin

ROUTE OF ADMINISTRATION: Oral

PURPOSE

EXPECTED PHARMACOLOGICAL ACTION
- Decrease mechanical obstruction of the urethra by relaxing smooth muscles of the bladder neck and prostate.
- Nonselective agents also cause vasodilation and can lower blood pressure. These agents are used for clients who have BPH and hypertension.

THERAPEUTIC USES
- BPH, thus increasing urinary flow
- Off-label use for women for treatment of urinary hesitancy or urinary retention

COMPLICATIONS

Hypotension, dizziness, nasal congestion, sleepiness, faintness

More likely with nonselective antagonists

NURSING CONSIDERATIONS
- Monitor blood pressure.
- Advise clients to rise slowly from sitting or lying position.
- Advise clients not to drive or operate machinery when starting therapy or with change in dose until response is known.

Problems with ejaculation

Failure, decreased volume with silodosin and tamsulosin

CLIENT EDUCATION: Advise clients of possible adverse effects.

Floppy iris syndrome following cataract surgery

NURSING CONSIDERATIONS: Hold the medication before cataract surgery.

CONTRAINDICATIONS/PRECAUTIONS

- Contraindicated in clients who have medication sensitivity. Qs
- Alfuzosin is contraindicated in women and in clients who have severe liver failure.
- Silodosin is contraindicated in clients who have renal failure or liver failure.
- Doxazosin should be used cautiously in clients who have liver impairment.
- Tamsulosin should be used cautiously in clients who have hepatic or renal impairment.

INTERACTIONS

Cimetidine can decrease clearance of tamsulosin.
NURSING CONSIDERATIONS: Use concurrently with caution.

Antihypertensives, PDE5 inhibitors, and nitroglycerin used concurrently with nonselective agents can cause severe hypotension.
NURSING CONSIDERATIONS
- Use with caution.
- Monitor blood pressure.

Erythromycin and HIV protease inhibitors (ritonavir) will increase levels of alfuzosin and silodosin when used concurrently.
NURSING CONSIDERATIONS: Avoid concurrent use.

NURSING ADMINISTRATION

- Monitor blood pressure, especially at the start of therapy and with changes of dose. Qpcc
- Advise clients to take medication daily as prescribed:
  - Tamsulosin: 30 min after a meal at the same time each day
  - Silodosin: With the same meal each day
  - Alfuzosin: Right after the same meal each day
  - Terazosin: At bedtime
  - Doxazosin: At the same time each day

NURSING EVALUATION OF MEDICATION EFFECTIVENESS

Depending on therapeutic intent, effectiveness is evidenced by improved urinary flow with minimal adverse effects.

Phosphodiesterase type 5 inhibitors

SELECT PROTOTYPE MEDICATIONS: Sildenafil

OTHER MEDICATIONS
- Tadalafil
- Vardenafil

PURPOSE

EXPECTED PHARMACOLOGICAL ACTION: Augments the effects of nitric oxide released during sexual stimulation, resulting in enhanced blood flow to the corpus cavernosum and penile erection

THERAPEUTIC USES: Erectile dysfunction

COMPLICATIONS

MI, sudden death

NURSING CONSIDERATIONS: Monitor risk factors and history with regard to cardiovascular health.

Priapism

CLIENT EDUCATION: Instruct clients to notify the provider if erection lasts more than 4 hr.

Sudden hearing loss

CLIENT EDUCATION: Advise clients to discontinue medication if hearing is affected.

CONTRAINDICATIONS/PRECAUTIONS

- Contraindicated in clients taking any medications in the nitrate family, such as nitroglycerin.
- Use cautiously in clients who have cardiovascular disease, including QT prolongation. Qs
- Advise clients that grapefruit juice can increase plasma concentrations and possible adverse effects of medication.

INTERACTIONS

Organic nitrates, such as nitroglycerin and isosorbide dinitrate, can lead to fatal hypotension.
NURSING CONSIDERATIONS: Do not use with organic nitrates or alpha blockers.

Ketoconazole, erythromycin, cimetidine, ritonavir, and grapefruit juice inhibit metabolism of sildenafil, thereby increasing plasma levels of medication.
NURSING CONSIDERATIONS: Use these medications cautiously in clients taking PDE5 inhibitors.

NURSING ADMINISTRATION

- Administer orally, 30 min to 4 hr before sexual activity, depending on dosage. Qpcc
- Instruct clients that tadalafil is approved to be taken daily or prior to sexual activity.

NURSING EVALUATION OF MEDICATION EFFECTIVENESS

Depending on therapeutic intent, effectiveness is evidenced by erection sufficient for sexual intercourse.

Application Exercises

1. A nurse is reviewing the health care record of a client who is asking about conjugated equine estrogens. The nurse should inform the client this medication is contraindicated in which of the following conditions?

   A. Atrophic vaginitis

   B. Dysfunctional uterine bleeding

   C. Osteoporosis

   D. Thrombophlebitis

2. A nurse is providing teaching to a female client who is taking testosterone to treat advanced breast cancer. The nurse should tell the client that which of the following are adverse effects of this medication? (Select all that apply.)

   A. Deepening voice

   B. Weight gain

   C. Low blood pressure

   D. Dry mouth

   E. Facial hair

3. A nurse is explaining the mechanism of action of combination oral contraceptives to a group of clients. The nurse should tell the clients that which of the following actions occur with the use of combination oral contraceptives? (Select all that apply.)

   A. Thickening the cervical mucus

   B. Inducing maturation of ovarian follicle

   C. Increasing development of the corpus luteum

   D. Altering the endometrial lining

   E. Inhibiting ovulation

4. A nurse is providing teaching to a client who will start alfuzosin for treatment of benign prostatic hyperplasia. The nurse should instruct the client that which of the following is an adverse effect of this medication?

   A. Bradycardia

   B. Edema

   C. Hypotension

   D. Tremor

5. A nurse is caring for a client who has angina and asks about obtaining a prescription for sildenafil to treat erectile dysfunction. Which of the following medications is contraindicated with sildenafil?

   A. Aspirin

   B. Isosorbide

   C. Clopidogrel

   D. Atorvastatin

PRACTICE Active Learning Scenario

A nurse in a provider's office is instructing a client who has a new prescription for finasteride to treat benign prostatic hyperplasia. Use the ATI Active Learning Template: Medication to complete this item.

EXPECTED PHARMACOLOGICAL ACTION

COMPLICATIONS: Identify two adverse effects.

Application Exercises Key

1. A. Atrophic vaginitis occurs when there is estrogen deficiency. This medication is used to treated atrophic vaginitis.

    B. Dysfunctional uterine bleeding can occur when there is estrogen deficiency. This medication is used to treat dysfunctional uterine bleeding.

    C. Women are at risk for osteoporosis after the onset of menopause. Estrogen is used to slow the progression of osteoporosis.

    D. **CORRECT**: Estrogen increases the risk of thrombolytic events. Estrogen use is contraindicated for a client who has a history of thrombophlebitis.

    Ⓝ *NCLEX® Connection: Pharmacological and Parenteral Therapies, Adverse Effects/Contraindications/Side Effects/Interactions*

2. A. **CORRECT**: Virilization, the development of adult male characteristics in a female, is an adverse effect of testosterone. The nurse should tell the client that a deepening voice is an adverse effect of testosterone.

    B. **CORRECT**: Edema and weight gain are adverse effects of testosterone.

    C. High blood pressure is an adverse effect of this medication.

    D. Nasal congestion is an adverse effect of this medication, not dry mouth.

    E. **CORRECT**: Virilization is an adverse effect of testosterone. The nurse should tell the client that the development of facial hair is an adverse effect of testosterone.

    Ⓝ *NCLEX® Connection: Pharmacological and Parenteral Therapies, Adverse Effects/Contraindications/Side Effects/Interactions*

3. A. **CORRECT**: Oral contraceptives cause thickening of the cervical mucus, which slows sperm passage.

    B. Inducing maturation of ovarian follicle is not an action of oral contraceptives.

    C. Increasing the development of the corpus luteum is not an action of oral contraceptives.

    D. **CORRECT**: Oral contraceptives alter the lining of the endometrium, which inhibits implantation of the fertilized egg.

    E. **CORRECT**: Oral contraceptives prevent pregnancy by inhibiting ovulation.

    Ⓝ *NCLEX® Connection: Pharmacological and Parenteral Therapies, Medication Administration*

4. A. Alfuzosin can cause tachycardia.

    B. Alfuzosin can cause diarrhea or constipation. Edema is not an adverse effect of this mediation.

    C. **CORRECT**: Alfuzosin relaxes muscle tone in veins and cardiac output decreases, which leads to hypotension. Clients taking this medication are advised to rise slowly from a sitting or lying position.

    D. Alfuzosin can cause dizziness. Tremor is not an adverse effect of this medication.

    Ⓝ *NCLEX® Connection: Pharmacological and Parenteral Therapies, Adverse Effects/Contraindications/Side Effects/Interactions*

5. A. Aspirin is contraindicated in clients who have a bleeding disorder, but there are no contradictions for concurrent use of sildenafil.

    B. **CORRECT**: Isosorbide is an organic nitrate that manages pain from angina. Concurrent use of it is contraindicated because fatal hypotension can occur. The client should avoid taking a nitrate medication for 24 hr after taking isosorbide.

    C. Clopidogrel is contraindicated in clients who are actively bleeding, but there is no contradiction for concurrent use of clopidogrel and sildenafil.

    D. Atorvastatin is contraindicated in clients who have hepatic disease, but there is no contradiction for concurrent use of atorvastatin and sildenafil.

    Ⓝ *NCLEX® Connection: Pharmacological and Parenteral Therapies, Adverse Effects/Contraindications/Side Effects/Interactions*

PRACTICE Answer

Using the ATI Active Learning Template: Medication

EXPECTED PHARMACOLOGICAL ACTION: Finasteride slows the production of testosterone, which reduces the size of the prostate and subsequently promotes urinary elimination.

COMPLICATIONS
- Decreased libido
- Decreased ejaculate volume
- Gynecomastia
- Orthostatic hypotension

Ⓝ *NCLEX® Connection: Pharmacological and Parenteral Therapies, Medication Administration*

CHAPTER 32 *Medications Affecting Labor and Delivery*

Understanding medications affecting labor and delivery is imperative to promote positive maternal and fetal outcomes. These include medications used to induce or augment labor, and medication used in the management of preterm labor.

Uterine stimulants: Oxytocics

SELECT PROTOTYPE MEDICATION: Oxytocin

OTHER MEDICATIONS
- Dinoprostone
- Methylergonovine

PURPOSE

EXPECTED PHARMACOLOGICAL ACTION

Uterine stimulants increase the strength, frequency, and length of uterine contractions.

THERAPEUTIC USES

Oxytocin
- Induction of labor (postterm pregnancy, premature rupture of membranes, preeclampsia)
- Enhancement of labor, such as with dysfunctional labor
- Delivery of placenta (postpartum, miscarriage)
- Management of postpartum hemorrhage
- Stress testing

Dinoprostone is a prostaglandin used to promote cervical ripening and to stimulate uterine contractions.

Methylergonovine contracts the uterus and is used for emergency intervention for serious postpartum hemorrhage.

COMPLICATIONS

OXYTOCIN

Uterine rupture, uterine tachysystole, placental abruption, hyponatremia

NURSING CONSIDERATIONS
- Preassess risk factors, such as multiple deliveries.
- Monitor the length, strength, and duration of contractions.
- Assess fetal status.
- Monitor vital signs.
- Monitor I&O.

DINOPROSTONE

Uterine tachysystole

NURSING CONSIDERATIONS
- Monitor the length, strength, and duration of contractions.
- Assess fetal status.
- Monitor vital signs.

METHYLERGONOVINE

Hypertensive crisis

NURSING CONSIDERATIONS
- Monitor vital signs
- Monitor for manifestations of hypertensive crisis (headache, nausea, vomiting, increased blood pressure).
- Monitor for uterine tone and vaginal bleeding.
- Provide emergency interventions.

CONTRAINDICATIONS/PRECAUTIONS

OXYTOCIN

Maternal factors: Sepsis, an unripe cervix, active genital herpes, history of multiple births, uterine surgery Qs

Fetal factors: Immature lungs, cephalopelvic disproportion, fetal malpresentation, prolapsed umbilical cord, fetal distress, placental abnormalities, threatened spontaneous abortion

DINOPROSTONE

Cesarean birth, fetal distress, vaginal bleeding
NURSING CONSIDERATIONS: Use with caution with maternal history of hypotension, hypertension, and asthma.

METHYLERGONOVINE

Hypertension, preeclampsia, asthma and cardiac disease
NURSING CONSIDERATIONS
- Use with caution with maternal history of severe renal or hepatic disease, diabetes mellitus, sepsis, and epilepsy.
- Use only after delivery, and not during labor.

INTERACTIONS

OXYTOCIN

CNS depressants increase effects. MAOIs cause unpredictable effects.
NURSING CONSIDERATIONS
• Avoid concurrent use.
• Monitor vital signs, uterine activity, and fetal status.

DINOPROSTONE

Other oxytocics increase effects.
NURSING CONSIDERATIONS
• Avoid concurrent use.
• Monitor vital signs, uterine activity, and fetal status.

METHYLERGONOVINE

Vasopressors, ergots increase effects.
NURSING CONSIDERATIONS
• Avoid concurrent use.
• Monitor vital signs.

NURSING ADMINISTRATION

• Use an infusion pump to administer IV oxytocin. Gradually increase the flow rate per prescribed parameters, such as 1 milliunits/min every 30 to 60 min. Q EBP
• Monitor blood pressure, respiratory rate, and pulse every 30 to 60 min and with every dosage change.
• Carefully monitor uterine contractions (frequency and duration) every 15 min and with every dosage change during the first stage of labor and every 5 min the second stage of labor. Generally, the goal is contractions that last 1 min or less every 2 to 3 min.
• Monitor for uterine tachysystole (more than five contractions in 10 min, contractions occurring within 1 min of each other, or a series of single contractions lasting greater than 2 min).
• Continuously monitor the fetal heart rate and rhythm. Report findings of fetal distress.

NURSING EVALUATION OF MEDICATION EFFECTIVENESS

Depending on therapeutic intent, effectiveness can be evidenced by the following.
• Effective contractions (lasting less than 60 seconds and occurring every 2 to 3 min)
• Increase in uterine tone and no evidence of postpartum hemorrhage

Tocolytic medications

SELECT PROTOTYPE MEDICATION
• Terbutaline
• Hydroxyprogesterone caproate

OTHER MEDICATIONS
• Nifedipine
• Indomethacin
• Magnesium sulfate

PURPOSE

EXPECTED PHARMACOLOGICAL ACTION

• Terbutaline selectively activates beta$_2$-adrenergic receptors (beta$_2$-adrenergic agonist), resulting in uterine smooth muscle relaxation.
• Hydroxyprogesterone caproate is a progestin hormone and the only FDA-approved medication to prevent preterm labor. Its mechanism of action is unknown. It is only for use in women with a single fetus.

THERAPEUTIC USES

• Subcutaneous terbutaline can be used for up to 24 hr to delay but not to prevent preterm labor.
• Hydroxyprogesterone caproate decreases the risk of recurrent preterm births.
• Nifedipine, a calcium channel blocker, is as equally effective as terbutaline in suppressing preterm labor.
• Indomethacin acts to suppress labor by inhibiting synthesis of prostaglandins.
• Magnesium sulfate is a central nervous system depressant and relaxes smooth muscles. Its primary use is to prevent seizures in clients who have preeclampsia. It has significant adverse maternal effects and increases fetal mortality.

COMPLICATIONS

TERBUTALINE

Multiple effects

Maternal
• Tachycardia, palpitations, chest pain, hypotension, hypokalemia, hyperglycemia
• Intolerable: Blood pressure less than 90/60 mm Hg, heart rate greater than 130/min, chest pain, pulmonary edema, cardiac arrhythmias

Fetal: Tachycardia

NURSING CONSIDERATIONS
• Monitor vital signs, blood glucose, and potassium levels.
• Notify the provider for intolerable adverse effects.
• Have propranolol available.

HYDROXYPROGESTERONE CAPROATE

Injection-site reactions

NURSING CONSIDERATIONS: Monitor for pain, swelling, itching, and appearance of hives.

NIFEDIPINE

Hypotension, headache, dizziness, nausea

NURSING CONSIDERATIONS: Monitor for manifestations of adverse effects.

INDOMETHACIN

Multiple effects

Maternal: Nausea, vomiting, heartburn, GI bleed, thrombocytopenia

Fetal: Neonatal pulmonary hypertension, oligohydramnios

NURSING CONSIDERATIONS: Monitor for manifestations of adverse effects.

MAGNESIUM SULFATE

Maternal
- Hypocalcemia, hot flashes, dyspnea, transient hypotension
- Intolerable: Respirations less than 12/min, pulmonary edema, altered level of consciousness, severe hypotension, urine output less than 25 mL/hr, serum magnesium level 10mEq/L or greater

Fetal: Nonreactive NST, reduced fetal heart rate (FHR) variability

NURSING CONSIDERATIONS
- Obtain vital signs.
- Monitor serum magnesium level.
- Limit IV fluids to 125 mL/hr.
- Have calcium gluconate available.
- Discontinue infusion with any intolerable adverse effects.

CONTRAINDICATIONS/PRECAUTIONS

TERBUTALINE

Hypersensitivity
NURSING CONSIDERATIONS: Use caution with chronic/active hepatic disease, renal disease.

HYDROXYPROGESTERONE CAPROATE

Uncontrolled hypertension, liver disease, history of thrombosis, breast cancer

NIFEDIPINE

Hypersensitivity
NURSING CONSIDERATIONS: Use caution with hypotension, hepatic or renal disease, or acute MI. Avoid concurrent use with magnesium sulfate or terbutaline.

INDOMETHACIN

GI bleeding, hypersensitivity
NURSING CONSIDERATIONS
- Use caution with seizures, renal/hepatic disease, GI disorders, cardiac disorders, depression, and diabetes mellitus.
- Use for clients less than 32 weeks of gestation.
- Administer for no more than 48 hr.

MAGNESIUM SULFATE

Hypersensitivity, abdominal pain, heart block
NURSING CONSIDERATIONS: Avoid concurrent use with nifedipine.

INTERACTIONS

TERBUTALINE

Increase effect: MAOIs, green tea

Decrease effect: Beta-blockers

NURSING CONSIDERATIONS
- Monitor for hypertensive crisis.
- Avoid using with beta-blockers.

NIFEDIPINE

Increase effect: Level of digoxin, phenytoin, beta-blockers, antihypertensives, ginkgo biloba, ginseng, grapefruit juice

Increase toxicity: Cimetidine, ranitidine, St. John's wort, melatonin

NURSING CONSIDERATIONS: Avoid using with grapefruit juice, ginkgo biloba, ginseng, melatonin, and St. John's wort.

INDOMETHACIN

Increase: Bleeding risk with anticoagulants, hyperkalemia with potassium sparing diuretics, toxicity with lithium, cyclosporine

NURSING CONSIDERATIONS
- Avoid NSAIDs, alcohol, and salicylates.
- Monitor for toxicity (blurred vision, ringing in the ears).

MAGNESIUM SULFATE

Increase: Antihypertensives, calcium channel blockers, neuromuscular blockers

Decrease effect: Digoxin

NURSING CONSIDERATIONS
- Monitor blood pressure.
- Monitor for toxicity (thirst, confusion, decreased reflexes).

NURSING ADMINISTRATION

- Terbutaline is administered subcutaneously. Monitor injection site for infection.
- Monitor FHR, uterine contractions, pulse, blood pressure, respirations, lung sounds, and daily weights.
- Withhold the medication and contact the provider for reports of chest pain, maternal heart rate greater than 120/min, or presence of cardiac arrhythmias.
- Limit fluid intake to 2,500 to 3,000 mL/day.
- Notify the provider if contractions persist or increase in frequency or duration.
- Monitor for magnesium sulfate toxicity and discontinue for any of the following adverse effects: loss of deep tendon reflexes, urinary output less than 25 to 30 mL/hr or 100 mL/4 hr, respirations less than 12/min, pulmonary edema, severe hypotension, or chest pain. Calcium gluconate should be available to administer as an antidote for magnesium sulfate toxicity.
- Monitor blood glucose of clients who have diabetes mellitus and gestational diabetes.

NURSING EVALUATION OF MEDICATION EFFECTIVENESS

Depending on therapeutic intent, effectiveness can be evidenced by cessation of preterm labor (20 to 36 weeks).

Glucocorticoid medications

SELECT PROTOTYPE MEDICATIONS
- Betamethasone
- Dexamethasone

PURPOSE

EXPECTED PHARMACOLOGICAL ACTION: Releases enzymes that produce and release lung surfactant to stimulate lung maturity in a fetus

THERAPEUTIC USES: Reduce neonatal respiratory distress syndrome, intraventricular hemorrhage, necrotizing enterocolitis and death

COMPLICATIONS

Fetal decreased breathing and body movements

Transient

NURSING CONSIDERATIONS: Maintain continuous fetal monitoring.

NURSING ADMINISTRATION

- Administer betamethasone 12 mg IM for two doses 24 hr apart.
- Administer dexamethasone 6 mg IM for four doses 12 hr apart.
- Administer between 24 and 34 weeks of gestation.
- Administer deep IM using ventral gluteal or vastus lateralis muscle.

NURSING EVALUATION OF MEDICATION EFFECTIVENESS

Depending on therapeutic intent, effectiveness can be evidenced by fetal lung maturity at birth.

Opioid analgesics

SELECT PROTOTYPE MEDICATION: Fentanyl

OTHER MEDICATIONS
- Butorphanol
- Nalbuphine

PURPOSE

EXPECTED PHARMACOLOGICAL ACTION

These medications act in the central nervous system to decrease the perception of pain without the loss of consciousness.

THERAPEUTIC USES

- The client can be given opioid analgesics IM or IV, but the IV route is recommended during labor because of its quicker action.
- Butorphanol and nalbuphine provide pain relief without causing significant respiratory depression in the mother or fetus.

COMPLICATIONS

Dry mouth

NURSING CONSIDERATIONS: Provide ice chips.

Nausea and vomiting

NURSING CONSIDERATIONS: Administer antiemetic as prescribed.

Neonatal depression

NURSING CONSIDERATIONS: Have naloxone available at birth.

Tachycardia, hypotension, decreased FHR variability

NURSING CONSIDERATIONS: Monitor vital signs and FHR per facility protocol.

Sedation

NURSING CONSIDERATIONS: Provide safety.

CONTRAINDICATIONS/PRECAUTIONS

- Delivery within 1 to 4 hr of administration.
- If the opioid is given too soon, it can delay the progression of labor. If given too late, it can depress neonatal respirations.

NURSING ADMINISTRATION

- Prior to administering analgesic or anesthetic pain relief, the nurse should verify that labor is well established by performing a vaginal exam showing cervical dilation to be at least 4 cm with the fetus engaged. Q EBP
- Naloxone is administered only in cases of severe respiratory depression in the newborn. Q s
- Administer antiemetics as prescribed.
- Monitor vital signs and uterine contraction pattern. Provide continuous FHR monitoring.
- Explain to the client that the medication will cause drowsiness.
- Instruct the client to request assistance with ambulation.

NURSING EVALUATION OF MEDICATION EFFECTIVENESS

Depending on therapeutic intent, effectiveness can be evidenced by decreased pain during labor.

PRACTICE Active Learning Scenario

A nurse is reviewing a new prescription for methylergonovine for a client who is postpartum. What information should the nurse include in this review? Use the ATI Active Learning Template: Medication to complete this item.

THERAPEUTIC USES

COMPLICATIONS: Describe one adverse effect.

CONTRAINDICATIONS/PRECAUTIONS: Describe one contraindication.

NURSING INTERVENTIONS: Describe at least three.

Application Exercises

1. A nurse is teaching a client about terbutaline. Which of the following statements by the client indicates understanding of the teaching?

   A. "This medication will stop my contractions."

   B. "This medication will prevent vaginal bleeding."

   C. "This medication will promote blood flow to my baby."

   D. "This medication will increase my prostaglandin production."

2. A nurse is caring for a client who has preeclampsia and is receiving magnesium sulfate IV continuous infusion. Which of the following findings should the nurse report to the provider?

   A. 2+ deep tendon reflexes

   B. 2+ pedal edema

   C. 24 mL/hr urinary output

   D. Respirations 12/min

3. A nurse is caring for a client who has a new prescription for oxytocin to stimulate uterine contractions. Which of the following interventions should the nurse make? (Select all that apply.)

   A. Use an infusion pump for medication administration.

   B. Obtain vital signs frequently and with every dosage change.

   C. Stop infusion if uterine contractions occur every 4 min and last 45 seconds.

   D. Increase medication infusion rate rapidly.

   E. Monitor fetal heart rate continuously.

4. A nurse is caring for a client who is in labor and receiving IV opioid analgesics. Which of the following actions should the nurse take?

   A. Instruct the client to self-ambulate every 2 hr.

   B. Offer oral hygiene every 2 hr.

   C. Anticipate medication administration 2 hr prior to delivery.

   D. Monitor fetal heart rate every 2 hr.

5. A nurse is reviewing a new prescription for terbutaline with a client who has a history of preterm labor. Which of the following client statements indicates understanding of the teaching?

   A. "I can increase my activity now that I've started on this medication."

   B. "I will increase my daily fluid intake to 3 quarts."

   C. "I will report increasing intensity of contractions to my doctor."

   D. "I am glad this will prevent preterm labor."

Application Exercises Key

1. A. **CORRECT:** Terbutaline blocks beta₂-adrenergic receptors, which causes uterine smooth muscle relaxation.

   B. Terbutaline is used to suppress preterm labor and does not prevent bleeding.

   C. Terbutaline causes smooth muscle relaxation and does not promote placental blood flow.

   D. Terbutaline suppresses uterine contractions and does not increase prostaglandin production.

   Ⓝ NCLEX® Connection: Pharmacological and Parenteral Therapies, Expected Actions/Outcomes

2. A. This is an expected finding and does not need to be reported to the provider.

   B. This is an expected finding and does not need to be reported to the provider.

   C. **CORRECT:** Urine output less than 25 to 30 mL/hr is associated with magnesium sulfate toxicity and should be reported to the provider.

   D. A respiratory rate of 12/min is an expected finding and does not need to be reported to the provider.

   Ⓝ NCLEX® Connection: Pharmacological and Parenteral Therapies, Expected Actions/Outcomes

3. A. **CORRECT:** Oxytocin must be administered by an infusion pump to ensure precise dosage.

   B. **CORRECT:** Vital signs are monitored to assess for hypertension, an adverse effect of oxytocin.

   C. Infusion should not be stopped because therapeutic effect has not been achieved.

   D. Oxytocin rate is increased gradually to prevent hypertonic uterine contractions.

   E. **CORRECT:** Continuous FHR monitoring is required to assess for fetal distress.

   Ⓝ NCLEX® Connection: Pharmacological and Parenteral Therapies, Medication Administration

4. A. Clients should be assisted with ambulation due to the sedative effect of opioid analgesics.

   B. **CORRECT:** Oral hygiene should be offered on a regular basis to a client receiving opioid analgesics due to the adverse effects of dry mouth, nausea, and vomiting.

   C. Opioid analgesics should not be administered within 4 hr of delivery.

   D. Fetal heart rate should be monitored continuously in a client receiving opioid analgesics.

   Ⓝ NCLEX® Connection: Pharmacological and Parenteral Therapies, Parenteral/Intravenous Therapies

5. A. The action of terbutaline is to relax uterine smooth muscle. Clients taking this medication are instructed to limit activity, which stimulates smooth muscle, to delay preterm labor.

   B. Fluid intake should be limited to 2,400 mL/day.

   C. **CORRECT:** The client should report increasing intensity, frequency, or duration of contractions to the provider because these are manifestations of preterm labor.

   D. Terbutaline delays preterm labor; it does not prevent it.

   Ⓝ NCLEX® Connection: Pharmacological and Parenteral Therapies, Medication Administration

---

PRACTICE Answer

Using the ATI Active Learning Template: Medication

THERAPEUTIC USES: Prevent postpartum hemorrhage

COMPLICATIONS: Hypertensive crisis

CONTRAINDICATIONS/PRECAUTIONS: Hypertension, preeclampsia, asthma and cardiac disease: Use with caution with maternal history of severe renal or hepatic disease, diabetes mellitus, sepsis, and epilepsy.

NURSING INTERVENTIONS
- Monitor vital signs for increase in blood pressure.
- Monitor for manifestations of hypertensive crisis (headache, nausea, vomiting, and increased blood pressure).
- Monitor for uterine tone and vaginal bleeding.
- Provide emergency interventions.

Ⓝ NCLEX® Connection: Pharmacological and Parenteral Therapies, Medication Administration

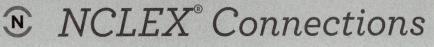
When reviewing the following chapters, keep in mind the relevant topics and tasks of the NCLEX outline, in particular:

Client Needs: Pharmacological and Parenteral Therapies

ADVERSE EFFECTS/CONTRAINDICATIONS/SIDE EFFECTS/ INTERACTIONS: Monitor for anticipated interactions among the client prescribed medications and fluids.

EXPECTED ACTIONS/OUTCOMES: Evaluate the client's use of medications over time.

MEDICATION ADMINISTRATION: Administer and document medications given by common routes.

UNIT 8   MEDICATIONS FOR JOINT AND
BONE CONDITIONS

CHAPTER 33 *Connective Tissue Disorders*

Rheumatoid arthritis (RA) is a chronic disorder with autoimmune and inflammatory components. Pharmacological management provides symptomatic relief and some delay in progression of the disorder without resulting in cure. Categories of medications in this section include disease-modifying antirheumatic medications (DMARDs), glucocorticoids, immunosuppressants, and nonsteroidal anti-inflammatory drugs (NSAIDs), which can be used individually or in combination to manage RA.

Gout (aka gouty arthritis) is a painful type of arthritis that is caused by elevated levels of uric acid, which can accumulate and cause localized inflammation in synovial areas. Antigout medications act either by reducing inflammation or decreasing serum uric acid levels. Categories of medications in this section include anti-inflammatory agents, NSAIDs, glucocorticoids, and agents for hyperuricemia.

Systemic lupus erythematous (SLE) is an autoimmune condition that can cause damage to joints, skin, blood vessels, and organs. Medications for treating lupus include anti-inflammatory medications, NSAIDs, corticosteroids, antimalarials, immunomodulators, and monoclonal antibodies. Topical cortisone can reduce inflammation of the typical skin rash of SLE.

Fibromyalgia is a syndrome characterized by muscle pain and fatigue. There are three FDA-approved medications for treating this syndrome: pregabalin, duloxetine, and milnacipran. Other medications used to treat fibromyalgia syndrome (but not FDA-approved for this use) include amitriptyline, cyclobenzaprine, tramadol, NSAIDs, and opioids. In addition, medications that facilitate sleep, such as zolpidem, and treat restless leg syndrome, such as gabapentin, are sometimes prescribed for manifestations of this condition.

Disease-modifying antirheumatic drugs

DMARDs I: Major nonbiologic DMARDs
- Immunomodulator medications: methotrexate, leflunomide
- Antimalarial agent: hydroxychloroquine
- Anti-inflammatory medication: sulfasalazine
- Tetracycline antibiotic: minocycline

DMARDs II: Major biologic DMARDs
- Tumor necrosis factor antagonists
  - Etanercept
  - Infliximab
  - Adalimumab
- B–lymphocyte-depleting agent: Rituximab
- Interleukin–1 receptor antagonist: Abatacept

DMARDs III: Minor nonbiologic and nonbiologic DMARDs
- Gold salts: Auranofin
- Penicillamine
- Immunosuppressant medications
  - Azathioprine
  - Cyclosporine

GLUCOCORTICOIDS
- Prednisone
- Prednisolone

NSAIDs
- Aspirin
- Ibuprofen
- Diclofenac
- Indomethacin
- Meloxicam
- Naproxen
- Celecoxib

PURPOSE

EXPECTED PHARMACOLOGICAL ACTION

- DMARDs slow joint degeneration and progression of rheumatoid arthritis.
- Glucocorticoids provide symptomatic relief of inflammation and pain.
- NSAIDs provide rapid, symptomatic relief of inflammation and pain.

THERAPEUTIC USES

- Analgesia for pain, swelling, and joint stiffness
- Maintenance of joint function
- Slow/delay the worsening of the disease (DMARDs, glucocorticoids)
- Short-term therapy (with NSAIDs, glucocorticoids) until long-acting DMARDs take effect
- Prevention of organ rejection in clients who have transplants such as kidney, liver, and heart transplants (glucocorticoids, immunosuppressants)
- Management of inflammatory bowel disease (glucocorticoids, immunosuppressants, DMARDs)

COMPLICATIONS

Cytotoxic agent/immunomodulator: methotrexate

Increased risk of infection
NURSING CONSIDERATIONS: Advise clients to notify the provider immediately for manifestations of infection, such as fever or sore throat.

Hepatic fibrosis and toxicity
NURSING CONSIDERATIONS
- Monitor liver function tests.
- Advise clients to observe for anorexia, abdominal fullness, and jaundice, and to notify the provider if symptoms occur.

Bone marrow suppression
NURSING CONSIDERATIONS: Obtain baseline CBC, including platelet counts. Repeat every 3 to 6 months.

Ulcerative stomatitis/other GI ulcerations
- Early finding with toxicity
- NURSING CONSIDERATIONS
  ○ Inspect mouth, gums, and throat daily for ulcerations, bleeding, or color changes.
  ○ Advise clients to take the medication with food or 8 oz of water.
  ○ Stop the medication if symptoms occur.

Fetal death/congenital abnormalities
NURSING CONSIDERATIONS
- Avoid use during pregnancy.
- Advise clients to use adequate contraception if taking this medication.

Gold salts: auranofin

Toxicity (severe pruritus, rashes, stomatitis)
NURSING CONSIDERATIONS: Notify the provider if these manifestations occur.

Renal toxicity, such as proteinuria
NURSING CONSIDERATIONS: Monitor I&O, BUN, creatinine, and UA.

Blood dyscrasias
- Thrombocytopenia, leukopenia, agranulocytosis, aplastic anemia
- NURSING CONSIDERATIONS
  ○ Monitor CBC, WBC, and platelet counts periodically.
  ○ Advise clients to observe for bruising and gum bleeding, and to notify the provider if these occur.

Hepatitis
NURSING CONSIDERATIONS: Monitor liver function tests.

GI discomfort (nausea, vomiting, abdominal pain)
NURSING CONSIDERATIONS: Observe for manifestations, and notify the provider if they occur.

Sulfasalazine

GI discomfort
- Nausea, vomiting, diarrhea, abdominal pain
- NURSING CONSIDERATIONS: Use an enteric-coated preparation, and divide dosage daily.

Hepatic dysfunction
NURSING CONSIDERATIONS: Monitor liver function tests.

Bone marrow suppression
NURSING CONSIDERATIONS: Monitor CBC, including platelet counts.

Antimalarial agent: hydroxychloroquine

Retinal damage (blindness)
NURSING CONSIDERATIONS
- Advise clients to have baseline eye examination and follow-up eye exams every 6 months with an ophthalmologist.
- Stop the medication and notify the provider if blurred vision occurs.

Tumor necrosis factor antagonists: etanercept, infliximab

Subcutaneous injection-site irritation
- Redness, swelling, pain, itching
- NURSING CONSIDERATIONS: Monitor the injection site, and stop the medication if signs of irritation occur.

IV infusion reactions (infliximab)
- Flu-like findings, hypotension, possible anaphylaxis
- NURSING CONSIDERATIONS
  ○ Stop infusion and notify provider immediately for severe reaction.
  ○ Continue to monitor for reaction 2 hr after IV infusion.

Risk of infection

- Especially TB and reactivation of hepatitis B
- NURSING CONSIDERATIONS
  - Instruct clients to monitor for infection (fever, sore throat, inflammation) and notify the provider if symptoms occur. Medication should be discontinued.
  - Test for hepatitis B and TB.

Severe skin reactions

- Including Stevens-Johnson syndrome
- NURSING CONSIDERATIONS: Instruct clients to monitor for adverse skin reactions and notify the provider if symptoms occur. Medication should be discontinued.

Heart failure

NURSING CONSIDERATIONS: Monitor for development or worsening of heart failure (distended neck veins, crackles in lungs, dyspnea). Medication should be discontinued.

Blood dyscrasias

NURSING CONSIDERATIONS: Monitor for signs of bleeding, bruising, or fever. Medication should be discontinued.

Penicillamine

Bone marrow suppression

NURSING CONSIDERATIONS: Obtain baseline CBC including platelet counts, and repeat every 3 to 6 months.

Toxicity (severe pruritus, rashes)

NURSING CONSIDERATIONS

- Stop the medication.
- Notify the provider if symptoms occur.

Cyclosporine

Risk of infection

- Flu-like symptoms, painful urination
- NURSING CONSIDERATIONS: Advise clients to notify the provider immediately if symptoms occur.

Hepatotoxicity (jaundice)

NURSING CONSIDERATIONS: Monitor liver function, and adjust dosage.

Nephrotoxicity

NURSING CONSIDERATIONS

- Monitor BUN and creatinine throughout treatment.
- Monitor I&O.

Hirsutism

NURSING CONSIDERATIONS: This effect is reversible with discontinuation of the medication.

Gingival hyperplasia

NURSING CONSIDERATIONS: Advise clients on importance of good dental hygiene and regular dental check-ups.

Glucocorticoids: prednisone

Risk of infection (fever and/or sore throat)

CLIENT EDUCATION: Advise clients to notify the provider immediately if symptoms occur.

Osteoporosis

CLIENT EDUCATION: Advise clients to take calcium supplements, vitamin D, and/or bisphosphonate (etidronate).

Adrenal suppression

- Nausea, vomiting, hypotension, and confusion can occur if glucocorticoids are stopped abruptly.
- NURSING CONSIDERATIONS
  - Advise clients to observe for manifestations, and to notify the provider if manifestations occur.
  - Administer IV fluids, such as 0.9% sodium chloride and hydrocortisone. Advise clients not to discontinue the medication suddenly.
  - Increase in glucocorticoid dosage can be needed during times of stress (e.g., surgery, acute illness).

Fluid retention

NURSING CONSIDERATIONS: Monitor for signs of fluid excess, such as crackles, weight gain, and edema.

GI discomfort/gastric ulceration

NURSING CONSIDERATIONS

- Advise clients to observe for symptoms and to notify the provider if symptoms occur.
- H_2-receptor antagonists can be used prophylactically.
- Advise clients to report symptoms of GI bleeding (coffee-ground emesis or black, tarry stools).

Hyperglycemia

NURSING CONSIDERATIONS: Monitor blood glucose level. Clients who have diabetes mellitus might need to adjust hypoglycemic agent.

Hypokalemia

NURSING CONSIDERATIONS

- Monitor serum potassium levels.
- Advise clients to eat potassium-rich foods.
- Administer potassium supplements.

CONTRAINDICATIONS/PRECAUTIONS

Methotrexate

- This medication is Pregnancy Risk Category X. **Qs**
- Methotrexate is contraindicated in clients who have liver failure, alcohol use disorder, or blood dyscrasias.
- Use with caution in clients who have liver or kidney dysfunction, cancer and suppressed bone marrow function, peptic ulcer disease, ulcerative colitis, impaired nutritional status, or infections.
- Use cautiously with children, or women who are breastfeeding.

Etanercept is contraindicated in clients who have malignancies, active infection, hematologic disorder, or during lactation. Use caution in clients who have heart failure, CNS demyelinating disorders such as multiple sclerosis, or blood dyscrasias.

Cyclosporine is contraindicated in pregnancy, recent vaccination with live virus vaccines, and recent contact with or active infection of chickenpox or herpes zoster.

Glucocorticoids

- Glucocorticoids are contraindicated in systemic fungal infections and live virus vaccines.
- Warn clients against abrupt discontinuation of glucocorticoids. Dosage of glucocorticoids is always adjusted and withdrawn gradually.

INTERACTIONS

Methotrexate

- Salicylates, other NSAIDs, sulfonamides, penicillin, and tetracyclines can cause methotrexate toxicity. Monitor for toxic effects.
- Folic acid changes the body's response to methotrexate, decreasing its effect. Avoid folic acid supplements or vitamins containing folic acid (even though folic acid can reduce GI toxicity).

Etanercept

- Concurrent use of etanercept with a live vaccine increases the risk of getting or transmitting infection. Avoid live vaccines.
- Concurrent use with immunosuppressants increases the client's chance of serious infection. Use precautions against illness if taking immunosuppressants.

Cyclosporine

- Concurrent use of phenytoin, phenobarbital, rifampin, carbamazepine, and trimethoprim-sulfamethoxazole decreases cyclosporine level, which can lead to organ rejection. Monitor cyclosporine levels, and adjust dosage accordingly.
- Concurrent use of ketoconazole, erythromycin, and amphotericin B can increase cyclosporine level, leading to toxicity. Monitor cyclosporine dosage, and adjust accordingly to prevent toxicity.
- Amphotericin B, aminoglycoside, and NSAIDs are nephrotoxic. Concurrent use with cyclosporine increases the risk for kidney dysfunction. Monitor BUN, creatinine, and I&O.
- Consumption of grapefruit juice increases cyclosporine levels by 50%, which poses an increased risk of toxicity. Advise clients to avoid drinking grapefruit juice.

Glucocorticoids

- Diuretics that promote potassium loss increase the risk of hypokalemia. Monitor potassium level, and administer supplements as needed.
- Because of the risk for hypokalemia, concurrent use of glucocorticoids with digoxin increases the risk of digoxin-induced dysrhythmias. Monitor for digoxin-induced dysrhythmias. Monitor potassium levels.
- NSAIDs increase the risk of GI ulceration. Advise clients to avoid use of NSAIDs. If GI distress occurs, instruct clients to notify the provider.
- Glucocorticoids promote hyperglycemia, thereby counteracting the effects of insulin and oral hypoglycemics. The dose of hypoglycemic medications might need to be increased.

NURSING ADMINISTRATION

- Advise clients that effects of DMARDs are delayed and can take 3 to 6 weeks, with full therapeutic effect taking several months. Qᴘᴄᴄ
- Administer adalimumab subcutaneously every 2 weeks.
- Administer etanercept by subcutaneous injection once per week. Ensure solution is clear without particles present.
- Glucocorticoids can be used as oral agents or as intra-articular injections. Short-term therapy can be used to control exacerbations of symptoms and also can be used while waiting for the effects of DMARDs to develop.

Cyclosporine

- Administer the initial IV dose of cyclosporine over 2 to 6 hr.
- Monitor for hypersensitivity reactions. Stay with clients for 30 min after administration of cyclosporine.
- Mix oral cyclosporine with milk or orange juice right before ingestion to increase palatability.
- Instruct clients regarding the importance of lifelong therapy if used to prevent organ rejection.

NURSING EVALUATION OF MEDICATION EFFECTIVENESS

Depending on the therapeutic intent, effectiveness can be evidenced by the following.
- Improvement of symptoms of rheumatoid arthritis (reduced swelling of joints, absence of joint stiffness, ability to maintain joint function, absence of pain)
- Decrease in systemic complications, such as weight loss and fatigue

Antigout medication

ANTI-INFLAMMATORY AGENTS

SELECT PROTOTYPE MEDICATION: Colchicine
Once considered drug of choice for acute gout, colchicine is now usually reserved for clients who do not respond to or cannot tolerate safer agents.

OTHER MEDICATIONS
- NSAIDs
  - Indomethacin
  - Naproxen
  - Diclofenac
- Glucocorticoids: Prednisone

PURPOSE

EXPECTED PHARMACOLOGICAL ACTION
- Colchicine is only effective for inflammation caused by gout.
- These medications decrease inflammation.

THERAPEUTIC USES
- Abort an acute gout attack in response to precursor symptoms.
- Treatment of acute attacks.
- Decrease incidence of acute attacks for clients who have chronic gout.
- Prednisone is used for clients who have acute gout who are unable to take or unresponsive to NSAIDs. This medication is not for clients who have hyperglycemia.

ROUTE OF ADMINISTRATION: **Colchicine:** Oral

AGENTS FOR HYPERURICEMIA

For clients who have chronic gout or frequent gout attacks

SELECT PROTOTYPE MEDICATION: Allopurinol

OTHER MEDICATIONS: Febuxostat, probenecid

PURPOSE

EXPECTED PHARMACOLOGICAL ACTION: Allopurinol and febuxostat inhibit uric acid production. Probenecid inhibits uric acid reabsorption by renal tubules

THERAPEUTIC USES: Hyperuricemia due to chronic gout or secondary to cancer chemotherapy.

ROUTE OF ADMINISTRATION
- Allopurinol (oral, IV)
- Colchicine (oral)

COMPLICATIONS

Colchicine

Mild GI distress, which can progress to GI toxicity
- Abdominal pain, diarrhea, nausea, vomiting
- NURSING CONSIDERATIONS
  - Take oral medications with food.
  - Provide antidiarrheal agents as prescribed.
  - If severe GI distress occurs, stop colchicine and notify provider.

Thrombocytopenia, suppressed bone marrow
NURSING CONSIDERATIONS: Advise clients to notify the provider of bleeding, bruising or sore throat.

Sudden onset of muscle pain, tenderness
- Rhabdomyolysis
- CLIENT EDUCATION: Advise clients to notify provider for new onset of these findings.

Probenecid

Renal calculi and renal injury
- Occur with higher excretion of uric acid
- NURSING CONSIDERATIONS: Advise client to drink 2.5 to 3 L fluid daily to decrease risk.

Gastrointestinal effects
NURSING CONSIDERATIONS: Take medication with food to decrease GI effects.

Hypersensitivity reactions (e.g., rash)
NURSING CONSIDERATIONS: Advise clients to report any rash to provider.

Allopurinol

Hypersensitivity reaction, fever, rash, and kidney and liver damage
NURSING CONSIDERATIONS: If administering IV, stop infusion. Severe reaction can require hemodialysis or glucocorticoids.

Kidney injury
NURSING CONSIDERATIONS: Alkalinize the urine and encourage intake of 2 to 3 L of fluids/day. Monitor I&O, BUN, and creatinine.

Hepatitis
NURSING CONSIDERATIONS: Monitor liver enzymes.

GI distress (nausea and vomiting)
NURSING CONSIDERATIONS: Administer with food.

Increase in gout attacks
- During the first months of treatment
- NURSING CONSIDERATIONS: Instruct client to report increased gout attacks to provider. Colchicine or an NSAID can be prescribed along with allopurinol to prevent this.

CONTRAINDICATIONS/PRECAUTIONS

Colchicine

- Pregnancy Risk Category C
- Contraindicated for clients who have severe renal, cardiac, hepatic, or gastrointestinal dysfunction.
- Use cautiously in older adults and clients who are debilitated or have blood disorders or mild to moderate hepatic dysfunction. ©

Probenecid

- Pregnancy Risk Category C
- Can precipitate acute gout. Do not give within 2 to 3 weeks of an acute attack.

Allopurinol

- Pregnancy Risk Category C
- This medication is contraindicated in clients who have medication hypersensitivity or idiopathic hemochromatosis.
- Rhabdomyolysis is most likely with long-term use. Risk is higher in clients taking statins for high cholesterol and those who have impaired kidneys or liver.

INTERACTIONS

Colchicine

Grapefruit or grapefruit juice can increase adverse effects. Advise clients to avoid eating grapefruit or drinking grapefruit juice when taking colchicine.

Probenecid

- Salicylates can lessen the effectiveness of probenecid and can precipitate gout. Advise clients not to use salicylates during colchicine/probenecid therapy.
- Salicylates, such as aspirin, interfere with probenecid's therapeutic effect. Avoid concurrent use of salicylates with probenecid.

Allopurinol

Allopurinol slows the metabolism of warfarin within the liver, which places clients at risk for bleeding.
- Instruct clients to observe for signs of bleeding (bruising, petechiae, hematuria).
- Monitor prothrombin time and INR levels, and adjust warfarin dosages accordingly.

NURSING ADMINISTRATION

- When clients are taking medications for gout, monitor uric acid levels, CBC, urinalysis, and liver and kidney function tests.
- Allopurinol IV should be well diluted and administered as an infusion over 30 to 60 min.
- Advise clients to take oral gout medication with food or after meals to minimize GI distress.
- **Allopurinol and probenecid:** If a rash develops, advise clients to stop the medication and report the occurrence to the provider.
- Instruct clients to concurrently take preventive measures, such as avoiding alcohol and foods high in purine (red meat, scallops). Assist clients in determining what foods precipitate their gout attacks and in avoiding these foods. Clients should ensure an adequate intake of water, exercise regularly, and maintain an appropriate body weight. Qᴘᴄᴄ

NURSING EVALUATION OF MEDICATION EFFECTIVENESS

Depending on the therapeutic intent, effectiveness can be evidenced by the following.
- Improvement of pain caused by a gout attack (decrease in joint swelling, redness, uric acid levels)
- Decrease in number of gout attacks
- Decrease in uric acid levels

Medication for systemic lupus erythematosus

MONOCLONAL ANTIBODY MEDICATION: Belimumab

PURPOSE

EXPECTED PHARMACOLOGICAL ACTION: Disrupts activation of B-lymphocytes through interference with BLyS, a protein needed for B-cell activation

THERAPEUTIC USES: SLE

COMPLICATIONS

GI effects (nausea, vomiting, diarrhea)

NURSING CONSIDERATIONS: Advise client on natural GI remedies (e.g., ginger tea or hard candy). If severe GI distress occurs, notify provider.

Headache, depressed mood

NURSING CONSIDERATIONS: If suicidal thoughts are present, notify the provider.

Insomnia

NURSING CONSIDERATIONS: Advise clients on strategies to promote adequate sleep. (Make sure bedroom is quiet, dark, and relaxing. Avoid large meals before bedtime.)

Infusion reaction

- Erythema, edema, pruritus around IV site.
- Anaphylaxis can occur.

NURSING CONSIDERATIONS

- Infuse slowly over an hour. If anaphylaxis occurs, discontinue infusion and begin emergency treatment.
- Premedication might be prescribed to minimize hypersensitivity reactions.

Increased risk of infection

NURSING CONSIDERATIONS: Advise client to avoid being around sick people, not receive live virus vaccines within 30 days of medication, and notify provider if fever, painful urination, or bloody diarrhea is present.

CONTRAINDICATIONS/PRECAUTIONS

- Pregnancy Risk Category C. Avoid breastfeeding.
- Not for clients who have severe renal impairment or SLE affecting CNS.
- Use caution in older adult clients, and clients who have depression, cardiac disorders, or infections. Ⓖ

INTERACTIONS

Cyclophosphamide or immune suppressants increase risk for infection.
CLIENT EDUCATION: Advise clients to avoid being around sick people, no live virus vaccines within 30 days of medication, and notify provider if fever, painful urination, or bloody diarrhea is present.

NURSING ADMINISTRATION

- Reconstitute with sterile water, and dilute only with 0.9% saline solution. Ⓠ**EBP**
- Refrigerate solution no longer than 8 hr after reconstitution. Allow solution to stand at room temperature for 10 to 15 min before using.
- Administered by IV infusion, and given slowly, over about 1 hr. Monitor closely for infusion reactions and hypersensitivity.
- Discard unused solution.
- No administration of live virus vaccines within 30 days.

NURSING EVALUATION OF MEDICATION EFFECTIVENESS

Decrease in manifestations of SLE

Medications for fibromyalgia

SEROTONIN-NOREPINEPHRINE REUPTAKE INHIBITORS
- Duloxetine
- Milnacipran

GAMMA-AMINOBUTYRIC ACID ANALOGUE (GABA):
Pregabalin

PURPOSE

Serotonin-norepinephrine reuptake inhibitors

EXPECTED PHARMACOLOGICAL ACTION: Restores balance of neurotransmitters, serotonin and norepinephrine

THERAPEUTIC USES
- Fibromyalgia (duloxetine and milnacipran)
- Depression (duloxetine)
- Diabetic peripheral neuropathy (duloxetine)

GABA

EXPECTED PHARMACOLOGICAL ACTION: It is thought that pregabalin binds to alpha-2-delta in CNS tissue.

THERAPEUTIC USES: Fibromyalgia, seizures, neuropathic pain

COMPLICATIONS

Serotonin-norepinephrine reuptake inhibitors

Drowsiness, dizziness, blurred vision
CLIENT EDUCATION
- Instruct clients to not drive or operate heavy machinery while taking this medication.
- Advise clients to change positions slowly.
- Employ fall prevention strategies (e.g., sensible shoes, removing home hazards).

Nausea, anorexia, weight loss
NURSING CONSIDERATIONS: Monitor weight and food intake.

Headache, insomnia, anxiety
NURSING CONSIDERATIONS: Monitor for these findings.

Hypertension, tachycardia
NURSING CONSIDERATIONS: Monitor vital signs, and report changes.

Withdrawal syndrome
- Results in headache, nausea, visual disturbances, anxiety, dizziness, and tremors
- NURSING CONSIDERATIONS: Instruct clients to withdraw from medication gradually.

Sexual dysfunction
- No orgasm, decreased libido, impotence, menstrual changes
- NURSING CONSIDERATIONS: Instruct clients to report sexual dysfunction to the provider.

GABA

Drowsiness, fatigue, dizziness, blurred vision, lightheadedness
CLIENT EDUCATION: Teach the client to not drive or operate heavy machinery while taking this medication; change positions slowly; and employ fall prevention strategies (e.g., sensible shoes, removing home hazards).

Increased appetite, weight gain, constipation, abdominal pain
CLIENT EDUCATION
- Teach clients about ways to prevent weight gain, such as eating a balanced diet, eliminating high-fat, high-sugar foods from the diet.
- Develop an exercise plan.

Hypersensitivity reactions (angioedema)
CLIENT EDUCATION: Instruct clients to stop taking the medication and notify the provider or call 911 immediately for rash, hives, dyspnea, or swelling of the face or tongue.

Rhabdomyolysis
- Acute onset of severe muscle weakness and tenderness with elevation of serum creatinine kinase
- CLIENT EDUCATION: Instruct the client to notify the provider for manifestations. Medication will need to be discontinued if rhabdomyolysis occurs.

Erectile dysfunction and anorgasmia
CLIENT EDUCATION: Instruct clients to report manifestations of sexual dysfunction

CONTRAINDICATIONS/PRECAUTIONS

Serotonin-norepinephrine reuptake inhibitors

- Pregnancy Risk Category C
- Contraindicated in clients who have hepatic or renal impairment or those taking MAOI within 14 days
- Caution in clients who have cardiac problems, hypertension, diabetes, gastrointestinal disorders, and glaucoma

GABA

- Pregnancy Risk Category C
- Dose might need to be adjusted in older adult clients and clients who have renal impairment. Ⓒ
- Use with caution in clients who have cardiac problems, hypertension, diabetes, renal impairment, mental illness, angioedema, and thrombocytopenia.

INTERACTIONS

Serotonin-norepinephrine reuptake inhibitors

Antidepressants
NURSING CONSIDERATIONS
- SSRIs increase risk for serotonin syndrome.
- Notify provider if suicidal thoughts are present.

Anticoagulants, warfarin, and NSAIDs, which increase risk of bleeding (e.g., GI bleed)
NURSING CONSIDERATIONS: Notify provider for signs of internal bleeding (e.g., blood in stools).

Diuretics increase risk of low serum sodium levels.
NURSING CONSIDERATIONS: Monitor serum sodium levels.

GABA

- **ACE inhibitors** increase risk of angioedema. Advise cool compresses and notify provider.
- **Benzodiazepines** increase drowsiness. Do not drive or operate heavy machinery.
- **Thiazolidinedione** (antidiabetic agent) increases risk of weight gain and peripheral edema. Advise healthy, well balanced diet and regular activity to help counteract weight gain and elevating extremities for peripheral edema.
- **Alcohol** increases drowsiness and dizziness. Advise clients not to consume alcohol while taking this medication.

NURSING ADMINISTRATION

Serotonin-norepinephrine reuptake inhibitors

- Administered orally without regard to food.
- Swallow capsule whole.
- Taper withdrawal gradually over 2 weeks.

GABA

- Administered orally with or without food.
- Notify provider if suicidal thoughts are present. Qs
- Taper withdrawal gradually over at least 1 week.

NURSING EVALUATION OF MEDICATION EFFECTIVENESS

Decrease in manifestations of fibromyalgia

Application Exercises

1. A nurse is providing teaching for a client who has gout and a new prescription for allopurinol. For which of the following adverse effects should the client be taught to monitor? (Select all that apply.)

   A. Stomatitis

   B. Insomnia

   C. Nausea

   D. Rash

   E. Increased gout pain

2. A nurse is caring for a client who has a new prescription for adalimumab for rheumatoid arthritis. Based on the route of administration of adalimumab, which of the following should the nurse plan to monitor?

   A. The vein for thrombophlebitis during IV administration

   B. The subcutaneous site for redness following injection

   C. The oral mucosa for ulceration after oral administration

   D. The skin for irritation following removal of transdermal patch

3. A nurse is preparing to administer belimumab for a client who has systemic lupus erythematosus. Which of the following actions should the nurse plan to take?

   A. Warm the medication to room temperature over 1 hr before administering.

   B. Administer the medication by IV bolus over 5 min.

   C. Dilute the medication in 5% dextrose and water solution.

   D. Monitor the client for hypersensitivity reactions.

4. A nurse is caring for a client who has a new diagnosis of fibromyalgia. Which of the following medications should the nurse anticipate being prescribed for this client?

   A. Colchicine

   B. Hydroxychloroquine

   C. Auranofin

   D. Duloxetine

5. A nurse is evaluating teaching for a client who has rheumatoid arthritis and a new prescription for methotrexate. Which of the following statements by the client indicates understanding of the teaching?

   A. "I will be sure to return to the clinic at least once a year to have my blood drawn while I'm taking methotrexate."

   B. "I will take this medication on an empty stomach."

   C. "I'll let the doctor know if I develop sores in my mouth while taking this medication."

   D. "I should stop taking oral contraceptives while I'm taking methotrexate."

PRACTICE Active Learning Scenario

A nurse is teaching a client who has rheumatoid arthritis (RA) about his new prescription for etanercept. What should the nurse teach the client about this medication? Use the ATI Active Learning Template: Medication to complete this item.

THERAPEUTIC USES: Describe the therapeutic use for etanercept in this client.

COMPLICATIONS: Describe at least three adverse effects the client should monitor for.

NURSING INTERVENTIONS: Describe one for each of the adverse effects above.

MEDICATION ADMINISTRATION: Describe at least three important factors.

Application Exercises Key

1. A. Stomatitis occurs with medications that increase the risk of infection, such as many of the DMARDs used to treat rheumatoid arthritis. Allopurinol does not increase a client's risk for infection.

    B. Insomnia is not an adverse effect caused by allopurinol.

    C. **CORRECT:** Nausea and vomiting are adverse effects that can be caused by allopurinol.

    D. **CORRECT:** Rash and other hypersensitivity reactions can be caused by allopurinol. The client should be taught to contact the provider for any manifestation of hypersensitivity so that the medication can be discontinued.

    E. **CORRECT:** An increase in gout attacks can occur during the first few months in a client who is taking allopurinol.

    Ⓝ *NCLEX® Connection: Pharmacological and Parenteral Therapies, Adverse Effects/Contraindications/Side Effects/Interactions*

2. A. Adalimumab is not administered IV. Assessing for thrombophlebitis during administration is not necessary.

    B. **CORRECT:** Adalimumab is administered subcutaneously, and injection-site redness and swelling are common. It is appropriate for the nurse to assess the site for redness following injection.

    C. Adalimumab is not administered orally. Assessing oral mucosa for ulceration following administration is not necessary.

    D. Adalimumab is not administered transdermally. Inspecting the skin for irritation is not necessary.

    Ⓝ *NCLEX® Connection: Pharmacological and Parenteral Therapies, Medication Administration*

3. A. The solution of belimumab should be carefully refrigerated and allowed to sit at room temperature for only 10 to 15 min after being taken from the refrigerator.

    B. Belimumab is administered by intermittent IV infusion over 1 hr.

    C. Belimumab should be diluted only in 0.9% saline solution.

    D. **CORRECT:** Belimumab can cause severe infusion reactions and can cause anaphylaxis. The nurse should carefully monitor the client during infusion of this medication and be prepared to slow or stop the medication if a reaction occurs.

    Ⓝ *NCLEX® Connection: Pharmacological and Parenteral Therapies, Adverse Effects/Contraindications/Side Effects/Interactions*

4. A. Colchicine is an anti-inflammatory medication used to treat gout.

    B. Hydroxychloroquine is an anti-malarial medication used as a DMARD along with methotrexate to treat rheumatoid arthritis.

    C. Auranofin is a gold salt used to relief joint pain and stiffness in clients who have rheumatoid arthritis.

    D. **CORRECT:** Duloxetine is a serotonin-norepinephrine reuptake inhibitor used to treat fibromyalgia. Other uses for this medication include treating depression and diabetic peripheral neuropathy.

    Ⓝ *NCLEX® Connection: Pharmacological and Parenteral Therapies, Medication Administration*

5. A. CBC including platelet count, and liver and kidney function tests will be monitored at baseline and frequently during treatment with methotrexate to check for adverse effects.

    B. Methotrexate should be taken with food to decrease gastrointestinal distress.

    C. **CORRECT:** Ulcerations in the mouth, tongue, or throat are often the first signs of methotrexate toxicity and should be reported to the provider immediately.

    D. Methotrexate is a Pregnancy Category X medication and can cause severe fetal damage. The client should have a pregnancy test before starting the medication and should use a reliable form of birth control during methotrexate therapy. Oral contraceptives are not contraindicated with methotrexate therapy.

    Ⓝ *NCLEX® Connection: Pharmacological and Parenteral Therapies, Medication Administration*

PRACTICE Answer

Using the ATI Active Learning Template: Medication

THERAPEUTIC USES: Etanercept is a biologic DMARD classified as a tumor necrosis factor antagonist. It suppresses manifestations of moderate to severe RA and slows the progression of the disorder.

COMPLICATIONS

- Severe infections, including tuberculosis or reactivation of hepatitis B
- Heart failure
- Severe skin reactions, such as Stevens-Johnson syndrome
- Hematologic disorders

NURSING INTERVENTIONS

- Instruct clients to monitor for infection, and to report sore throat and other manifestations.
- Discuss reasons for TB testing and possible hepatitis B testing.
- Clients should notify the provider for edema, shortness of breath, and other signs of heart failure.
- Report skin rash to provider.
- Report easy bruising, bleeding, or unusual fatigue to provider.

MEDICATION ADMINISTRATION

- Teach clients to administer by subcutaneous injection twice weekly.
- Discard solutions that are discolored or that contain particulate matter.
- Monitor for injection-site reactions, and report them to provider.
- Rotate injection sites.
- Avoid skin areas that are bruised or reddened when injecting.

Ⓝ *NCLEX® Connection: Pharmacological and Parenteral Therapies, Medication Administration*

UNIT 8 MEDICATIONS FOR JOINT AND
BONE CONDITIONS

CHAPTER 34 *Bone Disorders*

Calcium is necessary for the proper functioning of the heart, bones, nerves, muscles, and blood coagulation. It can be given as a supplement when dietary intake is insufficient. Other medications are also used for prevention and treatment of osteoporosis and prevention of fractures.

Medication classifications include calcium supplements, selective estrogen receptor modulators (also known as estrogen agonist/antagonists), bisphosphonates, and calcitonin.

Calcium supplements

SELECT PROTOTYPE MEDICATION: Calcium citrate

OTHER MEDICATIONS
- Calcium carbonate
- Calcium acetate
- **For IV administration**
  - Calcium chloride
  - Calcium gluconate

PURPOSE

EXPECTED PHARMACOLOGICAL ACTION

Maintenance of musculoskeletal, neurological, and cardiovascular function

THERAPEUTIC USES

- Oral calcium supplements are used for clients who have hypocalcemia or deficiencies of parathyroid hormone, vitamin D, or dietary calcium.
- Oral dietary supplements are used for adolescents, older adults, and women who are postmenopausal, pregnant, or breastfeeding. Ⓖ
- IV medications are used for clients who have critically low levels of calcium.

COMPLICATIONS

Hypercalcemia

Calcium level greater than 10.5 mg/dL

FINDINGS: Initially, tachycardia and elevated blood pressure eventually leading to bradycardia and hypotension. Other findings include muscle weakness, hypotonia, constipation, nausea, vomiting, abdominal pain, lethargy, and confusion.

NURSING CONSIDERATIONS
- Instruct clients to monitor for manifestations and report them to the provider.
- Monitor serum calcium levels to maintain between 9 and 10.5 mg/dL.
- Infuse 0.9% sodium chloride IV.
- Medications used to reverse hypercalcemia include IV furosemide, and calcium chelators (plicamycin).
- Medications used to prevent hypercalcemia include bisphosphonates, such as alendronate and oral inorganic phosphates.

CONTRAINDICATIONS/PRECAUTIONS

- Calcium supplements are contraindicated in clients who have hypercalcemia, renal calculi, hypophosphatemia, digoxin toxicity, and ventricular fibrillation. ⒬s
- Use cautiously in clients who have kidney disease or a decrease in GI function.

INTERACTIONS

Concurrent use of glucocorticoids reduces absorption of calcium.
NURSING CONSIDERATIONS: Give at least 1 hr apart.

Concurrent use of calcium decreases absorption of tetracyclines and thyroid hormone.
NURSING CONSIDERATIONS: Ensure 1 hr between administration of medications.

Concurrent administration of thiazide diuretics increases risk of hypercalcemia.
NURSING CONSIDERATIONS
- Assess for hypercalcemia.
- Avoid concurrent use.

Spinach, rhubarb, beets, bran, and whole grains can decrease calcium absorption.
NURSING CONSIDERATIONS
- Do not administer calcium with foods that decrease absorption.
- Instruct clients to avoid consuming these foods at the same time as taking calcium.

IV calcium precipitates with phosphates, carbonates, sulfates, and tartrates.
NURSING CONSIDERATIONS: Do not mix parenteral calcium with compounds that cause precipitation.

Concurrent use of digoxin and parenteral calcium can lead to severe bradycardia.
NURSING CONSIDERATIONS: IV injection of calcium must be given slowly with careful monitoring of client cardiac status. ⒬s

NURSING ADMINISTRATION

- Instruct clients to take a calcium supplement at least 1 hr apart from glucocorticoids, tetracyclines, or thyroid hormone.
- Chewable tablets provide more consistent bioavailability.
- Recommended doses of oral calcium vary widely depending on the specific calcium preparation. Instruct the client to follow the prescription.
- Advise clients to take oral calcium with an 8 oz glass of water.
- Prior to administration, warm IV infusions of calcium to body temperature.
- Administer IV injections at 0.5 to 2 mL/min.

NURSING EVALUATION OF MEDICATION EFFECTIVENESS

Depending on therapeutic intent, effectiveness is evidenced by serum calcium level within expected reference range: 9.0 to 10.5 mg/dL.

Selective estrogen receptor modulator (agonist/antagonist)

SELECT PROTOTYPE MEDICATION: Raloxifene

PURPOSE

EXPECTED PHARMACOLOGICAL ACTION

- Works as endogenous estrogen in bone, lipid metabolism, and blood coagulation
- Decreases bone resorption, which slows bone loss and preserves bone mineral density
- Works as an antagonist to estrogen on breast and endometrial tissue
- Can decrease plasma levels of cholesterol

THERAPEUTIC USES

- Prevent and treat postmenopausal osteoporosis to prevent spinal fractures in female clients.
- Protect against breast cancer.

COMPLICATIONS

Increased risk for pulmonary embolism and deep-vein thrombosis (DVT)

NURSING CONSIDERATIONS
- Medication should be stopped prior to scheduled immobilization, such as surgery. Medication can be resumed when the client is fully mobile.
- Monitor for manifestations of DVT, such as red, swollen calf.
- Discourage long periods of sitting and inactivity.

Hot flashes

CLIENT EDUCATION: Inform clients that the medication can exacerbate hot flashes.

CONTRAINDICATIONS/PRECAUTIONS

- Raloxifene is Pregnancy Risk Category X.
- This medication is contraindicated in clients who have a history of venous thrombosis.
- The medication should be stopped 3 days before periods in which risk of DVT is high (such as before surgical procedures). Qs

INTERACTIONS

Concurrent use with estrogen hormone therapy is discouraged.

NURSING ADMINISTRATION

- For maximum benefit of the medication, encourage clients to consume adequate amounts of calcium (such as from dairy products) and vitamin D (such as from egg yolks). Inadequate amounts of dietary calcium and vitamin D cause release of parathyroid hormone, which stimulates calcium release from the bone.
- Take medication with or without food once per day.
- Monitor bone density. Clients should undergo a bone density scan every 12 to 18 months.
- Monitor serum calcium. Expected reference range is 9 to 10.5 mg/dL.
- Monitor liver function tests. Raloxifene levels can increase in clients who have hepatic impairment.
- Encourage clients to perform weight-bearing exercises daily, such as walking 30 to 40 min each day.

NURSING EVALUATION OF MEDICATION EFFECTIVENESS

Depending on therapeutic intent, effectiveness is evidenced by the following.
- Increase in bone density
- No fractures

Bisphosphonates

SELECT PROTOTYPE MEDICATION: Alendronate

OTHER MEDICATIONS
- Ibandronate
- Risedronate
- **For IV infusion:** Zoledronic

PURPOSE

EXPECTED PHARMACOLOGICAL ACTION

Bisphosphonates decrease the number and action of osteoclasts, and inhibit bone resorption.

THERAPEUTIC USES

- Prophylaxis and treatment of postmenopausal osteoporosis
- For male clients who have osteoporosis
- Prophylaxis and treatment of osteoporosis produced by long-term glucocorticoid use
- For clients who have Paget's disease of the bone

COMPLICATIONS

Esophagitis, esophageal ulceration (oral formulations)

NURSING CONSIDERATIONS
- Instruct the client to sit upright or ambulate for 30 min after taking this medication orally. ○EBP
- Clients taking ibendronate must remain upright and not ingest food or other medications for 1 hr after taking the medication orally.
- Instruct the client to take tablets with at least 240 mL (8 oz) water and liquid formulation with at least 60 mL (2 oz).
- Discontinue the medication and contact the provider for difficulty swallowing or new heartburn.

GI disturbances (all bisphosphonates)

Such as abdominal pain, nausea, diarrhea, constipation

NURSING CONSIDERATIONS: Notify provider for GI problems that prevent adequate intake.

Musculoskeletal pain

CLIENT EDUCATION
- Advise the client to take a mild analgesic.
- Instruct the client to notify the provider if pain persists. Alternate medication can be prescribed.

Visual disturbances

Such as blurred vision and eye pain

CLIENT EDUCATION: Instruct clients to watch for manifestations and report them to the provider. Medication should be discontinued.

Bisphosphonate-related osteonecrosis of the jaw

With IV infusion

NURSING CONSIDERATIONS: See dentist prior to beginning treatment. Avoid dental work during administration of medication.

Kidney toxicity with IV infusion

NURSING CONSIDERATIONS: Monitor kidney function and hydration status.

CONTRAINDICATIONS/PRECAUTIONS

- Most bisphosphonates are Pregnancy Risk Category C. Zoledronic acid is Pregnancy Risk Category D.
- These medications are contraindicated for clients who have dysphagia, esophageal stricture, esophageal disorders, serious kidney impairment, and hypocalcemia. This medication should not be administered to clients who cannot sit upright or stand for at least 30 min after medication administration.
- Use cautiously for women who are lactating, and in clients who have upper GI disorders, infection, and liver impairment.
- Older adults are at slight risk for femoral fractures, which can occur without trauma while taking bisphosphonates. ©

INTERACTIONS

Alendronate absorption decreases when taken with calcium, iron, magnesium supplements, antacids, orange juice, and caffeine.
NURSING CONSIDERATIONS
- Advise clients to take the medication on an empty stomach with at least 240 mL (8 oz) water.
- Wait 30 min after administration to take antacids or supplements.

NURSING ADMINISTRATION

- Tablets are prescribed once daily or once a week. The liquid form is prescribed once a week.
- Monitor bone density. Clients should have a bone density scan every 12 to 18 months.
- Monitor serum calcium. Expected reference range is 9 to 10.5 mg/dL.

- Take the medication first thing in the morning after getting out of bed.
- Take oral medication on an empty stomach, drinking at least 240 mL (8 oz) water with tablets and at least 60 mL (2 oz) water with liquid formulation.
- Sit or ambulate for 30 min after taking the medication.
- Avoid all calcium-containing foods and liquids or any medications within 30 min of taking alendronate.
- Avoid chewing or sucking on the tablet.
- Perform weight-bearing exercises daily, such as walking 30 to 40 min each day.
- Notify the provider of difficulty swallowing, painful swallowing, or new or worsening heartburn.
- If a dose is skipped, wait until the next day 30 min before eating breakfast to take the dose. Do not take two tablets on the same day.
- For maximum benefit of the medication, consume adequate amounts of calcium and vitamin D.

NURSING EVALUATION OF MEDICATION EFFECTIVENESS

Depending on therapeutic intent, effectiveness is evidenced by the following.
- Increase in bone density
- No fractures

Calcitonin

SELECT PROTOTYPE MEDICATION: Calcitonin-salmon

PURPOSE

EXPECTED PHARMACOLOGICAL ACTION

- Decreases bone resorption by inhibiting the activity of osteoclasts in osteoporosis
- Increases renal calcium excretion by inhibiting tubular resorption

THERAPEUTIC USES

Treats (but does not prevent) postmenopausal osteoporosis, moderate to severe Paget's disease, hypercalcemia caused by hyperparathyroidism, and cancer

COMPLICATIONS

Nausea

CLIENT EDUCATION: Advise clients that nausea is usually self-limiting.

Nasal dryness and irritation with intranasal route

NURSING CONSIDERATIONS
- Instruct clients to alternate nostrils daily.
- Inspect nasal mucosa periodically for ulceration.

CONTRAINDICATIONS/PRECAUTIONS

- This medication is Pregnancy Risk Category C.
- The medication is contraindicated in clients who have hypersensitivity to the medication or fish protein. Perform an allergy skin test prior to administration if the client is at risk.
- Use cautiously with children, women who are lactating, and clients who have kidney disease.
- Intranasal spray is only approved for treatment of postmenopausal osteoporosis.

INTERACTIONS

Concurrent use with lithium can decrease serum lithium levels.
NURSING CONSIDERATIONS: Monitor lithium levels closely.

NURSING ADMINISTRATION

- Calcitonin-salmon is most commonly given by nasal spray. It can also be given IM or subcutaneously. Rotate injection sites to prevent inflammation. Qᴘᴄᴄ
- Keep the container in an upright position.
- Teach clients to alternate nostrils daily.
- Check for Chvostek's or Trousseau's signs to monitor for hypocalcemia.
- Monitor bone density scans periodically.
- Encourage clients to consume a diet high in calcium and vitamin D.

NURSING EVALUATION OF MEDICATION EFFECTIVENESS

Depending on therapeutic intent, effectiveness is evidenced by the following.
- Increase in bone density
- Serum calcium level within the expected reference range of 9 to 10.5 mg/dL

Application Exercises

1. A nurse is providing teaching to a client who is taking raloxifene to prevent postmenopausal osteoporosis. The nurse should advise the client that which of the following are adverse effects of this medication? (Select all that apply.)

   A. Hot flashes

   B. Lump in breast

   C. Swelling or redness in calf

   D. Shortness of breath

   E. Difficulty swallowing

2. A nurse is teaching a client who has osteoporosis and a new prescription for alendronate. Which of the following instructions should the nurse provide? (Select all that apply.)

   A. Take medication in the morning before eating.

   B. Chew tablets to increase bioavailability.

   C. Drink an 8 oz glass of water with each tablet.

   D. Take medication with an antacid if heartburn occurs.

   E. Avoid lying down after taking this medication.

3. A nurse is caring for a client who has a new prescription for calcitonin-salmon for osteoporosis. Which of the following tests should the nurse tell the client to expect before beginning this medication?

   A. Skin test for allergy to the medication

   B. ECG to rule out cardiac dysrhythmias

   C. Mantoux test to rule out exposure to tuberculosis

   D. Liver function tests to assess risk for medication toxicity

4. A nurse is caring for a young adult client whose serum calcium is 8.8 mg/dL. Which of the following medications should the nurse anticipate administering to this client?

   A. Calcitonin-salmon

   B. Calcium carbonate

   C. Zoledronic acid

   D. Ibandronate

5. A nurse is providing instruction to a client who has a new prescription for calcitonin-salmon for postmenopausal osteoporosis. Which of the following instructions should the nurse include in the teaching?

   A. Swallow tablets on an empty stomach with plenty of water.

   B. Watch for skin rash and redness when applying calcitonin-salmon topically.

   C. Mix the liquid medication with juice and take it after meals.

   D. Alternate nostrils each time calcitonin-salmon is inhaled.

PRACTICE Active Learning Scenario

A nurse in a provider's office is teaching a client who is postmenopausal and at high risk for osteoporosis about her new prescription for alendronate. What should the nurse teach the client about this medication? Use the ATI Active Learning Template: Medication to complete this item.

THERAPEUTIC USES: Identify the therapeutic use for alendronate.

COMPLICATIONS: List two adverse effects of this medication.

NURSING INTERVENTIONS
- Describe two diagnostic tests to monitor.
- Describe two nursing actions.

Application Exercises Key

1. A. **CORRECT:** Raloxifene can cause hot flashes or increase existing hot flashes.

   B. Raloxifene does not cause breast lumps. It is used therapeutically to protect against breast and endometrial cancer.

   C. **CORRECT:** Raloxifene increases the risk for thrombophlebitis, which can cause swelling or redness in the calf.

   D. **CORRECT:** Raloxifene increases the risk for pulmonary embolism, which can cause shortness of breath.

   E. Difficulty swallowing due to esophagitis is an adverse effect of bisphosphonates, such as alendronate, but is not an adverse effect of taking raloxifene.

   Ⓝ *NCLEX® Connection: Pharmacological and Parenteral Therapies, Adverse Effects/Contraindications/Side Effects/Interactions*

2. A. **CORRECT:** Take alendronate first thing in the morning before eating to increase absorption.

   B. Chewing alendronate tablets can cause esophageal ulcers. Swallow the tablets whole.

   C. **CORRECT:** Clients should drink at least 240 mL (8 oz) water with alendronate tablets.

   D. Do not take alendronate within 2 hr of an antacid.

   E. **CORRECT:** Clients should sit upright or stand for at least 30 min after taking alendronate.

   Ⓝ *NCLEX® Connection: Pharmacological and Parenteral Therapies, Medication Administration*

3. A. **CORRECT:** Anaphylaxis can occur if the client is allergic to calcitonin-salmon. A skin test to determine allergy might be done before starting this medication. The nurse also should ask the client about previous allergies to fish.

   B. An ECG to rule out cardiac dysrhythmias is not necessary before beginning calcitonin-salmon. This medication does not affect heart rhythm.

   C. A Mantoux test to rule out exposure to tuberculosis is not necessary before beginning calcitonin-salmon. This medication does not affect resistance to TB.

   D. Liver function tests are not necessary before beginning calcitonin-salmon. This medication is metabolized in the kidneys and does not affect the liver.

   Ⓝ *NCLEX® Connection: Pharmacological and Parenteral Therapies, Expected Actions/Outcomes*

4. A. Calcitonin-salmon increases excretion of calcium and should not be given to a client who has a serum calcium of 8.8 mg/dL.

   B. **CORRECT:** The client's serum calcium level is below the expected reference range. Calcium carbonate is an oral form of calcium used to increase serum calcium to the expected reference range.

   C. Zoledronic acid is an IV bisphosphonate used to treat osteoporosis. This medication can decrease serum calcium levels by inhibiting bone resorption of calcium, and should not be given to a client who has a serum calcium of 8.8. mg/dL.

   D. Ibandronate is a bisphosphonate used to treat osteoporosis. This medication can decrease serum calcium levels by inhibiting bone reabsorption of calcium. It should not be given to a client who has a serum calcium of 8.8 mg/dL.

   Ⓝ *NCLEX® Connection: Pharmacological and Parenteral Therapies, Expected Actions/Outcomes*

5. A. Clients should drink at least 240 mL (8 oz) water with alendronate tablets and take it on an empty stomach to promote absorption and prevent esophagitis.

   B. Calcitonin-salmon is not supplied as a topical preparation.

   C. Clients should drink at least 60 mL (2 oz) water with alendronate liquid solution.

   D. **CORRECT:** Calcitonin-salmon can be administered IM or subcutaneously, but is commonly administered intranasally for postmenopausal osteoporosis. The client should alternate nostrils daily.

   Ⓝ *NCLEX® Connection: Pharmacological and Parenteral Therapies, Medication Administration*

PRACTICE Answer

Using the ATI Active Learning Template: Medication

THERAPEUTIC USES: In this client who is at high risk for osteoporosis, the purpose of alendronate is to prevent osteoporosis from occurring by decreasing resorption of bone. The medication also is used to treat existing osteoporosis and Paget's disease.

COMPLICATIONS: Alendronate can cause esophagitis and esophageal ulceration; other GI effects, such as nausea, diarrhea, and constipation; muscle pain; and visual disturbances. Rarely, it can cause atraumatic femoral fracture.

NURSING INTERVENTIONS

Diagnostic tests: Serum calcium, bone density scans

Nursing interventions

- Assess the client's ability to follow administration directions (must be able to sit upright or stand for at least 30 min after taking alendronate).
- Teach the client to take this medication first thing in the morning with at least 240 mL (8 oz) water and wait 30 min before eating or drinking anything else or taking any other medications or supplements.
- Teach the client other ways to help prevent osteoporosis, such as performing weight-bearing exercises daily and obtaining adequate amounts of calcium and vitamin D.

Ⓝ *NCLEX® Connection: Pharmacological and Parenteral Therapies, Medication Administration*

NCLEX® Connections

When reviewing the following chapters, keep in mind the relevant topics and tasks of the NCLEX outline, in particular:

Client Needs: Pharmacological and Parenteral Therapies

MEDICATION ADMINISTRATION: Evaluate appropriateness and accuracy of medication order for client.

PARENTERAL/INTRAVENOUS THERAPIES: Monitor the use of an infusion pump.

PHARMACOLOGICAL PAIN MANAGEMENT: Administer pharmacological measures for pain management.

CHAPTER 35
Nonopioid Analgesics

Nonopioid analgesics can have anti-inflammatory, antipyretic, and analgesic actions. These medications include nonsteroidal anti-inflammatory drugs (NSAIDs) and acetaminophen.

Nonsteroidal anti-inflammatory drugs

SELECT PROTOTYPE MEDICATIONS

First-generation NSAIDs (COX-1 and COX-2 inhibitors)
- Aspirin
- Ibuprofen
- Naproxen
- Indomethacin
- Diclofenac
- Ketorolac
- Meloxicam

Second-generation NSAIDs (selective COX-2 inhibitor): Celecoxib

PURPOSE

EXPECTED PHARMACOLOGICAL ACTION

Inhibition of cyclooxygenase: Inhibition of COX-1 can result in decreased platelet aggregation and kidney damage while inhibition of COX-2 results in decreased inflammation, fever, and pain and does not decrease platelet aggregation.

THERAPEUTIC USES

- Inflammation suppression
- Analgesia for mild to moderate pain, such as with osteoarthritis and rheumatoid arthritis
- Fever reduction
- Dysmenorrhea
- Inhibition of platelet aggregation, which protects against ischemic stroke and myocardial infarction (aspirin)

COMPLICATIONS

Gastrointestinal discomfort

Dyspepsia, abdominal pain, heartburn, nausea

NURSING CONSIDERATIONS
- Damage to gastric mucosa can lead to gastrointestinal (GI) bleeding and perforation, especially with long-term use.
- Risk is increased in older adults, clients who smoke or have alcohol use disorder, and those who have a history of peptic ulcers or previous inability to tolerate NSAIDs.
- Advise clients to take medication with food or with an 8 oz glass of water or milk.
- Advise clients to avoid alcohol.
- Observe for indications of GI bleeding (passage of black or dark-colored stools, severe abdominal pain, nausea, vomiting).
- Administer a proton pump inhibitor, such as omeprazole, or an H_2 receptor antagonist, such as ranitidine, to decrease the risk of ulcer formation.
- Use prophylaxis agents, such as misoprostol.

Impaired kidney function

Decreased urine output, weight gain from fluid retention, increased BUN, and creatinine levels

NURSING CONSIDERATIONS
- Use cautiously with older adults and clients who have heart failure.
- Monitor I&O and kidney function (BUN, creatinine).

Increased risk of heart attack and stroke

With nonaspirin NSAIDs

NURSING CONSIDERATIONS: Use the smallest effective dose for clients who have cardiovascular disease.

Salicylism (can occur with aspirin)

MANIFESTATIONS: Tinnitus, sweating, headache, dizziness, and respiratory alkalosis

CLIENT EDUCATION: Advise clients to notify the provider and stop taking aspirin if manifestations occur.

Reye syndrome (rare but serious complication)

This occurs when aspirin is used for fever reduction in children and adolescents who have a viral illness, such as chickenpox or influenza.

CLIENT EDUCATION: Advise clients to avoid giving aspirin when a child or adolescent has a viral illness, such as chickenpox or influenza. Qs

Aspirin toxicity

Progresses from the mild findings in salicylism to sweating, high fever, acidosis, dehydration, electrolyte imbalances, coma, and respiratory depression

NURSING CONSIDERATIONS

- Aspirin toxicity should be managed as a medical emergency in the hospital.
- Activated charcoal may be given to decrease absorption.
- Hemodialysis can be indicated.
- Cool the client with tepid water.
- Correct dehydration and electrolyte imbalance with IV fluids.
- Reverse acidosis and promote salicylate excretion with bicarbonate.
- Perform gastric lavage.

CONTRAINDICATIONS/PRECAUTIONS

First-generation NSAIDs

- Pregnancy (Pregnancy Risk Category D)
- Peptic ulcer disease
- Bleeding disorders, such as hemophilia and vitamin K deficiency
- Hypersensitivity to aspirin and other NSAIDs
- Children and adolescents who have chickenpox or influenza (aspirin)

NURSING CONSIDERATIONS: Use NSAIDs cautiously in the following.
- Older adult clients Ⓖ
- Clients who smoke cigarettes
- Clients who have *Helicobacter pylori* infection, hypovolemia, asthma, chronic urticaria, bleeding disorders, or a history of alcohol use disorder
- Clients taking anticoagulants, glucocorticoids, ACE inhibitors, and ARBs

Ketorolac is contraindicated in clients who have advanced kidney disease. Use should be no longer than 5 days because of the risk for kidney damage. Ⓠs

Second-generation NSAIDs

Second-generation NSAIDs should be used cautiously in clients who have cardiovascular disease.

Celecoxib suppresses inflammation, relieves pain, decreases fever, and protects against colorectal cancer.
- Celecoxib, an NSAID COX-2 inhibitor, is a last-choice medication for chronic pain due to the increased risk of myocardial infarction (MI) and stroke due to secondary suppression of vasodilation.
- Celecoxib is contraindicated in clients who have an allergy to sulfonamides.

INTERACTIONS

Anticoagulants, such as heparin and warfarin, increase the risk of bleeding.
NURSING CONSIDERATIONS
- Monitor PTT, PT, and INR.
- Advise clients about the potential risk of bleeding when an NSAID is combined with an anticoagulant. Instruct clients to report indications of bleeding.

Glucocorticoids increase the risk of gastric bleeding.
NURSING CONSIDERATIONS: Advise clients to take antiulcer prophylaxis, such as misoprostol, to decrease the risk for gastric ulcer.

Alcohol increases the risk of bleeding.
NURSING CONSIDERATIONS: Advise clients to avoid consuming alcoholic beverages to decrease the risk of GI bleeding.

Ibuprofen decreases the antiplatelet effects of low-dose aspirin used to prevent MI.
NURSING CONSIDERATIONS: Advise clients not to take ibuprofen concurrently with aspirin.

Ketorolac and concurrent use of other NSAIDs increase the risk of known adverse effects.
NURSING CONSIDERATIONS: Ketorolac should not be used concurrently with other NSAIDs.

Over-the-counter interaction
NURSING CONSIDERATIONS: Advise the client to tell the provider about any over-the-counter medications, vitamins, or herbal supplements before taking them.

NURSING ADMINISTRATION

- Advise clients to stop aspirin 1 week before an elective surgery or expected date of childbirth. Ⓠebp
- Advise clients to take NSAIDs with food, milk, or an 8 oz glass of water to reduce gastric discomfort.
- Instruct clients not to chew or crush enteric-coated or sustained-release aspirin tablets.
- Advise clients to notify the provider if manifestations of gastric discomfort or ulceration occur.
- Advise clients to notify the provider if manifestations of salicylism occur. The medication should be discontinued until manifestations are resolved. The medication can be restarted at a lower dose.
- Ketorolac can be used for short-term treatment of moderate to severe pain such as that associated with postoperative recovery.
  - Concurrent use with opioids allows for lower dosages of opioids and thus minimizes adverse effects such as constipation and respiratory depression.
  - Ketorolac is usually first administered parenterally and then switched to oral doses. Use should not be longer than 5 days because of the risk for kidney damage.
- Administer IV ibuprofen as an infusion over 30 min. The client should be hydrated before infusion to prevent kidney damage.

NURSING EVALUATION OF MEDICATION EFFECTIVENESS

Depending on therapeutic intent, effectiveness can be evidenced by the following.
- Reduction in inflammation
- Reduction of fever
- Relief from mild to moderate pain
- Absence of injury

Acetaminophen

PURPOSE

EXPECTED PHARMACOLOGICAL ACTION: Slows the production of prostaglandins in the central nervous system.

THERAPEUTIC USES
- Analgesic (relief of pain) effect
- Antipyretic (reduction of fever) effects

COMPLICATIONS

Adverse effects are rare at therapeutic dosages.

Acute toxicity

Results in liver damage with early manifestations of nausea, vomiting, diarrhea, sweating, and abdominal discomfort progressing to hepatic failure, coma, and death

NURSING CONSIDERATIONS
- Advise clients to take acetaminophen as prescribed and not to exceed 4 g/day. Parents should carefully follow the provider's advice regarding administration to children.
- Undernourished clients should limit acetaminophen to 3 g/day.
- Advise clients who consume more than three alcoholic drinks per day to limit acetaminophen to 2 g/day.
- Limit over-the-counter dosage of acetaminophen when taking a prescription for combination analgesics that contain acetaminophen.
- Administer the antidote, acetylcysteine.

CONTRAINDICATIONS/PRECAUTIONS

Use cautiously in clients who consume three or more alcoholic drinks per day and those taking warfarin (interferes with metabolism), thus increasing the risk of bleeding. Qs

INTERACTIONS

Alcohol increases the risk of liver damage.
CLIENT EDUCATION: Advise clients about the potential risk of liver damage with consumption of alcohol.

Acetaminophen slows the metabolism of warfarin, leading to increased levels of warfarin. This places clients at risk for bleeding.
NURSING CONSIDERATIONS
- Instruct clients to observe for indications of bleeding (bruising, petechiae, hematuria).
- Monitor prothrombin time and INR levels, and adjust dosages of warfarin accordingly.

NURSING ADMINISTRATION

- Acetaminophen is a component of multiple prescribed and over-the-counter medications. Keep a running total of daily acetaminophen intake, and follow recommended dosages as prescribed by the provider to prevent toxicity, not to exceed 4 g/day. QEBP
- The U.S. Food and Drug Administration recommends that clients take only one product containing acetaminophen at a given time. Teach clients to read medication labels carefully to determine the amount of medication contained in each dose.
- In the event of an overdose, administer acetylcysteine, the antidote for acetaminophen, to prevent liver damage. Administer via an duodenal tube to prevent emesis and subsequent aspiration.

NURSING EVALUATION OF MEDICATION EFFECTIVENESS

Depending on therapeutic intent, effectiveness can be evidenced by the following.
- Relief of pain
- Reduction of fever

Application Exercises

1. A nurse is assessing a client who has salicylism. Which of the following findings should the nurse expect? (Select all that apply.)

   A. Dizziness

   B. Diarrhea

   C. Jaundice

   D. Tinnitus

   E. Headache

2. A nurse is admitting a toddler to the hospital after an acetaminophen overdose. Which of the following medications should the nurse anticipate administering to this client?

   A. Acetylcysteine

   B. Pegfilgrastim

   C. Misoprostol

   D. Naltrexone

3. A nurse is teaching a client about the a new prescription for celecoxib. Which of the following information should the nurse include in the teaching?

   A. Increases the risk for a myocardial infarction

   B. Decreases the risk of stroke

   C. Inhibits COX-1

   D. Increases platelet aggregation

4. A nurse is taking a history for a client who reports that he is taking aspirin about four times daily for a sprained wrist. Which of the following prescribed medications taken by the client is contraindicated with aspirin?

   A. Digoxin

   B. Metformin

   C. Warfarin

   D. Nitroglycerin

5. A nurse in an emergency department is performing an admission assessment for a client who has severe aspirin toxicity. Which of the following findings should the nurse expect?

   A. Body temperature 35° C (95° F)

   B. Lung crackles

   C. Cool, dry skin

   D. Respiratory depression

PRACTICE Active Learning Scenario

A nurse at a provider's office is providing teaching to a client who has osteoarthritis and is starting long-term therapy with NSAIDs. What should the nurse include in the teaching? Use the ATI Active Learning Template: Medication to complete this item.

THERAPEUTIC USES

COMPLICATIONS: Describe two adverse effects.

NURSING INTERVENTIONS: Describe three nursing actions, including two laboratory values the nurse should monitor.

Application Exercises Key

1. A. **CORRECT:** The client who has salicylism can have dizziness, which is an expected finding.

   B. The client who takes aspirin is not expected to develop diarrhea. However, the nurse should monitor the color of the client's stools to determine if the client has a gastric bleed from taking aspirin.

   C. The client who takes aspirin will metabolize the medication through the liver. Jaundice is not an expected finding in salicylism.

   D. **CORRECT:** The client who has salicylism can have tinnitus, which is an expected finding.

   E. **CORRECT:** The client who has salicylism can have a headache, which is an expected finding.

   Ⓝ *NCLEX® Connection: Pharmacological and Parenteral Therapies, Expected Actions/Outcomes*

2. A. **CORRECT:** The nurse should administer acetylcysteine, which is the antidote for acetaminophen overdose.

   B. To increase the body's production of neutrophils, the nurse should administer pegfilgrastim.

   C. To prevent the formation of gastric ulcers, the nurse should administer misoprostol, which is a prostaglandin hormone.

   D. To prevent alcohol craving, the nurse should administer naltrexone, which is an opioid antagonist.

   Ⓝ *NCLEX® Connection: Pharmacological and Parenteral Therapies, Expected Actions/Outcomes*

3. A. **CORRECT:** The client who takes celecoxib has an increased risk for a myocardial infarction secondary to suppressing vasodilation.

   B. The client who takes celecoxib has an increased risk for stroke secondary to suppressing vasodilation.

   C. Celecoxib inhibits COX-2, which suppresses inflammation, relieves pain, decreases fever, and protects against colorectal cancer.

   D. Celecoxib does not have an effect on platelet aggregation. However, the medication suppresses vasodilation.

   Ⓝ *NCLEX® Connection: Pharmacological and Parenteral Therapies, Dosage Calculation*

4. A. Digoxin does not interact with aspirin and therefore is not contraindicated.

   B. Metformin does not interact with aspirin and therefore is not contraindicated.

   C. **CORRECT:** The effect of warfarin and other anticoagulants is increased by aspirin, which inhibits platelet aggregation. This client would have an increased risk for bleeding. Use of aspirin generally is contraindicated for clients who take warfarin.

   D. Nitroglycerin does not interact with aspirin and therefore is not contraindicated.

   Ⓝ *NCLEX® Connection: Pharmacological and Parenteral Therapies, Adverse Effects/Contraindications/Side Effects/Interactions*

5. A. The nurse should expect hyperthermia as a manifestation of severe aspirin toxicity.

   B. The nurse should expect dehydration as a manifestation of severe aspirin toxicity. Lung crackles are not an expected finding.

   C. The nurse should expect diaphoresis as a manifestation of severe aspirin toxicity. Cool, dry skin is not an expected finding.

   D. **CORRECT:** Respiratory depression due to increasing respiratory acidosis is an expected manifestation of severe aspirin toxicity.

   Ⓝ *NCLEX® Connection: Pharmacological and Parenteral Therapies, Adverse Effects/Contraindications/Side Effects/Interactions*

PRACTICE Answer

Using ATI Active Learning Template: Medication

THERAPEUTIC USES: NSAIDs will treat mild to moderate joint pain and stiffness, and decrease inflammation in the client who has osteoarthritis.

COMPLICATIONS

- Gastrointestinal effects can occur, including anorexia, abdominal pain, nausea, vomiting, and heartburn.
- GI bleeding can occur because NSAIDs affect platelet function.
- Nephrotoxicity can occur.
- NSAIDs can cause CNS effects such as dizziness, headache, blurred vision, and tinnitus.
- Allergy can occur, including cross allergy with other NSAIDs, such as aspirin.

NURSING INTERVENTIONS

- Monitor Hgb/Hct and kidney function tests.
- Assess the client for previous allergy to NSAIDs.
- Assess the GI system, and ask about any history of GI bleed or peptic ulcer disease.
- Advise the client to take the medication with food, milk, or an 8 oz glass of water to prevent GI distress.
- Advise the client to tell provider about any over-the-counter medications, vitamins, or herbal supplements before taking them.

Ⓝ *NCLEX® Connection: Pharmacological and Parenteral Therapies, Medication Administration*

UNIT 9 MEDICATIONS FOR PAIN AND INFLAMMATION

CHAPTER 36 # Opioid Agonists and Antagonists

Opioid analgesics are medications used to treat moderate to severe pain. Most opioid analgesics reduce pain by attaching to a receptor in the central nervous system, altering perception and response to pain.

Opioids are classified as agonists, agonist-antagonists, and antagonists. An agonist attaches to a receptor and produces a response. An agonist-antagonist binds to one receptor, causing a response, and binds to another receptor, which prevents a response. An antagonist attaches to a receptor site and prevents a response.

The desired outcome is to reduce pain and increase activity with few adverse effects. Opioid agonists are listed as Schedule II under the Controlled Substances Act.

Opioid agonists

SELECT PROTOTYPE MEDICATION: Morphine

OTHER MEDICATIONS
- Fentanyl
- Meperidine
- Methadone
- Codeine
- Oxycodone
- Hydromorphone

ROUTE OF ADMINISTRATION
- Morphine: Oral, subcutaneous, IM, IV, epidural, intrathecal Qpcc
- Fentanyl: IV, IM, transmucosal, transdermal
- Meperidine: Oral, subcutaneous, IM, IV
- Codeine: Oral, subcutaneous, IM, IV
- Methadone: Oral, subcutaneous, IM
- Oxycodone: Oral, rectal
- Hydromorphone: Oral, subcutaneous, IM, IV

PURPOSE

EXPECTED PHARMACOLOGICAL ACTION: Opioid agonists and other morphine-like medications (fentanyl), act on the mu receptors, and to a lesser degree on kappa receptors. Activation of mu receptors produces analgesia, respiratory depression, euphoria, and sedation, whereas kappa receptor activation produces analgesia, sedation, and decreased GI motility. Activation of mu receptors can also be linked to physical dependence.

THERAPEUTIC USES
- Relief of moderate to severe pain (postoperative, myocardial infarction, following childbirth, cancer)
- Sedation
- Reduction of bowel motility
- Cough suppression (codeine)

COMPLICATIONS

Respiratory depression

NURSING CONSIDERATIONS
- Monitor vital signs.
- Stop opioids if the client's respiratory rate is less than 12/min, and notify the provider.
- Have naloxone and resuscitation equipment available.
- Avoid use of opioids with CNS depressant medications (barbiturates, benzodiazepines, consumption of alcohol).

Constipation

NURSING CONSIDERATIONS
- Teach the client to increase fluid/fiber intake and physical activity.
- Administer a stimulant laxative (such as bisacodyl) to counteract decreased bowel motility, or a stool softener (such as docusate sodium) to prevent constipation.
- For clients who have end-stage disorders, such as cancer or AIDS, administer an opioid antagonist, such as methylnaltrexone, designed to treat severe constipation in opioid-dependent clients.

Orthostatic hypotension

NURSING CONSIDERATIONS
- Advise clients to sit or lie down if lightheadedness or dizziness occur.
- Due to the dilation effect to the peripheral arterioles and veins, avoid sudden changes in position by slowly moving clients from a lying to a sitting or standing position.
- Provide assistance with ambulation as needed.

Urinary retention

NURSING CONSIDERATIONS
- Advise clients to void every 4 hr.
- Monitor I&O.
- Assess the bladder for distention by palpating the lower abdomen area every 4 to 6 hr because opioid medication can suppress awareness that the bladder is full.
- Advise the client that medications with anticholinergic properties (tricyclic antidepressants, antihistamines) can increase symptoms.

Cough suppression

NURSING CONSIDERATIONS
- Advise clients to cough at regular intervals to prevent accumulation of secretions in the airway.
- Auscultate the lungs for crackles, and instruct clients to increase intake of fluid to liquefy secretions.

Sedation

CLIENT EDUCATION: Advise clients to avoid hazardous activities, such as driving or operating heavy machinery.

Biliary colic

NURSING CONSIDERATIONS: Avoid giving morphine to clients who have a history of biliary colic. Use meperidine as an alternative.

Nausea/vomiting

NURSING CONSIDERATIONS: Administer an antiemetic

Opioid overdose triad

Coma, respiratory depression, and pinpoint pupils

NURSING CONSIDERATIONS
- Monitor vital signs.
- Provide mechanical ventilation.
- Administer naloxone, an opioid antagonist that reverses respiratory depression and other overdose manifestations.

CONTRAINDICATIONS/PRECAUTIONS

- Morphine is contraindicated after biliary tract surgery. Qs
- Morphine is contraindicated for premature infants during and after delivery because of respiratory depressant effects.
- Meperidine is contraindicated for clients who have kidney failure because of the accumulation of normeperidine, which can result in seizures and neurotoxicity.
- Use cautiously with the following.
  - Clients who have asthma, emphysema, or head injuries; infants; and older adult clients (risk of respiratory depression) Ⓒ
  - Clients who are pregnant (risk of physical dependence of the fetus)
  - Clients in labor (risk of respiratory depression in the newborn and inhibition of labor by decreasing uterine contractions)
  - Clients who are extremely obese (greater risk for prolonged adverse effects because of the accumulation of medication that is metabolized at a slower rate)
  - Clients who have inflammatory bowel disease (risk of megacolon or paralytic ileus)
  - Clients who have an enlarged prostate (risk of acute urinary retention)
  - Clients who have hepatic or renal disease

INTERACTIONS

CNS depressants (barbiturates, phenobarbital, benzodiazepines, alcohol) have additive CNS depression action.
CLIENT EDUCATION
- Warn clients about the use of these medications in conjunction with opioid agonists.
- Advise clients to avoid consumption of alcohol.

Anticholinergic agents (atropine or scopolamine), antihistamines (diphenhydramine), and tricyclic antidepressants (amitriptyline) have additive anticholinergic effects (constipation, urinary retention).
CLIENT EDUCATION: Advise clients to increase fluids and dietary fiber to prevent constipation.

Meperidine can interact with monoamine oxidase inhibitors (MAOIs) and cause hyperpyrexic coma, characterized by excitation, seizures, and respiratory depression.
NURSING CONSIDERATIONS: Avoid the use of meperidine with MAOIs to prevent occurrence of this syndrome.

Antihypertensives have additive hypotensive effects.
CLIENT EDUCATION: Warn clients to refrain from using opioids with antihypertensive agents.

Additional medications such as amphetamines, clonidine, and dextromethorphan can increase opioid-induced analgesia.
CLIENT EDUCATION: Instruct clients to avoid taking other medications that have a CNS effect with opioid medication.

NURSING ADMINISTRATION

- Assess pain level on a regular basis. Document the client's response. QEBP
- Take baseline vital signs. If the respiratory rate is less than 12/min, notify the provider and withhold the medication.
- Follow controlled substance procedures.
- Double-check opioid doses with another nurse prior to administration.
- Administer IV opioids slowly over 4 to 5 min. Have naloxone and resuscitation equipment available.
- Warn clients not to increase dosage without consulting the provider.
- For clients who have cancer, administer opioids on a fixed schedule around the clock. Administer supplemental doses as needed.
- Advise clients who have physical dependence not to discontinue opioids abruptly. Opioids should be withdrawn slowly, and the dosage should be tapered over a period of 3 days.
- Closely monitor patient-controlled analgesia (PCA) pump settings (dose, lockout interval, 4-hr limit). Reassure clients regarding safety measures that safeguard against self-administration of excessive doses. Encourage clients to use PCA prophylactically prior to activities likely to augment pain levels.

- When switching clients from PCA to oral doses of opioids, make sure the client receives adequate PCA dosing until the onset of oral medication takes place.
- The first administration of a transdermal fentanyl patch will take several hours to achieve the desired therapeutic effect. Administer short-acting opioids prior to onset of therapeutic effects and for breakthrough pain.

NURSING EVALUATION OF MEDICATION EFFECTIVENESS

Depending on the therapeutic intent, effectiveness can be evidenced by the following.
- Relief of moderate to severe pain (postoperative pain, cancer pain, myocardial pain)
- Cough suppression
- Resolution of diarrhea

Agonist-antagonist opioids

SELECT PROTOTYPE MEDICATION: Butorphanol

OTHER MEDICATION
- Nalbuphine
- Buprenorphine
- Pentazocine

ROUTE OF ADMINISTRATION
- Butorphanol: IV, IM, intranasal
- Nalbuphine: IV, IM, subcutaneous
- Buprenorphine: IV, sublingual, transdermal
- Pentazocine: IV, IM, subcutaneous

PURPOSE

EXPECTED PHARMACOLOGICAL ACTION

- These medications act as antagonists on mu receptors and agonists on kappa receptors, except for buprenorphine, whose agonist/antagonist activity is on opposite receptors.
- Compared to pure opioid agonists, agonist-antagonists have the following.
  - Low potential for abuse, causing little euphoria. In fact, high doses can cause adverse effects (anxiety, restlessness, mental confusion).
  - Less respiratory depression
  - Less analgesic effect

THERAPEUTIC USES

- Relief of moderate to severe pain
- Treatment of opioid dependence (buprenorphine)
- Adjunct to balanced anesthesia
- Relief of labor pain

COMPLICATIONS

Abstinence syndrome

Cramping, hypertension, vomiting, fever, and anxiety

NURSING CONSIDERATIONS
- This syndrome can be precipitated when these medications are given to clients who are physically dependent on opioid agonists.
- Advise clients to stop opioid agonists, such as morphine, before using agonist-antagonist medications, such as pentazocine.
- Avoid giving to clients if undisclosed opioid use is suspected.

Sedation, respiratory depression

NURSING CONSIDERATIONS
- Have naloxone and resuscitation equipment available.
- Monitor for respiratory depression.

Dizziness

CLIENT EDUCATION: Instruct the client to use caution in standing up and to avoid driving or using heavy machinery.

Headache

NURSING CONSIDERATIONS
- Monitor for headache.
- Assess level of consciousness.

CONTRAINDICATIONS/PRECAUTIONS

Use cautiously in clients who have a history of myocardial infarction, kidney or liver disease, respiratory depression, or head injury, and clients who are physically dependent on opioids. Qs

INTERACTIONS

CNS depressants and alcohol can cause additive effects.
NURSING CONSIDERATIONS
- Use together cautiously.
- Monitor respirations.

Opioid agonists can antagonize and reduce analgesic effects of the opioid.
NURSING CONSIDERATIONS: Do not use concurrently.

NURSING ADMINISTRATION

- Obtain baseline vital signs. If the respiratory rate is less than 12/min, withhold the medication and notify the provider. Q_{EBP}
- Have naloxone and resuscitation equipment available.
- Assess clients for opioid dependence prior to administration. Agonist-antagonists can trigger withdrawal symptoms.
- Warn clients not to increase dosage without consulting the provider.
- Advise clients to use caution when getting out of bed or standing. Clients should not operate heavy machinery or drive until CNS effects are known.
- Warn clients not to increase dosage without consulting the provider.

NURSING EVALUATION OF MEDICATION EFFECTIVENESS

Monitor for improvement of symptoms, such as relief of pain.

Opioid antagonists

SELECT PROTOTYPE MEDICATION: Naloxone

OTHER MEDICATIONS
- Naltrexone
- Methylnaltrexone
- Alvimopan

ROUTE OF ADMINISTRATION
- Naloxone: IV, IM, subcutaneous
- Naltrexone: Oral, IM
- Methylnaltrexone: Subcutaneous
- Alvimopan: Oral

PURPOSE

EXPECTED PHARMACOLOGICAL ACTION

Opioid antagonists interfere with the action of opioids by competing for opioid receptors. Opioid antagonists have no effect in the absence of opioids.

THERAPEUTIC USES

- Treatment of opioid abuse by preventing euphoria (naltrexone)
- Reversal of effects of opioids, such as respiratory depression (naloxone)
- Reversal of respiratory depression in an infant (naloxone)
- Reversal of severe opioid-caused constipation in clients who have late-stage cancer or other disorders (methylnaltrexone, alvimopan)

COMPLICATIONS

Tachycardia and tachypnea

NURSING CONSIDERATIONS
- Monitor heart rhythm (risk of ventricular tachycardia) and respiratory function.
- Have resuscitative equipment, including oxygen, on standby during administration.

Abstinence syndrome

Cramping, hypertension, vomiting, and reversal of analgesia

NURSING CONSIDERATIONS: These manifestations can occur when given to clients physically dependent on opioid agonists.

CONTRAINDICATIONS/PRECAUTIONS

- Opioid antagonists are Pregnancy Risk Category B Q_s
- Naloxone and naltrexone are contraindicated in clients who have opioid dependency.
- Naltrexone is contraindicated for clients who have acute hepatitis or liver failure and during lactation.

NURSING ADMINISTRATION

- Naloxone has rapid first-pass inactivation and should be administered IV, IM, or subcutaneously. Do not administer orally.
- Observe withdrawal symptoms or abrupt onset of pain. Be prepared to address the need for analgesia if given for postoperative opioid-related respiratory depression. Q_{EBP}
- Titrate naloxone dosage to achieve reversal of respiratory depression without full reversal of pain management effects.
- Rapid infusion of naloxone can cause hypertension, tachycardia, nausea, and vomiting.
- Half-life of opioid analgesic can exceed the half-life of naloxone (60 to 90 min).
- Monitor respirations for up to 2 hr after use to assess for reoccurrence of respiratory depression and the need for repeat dosage of naloxone.
- Alvimopan is only administered for a 7-day period due to increased risk for myocardial infarction in prolonged administration.

NURSING EVALUATION OF MEDICATION EFFECTIVENESS

- Reversal of respiratory depression
  - Respirations are regular.
  - Client is without shortness of breath.
  - Respiratory rate is 16 to 20/min in adults and 40 to 60/min in newborns.
- Reduced euphoria in alcohol dependency and decreased craving for alcohol in alcohol dependency (naltrexone)
- Severe opioid-caused constipation relieved (methylnaltrexone, alvimopan)

Application Exercises

1. A nurse is preparing to administer an opioid agonist to a client who has acute pain. Which of the following complications should the nurse monitor?

   A. Urinary retention

   B. Tachypnea

   C. Hypertension

   D. Irritating cough

2. A nurse is caring for a client who has end-stage cancer and is receiving morphine. The client's daughter asks why the provider prescribed methylnaltrexone. Which of the following responses should the nurse make?

   A. "The medication will increase your mother's respirations."

   B. "The medication will prevent dependence on the morphine."

   C. "The medication will relieve your mother's constipation."

   D. "The medication works with the morphine to increase pain relief."

3. A nurse is preparing to administer butorphanol to a client who has a history of substance use disorder. The nurse should identify which of the following information as true regarding butorphanol?

   A. Butorphanol has a greater risk for abuse than morphine.

   B. Butorphanol causes a higher incidence of respiratory depression than morphine.

   C. Butorphanol cannot be reversed with an opioid antagonist.

   D. Butorphanol can cause abstinence syndrome in opioid-dependent clients.

4. A nurse is planning to administer morphine IV to a client who is postoperative. Which of the following actions should the nurse take?

   A. Monitor for seizures and confusion with repeated doses.

   B. Protect the client's skin from the severe diarrhea that occurs with morphine.

   C. Withhold this medication if respiratory rate is less than 12/min.

   D. Give morphine intermittent via IV bolus over 30 seconds or less.

5. A nurse is reviewing the medication administration record for a client who is receiving transdermal fentanyl for severe pain. Which of the following medications should the nurse expect to cause an adverse effect when administered concurrently with fentanyl?

   A. Ampicillin

   B. Diazepam

   C. Furosemide

   D. Prednisone

PRACTICE Active Learning Scenario

A nurse is providing discharge teaching for a client who is postoperative and has a new prescription for an opioid medication for incisional pain. What should the nurse include in the teaching? Use the ATI Active Learning Template: Medication to complete this item.

THERAPEUTIC USES: Describe for oxycodone.

COMPLICATIONS: List three adverse effects for oxycodone.

NURSING INTERVENTIONS: List three.

Application Exercises Key

1. A. **CORRECT:** The nurse should monitor for urinary retention because morphine can suppress awareness that the bladder is full.

    B. The nurse should monitor for respiratory depression because the activation of mu receptors has an effect on respirations.

    C. The nurse should monitor for hypotension because opioid medications can lower blood pressure by dilating peripheral arterioles and veins.

    D. The nurse should administer an opioid medication to suppress a cough because opioid receptors affect the medulla.

    Ⓝ *NCLEX® Connection: Pharmacological and Parenteral Therapies, Adverse Effects/Contraindications/Side Effects/Interactions*

2. A. Methylnaltrexone does not decrease analgesia or increase a depressed respiratory rate.

    B. Methylnaltrexone does not prevent dependence on opioids, such as morphine.

    C. **CORRECT:** Methylnaltrexone is an opioid antagonist used for treating severe constipation that is unrelieved by laxatives in clients who are opioid-dependent. The medication blocks the mu opioid receptors in the GI tract.

    D. Methylnaltrexone is not an adjunct to opioids for pain relief.

    Ⓝ *NCLEX® Connection: Pharmacological and Parenteral Therapies, Medication Administration*

3. A. Butorphanol has less risk for misuse than morphine.

    B. Butorphanol is less likely to cause respiratory depression than morphine.

    C. Manifestations of butorphanol overdose can be reversed with an opioid antagonist if necessary.

    D. **CORRECT:** Opioid agonist/antagonist medications, such as butorphanol, can cause abstinence syndrome in opioid-dependent clients. Manifestations include abdominal pain, fever, and anxiety.

    Ⓝ *NCLEX® Connection: Pharmacological and Parenteral Therapies, Expected Actions/Outcomes*

4. A. When the nurse administers repeated doses of meperidine, a toxic metabolite can build up and cause severe CNS effects such as agitation, confusion, and seizures.

    B. The nurse should plan to monitor for constipation because morphine effects the mu opioid receptors in the GI tract.

    C. **CORRECT:** The nurse should withhold all opioids if the respiratory rate is 12/min or less, and notify the provider.

    D. The nurse should administer morphine IV bolus slowly over 3 to 5 min to determine the client's response, and monitor the respiratory rate and blood pressure.

    Ⓝ *NCLEX® Connection: Pharmacological and Parenteral Therapies, Medication Administration*

5. A. Ampicillin, an antibiotic, does not interact with fentanyl and should not cause an adverse effect.

    B. **CORRECT:** Diazepam, a benzodiazepine, is a CNS depressant, which can interact by causing the client to become severely sedated when administered concurrently with an opioid agonist or agonist/antagonist.

    C. Furosemide, a loop diuretic, does not interact with fentanyl and should not cause an adverse effect.

    D. Prednisone, a glucocorticoid, does not interact with fentanyl and should not cause an adverse effect.

    Ⓝ *NCLEX® Connection: Pharmacological and Parenteral Therapies, Adverse Effects/Contraindications/Side Effects/Interactions*

PRACTICE Answer

Using the ATI Active Learning Template: Medication

THERAPEUTIC USES:
Opioid medication is indicated for relief of moderate to severe pain.

COMPLICATIONS
- Sedation
- Nausea/vomiting
- Constipation
- Orthostatic hypotension
- Urinary retention

NURSING INTERVENTIONS
- Instruct the client not to drive or perform other hazardous activities while using this medication.
- Notify the provider for severe nausea or vomiting.
- Prevent constipation by increasing intake of liquids and foods with fiber. Consider use of a stool softener or laxatives if necessary.
- Move the client slowly from lying or sitting to standing to minimize effects of orthostatic hypotension.
- Instruct the client to void every 4 hr. Contact the provider for manifestations of dysuria.

Ⓝ *NCLEX® Connection: Pharmacological and Parenteral Therapies, Medication Administration*

UNIT 9   MEDICATIONS FOR PAIN AND INFLAMMATION

CHAPTER 37 *Adjuvant Medications for Pain*

Adjuvant medications for pain are used with a primary pain medication, usually an opioid agonist, to increase pain relief while reducing the dosage of the opioid agonist. Reduced dosage of the opioid results in reduced adverse reactions, such as respiratory depression, sedation, and constipation. Targeting pain stimulus using different types of medications often provides improved pain reduction.

Categories of medications include tricyclic antidepressants, anticonvulsants, CNS stimulants, antihistamines, glucocorticoids, bisphosphonates, and nonsteroidal anti-inflammatory drugs (NSAIDs). The use of these medications to assist in the alleviation of pain can be an off-label use.

SELECT PROTOTYPE MEDICATIONS

- **Tricyclic antidepressants:** Amitriptyline (oral)
- **Anticonvulsants:** Carbamazepine, gabapentin (oral)
- **CNS stimulants:** Methylphenidate (oral, transdermal)
- **Antihistamines:** Hydroxyzine (oral, IM)
- **Glucocorticoids:** Dexamethasone (oral, IV, IM)
- **Bisphosphonates:** Etidronate (oral)
- **NSAIDs:** Ibuprofen (oral, IV)

OTHER MEDICATIONS

- **Tricyclic antidepressants:** Imipramine (oral)
- **Anticonvulsants:** Phenytoin (oral, IV)
- **CNS stimulants:** Dextroamphetamine (oral)
- **Glucocorticoids:** Prednisone (oral)
- **Bisphosphonates:** Pamidronate (IV)
- **NSAIDs:** Ketorolac (oral, IM, IV, intranasal)

PURPOSE

EXPECTED PHARMACOLOGICAL ACTION

Adjuvant medications for pain enhance the effects of opioids. Q̇EBP

THERAPEUTIC USES

These medications are used in combination with opioids and cannot be used as a substitute for opioids.
- **Tricyclic antidepressants** are used to treat depression, fibromyalgia syndrome, and neuropathic pain, such as cramping, aching, burning, darting, and sharp, stabbing pain.
- **Anticonvulsants** are used to relieve neuropathic pain and neuralgia.
- **CNS stimulants** augment analgesia and decrease sedation.
- **Antihistamines** decrease anxiety, prevent insomnia, and relieve nausea and vomiting.
- **Glucocorticoids** improve appetite and decrease pain from intracranial pressure, spinal cord compression, and rheumatoid arthritis.
- **Bisphosphonates** manage hypercalcemia and bone pain.
- **NSAIDs** are used to treat inflammation and fever, and relieve mild to moderate pain and dysmenorrhea.

COMPLICATIONS

Tricyclic antidepressants: amitriptyline

Orthostatic hypotension
NURSING CONSIDERATIONS
- Advise clients to sit or lie down if lightheadedness or dizziness occurs, and to change positions slowly.
- Provide assistance with ambulation as needed.
- Monitor blood pressure while the client is lying, sitting, and standing.
- Withhold the medication and notify the provider for low blood pressure or increased heart rate.

Sedation
CLIENT EDUCATION: Advise clients to avoid hazardous activities, such as driving or operating heavy machinery.

Anticholinergic effects
- Dry mouth, urinary retention, constipation, and blurred vision
- NURSING CONSIDERATIONS
  ○ Advise clients to increase fluid intake, sip fluids throughout the day, chew sugarless gum or suck on sugarless hard candy, and use an alcohol-free mouthwash.
  ○ Advise clients to increase daily fiber intake.
  ○ Instruct clients to increase physical activity by engaging in a regular exercise routine.
  ○ Administer a stimulant laxative, such as bisacodyl, to counteract decreased bowel motility, and a stool softener, such as docusate sodium, to prevent constipation.
  ○ Advise clients to void just prior to taking medication and then every 4 hr. Clients should report urinary retention to the provider.
  ○ If blurred vision is present, instruct clients to avoid hazardous activities, wear dark glasses for intolerance to light, and report blurred vision to the provider.
  ○ Monitor I&O, and assess the bladder for distention by palpating the lower abdomen area every 4 to 6 hr.

Anticonvulsants: carbamazepine, gabapentin

Bone marrow suppression
NURSING CONSIDERATIONS
- Periodically monitor complete blood count, including platelets.
- Advise clients to observe for indications of bone marrow suppression, such as easy bruising and bleeding, fever, or sore throat, and to notify the provider if they occur.

Gastrointestinal distress
- Nausea, vomiting, diarrhea, and constipation
- CLIENT EDUCATION
  - Advise clients to take the medication with food.
  - If constipation occurs, instruct clients to increase physical activity and daily fluid and fiber intake, administer a stimulant laxative, such as bisacodyl, and a stool softener, such as docusate sodium.

Drowsiness
CLIENT EDUCATION: Avoid activities that require alertness.

Rash
NURSING CONSIDERATIONS: Hold the medication and notify the provider.

CNS stimulants: methylphenidate

Weight loss
NURSING CONSIDERATIONS
- Monitor the client's weight.
- Encourage good nutrition.

Insomnia
CLIENT EDUCATION
- Instruct clients to take the last dose of the day no later than 4 p.m.
- Advise clients to decrease caffeine consumption.

Antihistamines: hydroxyzine

Sedation
NURSING CONSIDERATIONS
- Advise clients to avoid hazardous activities, such as driving or operating heavy machinery.
- Reduce dosage in older adult clients. Ⓒ

Dry mouth
CLIENT EDUCATION: Advise clients to increase fluid intake, sip fluids throughout the day, and chew sugarless gum or suck on hard sugarless candy.

Glucocorticoids: dexamethasone

Adrenal insufficiency
- Hypotension, dehydration, infection, weakness, lethargy, vomiting, diarrhea associated with prolonged use
- CLIENT EDUCATION: Advise clients to observe for indications and to notify the provider if they occur.

Osteoporosis
CLIENT EDUCATION: Advise clients to take calcium supplements, vitamin D, and/or a bisphosphonate.

Fluid and electrolyte disturbances
- Hypokalemia, and sodium and water retention
- NURSING CONSIDERATIONS
  - Monitor potassium levels, and administer potassium supplements as needed.
  - Encourage intake of potassium-rich foods (potatoes, bananas, citrus fruits).
  - Restrict sodium intake.
  - Instruct clients to report fluid retention or edema to the provider.

Glucose intolerance
NURSING CONSIDERATIONS: Monitor blood glucose levels.

Peptic ulcer disease
NURSING CONSIDERATIONS
- Advise clients to take the medication with meals.
- Regularly check stools for occult blood.
- Instruct clients to report black, tarry stools.
- Encourage the use of an antiulcer medication.

Bisphosphonates: etidronate, pamidronate

Transient flu-like manifestations (pamidronate)
NURSING CONSIDERATIONS
- Monitor for fever.
- Advise clients to notify the provider if manifestations occur.

Abdominal cramps, nausea, diarrhea, esophagitis (etidronate)
NURSING CONSIDERATIONS
- Advise clients to administer this medication with a full glass of water and sit or stand upright for 30 to 60 min after taking. Qs
- For maximum absorption, clients should wait 2 hr before ingesting food, antacids, or vitamins.

Venous irritation at injection site (pamidronate)
NURSING CONSIDERATIONS: Monitor the injection site and infuse with sufficient IV fluids.

Hypocalcemia
NURSING CONSIDERATIONS
- Monitor calcium, magnesium, potassium, and phosphate levels. Instruct clients to report numbness/tingling around the mouth, spasms, or seizures to provider.
- Advise clients to take supplemental calcium and vitamin D.

NSAIDs: ibuprofen

Bone marrow suppression
NURSING CONSIDERATIONS
- Periodically monitor CBC, including platelets.
- Advise clients to observe for indications of easy bruising and bleeding, fever, or sore throat, and to notify the provider if they occur.

Gastrointestinal distress
- Abdominal pain, ulceration, nausea, vomiting, and diarrhea or constipation
- NURSING CONSIDERATIONS
  - Advise clients to take with food, milk, or antacid.
  - Monitor for GI bleeding (coffee-ground emesis; bloody or black tarry stools; abdominal pain).

MI or stroke

NURSING CONSIDERATIONS: Monitor cardiac and neurological status, especially in older adult clients and those who have a history of cardiac disease or risk factors for MI or stroke.

CONTRAINDICATIONS/PRECAUTIONS

Tricyclic antidepressants: amitriptyline

- These medications are contraindicated in clients recovering from an MI and within 14 days of taking a MAOI.
- Use caution with clients who have a seizure disorder, urinary retention, prostatic hyperplasia, angle-closure glaucoma, hyperthyroidism, and liver or kidney disease.

Anticonvulsants: carbamazepine, gabapentin

- These medications are contraindicated in clients who have bone marrow suppression and within 14 days of taking a MAOI.
- Avoid use in pregnancy.

CNS stimulants: methylphenidate

- Clients should not take methylphenidate within 14 days of taking a MAOI.
- Use caution with clients who have hypertension. Methylphenidate can result in hypertensive crisis.
- Use caution with clients who have agitation or tics.
- Use caution with clients who have a history of substance use disorder.

Antihistamines: hydroxyzine

- Clients who have acute asthma should not take hydroxyzine.
- Clients who are in the first trimester of pregnancy or breastfeeding should not take hydroxyzine.
- Use caution with older adults and those in the second or third trimester of pregnancy.

Glucocorticoids: dexamethasone

- Dexamethasone is contraindicated in clients who have fungal infection, seizure disorders, ulcerative colitis, or coagulopathy.
- Use caution with clients who have hypertension, hypothyroidism, diabetes mellitus, osteoporosis or liver disease.

Bisphosphonate: etidronate

- Etidronate is contraindicated in clients who have achalasia, esophageal structure, or osteomalacia.
- Use caution with clients who have kidney disease.

NSAIDs: ibuprofen

- Ibuprofen is contraindicated in clients who have a history of bronchospasms with aspirin or other NSAIDs, and those who have severe kidney/hepatic disease.
- Use caution with clients who have bleeding, GI, or cardiac disorders.
- Use caution with older adult clients.

INTERACTIONS

Tricyclic antidepressants: amitriptyline

Barbiturates, CNS depressants, antihistamines, over-the-counter (OTC) sleep aids, and alcohol can cause additive CNS depression.
NURSING CONSIDERATIONS: Do not use together.

Anticonvulsants: carbamazepine, gabapentin

Carbamazepine causes a decrease in the effects of oral contraceptives and warfarin.
NURSING CONSIDERATIONS
- Advise clients to discuss possible contraceptive changes with the provider.
- Monitor for therapeutic effects of warfarin with PT and INR. Dosage might need to be adjusted.

Carbamazepine can result in CNS toxicity with lithium, and a fatal reaction with MAOIs.
NURSING CONSIDERATIONS: Concurrent use should be avoided.

Grapefruit juice inhibits metabolism, and thus increases carbamazepine levels.
CLIENT EDUCATION: Advise clients to avoid intake of grapefruit juice.

Phenytoin and phenobarbital decrease the effects of carbamazepine.
NURSING CONSIDERATIONS: Concurrent use is not recommended.

CNS depression occurs with gabapentin and all other CNS depressants such as alcohol, sedatives, and antihistamines.
CLIENT EDUCATION: Advise clients to not use together.

CNS stimulants: methylphenidate

Alkalizing medications can cause increase in reabsorption.
NURSING CONSIDERATIONS: Monitor for increase in amphetamine effects.

Acidifying medications can increase excretion of amphetamine.
NURSING CONSIDERATIONS: Monitor for decrease in amphetamine effects.

Insulin and oral antidiabetic medications can decrease glucose level.
NURSING CONSIDERATIONS: Monitor glucose level.

Methylphenidate decreases the effect of antihypertensives.
NURSING CONSIDERATIONS: Monitor blood pressure. Check more frequently in clients who have cardiac disease.

MAOIs can cause severe hypertension.
NURSING CONSIDERATIONS: Avoid concurrent use.

Caffeine can increase stimulant effect.
CLIENT EDUCATION: Advise clients to avoid caffeine.

OTC medications with sympathomimetic action can lead to increased CNS stimulation.
CLIENT EDUCATION: Instruct clients to avoid use of OTC medications.

Antihistamines: hydroxyzine

Barbiturates, CNS depressants, and alcohol can cause additive CNS depression.
NURSING CONSIDERATIONS: Do not use together.

Glucocorticoids: dexamethasone

Glucocorticoids promote hyperglycemia, thereby counteracting the effects of insulin and oral hypoglycemics.
NURSING CONSIDERATIONS: The dose of hypoglycemic medications might need to be increased.

Concurrent use of salicylates and NSAIDs can increase the risk for GI bleed.
NURSING CONSIDERATIONS
- Monitor for GI bleed.
- Use together cautiously.

Because of the risk for hypokalemia, there is an increased risk of dysrhythmias caused by digoxin.
NURSING CONSIDERATIONS
- Monitor potassium and cardiac rhythm.
- Encourage clients to eat potassium-rich foods.
- Administer potassium supplements.

Diuretics that promote potassium loss increase the risk for hypokalemia.
NURSING CONSIDERATIONS
- Monitor serum potassium level.
- Encourage clients to eat potassium-rich foods.
- Administer potassium supplements.

Glucocorticoids decrease the antibody response to vaccines and increase the risk of infection from live virus vaccines.
NURSING CONSIDERATIONS: Clients should not receive immunizations while on glucocorticoid therapy.

Bisphosphonates: etidronate, pamidronate

Decreased absorption with calcium or iron supplements and high calcium foods
CLIENT EDUCATION: Advise clients to take etidronate on an empty stomach 2 hr before meals, with an 8 oz glass of water.

NSAIDs: ibuprofen

NSAIDs can reduce effectiveness of antihypertensives, furosemide, thiazide diuretics, and oral antidiabetic medications.
NURSING CONSIDERATIONS: Monitor for medication effectiveness.

Aspirin, corticosteroids, alcohol, and tobacco can increase GI effects.
CLIENT EDUCATION: Advise clients to not use together.

NSAIDs can increase levels of oral anticoagulants and lithium.
NURSING CONSIDERATIONS: Monitor medication levels.

There is an increased risk of bleeding with the use of other NSAIDs, thrombolytics, antiplatelets, anticoagulants, and salicylates.
NURSING CONSIDERATIONS
- Clients who take medications together should use caution.
- Monitor for bleeding.

NURSING ADMINISTRATION

- The client's self-report is the key element in the assessment of pain. Q PCC
- Clients should receive a pain management plan.
- Encourage clients who have cancer to voice fears and concerns about cancer, cancer pain, and pain treatment.
- Advise clients that pain medications should be given on a fixed schedule around the clock, and not as-needed. Q EBP
- Advise clients that physical dependence is not considered addiction.
- Older adult clients need careful monitoring because they are at risk for increased adverse effects and adverse medication interactions with pain medications.
- Because some medications used as adjuvants are an off-label use, it is important to explain to clients the medications are being given to reduce pain, and not for the original purpose.

NURSING EVALUATION OF MEDICATION EFFECTIVENESS

Depending on the therapeutic intent, effectiveness can be evidenced by the following.
- Relief of depression, seizures, dysrhythmias, and other manifestations that aggravate the client's pain level
- Decreased opioid adverse effects
- Relief of neuropathic pain
- Decreased cancer bone pain
- Relief of neuralgia

Application Exercises

1. A nurse is caring for a client who has cancer and is taking morphine and carbamazepine for pain. Which of the following effects should the nurse monitor for when giving the medications together? (Select all that apply.)

   A. Need for reduced dosage of the opioid

   B. Reduced adverse effects of the opioid

   C. Increased analgesic effects

   D. Enhanced CNS stimulation

   E. Increased opioid tolerance

2. A nurse is planning care for a client who has brain cancer and is experiencing headaches. Which of the following adjuvant medications are indicated for this client?

   A. Dexamethasone

   B. Methylphenidate

   C. Hydroxyzine

   D. Amitriptyline

3. A nurse is preparing to administer pamidronate to a client who has bone pain related to cancer. Which of the following precautions should the nurse take when administering pamidronate?

   A. Inspect the skin for redness and irritation when changing the intradermal patch.

   B. Assess the IV site for thrombophlebitis frequently during administration.

   C. Instruct the client to sit upright or stand for 30 min following oral administration.

   D. Watch for manifestations of anaphylaxis for 20 min after IM administration.

4. A nurse is planning care for a client who has cancer and is taking a glucocorticoid as an adjuvant medication for pain control. Which of the following interventions should the nurse include in the plan of care? (Select all that apply.)

   A. Monitor for urinary retention.

   B. Monitor serum glucose.

   C. Monitor serum potassium level.

   D. Monitor for gastric bleeding.

   E. Monitor for respiratory depression.

5. A nurse is administering amitriptyline to a client who is experiencing cancer pain. For which of the following adverse effects should the nurse monitor?

   A. Decreased appetite

   B. Explosive diarrhea

   C. Decreased pulse rate

   D. Orthostatic hypotension

PRACTICE Active Learning Scenario

A nurse in an acute care facility is teaching a client who has metastatic cancer and is receiving morphine and carbamazepine for pain. What information should the nurse provide about the use of these medications? Use the ATI Active Learning Template: Medication to complete this item.

THERAPEUTIC USES: Describe the therapeutic use for carbamazepine in this client.

COMPLICATIONS: Describe two adverse effects the client should monitor for.

INTERACTIONS: Describe two interactions with carbamazepine.

NURSING INTERVENTIONS: Describe two.

Application Exercises Key

1. A. **CORRECT:** Dosage of the opioid can be reduced when adjuvant medications are added for pain.

    B. **CORRECT:** Adverse effects of the opioid can be reduced when adjuvant medications are added for pain.

    C. **CORRECT:** Analgesic effects are increased when adjuvant medications are added for pain.

    D. CNS stimulation is not enhanced when morphine and carbamazepine are used together for pain relief.

    E. Opioid tolerance can be decreased when an adjuvant medication is added for pain.

    Ⓝ NCLEX® *Connection: Pharmacological and Parenteral Therapies, Pharmacological Pain Management*

2. A. **CORRECT:** Dexamethasone, a glucocorticoid, decreases inflammation and swelling. It is used to reduce cerebral edema and relieve pressure from the tumor.

    B. The use of methylphenidate as an adjuvant is to elevate mood and increase pain relief.

    C. The use of hydroxyzine as an adjuvant is to decrease anxiety and help the client sleep.

    D. The use of amitriptyline as an adjuvant is to relieve neuropathic pain and elevate mood.

    Ⓝ NCLEX® *Connection: Pharmacological and Parenteral Therapies, Pharmacological Pain Management*

3. A. This medication is not administered by the intradermal route.

    B. **CORRECT:** Pamidronate is administered by IV infusion. This medication is irritating to veins, and the nurse should assess for thrombophlebitis during administration.

    C. This medication is not administered orally.

    D. This medication is not administered by the IM route.

    Ⓝ NCLEX® *Connection: Pharmacological and Parenteral Therapies, Pharmacological Pain Management*

4. A. Monitoring for urinary retention is not necessary because glucocorticoids do not cause this effect.

    B. **CORRECT:** Monitoring serum glucose is important because glucocorticoids raise the glucose level, especially in clients who have diabetes mellitus.

    C. **CORRECT:** Monitoring serum potassium level is important because glucocorticoids can cause hypokalemia.

    D. **CORRECT:** Monitoring for gastric bleeding is important because glucocorticoids irritate the gastric mucosa and put the client at risk for a peptic ulcer.

    E. Monitoring for respiratory depression is not necessary because glucocorticoids do not depress respirations.

    Ⓝ NCLEX® *Connection: Pharmacological and Parenteral Therapies, Pharmacological Pain Management*

5. A. Amitriptyline can cause increased appetite and weight gain.

    B. Amitriptyline can cause constipation.

    C. Amitriptyline can cause increased pulse rate.

    D. **CORRECT:** Amitriptyline can cause orthostatic hypotension. The nurse should assess for this effect and instruct the client to move slowly from lying down or sitting after taking this medication.

    Ⓝ NCLEX® *Connection: Pharmacological and Parenteral Therapies, Adverse Effects/Contraindications/Side Effects/Interactions*

PRACTICE Answer

Using the ATI Active Learning Template: Medication

THERAPEUTIC USES: Carbamazepine relieves neuropathic (nerve) pain, which can be described as sharp, burning, or aching.

COMPLICATIONS: Adverse effects of carbamazepine include GI manifestations such as abdominal pain, nausea, and vomiting. It also can cause bone marrow suppression, affecting all blood cell types.

INTERACTIONS
- The medication can cause hypertensive crisis if taken within 14 days of an MAOI antidepressant.
- Toxicity can result if the client drinks grapefruit juice while taking carbamazepine.

NURSING INTERVENTIONS
- Monitor CBC, including platelet counts.
- Assess for abnormal bleeding, bruising, or infection.
- Monitor for GI manifestations, and advise the client to take the medication with food.

Ⓝ NCLEX® *Connection: Pharmacological and Parenteral Therapies, Medication Administration*

UNIT 9   MEDICATIONS FOR PAIN AND INFLAMMATION

CHAPTER 38 *Miscellaneous Pain Medications*

Pain is subjective and can be indicative of current or impending tissue injury. Pain can result from the release of chemical mediators, inflammation, or pressure.

Migraine headaches can be caused by the inflammation and vasodilation of cerebral blood vessels. Medications for migraine headaches can be used to stop a migraine (abortive) or prevent one from occurring (prophylactic). First-line treatment for migraine headaches includes nonspecific analgesics such as aspirin-like medications and migraine-specific medications such as serotonin receptor agonists (also known as triptans). Ergot alkaloids medications are second-line treatment for migraines, and prophylactic medications include beta-blockers, anticonvulsants, tricyclic antidepressants, and estrogens.

Local anesthetics block motor and sensory neurons to a specific area. They can be given topically; injected directly into an area; or given regionally, epidurally, or into the subarachnoid (spinal) space.

Migraine medications

SELECT PROTOTYPE MEDICATIONS
- **Aspirin-like medications:** Acetaminophen, NSAIDs (aspirin, naproxen)
- **Serotonin receptor agonists (triptans):** Sumatriptan (oral, subcutaneous, inhalation, transdermal)
- **Ergot alkaloids**
  - Ergotamine (oral, sublingual, rectal)
  - Dihydroergotamine (IV, IM, subcutaneous, intranasal)
- **Beta-blockers:** Propranolol (oral)
- **Anticonvulsants:** Divalproex (oral), topiramate
- **Tricyclic antidepressants:** Amitriptyline (oral)
- **Estrogens:** Estrogen (gel, patches)

OTHER MEDICATIONS
- **Triptans:** Almotriptan, frovatriptan, naratriptan, zolmitriptan
- **Ergot alkaloids:** Ergotamine and caffeine
- **Combination OTC analgesics:** Acetaminophen, aspirin, caffeine
- **Other combinations:** Isometheptene, dichloralphenazone/acetaminophen
  - Isometheptene relieves headaches through vasoconstriction of arterioles.
  - Dichloralphenazone has sedative properties.
  - Acetaminophen is a mild analgesic.

PURPOSE

EXPECTED PHARMACOLOGICAL ACTION: Migraine medications prevent inflammation and dilation of the intracranial blood vessels, thereby relieving migraine pain.

THERAPEUTIC USES
- Some medications are used as abortive therapy to stop a migraine after it begins or after prodromal manifestations start. These include nonsteroidal anti-inflammatory drugs (NSAIDs) and combination anti-inflammatory medications, triptans, and ergot alkaloids.
- Other medications are used as prophylactic therapy to help prevent a migraine headache. Preventive agents include beta-blockers, anticonvulsants, amitriptyline, and estrogens.

COMPLICATIONS

Aspirin-like drugs: NSAIDs, acetaminophen combination

Bone marrow suppression
NURSING CONSIDERATIONS
- Periodically monitor CBC, including platelets.
- Advise clients to observe for indications of easy bruising and bleeding, fever, or sore throat, and to notify the provider if they occur.

Gastrointestinal (GI) distress
- Abdominal pain, ulceration, nausea, vomiting, and diarrhea or constipation
- NURSING CONSIDERATIONS
  - Advise clients to take with food, milk, or antacid.
  - Monitor for GI bleeding (coffee-ground emesis; bloody or black tarry stools; abdominal pain).

Myocardial infarction (MI) or stroke
NURSING CONSIDERATIONS: Monitor cardiac status, especially in older adult clients and clients who have a history of cardiac disease.

Serotonin receptor antagonists (triptans): sumatriptan

Chest pressure (heavy arms or chest tightness)
CLIENT EDUCATION
- Warn clients about symptoms, and reassure that symptoms are self-limiting and not dangerous.
- Advise clients to notify the provider for continuous or severe chest pain.

Coronary artery vasospasm/angina
NURSING CONSIDERATIONS: Do not administer to a client who has or is at risk for coronary artery disease (CAD).

Dizziness or vertigo
CLIENT EDUCATION: Advise clients to avoid driving or operating machinery until medication effects are known.

Teratogenesis
NURSING CONSIDERATIONS: The medication should be avoided in clients who are pregnant, trying to become pregnant, or are not using adequate contraception.

Ergot alkaloids: ergotamine and dihydroergotamine

Gastrointestinal discomfort
- Such as nausea and vomiting
- NURSING CONSIDERATIONS: Administer an antiemetic, such as metoclopramide.

Acute or chronic overdose (ergotism)
- Muscle pain, paresthesias in fingers and toes; peripheral ischemia
- NURSING CONSIDERATIONS: Stop medication, and immediately notify the provider if symptoms occur.

Physical dependence
NURSING CONSIDERATIONS
- Advise clients not to exceed the prescribed dose.
- Medication should not be taken daily on a long-term basis.
- Inform clients regarding symptoms of withdrawal (headache, nausea, vomiting, restlessness).
- Notify the provider if symptoms occur.

Fetal harm or abortion
NURSING CONSIDERATIONS
- Avoid using this medication during pregnancy.
- Advise clients to use additional contraception while using the medication.

Beta-blockers: propranolol

Extreme tiredness, fatigue, depression, asthma exacerbation
CLIENT EDUCATION: Advise clients to observe for symptoms and notify the provider if they occur.

Bradycardia, hypotension
NURSING CONSIDERATIONS
- Monitor heart rate and blood pressure.
- Instruct client to take apical pulse prior to dosing.
- Notify the provider of significant change.

Anticonvulsants: divalproex

GI distress
- Nausea, vomiting, diarrhea, dyspepsia, indigestion
- NURSING CONSIDERATIONS: Report symptoms to the provider.

Neural tube defects
NURSING CONSIDERATIONS
- Avoid use during pregnancy.
- Advise client to use additional contraception if using this medication.

Hepatitis
NURSING CONSIDERATIONS
- Monitor liver enzymes.
- Notify the provider of lethargy or fever.

Pancreatitis
CLIENT EDUCATION: Instruct clients to report abdominal pain, nausea, vomiting, and anorexia. Medication should be discontinued.

Tricyclic antidepressants: amitriptyline

Anticholinergic effects

- Dry mouth, constipation, urinary retention, blurred vision, tachycardia
- NURSING CONSIDERATIONS
  - Advise clients to increase fluid intake, sip fluids throughout the day, chew sugarless gum or suck on sugarless hard candy, and use an alcohol-free mouthwash.
  - Increase daily fiber intake.
  - Increase physical activity by engaging in regular exercise.
  - Administer stimulant laxatives, such as bisacodyl to counteract reduced bowel motility, or stool softeners, such as docusate sodium to prevent constipation.
  - Advise clients to void just before taking medication and then every 4 hr. Clients should report urinary retention to the provider.
  - Advise clients to report blurred vision.

Drowsiness or dizziness
CLIENT EDUCATION: Advise clients to avoid driving or operating machinery until medication effects are known.

CONTRAINDICATIONS/PRECAUTIONS

Ergotamine

- Contraindicated in clients who have renal and/or liver dysfunction, sepsis, hypertension, history of myocardial infarction, and CAD, as well as during pregnancy.
- Pregnancy Risk Category X

Triptans

- Contraindicated in clients who have liver failure, ischemic heart disease, a history of myocardial infarction, uncontrolled hypertension, and other heart diseases.
- Pregnancy Risk Category C

Propranolol

- Contraindicated in clients who have greater than first-degree heart block, bradycardia, bronchial asthma, cardiogenic shock, or heart failure.
- Use with caution in clients taking other antihypertensives or who have liver or renal impairment, diabetes mellitus, or Wolff-Parkinson-White syndrome.
- Pregnancy Risk Category C

Divalproex

- Contraindicated in clients who have liver disease.
- Pregnancy Risk Category D

Amitriptyline

- Contraindicated in clients who have recent MI or within 14 days of a MAO inhibitor.
- Use with caution in clients who have seizure history, urinary retention, prostatic hyperplasia, angle-closure glaucoma, hyperthyroidism, and liver or kidney disease.
- Pregnancy Risk Category C

Aspirin-like drugs

- Contraindicated in clients who have severe renal/hepatic disease.
- Use caution with clients who have bleeding, or GI or cardiac disorders; and with older adult clients.

Acetaminophen

Should not be used alone, but only in combination with other medications.

INTERACTIONS

Aspirin-like medications: NSAIDs, acetaminophen combination

NSAIDs can reduce the effectiveness of antihypertensives, furosemide, thiazide diuretics, and oral antidiabetic medications.
NURSING CONSIDERATIONS: Monitor for medication effectiveness.

Corticosteroids, alcohol, and tobacco can increase GI effects.
NURSING CONSIDERATIONS: Advise clients to not use these together.

NSAIDs can increase levels of oral anticoagulants and lithium.
NURSING CONSIDERATIONS: Monitor medication levels.

There is an increased risk of bleeding with the use of other NSAIDs, thrombolytics, antiplatelets, anticoagulants, and salicylates.
NURSING CONSIDERATIONS

- Clients who take medications together should use caution.
- Monitor for bleeding.

Serotonin receptor antagonists (triptans): sumatriptan

Concurrent use of MAOIs can lead to MAO toxicity.
NURSING CONSIDERATIONS: Do not give triptans within 2 weeks of stopping MAOIs.

Concurrent use with ergotamine or another triptan can cause a vasospastic reaction.
NURSING CONSIDERATIONS: Avoid concurrent use of these medications.

Selective serotonin reuptake inhibitors (SSRIs) taken with triptans can cause serotonin syndrome (confusion, agitation, hyperthermia, diaphoresis, possible death).
NURSING CONSIDERATIONS: Do not use medications together.

Ergotamine and dihydroergotamine

Concurrent use with triptans can cause a vasospastic reaction.
NURSING CONSIDERATIONS: Triptans should be taken at least 24 hr apart from an ergotamine medication.

Some HIV protease inhibitors, antifungal medications, macrolide antibiotics, and grapefruit juice can increase ergotamine levels, causing increased vasospasm.
NURSING CONSIDERATIONS: Do not use together.

Beta-blockers: propranolol

Verapamil and diltiazem have additive cardiosuppression effects.
NURSING CONSIDERATIONS: If medications are used together, monitor ECG, heart rate, and blood pressure.

Diuretics and antihypertensive medications have additive hypotensive effects.
NURSING CONSIDERATIONS: Monitor blood pressure. Hold and notify the provider if systolic blood pressure is less than 90 mm Hg.

Propranolol can mask the hypoglycemic effect of insulin and prevent the breakdown of fat in response to hypoglycemia.
NURSING CONSIDERATIONS
- Use with caution.
- Monitor blood glucose.

Anticonvulsants: divalproex

NSAIDs, erythromycin, and salicylates can cause divalproex toxicity.
NURSING CONSIDERATIONS: Monitor medication levels.

Benzodiazepines, opioids, antihistamines, and alcohol can cause CNS depression.
NURSING CONSIDERATIONS: Do not use together.

Divalproex can increase levels of phenobarbital and phenytoin.
NURSING CONSIDERATIONS: Monitor medication levels.

Increase the effects of warfarin.
NURSING CONSIDERATIONS
- Monitor for therapeutic effects of warfarin with PT and INR. Dosage can need to be adjusted.
- Monitor for bleeding.

Tricyclic antidepressants: amitriptyline

Barbiturates, CNS depressants, antihistamines, over-the-counter sleep aids, and alcohol can cause additive CNS depression.
NURSING CONSIDERATIONS: Do not use together.

Cimetidine can increase amitriptyline levels.
NURSING CONSIDERATIONS: Monitor medication effects.

MAOIs can increase CNS excitation or cause seizures.
NURSING CONSIDERATIONS: Do not give amitriptyline within 2 weeks of stopping MAOIs.

NURSING ADMINISTRATION

- Advise clients that abortive medications should not be used more than 2 days a week.
- Advise clients who have migraines to avoid trigger factors that cause stress and fatigue, such as consumption of alcohol and tyramine-containing foods (wine, aged cheese).
- Advise clients that lying down in a dark, quiet place can help ease symptoms. Qᴘᴄᴄ
- Antiemetics, preferably metoclopramide, are useful as adjunct medications in migraine treatment.
- Advise clients to check apical pulse before dosage (propranolol).
- Clients can take dosage with food to reduce GI distress (divalproex) and increase absorption (propranolol).
- Advise clients to protect skin and eyes from sun (amitriptyline) and avoid driving or operating machinery until medication effects are known (amitriptyline, sumatriptan).
- Use caution in case of orthostatic hypotension (amitriptyline, propranolol).

NURSING EVALUATION OF MEDICATION EFFECTIVENESS

Depending on the therapeutic intent, effectiveness can be evidenced by the following.
- Reduction in intensity and frequency of migraine attacks
- Prophylaxis against migraine attacks
- Termination of migraine headaches
- Reduction in size and frequency of medication doses used

Local anesthetics

SELECT PROTOTYPE MEDICATIONS
- **Amide type:** Lidocaine

OTHER MEDICATIONS
- **Ester type:** Tetracaine, procaine
- **Amide type:** EMLA (eutectic mixture of 2.5% lidocaine/2.5% prilocaine)

PURPOSE

EXPECTED PHARMACOLOGICAL ACTION

These medications decrease pain by blocking conduction of pain impulses in a circumscribed area. Loss of consciousness does not occur.

THERAPEUTIC USES

PARENTERAL ADMINISTRATION
- Pain management for dental procedures, minor surgical procedures, labor and delivery, and diagnostic procedures
- Regional anesthesia (spinal, epidural)

TOPICAL ADMINISTRATION
- Skin and mucous membrane disorders
- Control laryngeal and esophageal reflexes prior to endoscopic procedures
- Minor procedures, such as IV insertion, injection (pediatric), and wart removal

COMPLICATIONS

CNS excitation

Seizures, followed by respiratory depression, leading to unconsciousness

NURSING CONSIDERATIONS
- Monitor for signs of seizure activity, sedation, and change in mental status (decrease in level of consciousness).
- Monitor vital signs and respiratory status.
- Have equipment ready for resuscitation.
- Administer benzodiazepines, such as midazolam or diazepam, to treat seizures.

Hypotension, cardiosuppression

Evidenced by bradycardia, heart block, and cardiac arrest (common in spinal anesthesia due to sympathetic block)

NURSING CONSIDERATIONS
- Monitor vital signs and ECG.
- If symptoms occur, administer treatment as prescribed.

Allergic reactions

More likely with ester-type agents, such as procaine

NURSING CONSIDERATIONS
- Clients who are allergic to one ester-type agent are likely allergic to all other ester-type agents.
- Amide-type anesthetic agents are less likely to cause allergic reactions, and therefore are used for injection.
- Observe for symptoms of allergy to anesthetics, such as allergic dermatitis or anaphylaxis.
- Treat with antihistamines or agency protocol.

Labor and delivery

- Labor can be prolonged due to a decrease in uterine contractility.
- Local anesthetics can cross the placenta and result in fetal bradycardia and CNS depression.

NURSING CONSIDERATIONS
- Use cautiously in women who are in labor.
- Monitor uterine activity for effectiveness.
- Monitor fetal heart rate for bradycardia and decreased variability.

Spinal headache

NURSING CONSIDERATIONS
- Monitor for signs of severe headache.
- Advise clients to remain flat in bed for 12 hr postprocedure.

Urinary retention

Can occur with spinal anesthesia

NURSING CONSIDERATIONS
- Monitor urinary output.
- Notify the provider if the client has not voided within 8 hr.

CONTRAINDICATIONS/PRECAUTIONS

- Local anesthetics are Pregnancy Risk Category B.
- Supraventricular dysrhythmias and/or heart block.
- Use cautiously in clients who have liver and kidney dysfunction, heart failure, and myasthenia gravis.
- Epinephrine added to the local anesthetic is contraindicated for use in fingers, nose, and other body parts with end arteries. Gangrene can result due to vasoconstriction.
- Advise clients to use caution against self-inflicted injury until the anesthetic effect wears off.

INTERACTIONS

Antihypertensive medications have additive hypotensive effects with parenteral administration of local anesthetics.
NURSING CONSIDERATIONS: Monitor heart rate and blood pressure.

NURSING ADMINISTRATION

- Advise clients to avoid hazardous activities when recovering from anesthesia.
- Maintain clients in a comfortable position during recovery.

Injection of local anesthetic

- Vasoconstrictors, such as epinephrine, often are used in combination with local anesthetics to prevent the spread of the local anesthetic.
  - Keeping the anesthetic contained prolongs the anesthesia and decreases the chance of systemic toxicity.
  - Epinephrine added to the local anesthetic is contraindicated for use in fingers, nose, and other body parts with end arteries.
  - Gangrene can result due to vasoconstriction.
- Prepare injection site for local anesthetic by cleansing and shaving if indicated.
- Monitor vital signs and level of consciousness.
- Maintain IV access for administration of emergency medications if necessary.
- Have equipment ready for resuscitation.
- For regional block, protect the area of numbness from injury.

Spinal or epidural nerve blocks

- Monitor during insertion for hypotension, anaphylaxis, seizure, and dura puncture. Q**EBP**
- Monitor for respiratory depression and sedation.
- Monitor insertion site for hematoma and signs of an infection.
- Assess level of sensory block. Evaluate leg strength prior to ambulating.
- Prepare IV fluids to administer to compensate for the sympathetic blocking effects of regional anesthetics.
- Have client lie supine for 12 hr following spinal anesthesia to minimize headache.
- Notify provider if the client is unable to void after 8 hr.

Topical cream (EMLA)

- Apply to intact skin 1 hr before routine procedures or superficial puncture and 2 hr before more extensive procedures or deep puncture.
- Apply to the smallest surface area needed to minimize systemic absorption. Avoid wrapping or heating the area.
- Prior to the procedure, remove the dressing and clean the skin with aseptic solution.
- Keep the client NPO following oral administration until normal pharyngeal sensation returns (approximately 1 hr). Monitor the client's first oral intake.
- EMLA can be applied at home prior to coming to a health care facility for a procedure.

CLIENT EDUCATION

- Advise clients to notify the provider for signs of infection, such as fever, swelling, and redness; increase in pain or severe headache; sudden weakness to lower extremities; or decrease in bowel or bladder control. Q**s**
- Notify the provider for signs of systemic infusion, such as a metallic taste, ringing in ears, perioral numbness, and seizures.
- Advise clients to sanitize hands before and after administration of topical anesthetic.

NURSING EVALUATION OF MEDICATION EFFECTIVENESS

Depending on the therapeutic intent, effectiveness can be evidenced by the following.
- Client undergoes procedure without experiencing pain
- Pain is relieved

Application Exercises

1. A nurse is providing teaching to a client who is experiencing migraine headaches. Which of the following instructions should the nurse provide? (Select all that apply.)

   A. Take ergotamine as a prophylaxis to prevent a migraine headache.

   B. Identify and avoid trigger factors.

   C. Lie down in a dark quiet room at the onset of a migraine.

   D. Avoid foods that contain tyramine.

   E. Avoid exercise that can increase heart rate.

2. A nurse is planning care for a client who is to receive tetracaine prior to a bronchoscopy. Which of the following actions should the nurse include in the plan of care?

   A. Keep the client NPO until pharyngeal response returns.

   B. Monitor the insertion site for a hematoma.

   C. Palpate the bladder to detect urinary retention.

   D. Maintain the client on bed rest for 12 hr following the procedure.

3. A nurse is caring for a client who receives a local anesthetic of lidocaine during the repair of a skin laceration. For which of the following adverse reactions should the nurse monitor the client?

   A. Seizures

   B. Tachycardia

   C. Hypertension

   D. Fever

4. A nurse is reviewing the health history of a client who has migraine headaches and is to begin prophylaxis therapy with propranolol. Which of the following findings in the client history should the nurse report to the provider?

   A. The client had a prior myocardial infarction.

   B. The client takes warfarin for atrial fibrillation.

   C. The client takes an SSRI for depression.

   D. An ECG indicates a first-degree heart block.

5. A nurse is providing teaching to a client who has migraine headaches and a new prescription for ergotamine. For which of the following adverse effects should the nurse instruct the client to stop taking the medication and notify the provider? (Select all that apply.)

   A. Nausea

   B. Visual disturbances

   C. Positive home pregnancy test

   D. Numbness and tingling in fingers

   E. Muscle pain

PRACTICE Active Learning Scenario

A nurse is teaching a client who has frequent migraine headaches about her new prescription for sumatriptan. What should the nurse teach the client about this medication? Use the ATI Active Learning Template: Medication to complete this item.

THERAPEUTIC USES: Describe the therapeutic use for sumatriptan in this client.

COMPLICATIONS: Describe two adverse effects the client should monitor for.

INTERACTIONS: Describe two interactions the nurse should teach the client about.

NURSING INTERVENTIONS: Describe two for this client.

Application Exercises Key

1. A. Ergotamine is used at the onset of a migraine to abort headache manifestations. It should not be used regularly because it can cause physical dependence and toxicity.

   B. **CORRECT:** Identifying and avoiding trigger factors is an important action that can help to prevent some migraines.

   C. **CORRECT:** Lying down in a dark, quiet room at the onset of a migraine can prevent the onset of more severe manifestations.

   D. **CORRECT:** Foods that contain tyramine can be a trigger for some migraines and should be avoided.

   E. Exercise should be encouraged between migraines because it can relieve stress, which can trigger headaches.

   Ⓝ *NCLEX® Connection: Pharmacological and Parenteral Therapies, Medication Administration*

2. A. **CORRECT:** The nurse should keep the client NPO following the procedure until normal pharyngeal sensation returns (approximately 1 hr) and should then monitor the client's first oral intake to ensure aspiration does not occur.

   B. The nurse should monitor the insertion site for a hematoma for the client who receives spinal anesthesia.

   C. The nurse should palpate the bladder to detect for urinary retention for the client who receives spinal anesthesia.

   D. The nurse should maintain the client on bed rest for 12 hr following the procedure for the client who receives spinal anesthesia.

   Ⓝ *NCLEX® Connection: Pharmacological and Parenteral Therapies, Pharmacological Pain Management*

3. A. **CORRECT:** Seizure activity is an adverse effect that can occur as a result of local anesthetic injection.

   B. Bradycardia can occur as a result of local anesthetic injection.

   C. Hypotension can occur as a result of local anesthetic injection.

   D. Fever is not an adverse effect of local anesthetic injection.

   Ⓝ *NCLEX® Connection: Pharmacological and Parenteral Therapies, Adverse Effects/Contraindications/Side Effects/Interactions*

4. A. A prior MI is not a contraindication to taking propranolol.

   B. Concurrent use of warfarin is not a contraindication to taking propranolol.

   C. Concurrent use of an SSRI is not a contraindication to taking propranolol. Taking sumatriptan with SSRIs can lead to serotonin syndrome. The medications should not be used together.

   D. **CORRECT:** Propranolol is contraindicated in clients who have a first-degree heart block. The nurse should report this finding to the provider.

   Ⓝ *NCLEX® Connection: Pharmacological and Parenteral Therapies, Medication Administration*

5. A. Nausea that occurs with a migraine is a common associated finding and does not warrant stopping the medication and notifying the provider. Nausea and vomiting also are common adverse effects of ergotamine, and the provider may prescribe an antiemetic.

   B. Visual disturbances, such as flashing lights, are common findings associated with migraine and do not warrant stopping the medication and notifying the provider.

   C. **CORRECT:** A client who has a positive home pregnancy test should stop taking ergotamine and notify the provider. Ergotamine is classified as Pregnancy Risk Category X and can cause fetal abortion.

   D. **CORRECT:** Numbness and tingling in fingers or toes can be a finding in ergotamine overdose. The medication should be stopped and the provider notified.

   E. **CORRECT:** Unexplained muscle pain can be a finding in ergotamine overdose. The medication should be stopped and the provider notified.

   Ⓝ *NCLEX® Connection: Pharmacological and Parenteral Therapies, Adverse Effects/Contraindications/Side Effects/Interactions*

PRACTICE Answer

Using the ATI Active Learning Template: Medication

THERAPEUTIC USES: Sumatriptan is used to abort a migraine headache and associated manifestations, such as nausea and vomiting, after it begins by causing cranial artery vasoconstriction.

COMPLICATIONS: The nurse should monitor for chest and arm heaviness/pressure, angina caused by coronary vasospasm, dizziness, and vertigo.

INTERACTIONS: Toxicity can result if sumatriptan is given concurrently or within 2 weeks of an MAOI antidepressant. Sumatriptan should not be given concurrently with other triptan medications or within 24 hr of ergotamine or dihydroergotamine.

NURSING INTERVENTIONS

- Teach clients to take sumatriptan at the first sign of migraine manifestations.
- Teach client how to administer sumatriptan if it is prescribed intranasally or by subcutaneous injection.
- Monitor cardiovascular risk factors and vital signs while taking this medication.
- Advise clients to notify the provider immediately for onset of angina pain. Teach clients to distinguish transient chest or arm heaviness caused by sumatriptan from angina pain.

Ⓝ *NCLEX® Connection: Pharmacological and Parenteral Therapies, Medication Administration*

NCLEX® Connections

When reviewing the following chapters, keep in mind the relevant topics and tasks of the NCLEX outline, in particular:

Client Needs: Pharmacological and Parenteral Therapies

ADVERSE EFFECTS/CONTRAINDICATIONS/ SIDE EFFECTS/INTERACTIONS: Identify actual and potential incompatibilities of prescribed client medications.

DOSAGE CALCULATION: Use clinical decision making/ critical thinking when calculating dosages.

MEDICATION ADMINISTRATION: Mix medications from two vials when necessary.

UNIT 10   MEDICATIONS AFFECTING THE
ENDOCRINE SYSTEM

CHAPTER 39 *Diabetes Mellitus*

Diabetes mellitus is a chronic illness that results from an absolute or relative deficiency of insulin, often combined with a cellular resistance to insulin's actions. Various insulins are available to manage diabetes. These medications differ in their onset, peak, and duration.

Oral antidiabetic medications work in various ways to increase available insulin or modify carbohydrate metabolism. Newer injectable medications are used to supplement insulin or oral agents to manage glucose control.

Insulin

SELECT PROTOTYPE MEDICATIONS
- **Rapid-acting:** Lispro insulin
  - ONSET: 15 to 30 min
  - PEAK: 0.5 to 2.5 hr
  - DURATION: 3 to 6 hr
- **Short-acting:** Regular insulin
  - ONSET: 0.5 to 1 hr
  - PEAK: 1 to 5 hr
  - DURATION: 6 to 10 hr
- **Intermediate-acting:** NPH insulin
  - ONSET: 1 to 2 hr
  - PEAK: 6 to 14 hr
  - DURATION: 16 to 24 hr
- **Long-acting:** Insulin glargine
  - ONSET: 70 min
  - PEAK: None
  - DURATION: 24 hr

OTHER MEDICATIONS
- **Rapid-acting**
  - Insulin aspart
  - Insulin glulisine
- **Short-acting:** Regular insulin
- **Intermediate-acting:** Insulin detemir is dose-dependent. The greater units/kg the client receives, the longer the duration of the insulin. In some cases, the client can receive up to 0.4 units/kg, resulting in a duration of 20 to 24 hr, making it a long-acting insulin.

PREMIXED INSULINS
- **70% NPH and 30% regular**: Mixture of intermediate- and short-acting insulin
- **75% insulin lispro protamine and 25% insulin lispro:** Mixture of intermediate- and rapid-acting insulin

PURPOSE

EXPECTED PHARMACOLOGICAL ACTION
- Promotes cellular uptake of glucose (decreases glucose levels)
- Converts glucose into glycogen
- Moves potassium into cells (along with glucose)

THERAPEUTIC USES
- Insulin is used for glycemic control of diabetes mellitus (type 1, type 2, gestational) to prevent complications.
- Clients who have type 2 diabetes mellitus can require insulin when:
  - Oral antidiabetic medications, diet, and exercise are unable to control blood glucose levels.
  - Severe renal or liver disease is present.
  - Painful neuropathy is present.
  - Undergoing surgery or diagnostic tests.
  - Experiencing severe stress such as infection and trauma.
  - Undergoing emergency treatment of diabetes ketoacidosis (DKA) and hyperosmolar hyperglycemic nonketotic syndrome.
  - Requiring treatment of hyperkalemia.

COMPLICATIONS

Hypoglycemia

- Hypoglycemia occurs when blood glucose is less than 70 mg/dL.
- Hypoglycemia can result from the following.
  - Overdose of insulin
  - Too little food
  - Vomiting and diarrhea
  - Alcohol intake
  - Strenuous exercise
  - Childbirth

NURSING CONSIDERATIONS
- Monitor clients for hypoglycemia. If abrupt onset, client will experience sympathetic nervous system (SNS) effects (tachycardia, palpitations, diaphoresis, shakiness). If gradual onset, client will experience parasympathetic (PNS) manifestations (headache, tremors, weakness, lethargy, disorientation).
- Administer glucose. For conscious clients, administer a snack of 15 g carbohydrate (4 oz orange juice, 2 oz grape juice, 8 oz milk, glucose tablets per manufacturer's suggestion to equal 15 g).
- If the client is not fully conscious, do not risk aspiration. Administer glucose parenterally, such as IV glucose, or subcutaneous/IM glucagon.
- Encourage clients to wear a medical alert bracelet and to always have a snack with glucose handy.

Lipohypertrophy

CLIENT EDUCATION: Instruct clients to systematically rotate injection sites and to allow 1 inch between injection sites.

INTERACTIONS

Sulfonylureas, meglitinides, beta-blockers, and alcohol have additive hypoglycemic effects with concurrent use.
NURSING CONSIDERATIONS: Monitor serum glucose levels for hypoglycemia (less than 70 mg/dL) and adjust insulin or oral antidiabetic dosages accordingly.

Concurrent use of thiazide diuretics and glucocorticoids can raise blood glucose levels and thereby counteract the effects of insulin.
NURSING CONSIDERATIONS: Monitor serum glucose levels for hyperglycemia, and adjust insulin doses accordingly. Higher insulin doses can be indicated.

Beta blockers can mask SNS response to hypoglycemia (tachycardia, tremors), making it difficult for clients to identify hypoglycemia
NURSING CONSIDERATIONS
- Advise clients of the importance of monitoring glucose levels and not relying on SNS symptoms as an alert to developing hypoglycemia.
- Instruct clients to maintain a regular eating schedule to ensure adequate glucose during times of hypoglycemic action.

NURSING ADMINISTRATION

- Adjust the insulin dosage to meet insulin needs.
  - The dosage can need to be increased in response to increase in caloric intake, infection, stress, growth spurts, and in the second and third trimesters of pregnancy. Qᴾᶜᶜ
  - The dosage can need to be decreased in response to level of exercise or first trimester of pregnancy.
- Ensure adequate glucose is available at the time of onset of insulin and during all peak times.
- When mixing short-acting insulin with longer-acting insulin, draw the short-acting insulin up into the syringe first, then the longer-acting insulin. This prevents the possibility of accidentally injecting some of the longer-acting insulin into the shorter-acting insulin vial. (This can pose a risk for unexpected insulin effects with subsequent uses of the vial.)
- For insulin suspensions, gently rotate the vial between the palms to disperse the particles throughout the vial prior to withdrawing insulin.
- NPH and premixed insulins should appear cloudy. Do not administer other insulins if they are cloudy or any insulins that are discolored or if a precipitate is present.
- Insulin glargine and insulin detemir are both clear in color, not administered IV, and should not be mixed in a syringe with any other insulin.
- Administer lispro, aspart, glulisine, and regular insulin by subcutaneous injection, continuous subcutaneous infusion, and IV route.
- Administer NPH by subcutaneous route.
- Instruct clients to administer subcutaneous insulin in one general area to have consistent rates of absorption. Absorption rates from subcutaneous tissue increase from thigh to upper arm to abdomen.

- Use only insulin-specific syringes that correspond to the concentration of insulin being administered. Administer U-100 insulin with a U-100 syringe; administer U-500 insulin with a U-500 syringe.
- Select an appropriate needle length to ensure insulin is injected into subcutaneous tissue vs. intradermal (too short) or intramuscular (too long).
- Encourage clients to enhance diabetes medication therapy with a proper diet and consistent activity.
- Ensure proper storage of insulin.
  - Unopened vials of a single type of insulin can be stored in the refrigerator until their expiration date. Qᴱᴮᴾ
  - Vials of premixed insulins can be stored for up to 3 months under refrigeration.
  - Insulins premixed in syringes can be kept for 1 to 2 weeks under refrigeration. Keep the syringes in a vertical position, with the needles pointing up. Prior to administration, the insulin should be resuspended by gently moving the syringe.
  - Store the vial that is in use at room temperature, avoiding proximity to sunlight and intense heat. Discard after 1 month.

Oral antidiabetics

Sulfonylureas

SELECT PROTOTYPE MEDICATIONS
- **1st generation:** Chlorpropamide
- **2nd generation:** Glipizide

OTHER MEDICATIONS
- **1st generation:** Tolzamide
- **2nd generation:** Glyburide, glimepiride

Meglitinides (glinides)

SELECT PROTOTYPE MEDICATION: Repaglinide

OTHER MEDICATION: Nateglinide

Biguanides

SELECT PROTOTYPE MEDICATION: Metformin

Thiazolidinediones (glitazones)

SELECT PROTOTYPE MEDICATION: Pioglitazone

Alpha-glucosidase inhibitors

SELECT PROTOTYPE MEDICATION: Acarbose

OTHER MEDICATIONS: Miglitol

DPP-4 inhibitors (gliptins)

SELECT PROTOTYPE MEDICATION: Sitagliptin

Sodium-glucose co-transporter 2 (SGLT-2) inhibitors

SELECT PROTOTYPE MEDICATION: Canagliflozin

OTHER MEDICATIONS: Dapagliflozin

PURPOSE

EXPECTED PHARMACOLOGICAL ACTION

Sulfonylureas: Insulin release from the pancreas

Meglitinides (glinides): Insulin release from the pancreas

Biguanides
- Reduces the production of glucose within the liver through suppression of gluconeogenesis
- Increases muscles' glucose uptake and use
- First choice medication for most clients who have type 2 diabetes

Thiazolidinediones (glitazones)
- Increases cellular response to insulin by decreasing insulin resistance
- Increases glucose uptake and decreased glucose production

Alpha-glucosidase inhibitors: Slows carbohydrate absorption and digestion

DPP-4 inhibitors (gliptins)
- Augments naturally occurring incretin hormones, which promote release of insulin and decrease secretion of glucagon
- Lowers fasting and postprandial blood glucose levels

SGLT-2 inhibitors
- Used in combination with insulin for type 1 diabetes
- Limits the rise of glucose postprandial
- Excretes glucose through the urine
- Promotes weight loss

THERAPEUTIC USES

- Antidiabetic agents control blood glucose levels in clients who have type 2 diabetes mellitus and are used in conjunction with diet and exercise lifestyle changes.
- Metformin is also used to treat polycystic ovary syndrome (PCOS) (off-label use).

COMPLICATIONS

Glipizide and repaglinide

Hypoglycemia
NURSING CONSIDERATIONS
- Monitor for signs of hypoglycemia. If abrupt onset, the client will experience SNS symptoms, such as tachycardia, palpitations, diaphoresis, and shakiness. If gradual onset, the client will experience PNS symptoms, such as headache, tremors, and weakness.
- Instruct clients to self-administer a snack of 15 g carbohydrate (4 oz orange juice, 2 oz grape juice, 8 oz milk, glucose tablets per manufacturer's suggestion to equal 15 g).
- Instruct clients to notify the provider if there is a recurrent problem.
- If severe hypoglycemia occurs, IV glucose might be needed.
- Encourage clients to wear a medical alert bracelet.

Weight gain
CLIENT EDUCATION: Encourage clients to adhere to a proper diet and to increase physical activity.

Metformin

Gastrointestinal effects
- Anorexia, nausea, and diarrhea, which frequently result in weight loss of 3 to 4 kg (6.6 to 8.8 lb)
- NURSING CONSIDERATIONS
  - Effects usually subside with use.
  - Monitor for severity of these effects.
  - Discontinue the medication if necessary.

Vitamin B_{12} and folic acid deficiency
- Caused by altered absorption
- NURSING CONSIDERATIONS: Provide supplements as needed.

Lactic acidosis
- Hyperventilation, myalgia, sluggishness, somnolence: 50% mortality rate
- NURSING CONSIDERATIONS
  - Instruct clients to withhold medication if these symptoms occur, and to inform the provider immediately.
  - Severe lactic acidosis can be treated with hemodialysis.

Pioglitazone

Fluid retention
NURSING CONSIDERATIONS: Monitor for edema, weight gain, and/or indications of heart failure.

Elevations in low density lipoproteins (LDL) cholesterol
NURSING CONSIDERATIONS: Monitor cholesterol levels.

Hepatotoxicity
NURSING CONSIDERATIONS
- Perform baseline and periodic liver function tests.
- Instruct clients to report any hepatotoxicity symptoms, such as jaundice or dark urine.

Acarbose

Gastrointestinal effects
- Abdominal distention and cramping, hyperactive bowel sounds, diarrhea, excessive gas
- NURSING CONSIDERATIONS
  - Monitor impact of these effects on the client.
  - Discontinue the medication if necessary.

Anemia due to the decrease of iron absorption
NURSING CONSIDERATIONS
- Monitor hemoglobin and iron levels.
- Discontinue the medication if necessary.

Hepatotoxicity with long-term use
NURSING CONSIDERATIONS
- Check baseline liver function and perform periodic liver function tests.
- Discontinue the medication if elevations occur.
- Liver function will return to normal after the medication is discontinued.

Sitagliptin

Generally well tolerated

Canagliflozin

Cystitis, candidiasis, and polyuria in women
NURSING CONSIDERATIONS: Monitor for signs of infection.

Dizziness and risk for hypotension
- In older adults with concurrent use of diuretics
- NURSING CONSIDERATIONS
  - Advise clients to rise slowly from a seated position and report episodes of dizziness to the provider.
  - Use caution if medications are given together.

CONTRAINDICATIONS/PRECAUTIONS

- PREGNANCY RISK CATEGORY C: Glipizide, repaglinide, pioglitazone, canagliflozin Qs
- PREGNANCY RISK CATEGORY B: Metformin, acarbose, sitagliptin. These oral agents are generally avoided in pregnancy and lactation, but the provider may prescribe them.
- Use cautiously in clients who have renal failure, hepatic dysfunction, or heart failure due to the risk of medication accumulation and resulting hypoglycemia. Severity of disease can indicate contraindication.
- All oral diabetic medications are contraindicated in the treatment of DKA.
- **Metformin** is contraindicated for clients who have severe infection, shock, and any hypoxic condition. The medication should not be used by clients who have alcohol use disorder.
- **Acarbose** is contraindicated for clients who have gastrointestinal disorders, such as inflammatory disease, ulceration, or obstruction.
- **Pioglitazone** is contraindicated for clients who have severe heart failure, history of bladder cancer, and active hepatic disease. Use cautiously in clients who have mild heart failure and in older adults. Ⓒ
- **Canagliflozin** is contraindicated for clients who have renal failure and are undergoing dialysis.

INTERACTIONS

Glipizide

Use of alcohol can result in disulfiram-like reaction (intense nausea and vomiting, flushing, palpitations).
CLIENT EDUCATION: Inform clients about the risk, and encourage them to avoid alcohol.

NSAIDs, sulfonamide antibiotics, ranitidine, and cimetidine have additive hypoglycemic effect.
NURSING CONSIDERATIONS
- Instruct clients to closely monitor glucose levels when these other agents are used concurrently.
- Dosage adjustment of the oral antidiabetic medication might be indicated.

Beta-blockers can mask SNS response to hypoglycemia (tachycardia, tremors, palpitations, diaphoresis), making it difficult for clients to identify hypoglycemia.
NURSING CONSIDERATIONS
- Advise clients of the importance of monitoring glucose levels and not relying on SNS symptoms as an alert to developing hypoglycemia.
- Instruct client to maintain a regular eating schedule to ensure adequate glucose during times of hypoglycemic action.

Beta-blockers decrease effectiveness by inhibiting insulin release.
CLIENT EDUCATION: Instruct clients to closely monitor glucose levels.

Repaglinide

Concurrent use of gemfibrozil results in inhibition of repaglinide metabolism, leading to an increased risk for hypoglycemia.
NURSING CONSIDERATIONS
- Avoid concurrent use of repaglinide or pioglitazone and gemfibrozil.
- Closely monitor for signs of hypoglycemia.

Pioglitazone

Use with insulin can lead to fluid retention.
NURSING CONSIDERATIONS: Avoid concurrent use.

Increased levels with atorvastatin and ketoconazole.
NURSING CONSIDERATIONS: Monitor glucose levels. Dosage of pioglitazone might need to be reduced.

Decreased levels with rifampin and cimetidine.
NURSING CONSIDERATIONS: Monitor glucose levels. Dosage of pioglitazone might need to be increased.

Metformin

Alcohol increases the risk of lactic acidosis with concurrent use.
CLIENT EDUCATION: Inform clients of the risks, and encourage clients to avoid consuming alcohol.

Concurrent use of iodine-containing contrast media can result in acute kidney failure.
NURSING CONSIDERATIONS: Clients taking metformin should discontinue medication 24 to 48 hr prior to procedure. They can resume medication 48 hr after test if lab results indicate normal kidney function.

Acarbose

Concurrent use of acarbose with sulfonylureas or insulin increases the risk for hypoglycemia.
NURSING CONSIDERATIONS: Monitor carefully for hypoglycemia.

Concurrent use of metformin causes additive gastrointestinal effects and risk for hypoglycemia.
NURSING CONSIDERATIONS: Monitor carefully for gastrointestinal effects and hypoglycemia.

Sitagliptin

No significant interactions

Canagliflozin

Decreased effect if used concurrently with rifampin, phenytoin, or phenobarbital
NURSING CONSIDERATIONS: Monitor glucose levels, as dosage might need to be increased.

Increases the effect of thiazide and loop diuretics
NURSING CONSIDERATIONS: Monitor for dehydration and hypotension. Use caution if medications are used together.

NURSING ADMINISTRATION

- Encourage clients to exercise consistently and to follow appropriate dietary guidelines.
- Encourage clients to maintain a log of glucose levels and to note patterns that affect glucose levels (increased dietary intake, infection).
- Consider referring clients to a registered dietitian or diabetic nurse educator. Qᴛᴄ
- Administer medications orally and at appropriate times.
  - **Glipizide:** Best taken with breakfast.
  - **Repaglinide:** Instruct clients to eat within 30 min of taking a dose of the medication, three times per day.
  - **Metformin:** Instruct clients to take immediate release tablets two times per day with breakfast and dinner and to take sustained-release tablets once daily with dinner.
  - **Pioglitazone:** Instruct clients to take once a day, with or without food.
  - **Acarbose:** Instruct clients to take with the first bite of food, three times per day. If a dose is missed, take the dose at the next meal but do not take two doses.
  - **Sitagliptin:** Instruct clients to take once a day with or without food.
  - **Canagliflozin:** Instruct clients to take once a day, before breakfast.
- Instruct clients that formulations can combine two medications.
- Instruct clients who are also taking insulin to monitor for signs of hypoglycemia.

Amylin mimetics

SELECT PROTOTYPE MEDICATION: Pramlintide

PURPOSE

EXPECTED PHARMACOLOGICAL ACTION

Pramlintide mimics the actions of the naturally occurring peptide hormone amylin, resulting in reduction of postprandial glucose levels from decreased gastric emptying time and inhibition of secretion of glucagon. There is also an increase in the sensation of satiety, which helps decrease caloric intake.

THERAPEUTIC USES

- Supplemental glucose control for clients who have type 1 or type 2 diabetes mellitus
- Can be used in conjunction with insulin or an oral antidiabetic medication, usually metformin and/or a sulfonylurea

COMPLICATIONS

Nausea
CLIENT EDUCATION: Instruct clients to report manifestations to the provider. Dose can be decreased.

Reaction at injection sites
Generally self-limiting.

CONTRAINDICATIONS/PRECAUTIONS

- Pregnancy Risk Category C. Qs
- This medication is contraindicated for clients who have kidney failure or are receiving dialysis.
- Use cautiously in clients who have thyroid disease, osteoporosis, or alcohol use disorder.

INTERACTIONS

Insulin increases the risk for hypoglycemia.
NURSING CONSIDERATIONS: Concurrent use can require a decrease in insulin dose, usually 50% of rapid- or short-acting insulin. Avoid use in clients unable to self-monitor blood glucose levels.

Concurrent use of pramlintide with medications that slow gastric emptying, such as opioids, or medications that delay food absorption, such as acarbose, can further slow gastric emptying time.
NURSING CONSIDERATIONS: Avoid concurrent use.

Oral medication absorption is delayed.
NURSING CONSIDERATIONS: Administer oral medications 1 hr before or 2 hr after injection of pramlintide.

NURSING ADMINISTRATION

- Administer subcutaneously prior to meals, using the thigh or abdomen. ⓠEBP
- Instruct clients to keep unopened vials in the refrigerator and not to freeze. Opened vials can be kept cool or at room temperature but should be discarded after 28 days. Keep vials out of direct sunlight.
- Instruct clients not to mix medication with insulin in the same syringe.

Incretin mimetics

SELECT PROTOTYPE MEDICATION: Exenatide

OTHER MEDICATIONS
- Liraglutide
- Albiglutide

PURPOSE

EXPECTED PHARMACOLOGICAL ACTION

Mimics the effects of naturally occurring glucagon-like peptide-1, and thereby promotes release of insulin, decreases secretion of glucagon, and slows gastric emptying. Fasting and postprandial blood glucose levels are lowered. Incretin mimetics decrease appetite which can lead to weight loss.

THERAPEUTIC USES

- Supplemental glucose control for clients who have type 2 diabetes
- Can be used in conjunction with an oral antidiabetic medication, usually metformin or a sulfonylurea

COMPLICATIONS

GI effects (nausea, vomiting, diarrhea)
CLIENT EDUCATION: Instruct the client to notify the provider if manifestations are intolerable.

Pancreatitis (severe and intolerable abdominal pain)
CLIENT EDUCATION: Instruct the client to withhold medication and to notify the provider.

CONTRAINDICATIONS/PRECAUTIONS

- Pregnancy Risk Category C. ⓠs
- Contraindicated for clients who have kidney failure, ulcerative colitis, Crohn's disease, or a history of pancreatitis.
- Use cautiously in older adult clients and clients who have renal impairment or thyroid disease. ⓖ

INTERACTIONS

Oral medication absorption is delayed, especially oral contraceptives, antibiotics, and acetaminophen.
NURSING CONSIDERATIONS: Administer oral medications 1 hr before injection of exenatide.

Concurrent use of sulfonylurea increases risk of hypoglycemia.
NURSING CONSIDERATIONS: Clients can require a lower dose of sulfonylurea. Instruct clients to monitor blood glucose levels.

NURSING ADMINISTRATION

- This medication is supplied in prefilled injector pens.
- Administer subcutaneously in the thigh, abdomen, or upper arm. ⓠEBP
- Give exenatide injection within 60 min before the morning and evening meal. Never administer after a meal. Exenatide is also available in a longer-acting formula that can be administered once weekly. Liraglutide is administered once a day without regard to meals. Albiglutide is administered once weekly.
- Instruct clients to keep the injection pen in the refrigerator and to discard after 30 days.

NURSING EVALUATION OF MEDICATION EFFECTIVENESS

Depending on therapeutic intent, effectiveness can be evidenced by the following.
- Preprandial glucose levels 90 to 130 mg/dL and postprandial levels less than 180 mg/dL
- HbA1c less than 7%

Hyperglycemic agent

SELECT PROTOTYPE MEDICATION: Glucagon

PURPOSE

EXPECTED PHARMACOLOGICAL ACTION

Increases blood glucose levels by increasing the breakdown of glycogen into glucose; decreasing glycogen synthesis enhances the synthesis of glucose

THERAPEUTIC USES

- Emergency management of hypoglycemic reactions, such as insulin overdose, in clients who are unable to take oral glucose
- Decrease in gastrointestinal motility in clients undergoing radiological procedures of the stomach and intestines

COMPLICATIONS

GI distress (nausea, vomiting)
NURSING CONSIDERATIONS: Turn clients onto the left side following administration to reduce the risk of aspiration if emesis occurs.

CONTRAINDICATIONS/PRECAUTIONS

- Glucagon is ineffective for hypoglycemia resulting from inadequate glycogen stores (starvation).
- Pregnancy Risk Category B. Qs
- Use cautiously in clients who have cardiovascular disease.

NURSING ADMINISTRATION

- Administer glucagon subcutaneously, IM, or IV immediately following reconstitution parameters. QEBP
- Provide food as soon as the client regains full consciousness and is able to swallow.
- Instruct clients to maintain access to a source of glucose and glucagon kit at all times.

NURSING EVALUATION OF MEDICATION EFFECTIVENESS

Depending on therapeutic intent, effectiveness can be evidenced by elevation in blood glucose level to greater than 70 mg/dL.

Application Exercises

1. A nurse is teaching clients in an outpatient facility about the use of insulin to treat type 1 diabetes mellitus. For which of the following types of insulin should the nurse tell the clients to expect a peak effect 1 to 5 hr after administration?

   A. Insulin glargine

   B. NPH insulin

   C. Regular insulin

   D. Insulin lispro

2. A nurse is caring for a client in an outpatient facility who has been taking acarbose for type 2 diabetes mellitus. Which of the following laboratory tests should the nurse plan to monitor?

   A. WBC

   B. Serum potassium

   C. Platelet count

   D. Liver function tests

3. A nurse is providing teaching to a client who has type 2 diabetes mellitus and is starting repaglinide. Which of the following statements by the client indicates understanding of the administration of this medication?

   A. "I'll take this medication after I eat."

   B. "I'll take this medicine 30 minutes before I eat."

   C. "I'll take this medicine just before I go to bed."

   D. "I'll take this medicine as soon as I wake up in the morning."

4. A nurse is providing teaching for a client who has a new prescription for metformin. Which of the following adverse effects of metformin should the nurse instruct the client to report to the provider?

   A. Somnolence

   B. Constipation

   C. Fluid retention

   D. Weight gain

5. A nurse is providing teaching to a client who has a prescription for pramlintide for type 1 diabetes mellitus. Which of the following should the nurse include in the teaching? (Select all that apply.)

   A. "Take oral medications 1 hr before injection."

   B. "Use upper arms as preferred injection sites."

   C. "Mix pramlintide with breakfast dose of insulin."

   D. "Inject pramlintide just before a meal."

   E. "Discard open vials after 28 days."

PRACTICE Active Learning Scenario

A nurse in an acute care facility is teaching a client who has type 2 diabetes mellitus and is taking exenatide along with an oral antidiabetic agent. What should the nurse teach the client about this medication? Use the ATI Active Learning Template: Medication to complete this item.

THERAPEUTIC USES: Identify the therapeutic use for exenatide in this client.

COMPLICATIONS: Identify two adverse effects the client should watch for.

NURSING INTERVENTIONS: Describe two laboratory tests the nurse should monitor.

CLIENT EDUCATION: Describe teaching points to give a client taking exenatide.

Application Exercises Key

1. A. Insulin glargine, a long-acting insulin, does not have a peak effect time, but is fairly stable in effect after metabolized.

   B. NPH insulin has a peak effect around 6 to 14 hr following administration.

   C. **CORRECT:** Regular insulin has a peak effect around 1 to 5 hr following administration.

   D. Insulin lispro has a peak effect around 30 min to 2.5 hr following administration.

   Ⓝ NCLEX® Connection: Pharmacological and Parenteral Therapies, Medication Administration

2. A. Infection is not an adverse effect of acarbose. It is not necessary to monitor WBC while the client is taking this medication.

   B. Acarbose does not affect potassium levels. It is not necessary to monitor serum potassium while the client is taking this medication.

   C. Acarbose does not affect the platelet levels. It is not necessary to monitor the platelet count while the client is taking this medication.

   D. **CORRECT:** Acarbose can cause liver toxicity when taken long-term. Liver function tests should be monitored periodically while the client takes this medication.

   Ⓝ NCLEX® Connection: Pharmacological and Parenteral Therapies, Expected Actions/Outcomes

3. A. Repaglinide is a meglitinide agent that is short-acting. It is taken prior to meals.

   B. **CORRECT:** Repaglinide causes a rapid, short-lived release of insulin. The client should take this medication within 30 min before each meal so that insulin is available when food is digested.

   C. Repaglinide should not be taken just before bedtime.

   D. Repaglinide is not taken upon awakening in the morning.

   Ⓝ NCLEX® Connection: Pharmacological and Parenteral Therapies, Medication Administration

4. A. **CORRECT:** Somnolence can indicate lactic acidosis, which is manifested by extreme drowsiness, hyperventilation, and muscle pain. It is a rare but very serious adverse effect caused by metformin and should be reported to the provider.

   B. Diarrhea is an adverse effect of metformin.

   C. Fluid retention is not an adverse effect caused by metformin.

   D. Anorexia and weight loss are adverse effects of metformin.

   Ⓝ NCLEX® Connection: Pharmacological and Parenteral Therapies, Adverse Effects/Contraindications/Side Effects/Interactions

5. A. Pramlintide delays oral medication absorption, so oral medications should be taken 1 to 2 hr after pramlintide injection.

   B. The thigh or abdomen, rather than the upper arms, are preferred sites for pramlintide injection.

   C. Pramlintide should not be mixed in a syringe with any type of insulin.

   D. **CORRECT:** Pramlintide can cause hypoglycemia, especially when the client also takes insulin, so it is important to eat a meal after injecting this medication.

   E. **CORRECT:** Unused medication in the open pramlintide vial should be discarded after 28 days.

   Ⓝ NCLEX® Connection: Pharmacological and Parenteral Therapies, Medication Administration

---

PRACTICE Answer

Using the ATI Active Learning Template: Medication

THERAPEUTIC USES: Exenatide is prescribed along with an oral antidiabetic medication, such as metformin or a sulfonylurea medication, for clients who have type 2 diabetes mellitus to improve diabetes control. Exenatide improves insulin secretion by the pancreas, decreases secretion of glucagon, and slows gastric emptying.

COMPLICATIONS
- GI effects, such as nausea and vomiting
- Pancreatitis manifested by acute abdominal pain and possibly severe vomiting
- Hypoglycemia, especially when taken concurrently with a sulfonylurea medication, such as glipizide

NURSING INTERVENTIONS: The nurse should monitor daily blood glucose testing by the client, periodic HbA1c tests, and periodic kidney function testing. Exenatide should be used cautiously in clients who have any renal impairment.

Ⓝ NCLEX® Connection: Pharmacological and Parenteral Therapies, Medication Administration

CLIENT EDUCATION
- Instruct the client how to inject exenatide subcutaneously.
- Teach the client to take exenatide within 60 min before the morning and evening meal but not following the meal.
- Advise the client to withhold exenatide and notify the provider for severe abdominal pain.
- Teach the client how to recognize and treat hypoglycemia.
- Teach the client that exenatide should not be given within 1 hr of oral antibiotics, acetaminophen, or an oral contraceptive due to its ability to slow gastric emptying.

CHAPTER 40 Endocrine Disorders

The endocrine system is made up of glands that secrete hormones, which act on specific receptor sites. Hormones target receptor sites to regulate response to stress, growth, metabolism, and homeostasis.

An endocrine disorder usually involves the oversecretion or undersecretion of hormones, or an altered response by the target area or receptor.

Medications used to treat disorders of the thyroid, anterior and posterior pituitary, and adrenal glands are discussed in this chapter.

Thyroid hormone

SELECT PROTOTYPE MEDICATION: Levothyroxine

OTHER MEDICATIONS
- Liothyronine
- Liotrix
- Thyroid USP

PURPOSE

EXPECTED PHARMACOLOGICAL ACTION: Thyroid hormones are a synthetic form of thyroxine (T_4), a form of liothyronine (T_3), or a combination of T_3 and T_4, that increase metabolic rate, protein synthesis, cardiac output, renal perfusion, oxygen use, body temperature, blood volume, and growth processes.

THERAPEUTIC USES
- Thyroid hormone replacement is used for treatment of hypothyroidism (all ages, all forms).
- Thyroid hormones are used for the emergency treatment of myxedema coma (IV route), a severe deficiency of thyroid hormone.

ROUTE OF ADMINISTRATION: Oral, IV (myxedema coma)

COMPLICATIONS

Overmedication

Overmedication can result in indications of hyperthyroidism (anxiety, tachycardia, palpitations, altered appetite, abdominal cramping, heat intolerance, fever, diaphoresis, weight loss, menstrual irregularities).

CLIENT EDUCATION: Instruct clients to report indications of overmedication to the provider.

Chronic overtreatment

Chronic overtreatment can cause atrial fibrillation and an increased risk of fractures from bone loss, especially in older adults.

NURSING CONSIDERATIONS: TSH levels should be monitored at least once a year.

CONTRAINDICATIONS/PRECAUTIONS

- Pregnancy Risk Category A.
- Use is contraindicated for clients who have thyrotoxicosis and adrenal insufficiency.
- Because of cardiac stimulant effects, use is contraindicated following a MI.
- Use cautiously in clients who have cardiovascular problems (hypertension, angina pectoris, ischemic heart disease) because of cardiac stimulant effects.
- Use cautiously in older adults. Ⓒ
- Use cautiously in clients who have diabetes.
- Thyroid hormone replacement is not for use in the treatment of obesity.

INTERACTIONS

Binding agents, antiulcer medications, calcium and iron supplements, and food reduce levothyroxine absorption with concurrent use.
- Binding agents include cholestyramine and colestipol. Antiulcer medications include sucralfate, cimetidine, lansoprazole, and antacids.
- NURSING CONSIDERATIONS: Allow at least 4 hr between medication administration.

Many antiseizure and antidepressant medications, including carbamazepine, phenytoin, phenobarbital, and sertraline, can increase levothyroxine metabolism.
NURSING CONSIDERATIONS: Monitor for therapeutic effects of levothyroxine. Dosages of levothyroxine might need to be increased.

Levothyroxine can increase the anticoagulant effects of warfarin by breaking down vitamin K.
NURSING CONSIDERATIONS
- Monitor prothrombin time (PT) and international normalized ratio (INR).
- Instruct clients to report signs of bleeding (bruising, petechiae).
- Decreased dosages of warfarin can be needed.

NURSING ADMINISTRATION

- Obtain baseline vital signs, weight, and height, and monitor periodically throughout treatment.
- Monitor and report signs of cardiac excitability (angina, chest pain, palpitations, dysrhythmias).
- Daily therapy begins with a low dose that increases gradually over several weeks. Full effect of medication can take 6 to 8 weeks.
- Monitor T_4 and TSH levels.
- Instruct clients to take the medication daily on an empty stomach 30 to 60 min before breakfast.
- Provide client education regarding the importance of lifelong replacement (even after improvement of symptoms). Advise clients not to discontinue the medication without checking with the provider.
- Instruct clients to check with the provider before switching to another brand of levothyroxine because some concerns regarding interchangeability of brands have been raised, and dosage adjustments can be necessary. Qᴛᴄ

NURSING EVALUATION OF MEDICATION EFFECTIVENESS

Depending on therapeutic intent, evidence of effectiveness can include the following.
- Decreased TSH levels
- T_4 levels within expected reference range
- Absence of hypothyroidism manifestations (depression, weight gain, bradycardia, anorexia, cold intolerance, dry skin, menorrhagia)

Thionamides

SELECT PROTOTYPE MEDICATION: Propylthiouracil

OTHER MEDICATION: Methimazole

PURPOSE

EXPECTED PHARMACOLOGICAL ACTION
- Blocks the synthesis of thyroid hormones
- Prevents the oxidation of iodide
- Blocks conversion of T_4 into T_3

THERAPEUTIC USES
- Treatment of Graves' disease
- Produces a euthyroid state prior to thyroid removal surgery
- As an adjunct to irradiation of the thyroid gland
- In the emergency treatment of thyrotoxicosis
- Methimazole is considered first-line therapy

ROUTE OF ADMINISTRATION: Oral

COMPLICATIONS

Hypothyroidism

Overmedication can result in indications of hypothyroidism (drowsiness, depression, weight gain, edema, bradycardia, anorexia, cold intolerance, dry skin, menorrhagia).

NURSING CONSIDERATIONS
- Instruct clients to report signs of overmedication to the provider.
- Reduced dosages and/or temporary administration of thyroid supplements can be needed.

Agranulocytosis

NURSING CONSIDERATIONS
- Monitor for early indications of agranulocytosis (sore throat, fever, fatigue), and instruct clients to report them promptly to provider.
- Monitor blood counts at baseline and periodically.
- If agranulocytosis occurs, stop treatment and monitor the client for reversal of agranulocytosis.
- Neupogen can be indicated to treat agranulocytosis.

Liver injury, hepatitis (propylthiouracil)

NURSING CONSIDERATIONS: Monitor for jaundice, dark urine, light-colored stools, and elevated liver function tests during treatment.

CONTRAINDICATIONS/PRECAUTIONS

- Use is contraindicated in pregnancy (Pregnancy Risk Category D) and during lactation due to the risk of neonatal hypothyroidism. Propylthiouracil is safer than methimazole during the first trimester of pregnancy and is considered safer during lactation if an antithyroid medication is necessary. Qs
- Use cautiously in clients who have bone marrow depression and/or immunosuppression, and in clients at risk for liver failure.

INTERACTIONS

Concurrent use of antithyroid medications and anticoagulants can increase anticoagulation.
NURSING CONSIDERATIONS: Monitor PT, INR, and activated partial thromboplastin time (aPTT), and adjust dosages of anticoagulants accordingly.

Concurrent use of antithyroid medications and digoxin can increase glycoside level.
NURSING CONSIDERATIONS: Monitor digoxin level and reduce digoxin dose as needed.

NURSING ADMINISTRATION

- Advise clients that therapeutic effects can take 1 to 2 weeks to be evident, while full benefit can take 3 to 12 weeks. Q**pcc**
- Propylthiouracil does not destroy the thyroid hormone that is present, but rather prevents continued synthesis of TH.
- Monitor vital signs, weight, and I&O at baseline and periodically.
- Instruct clients to take medication at consistent times each day and with meals to maintain a consistent therapeutic level and decrease gastric distress.
- Instruct clients not to discontinue the medication abruptly (risk of thyroid crisis due to stress response).
- Monitor for signs of hyperthyroidism (indicating inadequate medication).
- Clients who have hyperthyroidism may be given a beta-adrenergic antagonist, such as propranolol, to decrease tremors and tachycardia.
- Monitor for indications of hypothyroidism (indicating overmedication), such as drowsiness, depression, weight gain, edema, bradycardia, anorexia, cold intolerance, and dry skin.
- Monitor CBC for leukopenia or thrombocytopenia.
- Instruct clients to not take any OTC medications without consent of provider.
- Advise clients to avoid consumption of seafood, which contains iodine, and other iodine products.

NURSING EVALUATION OF MEDICATION EFFECTIVENESS

Depending on therapeutic intent, evidence of effectiveness can include the following.
- Weight gain
- Vital signs within expected reference range
- Decreased T_4 levels
- Absence of signs of hyperthyroidism (anxiety, tachycardia, palpitations, increased appetite, abdominal cramping, heat intolerance, fever, diaphoresis, weight loss, menstrual irregularities)

Radiopharmaceuticals

SELECT PROTOTYPE MEDICATION: Radioactive iodine (^{131}I)

PURPOSE

EXPECTED PHARMACOLOGICAL ACTION: Radioactive iodine is absorbed by the thyroid and destroys some of the thyroid producing cells. At high doses, thyroid-radioactive iodine destroys thyroid cells.

THERAPEUTIC USES
- At high doses:
  - Hyperthyroidism
  - Thyroid cancer
  - Clients who have not responded to other antithyroid treatments
- At low doses:
  - Thyroid function studies (Visualization of the degree of iodine uptake by the thyroid gland is helpful in the diagnosis of thyroid disorders.)

ROUTE OF ADMINISTRATION: Oral

COMPLICATIONS

Radiation sickness

NURSING CONSIDERATIONS
- Monitor for manifestations of radiation sickness (hematemesis, epistaxis, intense nausea, vomiting).
- Stop treatment and notify the provider.

Bone marrow depression

NURSING CONSIDERATIONS: Monitor for anemia, leukopenia, and thrombocytopenia.

Hypothyroidism

Intolerance to cold, edema, bradycardia, weight gain, depression

CLIENT EDUCATION: Instruct clients to report indications of hypothyroidism to the provider.

CONTRAINDICATIONS/PRECAUTIONS

Because of irradiating effects, use is contraindicated in pregnancy (Pregnancy Risk Category X), clients of childbearing age/intent, and during lactation. Q**s**

INTERACTIONS

Concurrent use of other antithyroid medications reduces uptake of radioactive iodine.
NURSING CONSIDERATIONS: Discontinue use of other antithyroid medications for a week prior to therapy.

NURSING ADMINISTRATION

Instruct clients regarding radioactivity precautions.
- Maintain a distance of 6 feet from others. Do not prepare food for others or share utensils. Qᴘᴄᴄ
- Limit contact with clients to 30 min/day/person.
- Encourage clients to increase fluid intake, usually 2 to 3 L/day.
- Instruct clients to dispose of body wastes per protocol.
- Instruct clients to avoid coughing and expectoration (source of radioactive iodine).

Iodine products

SELECT PROTOTYPE MEDICATION: Strong iodine solution: nonradioactive iodine

OTHER MEDICATIONS
- Sodium iodide
- Potassium iodide

PURPOSE

EXPECTED PHARMACOLOGICAL ACTION: Nonradioactive iodine creates high levels of iodide that will reduce iodine uptake (by the thyroid gland), inhibit thyroid hormone production, and block the release of thyroid hormones into the bloodstream.

THERAPEUTIC USES
- Nonradioactive iodine is used for the development of euthyroid state and reduction of thyroid gland size prior to thyroid removal surgery.
- Nonradioactive iodine is used for the emergency treatment of thyrotoxicosis.

ROUTE OF ADMINISTRATION: Oral

COMPLICATIONS

Iodism

- Due to corrosive property (metallic taste, stomatitis, sore teeth and gums, frontal headache, skin rash).
- Iodism (early toxicity) can progress to overdose (severe GI distress and swelling of the glottis).

NURSING CONSIDERATIONS
- Teach clients to notify provider for any manifestations of overdose.
- Prepare to administer sodium thiosulfate (to reverse effects of iodine). Assist with gastric lavage as needed.

CONTRAINDICATIONS/PRECAUTIONS

Use in pregnancy is contraindicated (Pregnancy Risk Category D). Qs

INTERACTIONS

Concurrent intake of foods high in iodine (iodized salt, seafood containing iodine) increases risk for iodism.
NURSING CONSIDERATIONS:
- Monitor for signs of iodism (brassy taste in mouth, burning sensation in mouth, sore teeth).
- Instruct clients regarding foods high in iodine.

Concurrent use of potassium-sparing diuretics, potassium supplements, and ACE inhibitors increases the risk of hyperkalemia.
NURSING CONSIDERATIONS: Do not use medications together.

NURSING ADMINISTRATION

- Nonradioactive iodine can be used in conjunction with other therapy because effects are not usually complete or permanent. Qᴘᴄᴄ
- Obtain baseline vital signs, weight, and I&O, and monitor periodically.
- Instruct clients to dilute strong iodine solution with juice to improve taste.
- Instruct clients to take at the same time each day to maintain therapeutic levels.
- Encourage clients to increase fluid intake, unless contraindicated.
- Instruct clients to not take any OTC medications that contain iodine.
- Instruct clients not to discontinue medication abruptly.

NURSING EVALUATION OF MEDICATION EFFECTIVENESS

Depending on therapeutic intent, effectiveness can be evidenced by the following.
- Weight gain
- Vital signs within expected reference range
- Decreased T_4 levels
- Reduction in size of thyroid gland
- Client will be able to get adequate sleep, achieve and maintain appropriate weight, maintain blood pressure and heart rate within expected reference range, and be free of complications of hyperthyroidism.

Anterior pituitary hormones/ growth hormones

SELECT PROTOTYPE MEDICATION: Somatropin

PURPOSE

EXPECTED PHARMACOLOGICAL ACTION: Anterior pituitary hormones/growth hormones stimulate overall growth and the production of protein, and decrease the use of glucose.

THERAPEUTIC USES
- Anterior pituitary hormones/growth hormones are used to treat growth hormone deficiencies (pediatric and adult growth hormone deficiencies, Turner's syndrome, Prader-Willi syndrome).
- AIDS wasting syndrome

ROUTES OF ADMINISTRATION: IM or subcutaneous (preferred route)

COMPLICATIONS

Hyperglycemia

NURSING CONSIDERATIONS
- Observe for indications of hyperglycemia (polyphagia, polydipsia, polyuria).
- Monitor glucose levels when used in clients who have diabetes. Insulin doses can need to be adjusted.

Hypercalciuria and renal calculi

CLIENT EDUCATION: Teach clients to monitor for flank pain, fever, and dysuria, and report these to the provider.

CONTRAINDICATIONS/PRECAUTIONS

- These medications are Pregnancy Risk Category B or C (depending on the brand prescribed). Qs
- Use is contraindicated in clients who are severely obese or have severe respiratory impairment (sleep apnea) because of higher risk of fatality.
- Use cautiously in clients who have diabetes because of the risk of hyperglycemia.
- Use cautiously in clients who have hypothyroidism, as thyroid function can be suppressed. Evaluate thyroid function prior to administering and periodically.
- Treatment should be stopped prior to epiphyseal closure.

INTERACTIONS

Concurrent use of glucocorticoids can counteract growth-promoting effects.
NURSING CONSIDERATIONS: Avoid concurrent use of glucocorticoids and somatrem if possible.

NURSING ADMINISTRATION

- Obtain baseline height and weight.
- Monitor growth patterns during medication administration, usually monthly. Qpcc
- Reconstitute medication per directions. Mix gently, and do not shake prior to administration. Do not administer if medication contains particulates or is discolored.
- Rotate injection sites. Abdomen (subcutaneous) and thighs (subcutaneous, IM) are preferred.

NURSING EVALUATION OF MEDICATION EFFECTIVENESS

Depending on therapeutic intent, effectiveness can be evidenced by the client increasing height and weight.

Antidiuretic hormone

SELECT PROTOTYPE MEDICATION: Vasopressin

OTHER MEDICATION: Desmopressin

PURPOSE

EXPECTED PHARMACOLOGICAL ACTION
- Antidiuretic hormone (ADH), produced by the hypothalamus and stored in the posterior pituitary, promotes reabsorption of water within the kidney.
- Natural ADH causes vasoconstriction due to the contraction of vascular smooth muscle. Vasopressin simulates the potent action of ADH, while desmopressin causes much less vasoconstriction.

THERAPEUTIC USES
- These hormones are used to treat diabetes insipidus (DI). Desmopressin is the agent of choice for DI.
- Antidiuretic hormone (vasopressin) is sometimes used during CPR to temporarily decrease blood flow to the periphery and increase flow to the brain and heart.

ROUTE OF ADMINISTRATION
- Desmopressin: Oral, intranasal, subcutaneous, IV
- Vasopressin: Subcutaneous, IM, IV

COMPLICATIONS

Reabsorption of too much water

NURSING CONSIDERATIONS
- Monitor for indications of overhydration (sleepiness, pounding headache). Instruct clients to notify the provider of symptoms.
- In general, clients should reduce fluid intake during therapy.
- Clients should use the smallest effective dose of desmopressin.

Myocardial ischemia

From excessive vasoconstriction (vasopressin)

NURSING CONSIDERATIONS: Monitor ECG and blood pressure. Advise clients to notify the provider of chest pain, tightness, or diaphoresis.

CONTRAINDICATIONS/PRECAUTIONS

- Use of vasopressin is contraindicated in clients who have coronary artery disease (risk for angina, MI), decreased peripheral circulation (risk for gangrene), or chronic nephritis. Qs
- Vasopressin is Pregnancy Risk Category C, and desmopressin is Pregnancy Risk Category B.
- Use caution in clients who have renal impairment, as risk of water intoxication is increased. ADH should not be administered to clients who have creatinine clearance less than 50 mL/min.

INTERACTIONS

Carbamazepine and tricyclic antidepressants can increase the antidiuretic action.
NURSING CONSIDERATIONS: Use cautiously together.

Concurrent use of alcohol, heparin, lithium, and phenytoin can decrease antidiuretic effects.
NURSING CONSIDERATIONS: Establish baseline I&O and weight, and monitor frequently.

NURSING ADMINISTRATION

- Monitor vital signs, central venous pressure, I&O, specific gravity, and laboratory studies (potassium, sodium, BUN, creatinine, specific gravity, osmolality).
- Monitor blood pressure and heart rate.
- Monitor for headache, confusion, or other indications of water intoxication.
- With IV administration of vasopressin, monitor the IV site carefully because extravasation can lead to gangrene.
- Intranasal desmopressin starts with a bedtime dose. I&O is monitored. When nocturia is controlled, doses are given twice daily.

NURSING EVALUATION OF MEDICATION EFFECTIVENESS

Depending on therapeutic intent, evidence of effectiveness can include the following.
- Reduction in the large volumes of urine output associated with diabetes insipidus to normal levels of urine output (1.5 to 2 L/24 hr)
- Cardiac arrest survival

Adrenal hormone replacement

SELECT PROTOTYPE MEDICATION: Hydrocortisone

OTHER MEDICATIONS
- Glucocorticoids
  - Prednisone
  - Dexamethasone
- Mineralocorticoid: Fludrocortisone

PURPOSE

EXPECTED PHARMACOLOGICAL ACTION: Mimic effect of natural steroid hormones

THERAPEUTIC USES
- Acute and chronic replacement therapy for adrenocortical insufficiency (Addison's disease, adrenal crisis).
- Nonendocrine disorders include cancer, inflammation, and allergic reactions.

ROUTE OF ADMINISTRATION: Oral, IV

COMPLICATIONS

Glucocorticoids: hydrocortisone

Osteoporosis
CLIENT EDUCATION: Advise clients to take calcium supplements, vitamin D, and/or bisphosphonate, and to get regular exercise.

Adrenal suppression
NURSING CONSIDERATIONS
- Advise clients to observe for manifestations (fatigue, muscle weakness, weight loss, hypotension), and to notify the provider if they occur.
- Increase dose with stress. Do not stop the medication suddenly. Taper dose to discontinue.

Peptic ulcer, GI discomfort
NURSING CONSIDERATIONS
- Advise clients to observe for manifestations (coffee-ground emesis, bloody or tarry stools, abdominal pain), and to notify the provider if they occur.
- Administer prophylactic H_2 receptor antagonists.

Infection
NURSING CONSIDERATIONS
- Advise clients to avoid contact with people who have a communicable disease.
- Monitor for any indications of infection, such as fever.

Cushing's syndrome
NURSING CONSIDERATIONS: Risks are associated with long-term use of glucocorticoids and excessive doses. Advise clients to observe for manifestations (muscle weakness, moon face, buffalo hump, cutaneous striations), and to notify the provider if they occur.

Mineralocorticoid: fludrocortisone

Retention of sodium and water
This can lead to hypertension, edema, heart failure and hypokalemia.

NURSING CONSIDERATIONS
- Monitor weight, blood pressure, and serum potassium. Monitor breath sounds and urine output.
- Educate clients on manifestations of sodium and water retention (weight gain, peripheral edema) and hypokalemia (muscle weakness, irregular pulse), and to notify provider if they occur.

CONTRAINDICATIONS/PRECAUTIONS

- Hydrocortisone and fludrocortisone are Pregnancy Risk Category C. Qs
- Use is contraindicated in clients who have a viral, bacterial, or fungal infection not controlled by antibiotics.
- Use with caution in clients who have had a recent MI, gastric ulcer, hypertension, kidney disorder, osteoporosis, diabetes mellitus, hypothyroidism, myasthenia gravis, glaucoma, or seizure disorder.

INTERACTIONS

Glucocorticoids: hydrocortisone

NSAIDs, acetaminophen, or alcohol use can cause increased gastric distress or bleed.
NURSING CONSIDERATIONS: Use together with caution.

Concurrent use with oral anticoagulants can increase or decrease anticoagulation.
NURSING CONSIDERATIONS: Monitor coagulation studies and medication levels.

Concurrent use with potassium depleting agents can cause increased potassium loss.
NURSING CONSIDERATIONS: Monitor serum potassium and ECG.

Concurrent use with vaccines and toxoids can reduce the antibody response.
NURSING CONSIDERATIONS: Do not use together.

Mineralocorticoid: fludrocortisone

Barbiturates and phenytoin can reduce effects of fludrocortisone.
NURSING CONSIDERATIONS: Monitor for reduced medication effects.

Antidiabetic effects of insulin and sulfonylureas decrease with concurrent use of fludrocortisone.
NURSING CONSIDERATIONS: Closely monitor blood glucose levels in clients who have diabetes mellitus.

NURSING ADMINISTRATION

- Monitor weight, blood pressure, and electrolytes.
- Give with food to reduce gastric distress.
- Advise clients to observe for indications of peptic ulcer (coffee-ground emesis, bloody or tarry stools, abdominal pain) and to notify the provider if they occur.
- Do not stop the medication suddenly. Taper dosage if discontinuing.
- Instruct clients to notify the provider of indications of acute adrenal insufficiency (fever, muscle and joint pain, weakness, fatigue).
- Instruct clients that dosages need to be increased during times of stress (infection, surgery, trauma).
- Advise clients that replacement therapy for Addison's disease must continue for life.
- Instruct clients to carry an extra supply of glucocorticoids for emergencies and to wear medical identification at all times.

NURSING EVALUATION OF MEDICATION EFFECTIVENESS

Depending on therapeutic intent, evidence of effectiveness can include relief of effects of adrenocortical deficiency, such as weakness, hypoglycemia, hyperkalemia, and fatigue, with minimal adverse effects.

Hyperpituitarism medications

SELECT PROTOTYPE MEDICATION: Octreotide

OTHER MEDICATIONS
- Lanreotide
- Pegvisomant

PURPOSE

EXPECTED PHARMACOLOGICAL ACTION: Suppresses growth hormone release

THERAPEUTIC USES: Gigantism in children, acromegaly in adults

ROUTE OF ADMINISTRATION
- Octreotide (IM, subcutaneous)
- Lanreotide (subcutaneous)
- Pegvisomant (subcutaneous)

COMPLICATIONS

Octreotide

Gastrointestinal disturbances
- Nausea, cramps, diarrhea, flatulence
- NURSING CONSIDERATIONS
  - Advise clients that symptoms usually subside in 1 to 2 weeks.
  - Give injections without food or at bedtime to minimize symptoms.

Hypo/hyperglycemia
NURSING CONSIDERATIONS: Monitor glucose levels regularly.

Lanreotide

Gastrointestinal disturbances
- Abdominal pain, diarrhea, nausea, vomiting, flatulence, cholelithiasis
- CLIENT EDUCATION: Advise client to notify the provider of symptoms.

Hypo/hyperglycemia
NURSING CONSIDERATIONS: Monitor glucose levels regularly.

Pegvisomant

Nausea, diarrhea
CLIENT EDUCATION: Advise the client to notify the provider of symptoms.

Hypoglycemia
NURSING CONSIDERATIONS: Monitor glucose levels regularly.

Liver injury
NURSING CONSIDERATIONS
- Advise clients to discontinue the medication and notify the provider if jaundice appears.
- Monitor liver function studies.

Chest pain
CLIENT EDUCATION: Advise clients to notify the provider of symptoms promptly.

Flu-like symptoms
CLIENT EDUCATION: Advise clients to notify the provider of signs of infection.

CONTRAINDICATIONS/PRECAUTIONS

Octreotide
- Pregnancy Risk Category B. Qs
- Use cautiously in clients who have diabetes, hypothyroidism, and renal disease, and in older adult clients.

Lanreotide
- Pregnancy Risk Category C.
- Use cautiously in clients who have gallbladder, liver, or renal disease; diabetes; hypothyroidism; and cardiac disease.

Pegvisomant
- Pregnancy Risk Category B.
- Use cautiously in clients who have liver or renal disease, diabetes, pituitary tumors, or neoplastic disease.

INTERACTIONS

Octreotide: Conduction delays can occur if used with antidysrhythmics.
NURSING CONSIDERATIONS: Monitor cardiac status.

Lanreotide: Bradycardia can occur with concurrent use of medications that affect heart rate.
NURSING CONSIDERATIONS: Monitor cardiac status.

Pegvisomant: Concurrent use with opioids can reduce the effect of pegvisomant.
NURSING CONSIDERATIONS: Dosage can need to be increased.

NURSING ADMINISTRATION
- Teach clients proper technique for subcutaneous injection. Qs
- Minimize injection site pain by rotating sites. The abdomen, hip, and thigh are the preferred sites.
- IM injection of octreotide should be to a large muscle. Teach clients to minimize injection site pain by administering slowly, after the medication reaches room temperature.

NURSING EVALUATION OF MEDICATION EFFECTIVENESS

Depending on therapeutic intent, evidence of effectiveness can include the suppression of excess growth hormone for the management of acromegaly when surgery or radiation has failed.

Application Exercises

1. A nurse is caring for a client who is taking propylthiouracil. For which of the following adverse effects of this medication should the nurse monitor?

   A. Bradycardia

   B. Insomnia

   C. Heat intolerance

   D. Weight loss

2. A nurse is teaching a client who has Graves' disease about her prescribed medications. Which of the following statements by the client indicates an understanding of the use of propranolol in the treatment of Graves' disease?

   A. "Propranolol helps increase blood flow to my thyroid gland."

   B. "Propranolol is used to prevent excess glucose in my blood."

   C. "Propranolol will decrease my tremors and fast heart beat."

   D. "Propranolol promotes a decrease of thyroid hormone in my body."

3. A nurse is caring for an older adult client in a long-term care facility who has hypothyroidism and a new prescription for levothyroxine. Which of the following dosage schedules should the nurse expect for this client?

   A. The client will start at a high dose, and the dose will be tapered as needed.

   B. The client will remain on the initial dosage during the course of treatment.

   C. The client's dosage will be adjusted daily based on blood levels.

   D. The client will start on a low dose, which will be gradually increased.

4. A nurse is caring for a client who is taking for somatropin to stimulate growth. The nurse should plan to monitor the client's urine for which of the following?

   A. Bilirubin

   B. Protein

   C. Potassium

   D. Calcium

5. A nurse is assessing a client who takes desmopressin for diabetes insipidus. For which of the following adverse effects should the nurse monitor?

   A. Hypovolemia

   B. Hypercalcemia

   C. Agitation

   D. Headache

6. A nurse is admitting a client to an acute care facility for a total hip arthroplasty. The client takes hydrocortisone for Addison's disease. Which of the following actions is the nurse's priority?

   A. Administering a supplemental dose of hydrocortisone

   B. Instructing the client about coughing and deep breathing

   C. Collecting additional information from the client about his history of Addison's disease

   D. Inserting an indwelling urinary catheter

PRACTICE Active Learning Scenario

A nurse in a provider's office is providing instructions to a client who has a new prescription for levothyroxine to treat hypothyroidism. Use the ATI Active Learning Template: Medication to complete this item.

THERAPEUTIC USES: Describe the therapeutic use of levothyroxine in this client.

COMPLICATIONS: Identify two adverse effects of this medication.

NURSING INTERVENTIONS: Describe two laboratory tests the nurse should monitor.

CLIENT TEACHING: Describe teaching points for a client taking levothyroxine.

Application Exercises Key

1. A. **CORRECT:** Bradycardia is an adverse effect of propylthiouracil. The nurse should monitor for bradycardia.

   B. Drowsiness, rather than insomnia, is an adverse effect of propylthiouracil.

   C. Cold intolerance rather than heat intolerance is an adverse effect of propylthiouracil.

   D. Weight gain, rather than weight loss, is an adverse effect of propylthiouracil.

   Ⓝ NCLEX® Connection: Pharmacological and Parenteral Therapies, Adverse Effects/Contraindications/Side Effects/Interactions

2. A. Propranolol lowers blood pressure, but does not increase blood flow to the thyroid gland.

   B. Propranolol does not help prevent hyperglycemia.

   C. **CORRECT:** Propranolol is a beta-adrenergic antagonist that decreases heart rate and controls tremors.

   D. Propranolol does not promote a decrease of thyroid hormone.

   Ⓝ NCLEX® Connection: Pharmacological and Parenteral Therapies, Medication Administration

3. A. The nurse should not expect that the levothyroxine will be started at a high dose.

   B. The nurse should not expect that the client's dosage will remain the same throughout treatment.

   C. The nurse should not expect that the client's dosage will be adjusted daily based on blood levels.

   D. **CORRECT:** The nurse should expect that levothyroxine will be started at a low dose and gradually increased over several weeks. This is especially important in older adult clients to prevent toxicity.

   Ⓝ NCLEX® Connection: Pharmacological and Parenteral Therapies, Expected Actions/Outcomes

4. A. Bilirubin can be present in the urine with liver or biliary disorders, but is not monitored during somatropin therapy.

   B. Protein can be present in the urine during stress, infection, or glomerular disorders, but is not monitored during somatropin therapy.

   C. Potassium is not expected to be present in a urine specimen.

   D. **CORRECT:** A large amount of calcium can be present in the urine of a client who takes somatropin. This puts the client at risk for renal calculi.

   Ⓝ NCLEX® Connection: Pharmacological and Parenteral Therapies, Adverse Effects/Contraindications/Side Effects/Interactions

5. A. Edema and hypervolemia, rather than hypovolemia, are adverse effects of desmopressin.

   B. Calcium imbalance is not an adverse effect of desmopressin.

   C. Sleepiness, rather than agitation, is an adverse effect of desmopressin, which can indicate water intoxication.

   D. **CORRECT:** Headache during desmopressin therapy is an indication of water intoxication.

   Ⓝ NCLEX® Connection: Pharmacological and Parenteral Therapies, Adverse Effects/Contraindications/Side Effects/Interactions

6. A. **CORRECT:** Acute adrenal insufficiency (adrenal crisis) is the greatest risk to a client who has Addison's disease, is taking a glucocorticoid, and is undergoing surgery. To prevent acute adrenal insufficiency, supplemental doses are administered during times of increased stress.

   B. Instruction on coughing and deep breathing is important, but is not the nurse's priority for this client.

   C. Obtaining additional data from the client about past medical history is important, but is not the nurse's priority for this client.

   D. Inserting an indwelling urinary catheter is important, but is not the nurse's priority for this client.

   Ⓝ NCLEX® Connection: Pharmacological and Parenteral Therapies, Medication Administration

---

PRACTICE Answer

Using the ATI Active Learning Template: Medication

THERAPEUTIC USES: Levothyroxine replaces T4 and is used as thyroid hormone replacement therapy. Replacement of T4 also raises T3 levels, because some T4 is converted into T3.

COMPLICATIONS: Adverse effects are essentially the same as manifestations of hyperthyroidism: cardiac symptoms, such as hypertension and angina pectoris; insomnia; anxiety; weight loss; heat intolerance; increased body temperature; tremors; and menstrual irregularities.

NURSING INTERVENTIONS: The nurse should monitor thyroid function tests: T3, T4, and TSH.

CLIENT TEACHING
- Teach the client to take levothyroxine on an empty stomach, usually 1 hr before breakfast.
- Teach the client that thyroid replacement therapy is usually for life
- Monitor for adverse effects that indicate that the dosage needs to be adjusted.
- Adverse effects include cardiac effects, chest pain, hypertension, and palpitations, especially in older adults.

Ⓝ NCLEX® Connection: Pharmacological and Parenteral Therapies, Medication Administration

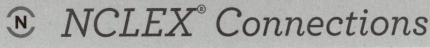

NCLEX® Connections

When reviewing the following chapters, keep in mind the relevant topics and tasks of the NCLEX outline, in particular:

Client Needs: Pharmacological and Parenteral Therapies

ADVERSE EFFECTS/CONTRAINDICATIONS/SIDE EFFECTS/ INTERACTIONS: Identify a contraindication to the administration of a medication to the client.

EXPECTED ACTIONS/OUTCOMES: Obtain information on a client's prescribed medications.

MEDICATION ADMINISTRATION: Administer and document medications given by parenteral routes.

CHAPTER 41

CHAPTER 41 *Immunizations*

Administration of a vaccine causes the immune system to produce antibodies that target a specific microbe. Vaccines are made from killed viruses or live, attenuated (weakened) viruses.

IMMUNITY

Active immunity develops when the immune system produces antibodies in response to the entry of antigens into the body.

- **Artificial active immunity** develops when a vaccine is administered and the body produces antibodies in response to exposure to a killed or attenuated virus.
- **Natural active immunity** develops when an antigen enters the body naturally, without human assistance, stimulating the immune system to produce antibodies to the antigen.

Passive immunity is temporary, and develops when antibodies are created by another human or animal and then transferred to the client.

- **Natural passive immunity** develops when antibodies are passed from a mother to her fetus through the placenta, and then to the newborn/infant via the colostrum and breast milk.
- **Artificial passive immunity** develops after antibodies in the form of immune globulins are administered to an individual who requires immediate protection against a disease after exposure has occurred.

RECOMMENDED CHILDHOOD IMMUNIZATIONS

See www.cdc.gov for updates. ⃝EBP

Diphtheria and tetanus toxoids and acellular pertussis vaccine (DTaP): Administer doses at 2, 4, 6, 15 to 18 months, and 4 to 6 years.

Tetanus and diphtheria toxoids and pertussis vaccine (Tdap): Administer one dose at 11 to 12 years.

Tetanus and diphtheria (Td) booster: Administer one dose every 10 years following Tdap.

Haemophilus influenzae **type B (Hib):** Administer doses at 2, 4, 6 (if a four-dose series), and 12 to 15 months.

Rotavirus (RV) oral vaccine

- Two formulations are available. The infant may receive either formulation. The first dose of either form should not be initiated for infants 15 weeks, 0 days or older.
  - RV-5 vaccine should be administered as a three-dose series at ages 2, 4, and 6 months.
  - RV-1 vaccine should be administered as two-dose series at 2 and 4 months.
- Maximum age for the final dose of RV vaccine is 8 months, 0 days.

Inactivated poliovirus vaccine (IPV): Administer doses at 2, 4, and 6 to 18 months, and 4 to 6 years.

Measles, mumps, and rubella vaccine (MMR): Administer doses at 12 to 15 months and 4 to 6 years.

Varicella vaccine: Administer one dose at 12 to 15 months and 4 to 6 years or two doses administered a minimum of 4 weeks apart if administered after age 13 years.

Pneumococcal conjugate vaccine (PCV13): Administer doses at 2, 4, 6, and 12 to 15 months.

Hepatitis A: Administer the first dose between 12 and 23 months. Administer the second dose 6 to 18 months after the first.

Hepatitis B: Administer within 12 hr after birth with additional doses at age 1 to 2 months and 6 to 18 months. The third dose should not be given prior to 24 weeks of age.

Seasonal influenza vaccine

- Annually, beginning at age 6 months, administer inactivated influenza vaccine (IIV).
- Starting at age 2 years the live, attenuated influenza vaccine (LAIV) nasal spray can be used. LAIV is contraindicated for children age 2 to 17 years who are receiving aspirin-containing products, children age 2 to 4 years who have asthma or have had wheezing during the past year, or anyone who has taken an antiviral medication in the 48 hr prior to vaccine administration.
- Administration recommendations can change yearly because the vaccine is created with different influenza strains each year. The vaccine is typically available beginning in early fall.

Meningococcal vaccine (MenACWY): Administer first dose at age 11 to 12 years (earlier if specific risk factors are present). Administer a booster dose at age 16 years.

Human papillomavirus (HPV2, HPV4, or HPV9): Administer three doses over a 6-month period for males and females 11 to 12 years of age (minimum age of 9 years). Administer males only HPV4 or HPV9; administer females HPV2, HPV4 or HPV9. The second dose is administered 1 to 2 months after the first dose, and the third dose is administered 16 weeks after the second dose.

RECOMMENDED ADULT IMMUNIZATIONS

- For adults age 19 and older.
- See www.cdc.gov for updates.

Td/Tdap: Administer one dose of Tdap instead of Td, and then give Td booster every 10 years. Give one dose of Tdap to women who are pregnant (with each pregnancy) between 27 and 36 weeks gestation.

MMR: Follow recommendations for administering one or two doses to clients between the ages of 19 and 49 who lack documentation of immunization or prior infection, or laboratory proof of immunity.

Varicella vaccine: Administer two doses to adults who do not have evidence of immunity. Administer a second dose to adults who had only one previous dose and lack evidence of immunity. Pregnant women needing protection against varicella should wait until the postpartum period for immunization.

Pneumococcal polysaccharide vaccine (PPSV23) and pneumococcal conjugate vaccine (PCV13): Follow recommendations for administration to adults who are immunocompromised, have certain chronic diseases, smoke cigarettes, or live in a long-term care facility. For adults 65 years and older who have not been immunized with PCV13 or PPSV23, administer PCV13 first and then give PPSV23 in 6 to 12 months; do not administer both during the same visit. For adults who received a dose of PPSV23 at age 65 or older, an additional dose is not indicated. Ⓒ

Hepatitis A: Administer single-antigen vaccines as two doses spaced 6 to 12 months, or 6 to 18 months apart to high-risk individuals.

Hepatitis B: Administer three doses to high-risk individuals who lack completion of the series. There must be at least 1 month between doses one and two, and at least 2 months between doses two and three. A minimum of 4 months are required between doses one and three.

Influenza vaccine
- One dose annually is recommended for all adults.
- IIV is approved for individuals 6 months of age or older, including those who are pregnant.
- Recombinant influenza vaccine (RIV) is approved for adults 18 years of age and older.
- LAIV is a nasal spray and is approved for individuals between aged 2 to 49 years who are healthy and not pregnant.

Meningococcal polysaccharide vaccine (MPSV4) and Meningococcal (MenACWY) vaccine: Administer a dose of MenACWY to students up to age 21 years entering college and living in dormitories if a dose was not received on or after the 16th birthday. Two doses of MenACWY at least 2 months apart are recommended for individuals who have anatomical or functional asplenia, and one dose is recommended for military recruits, and those traveling or living in areas of hyperendemic or epidemic rates of meningococcal disease. MPSV4 is preferred for adults who are 56 years of age or older, require a single dose, and have not had MenACWY previously. Reimmunization with MenACWY is recommended every 5 years for adults who remain at high risk for infection and were previously immunized with MenACWY or MPSV4.

HPV2, HPV4, or HPV9: Three doses are recommended for females up to age 26 years who were not immunized as children. Females can receive HPV2, HPV4, or HPV9. If not immunized as children, HPV4 or HPV9 is recommended for males age 19 to 21 years, and for males age 22 to 26 years who have a high risk for human papilloma virus.

Zoster vaccine: A one-time dose is recommended for all adults 60 years or older.

PURPOSE

EXPECTED PHARMACOLOGICAL ACTION

Vaccines cause the immune system to produce antibodies that provide passive active immunity. Immunizations can take months to have an effect but confer long-lasting protection against infectious diseases.

THERAPEUTIC USES

- Eradication of infectious diseases (polio, smallpox)
- Prevention of childhood and adult infectious diseases (measles, diphtheria, mumps, rubella, tetanus, *H. influenzae*) and their complications

COMPLICATIONS, CONTRAINDICATIONS, AND PRECAUTIONS

- Anaphylactic reaction to a vaccine is a contraindication for further doses of that vaccine. Ⓠs
- Anaphylactic reaction to any component of a vaccine is a contraindication to use of subsequent vaccines containing that substance.
- Do not administer live virus vaccines, such as varicella or MMR, to a client who is severely immunocompromised. Severe febrile illness is a contraindication to all immunizations.
- Precautions to immunizations require the provider to analyze data and weigh the risks that come with immunizing or not immunizing. Ⓠ𝗉𝖼𝖼
- Moderate or severe illnesses with or without fever are precautions to receiving immunizations.
- The common cold and other minor illnesses are not a contraindication or precaution for receiving immunizations.

DTaP

ADVERSE EFFECTS
- **Mild**
  - Redness, swelling, and tenderness at the injection site
  - Low fever
  - Behavioral changes (drowsiness, irritability, anorexia)
- **Moderate**
  - Inconsolable crying for 3 hr or more
  - Fever 40.6° C (105° F) or greater
  - Seizures (with or without fever)
  - Shock-like state
- **Severe:** Acute encephalopathy (rare)

CONTRAINDICATIONS: Occurrence of encephalopathy within 7 days following prior dose of the vaccine

PRECAUTIONS
- Occurrence of Guillain-Barré syndrome within 6 weeks of prior dose of tetanus toxoid
- Progressive neurologic disorders; uncontrolled seizures
- Fever 40.6° C (105° F) or greater within 48 hr of prior dose
- Shock-like state within 48 hr of prior dose
- Seizures within 3 days of prior dose
- Inconsolable crying for 3 hr or more within 48 hr of prior dose

Haemophilus influenzae type B

ADVERSE EFFECTS
- Redness, swelling, warmth, and tenderness at the injection site
- Fever greater than 37.8° C (101° F), vomiting, diarrhea, and crying

CONTRAINDICATION: Age less than 6 weeks

Rotavirus

ADVERSE EFFECTS
- Irritability
- Mild, temporary diarrhea or vomiting
- Intussusception

CONTRAINDICATIONS
- History of intussusception
- Severe combined immunodeficiency (SCID), which is a rare disorder that is inherited

PRECAUTIONS
- Chronic gastrointestinal disease
- Spina bifida
- Bladder exstrophy
- Immunocompromised (other than SCID)

Inactivated poliovirus vaccine

ADVERSE EFFECTS: Tenderness at the injection site

CONTRAINDICATION: Anaphylactic reaction to neomycin, streptomycin, or polymyxin B

PRECAUTION: Pregnancy

Measles, mumps, and rubella

ADVERSE EFFECTS
- **Mild:** Local reactions (rash; fever; swollen glands in cheeks or neck)
- **Moderate**
  - Joint pain and stiffness lasting for days to weeks
  - Febrile seizure
  - Low platelet count
- **Severe**
  - Transient thrombocytopenia
  - Deafness
  - Long-term seizures
  - Brain damage

CONTRAINDICATION: Pregnancy

PRECAUTIONS
- History of thrombocytopenia or thrombocytopenic purpura
- Anaphylactic reaction to eggs, gelatin, or neomycin
- Transfusion with blood product containing antibodies within the prior 11 months
- Simultaneous tuberculin skin testing

Varicella

ADVERSE EFFECTS
- **Mild**
  - Tenderness and swelling at injection site
  - Fever
  - Rash (mild) for up to 1 month after immunization
- **Moderate:** Seizures
- **Severe**
  - Pneumonia
  - Low blood count (extremely rare)
  - Severe brain reactions (extremely rare)

CONTRAINDICATIONS
- Pregnancy
- Anaphylactic reaction to gelatin or neomycin

PRECAUTIONS
- Transfusion with blood product containing antibodies within the prior 11 months
- Treatment with antiviral medication within 24 hr prior to immunization (avoid taking antivirals for 14 days following immunization)
- Extended use (2 weeks or longer) of corticosteroids or other medications that affect the immune system
- Cancer

Pneumococcal conjugate vaccine

ADVERSE EFFECTS
- Swelling, redness and tenderness at site of injection
- Fever
- Irritability
- Drowsiness
- Anorexia

CONTRAINDICATION: Anaphylactic reaction to any vaccine containing diphtheria toxoid

Pneumococcal polysaccharide vaccine

ADVERSE EFFECTS
- Redness and tenderness at site of injection
- Fever
- Myalgia

CONTRAINDICATION: Age less than 2 years

PRECAUTION: Pregnancy

Hepatitis A

ADVERSE EFFECTS
- Tenderness at the injection site
- Headache
- Anorexia
- Malaise

CONTRAINDICATION: Severe allergy to latex

PRECAUTION: Pregnancy

Hepatitis B

ADVERSE EFFECTS
- Tenderness at the injection site
- Temperature of 37.7° C (99.9° F) or greater

CONTRAINDICATION: Anaphylactic allergy to yeast

PRECAUTION: Infant weight less than 2 kg (4 lb, 6.5 oz)

Inactivated influenza vaccine

ADVERSE EFFECTS
- Swelling, redness and tenderness at the injection site
- Hoarseness
- Fever
- Malaise
- Headache
- Cough
- Aches
- Increased risk for Guillain-Barré syndrome
- Increased risk of seizures in children receiving PCV13 or DTaP simultaneously

PRECAUTIONS: Occurrence of Guillain-Barré syndrome within 6 weeks of prior influenza vaccine

Live, attenuated influenza vaccine

ADVERSE EFFECTS
- Vomiting, diarrhea
- Cough
- Fever
- Headache
- Myalgia
- Nasal congestion/runny nose

CONTRAINDICATIONS
- Age less than 2 years
- Age 50 years or older
- Pregnancy

PRECAUTIONS
- Occurrence of Guillain-Barré syndrome within 6 weeks of prior influenza vaccine
- Treatment with antiviral medication within 48 hr prior to immunization (avoid taking antivirals for 14 days following immunization)
- Some chronic conditions
- The Advisory Committee on Immunization Practices recommends the option of the live-attenuated influenza vaccine to clients regardless of the severity of egg allergy. Clients who have a history of an egg allergy, other than a hive-only reaction, should receive the immunization where a provider is present and emergency equipment is available. (At the time of publication, these recommendations were awaiting approval by the CDC. Please refer to www.cdc.gov for current approval status.)

Meningococcal ACWY

ADVERSE EFFECTS
- Redness and tenderness at the injection site
- Fever

HPV4 and HPV9

ADVERSE EFFECTS
- Redness, swelling and tenderness at the injection site
- Mild to moderate fever
- Headache
- Fainting (shortly after receiving the vaccine)

CONTRAINDICATIONS
- Pregnancy
- Severe allergy to yeast

HPV2

ADVERSE EFFECTS
- Redness, swelling and tenderness at the injection site
- Temperature 37.7° C (99.9° F) or greater
- Headache
- Fatigue
- Nausea, vomiting, abdominal pain
- Myalgia
- Fainting (shortly after receiving the vaccine)

CONTRAINDICATIONS
- Pregnancy
- Severe allergy to latex

Zoster

ADVERSE EFFECTS
- Redness, edema, itching, and tenderness at the injection site
- Headache

CONTRAINDICATIONS
- Immunosuppression
- Pregnancy
- Treatment with medications that alter the immune system

INTERACTIONS

None significant

NURSING ADMINISTRATION

FOR INFANTS AND CHILDREN

- Obtain informed consent from the legal guardian prior to administration.
- Administer IM immunizations in the vastus lateralis or ventrogluteal muscle in infants and young children, and in the deltoid muscle for older children and adolescents.
- Administer subcutaneous injections in the outer aspect of the upper arm or anterolateral thigh.
- Use the appropriate size needle for route, site, age, and amount of medication. Adequate needle length reduces the incidence of swelling and tenderness at the injection site. Qpcc
- Use strategies to minimize discomfort, such as providing distraction, applying a topical anesthetic prior to injection, and giving infants a concentrated oral sucrose solution 2 min prior to, during, and 3 min after immunization administration.
- Do not allow the child to delay the procedure.
- Encourage caregivers to use comforting measures such as cuddling and pacifiers during procedure, and measures such as application of cool compresses to injection site or gentle movement of the involved extremity after the procedure.
- Provide praise afterward.
- Apply a colorful bandage if appropriate.
- Instruct parents to avoid administration of aspirin to children to treat fever or local reaction following administration of a live virus vaccine due to the risk of developing Reye syndrome.

FOR ADULTS

- Administer subcutaneous immunizations in the outer aspect of the upper arm or anterolateral thigh.
- Administer IM immunizations into the deltoid muscle.

FOR CLIENTS OF ALL AGES

- Have emergency medications and equipment on standby in case the client experiences an allergic response such as anaphylaxis.
- Provide written vaccine information sheets (VIS) and review the content with legal guardians or clients. Include the publication date of each VIS given in documentation.
- Instruct parents and clients to observe for complications and to notify the provider if adverse effects occur.
- Document the administration of the vaccine, including the date, route, and site of immunization; type, manufacturer, lot number, and expiration date of the vaccine; evidence of informed consent from the legal guardian, and; name, address and title of the administering nurse. Qℓ

NURSING EVALUATION OF MEDICATION EFFECTIVENESS

Depending on therapeutic intent, effectiveness can be evidenced by the following.

- Improvement of local reaction to immunization with absence of pain, fever, and swelling at the site of injection
- Development of immunity

Application Exercises

1. A nurse is caring for several clients who came to the clinic for a seasonal influenza immunization. The nurse should identify that which of the following clients is a candidate to receive the vaccine via nasal spray rather than an injection?

   A. 1-year-old who has no health problems

   B. 17-year-old who has a hypersensitivity to penicillin

   C. 25-year-old who is pregnant

   D. 52-year-old who takes a multivitamin supplement

2. A nurse is teaching a group of new parents about immunizations. The nurse should instruct the parents that the series for which of the following vaccines is completed prior to the first birthday?

   A. Pneumococcal conjugate vaccine

   B. Meningococcal conjugate vaccine

   C. Varicella vaccine

   D. Rotavirus vaccine

3. A nurse at a provider's office is preparing to administer RV, DTaP, Hib, PCV13, and IPV immunizations to a 4-month-old infant. Which of the following actions should the nurse plan to take? (Select all that apply.)

   A. Administer IPV orally.

   B. Administer subcutaneous injections in the anterolateral thigh.

   C. Administer IM injections in the deltoid muscle.

   D. Give the infant his pacifier during vaccine injections.

   E. Teach parents to give aspirin on a schedule for 24 hr after immunization.

4. A 12-month-old child just received the first measles, mumps, and rubella (MMR) vaccine. For which of the following possible reactions to this vaccine should the nurse teach the parents to monitor? (Select all that apply.)

   A. Rash

   B. Swollen glands

   C. Bruising

   D. Headache

   E. Inconsolable crying

5. A nurse is caring for a group of clients who are not protected against varicella. The nurse should prepare to administer the varicella vaccine at this time to which of the following clients?

   A. 24-year-old woman in the third trimester of pregnancy

   B. 12-year-old child who has a severe allergy to neomycin

   C. 2-month-old infant who has no health problems

   D. 32-year-old man who has essential hypertension

Application Exercises Key

1. A. Children younger than 2 years of age are not eligible to receive the live, attenuated influenza vaccine (LAIV). The 1-year-old should instead receive the inactivated influenza vaccine by injection.

   B. **CORRECT:** A 17-year-old can be immunized for influenza with the LAIV via nasal spray. A hypersensitivity to penicillin is not a contraindication for an influenza immunization.

   C. The LAIV is contraindicated during pregnancy. Instead, this client should receive the inactivated influenza vaccine by injection.

   D. Clients older than age 50 are not eligible for the LAIV. Instead, this client should receive the inactivated influenza vaccine by injection.

   Ⓝ *NCLEX® Connection: Pharmacological and Parenteral Therapies, Expected Actions/Outcomes*

2. A. Pneumococcal conjugate vaccine (PCV13) is a four-dose series with the final dose given between the ages of 12 to 15 months. A one-time dose of PCV13 followed by a dose of pneumococcal polysaccharide vaccine (PPSV23) in 6 to 12 months is also recommended for adults 65 years or older.

   B. Meningococcal conjugate vaccine is recommended for children at age 11 to 12 years, followed by a booster dose at 16 to 18 years. It is also recommended for adults at high risk for meningococcal disease.

   C. The two-dose series of varicella vaccine is given at the age of 12 to 15 months, and 4 to 6 years. It is also recommended for adults who have no evidence of immunity.

   D. **CORRECT:** Rotavirus vaccine is administered only to infants less than 8 months, 0 days of age.

   Ⓝ *NCLEX® Connection: Pharmacological and Parenteral Therapies, Medication Administration*

3. A. The nurse should administer IPV subcutaneously. An oral polio vaccine is no longer used in the U.S.

   B. **CORRECT:** Subcutaneous immunizations may be administered in either the anterolateral thigh or the outer aspect of the upper arm to infants and children.

   C. The deltoid muscle is not fully developed in infants and generally should not be used for IM injections until the approximate age of 18 months. The nurse should use the vastus lateralis muscle for immunizations in the infant.

   D. **CORRECT:** Giving the infant a pacifier during injections is a comfort measure that should be encouraged by the nurse.

   E. The nurse should not teach the parents to give aspirin to the infant on a schedule because this can increase the risk of developing Reye syndrome.

   Ⓝ *NCLEX® Connection: Pharmacological and Parenteral Therapies, Medication Administration*

4. A. **CORRECT:** A rash and fever can develop in children 1 to 2 weeks following MMR immunization.

   B. **CORRECT:** Swollen glands can develop in children 1 to 2 weeks following MMR immunization.

   C. **CORRECT:** A temporary low platelet count, causing bruising or bleeding, can occur occasionally following MMR immunization.

   D. Headache is an adverse reaction that can occur following immunization with the IIV or LAIV influenza vaccine.

   E. Inconsolable crying can occur in some infants following the DTaP immunization.

   Ⓝ *NCLEX® Connection: Pharmacological and Parenteral Therapies, Adverse Effects/Contraindications/Side Effects/Interactions*

5. A. A woman in the third trimester of pregnancy should wait until the postpartum period for varicella immunization. This is a live vaccine that is not safe for pregnant women.

   B. The varicella vaccine is contraindicated for clients who have a severe allergy to neomycin.

   C. A 2-month-old infant is too young to receive the varicella vaccine, which is a two-dose series recommended at age 12 to 15 months and 4 to 6 years.

   D. **CORRECT:** A 32-year-old man who has essential hypertension and did not receive two doses of varicella vaccine earlier in life should be immunized. Essential hypertension is not a contraindication for this vaccine.

   Ⓝ *NCLEX® Connection: Pharmacological and Parenteral Therapies, Expected Actions/Outcomes*

PRACTICE Active Learning Scenario

A nurse at a community health clinic is planning to administer the human papilloma virus (HPV4) vaccine to an 11-year-old female client. Use the ATI Active Learning Template: Medication to complete this item.

COMPLICATIONS: Identify two adverse effects the client should monitor for.

CONTRAINDICATIONS/PRECAUTIONS: Identify contraindications to receiving the HPV vaccine.

CLIENT EDUCATION: Describe two teaching points for a client who receives a first dose of the HPV vaccine.

PRACTICE Answer

Using the ATI Active Learning Template: Medication

COMPLICATIONS
- The HPV4 vaccine can cause redness, tenderness, and swelling at the injection site.
- It has caused fainting in some clients shortly after the vaccine is administered.
- Headache and mild to moderate fever are also possible adverse effects the client should monitor for.

CONTRAINDICATIONS/PRECAUTIONS: Contraindications to receiving HPV include pregnancy and a severe allergy to yeast.

CLIENT EDUCATION
- Teach the client and family about the possible adverse effects, and tell them that the common adverse effects are mild and temporary.
- Tell the client and family that three doses of the vaccine are administered within 6 months. The second dose is administered 1 to 2 months after the first dose, and the third dose is administered 16 weeks after the second dose.

Ⓝ *NCLEX® Connection: Pharmacological and Parenteral Therapies, Medication Administration*

CHAPTER 42

CHAPTER 42
Chemotherapy Agents

Chemotherapy is used to cure some cancers, augment the treatment of other cancers, and attempt to increase a client's survival rate and time. Depending on the agent, it can be given orally, parentally, intravenous, intracavitary, or intrathecal. Specific training/certification is necessary for administration of some agents.

Combination chemotherapy uses more than one chemotherapy agent to treat the cancer. Medications used for combination chemotherapy should act in different phases of the cell cycle. Combination therapy is used to reduce medication resistance, increase effectiveness, and, ideally, reduce toxic effects to healthy cells.

Personnel preparing and administering chemotherapeutic agents should follow safe handling procedures to prevent absorption through the skin.

If a chemotherapy spill occurs, follow institutional procedures. Generally, small spills can be handled by following procedures and using supplies contained in a chemotherapy spill kit (goggles, mask, protective clothing, shoe covers, absorbent pads, detergent cleansers, and chemotherapy waste disposal bags). For large spills, contact the Occupational Safety and Health Administration. Qs

Cytotoxic chemotherapy agents

Cytotoxic chemotherapy agents are toxic to cancer cells.
- Cytotoxic chemotherapy agents kill fast-growing cancer cells as well as healthy cells, including skin, hair, intestinal mucosa, and hematopoietic cells. Many of the adverse effects of chemotherapeutic agents are related to the unintentional harm done to healthy rapidly proliferating cells, such as those found in the gastrointestinal (GI) tract, hair follicles, and bone marrow.
- Common adverse effects of cytotoxic chemotherapy agents include nausea, vomiting, myelosuppression, and alopecia. Many cytotoxic agents are vesicants and can cause severe damage if there is leakage into tissue. Extravasation of agents that are vesicants requires immediate attention to minimize tissue damage. Selection of the neutralizing solution is dependent on vesicant. Qs

PURPOSE

EXPECTED PHARMACOLOGICAL ACTION

Antimetabolites: Kill cancer cells by interrupting a specific phase of cell reproduction: known as S-phase specific

Antitumor antibiotics: Kill cancer cells by stopping the synthesis of RNA, DNA, or proteins

Antimitotics: Kill cancer cells by inhibiting mitosis and preventing cell division

Alkylating agents: Kill fast-growing cancer cells by altering DNA structure and preventing cell reproduction

Topoisomerase inhibitors: Kill cancer cells by interrupting DNA synthesis

Other: Kill cells by various mechanisms including interrupting DNA and RNA synthesis in leukemia cells

Antimetabolites

Folic acid analog

SELECT PROTOTYPE MEDICATION: Methotrexate (oral, IV, IM, intrathecal)

OTHER MEDICATIONS
- Pemetrexed (IV infusion)
- Pralatrexate (IV bolus)

Pyrimidine analog

SELECT PROTOTYPE MEDICATION: Cytarabine (IV, subcutaneous, intrathecal)

OTHER MEDICATIONS
- Fluorouracil (continuous IV)
- Floxuridine (infusion directly into the hepatic artery)
- Capecitabine (oral)
- Gemcitabine (IV infusion)

Purine analogs

SELECT PROTOTYPE MEDICATION: Mercaptopurine (oral)

OTHER MEDICATIONS
- Thioguanine (oral)
- Pentostatin (IV bolus or infusion)
- Fludarabine (IV infusion)

PURPOSE

EXPECTED PHARMACOLOGICAL ACTION

Folic acid analog

Methotrexate
- Stops cell reproduction needed for the synthesis of DNA by inhibiting folic acid conversion
- S-phase specific

Pemetrexed
- Suppresses synthesis of DNA, RNA, and proteins
- S-phase specific

Pralatrexate
- Disrupts synthesis of DNA
- S-phase specific

Pyrimidine analog

Cytarabine
- Incorporates into DNA, then inhibits DNA and RNA synthesis of cancer cells
- S-phase specific

Fluorouracil, floxuridine
- Destroys cells mainly in the S-phase specificity
- Derivative of uracil

Capecitabine
- Active only against divided cells
- Has S-phase specificity

Gemcitabine: Has S-phase specificity

Purine analogs

Mercaptopurine
- Interrupts the action of adenine and guanine present in DNA and RNA for the synthesis of the purine nucleotides needed to incorporate into the nucleic acid molecules.
- All the medications are administered to interrupt the synthesis of both DNA and RNA.
- S-phase specific

Thioguanine
- Inhibits purine synthesis and DNA, and the interconversion of nucleotides
- S-phase specific

Pentostatin: Blocks DNA synthesis

Fludarabine: Inhibits DNA replication, impairs RNA function, and promotes apoptosis (destruction by a suppressive agent to eliminate cells)

THERAPEUTIC USES

Folic acid analog

Methotrexate: Choriocarcinoma, solid tumors (such as breast and lung), head and neck sarcomas, osteogenic sarcoma, acute lymphocytic leukemia, non-Hodgkin's lymphoma, T-cell lymphoma

Pemetrexed: Malignant pleural mesothelioma, non-small cell lung cancer

Pralatrexate: Peripheral T-cell lymphoma, non-Hodgkin's lymphoma

Pyrimidine analog

Cytarabine: Acute myelogenous leukemia, non-Hodgkin's lymphomas

Fluorouracil: Solid tumors: Colon, rectal, breast esophageal, head and neck, cervical, and renal cancer.

Floxuridine: GI adenoma metastatic to the liver

Capecitabine: Metastatic colorectal and breast cancer

Gemcitabine: Pancreatic, non-small cell lung, and bladder cancer; advanced ovarian and breast cancer

Purine analogs

Mercaptopurine, thioguanine
- Acute and chronic lymphocytic leukemia
- Acute nonlymphocytic leukemias
- Low-grade non-Hodgkin's lymphoma and acute myelogenous leukemia

Pentostatin: Hairy cell leukemia

Fludarabine: Chronic lymphocytic leukemia, low-grade non-Hodgkin's lymphoma, acute myelogenous leukemia

COMPLICATIONS

Bone marrow suppression
- Low WBC count or neutropenia, bleeding caused by thrombocytopenia or low platelet count, and anemia or low RBCs
- NURSING CONSIDERATIONS
  - Monitor WBC, absolute neutrophil count, platelet count, Hgb, and Hct.
  - Assess clients for bruising and bleeding gums.
  - Instruct clients to avoid crowds and contact with infectious individuals.

GI discomfort (nausea and vomiting)
NURSING CONSIDERATIONS: Administer antiemetic such as ondansetron in combination with dexamethasone, granisetron, or metoclopramide before beginning chemotherapy.

Methotrexate

Mucositis (GI tract), gastric ulcers, perforation
NURSING CONSIDERATIONS
- Monitor for GI bleed (coffee-ground emesis or tarry black stools). Assess the mouth for sores.
- Provide frequent oral hygiene using soft toothbrushes and avoid alcohol mouthwashes.

Reproductive toxicity (congenital abnormalities)
NURSING CONSIDERATIONS: Advise female clients against becoming pregnant while taking these medications and for 6 months after.

Renal damage
Due to hyperuricemia or elevated levels of uric acid
NURSING CONSIDERATIONS
- Monitor kidney function, BUN, creatinine, and I&O.
- Encourage adequate fluid intake of 2 to 3 L/day.
- Administer allopurinol if uric acid level is elevated.

Cytarabine

Liver disease
NURSING CONSIDERATIONS
- Monitor liver enzymes.
- Monitor for indications of jaundice.

Pulmonary edema
NURSING CONSIDERATIONS
- Monitor breath sounds.
- Advise clients to notify the provider of shortness of breath.

Arachnoiditis
Indications include nausea, headache, and fever.
NURSING CONSIDERATIONS
- Advise clients to notify the provider of nausea, vomiting, headache, or fever.
- Manifestations can be treated with dexamethasone.

Mercaptopurine

Liver toxicity
NURSING CONSIDERATIONS
- Monitor liver enzymes.
- Monitor for signs of jaundice.

Mucositis (GI tract), gastric ulcers, perforation
NURSING CONSIDERATIONS
- Monitor for GI bleed, such as coffee-ground emesis or tarry black stools.
- Assess mouth for sores.
- Provide frequent oral hygiene using soft toothbrushes and avoiding alcohol mouthwashes.

Reproductive toxicity
- Such as congenital abnormalities
- NURSING CONSIDERATIONS: Advise female clients against becoming pregnant while taking these medications and for 6 months after.

CONTRAINDICATIONS/PRECAUTIONS

Methotrexate

- Pregnancy Risk Category X
- Contraindicated in renal or hepatic failure, blood dyscrasias, or lactation.
- Use with caution in clients who have liver or kidney dysfunction, suppressed bone marrow, leukopenia, thrombocytopenia, anemia, or gastric ulcers, and in older adult clients.

Cytarabine

- Pregnancy Risk Category D
- Use with caution in clients who have liver disease.

Mercaptopurine

- Pregnancy Risk Category D
- Contraindicated in clients who are resistant to the medication.

INTERACTIONS

Methotrexate

Salicylates, other NSAIDs, sulfonamides, penicillin, and tetracyclines can cause methotrexate toxicity.
NURSING CONSIDERATIONS: Monitor for toxic effects.

Folic acid changes the body's response to methotrexate, decreasing its effect.
NURSING CONSIDERATIONS: Avoid folic acid supplements or vitamins containing folic acid.

Proton pump inhibitors
NURSING CONSIDERATIONS
- Avoid concurrent use.
- Monitor BUN and creatinine.

Cytarabine

Cytarabine can reduce the absorption of digoxin.
NURSING CONSIDERATIONS: Monitor digoxin level and ECG.

Live virus vaccines
NURSING CONSIDERATIONS: Avoid concurrent use.

Cytarabine can place the client at risk for bleeding if used with anticoagulants, salicylates, thrombolytics, NSAIDs, and platelet inhibitors.
NURSING CONSIDERATIONS: Monitor bleeding times and for signs of bleeding.

Mercaptopurine

Allopurinol can reduce breakdown of mercaptopurine.
NURSING CONSIDERATIONS: Reduce medication dosage.

Mercaptopurine can either increase or decrease anticoagulant effect of warfarin.
NURSING CONSIDERATIONS: Monitor PT and INR.

NURSING ADMINISTRATION

- Reduce dosage in clients who have renal disease.
- Encourage 2 to 3 L of daily fluid intake from food and beverage sources. Qᴘᴄᴄ
- Give with sodium bicarbonate capsules to alkalinize urine.
- Advise female clients to use birth control during treatment.
- Advise clients to avoid use of alcohol during treatment.
- Monitor for bleeding (bruising) and infection (fever, sore throat).
- Monitor CBC, BUN, creatinine, and liver enzymes.
- Monitor I&O. Monitor uric acid.
- Monitor the skin for jaundice. Advise clients to monitor for dark urine and clay-colored stools.
- Give an antiemetic for nausea and vomiting.
- Advise clients to practice good oral hygiene and to avoid mouthwash with alcohol.

For methotrexate

- Administer with leucovorin rescue to reduce toxicity to healthy cells. Leucovorin is a folic acid derivative. It enters healthy cells and blocks methotrexate.
- Instruct clients to take the medication on an empty stomach.
- Advise clients to protect the skin from sunlight.
- Advise female clients to use birth control during and for 6 months after completing treatment (Pregnancy Risk Category X).

For cytarabine: Monitor for indications of neurotoxicity, such as nystagmus.

Antitumor antibiotics

Anthracyclines

SELECT PROTOTYPE MEDICATION: Doxorubicin (IV)

OTHER MEDICATIONS
- Liposomal doxorubicin (IV infusion over 30 min)
- Daunorubicin (conventional or liposomal; IV infusion)
- Epirubicin (IV infusion)
- Idarubicin (IV infusion)
- Valrubicin (intravesical)
- Mitoxantrone (IV infusion)

Nonanthracyclines

SELECT PROTOTYPE MEDICATION: Dactinomycin (IV infusion)

OTHER MEDICATIONS
- Bleomycin (IM, IV, subcutaneous, intrapleural)
- Mitomycin (IV infusion)

PURPOSE

EXPECTED PHARMACOLOGICAL ACTION

Anthracyclines

Doxorubicin, daunorubicin, epirubicin, idarubicin
- Binds to DNA, altering its structure; therefore, inhibits synthesis of DNA and RNA (intercalation)
- Cell cycle phase nonspecific

Liposomal doxorubicin: Medication encapsulated within lipid vesicles (liposomes) to increase uptake to cancer cells and decrease uptake to healthy cells.

Valrubicin: Administered directly in to the bladder and it stops cell growth by disrupting, not intercalating, with DNA.

Mitoxantrone
- Intercalates DNA and DNA strand breakage
- Cell-cycle phase nonspecific

Nonanthracyclines

Dactinomycin
- Binds to DNA, altering its structure, which inhibits RNA synthesis
- Cell cycle phase nonspecific

Bleomycin: Binds to DNA

Mitomycin: Blockade of DNA synthesis

THERAPEUTIC USES

Anthracyclines

Doxorubicin: Includes solid tumors, such as lung, bone, stomach, and breast cancers; Hodgkin's and non-Hodgkin's lymphomas; sarcomas of soft tissue and bone; and carcinoma of ovaries, testes, and thyroid

Liposomal doxorubicin: AIDS-related Kaposi's sarcoma, metastatic ovarian and breast cancer, multiple myeloma

Daunorubicin: HIV-associated Kaposi's sarcoma, leukemia

Epirubicin: Breast cancer

Idarubicin: Acute myelogenous leukemia

Valrubicin: Bladder cancer

Mitoxantrone: Prostate cancer, acute nonlymphocytic leukemias

Nonanthracyclines

Dactinomycin: Includes Wilms' tumor, rhabdomyosarcoma, choriocarcinoma, Ewing's sarcoma, testicular cancer, and Kaposi's sarcoma

Bleomycin: Testicular carcinomas, lymphomas, squamous cell carcinomas, Hodgkin's disease

Mitomycin: Disseminated adenocarcinoma of the stomach and pancreas; carcinomas of the colon, rectum, esophagus, lung, breast, cervix, and bladder

COMPLICATIONS

Bone marrow suppression
- Low WBC or neutropenia, bleeding caused by thrombocytopenia or low platelet count, and anemia or low RBCs
- NURSING CONSIDERATIONS
  - Monitor WBC, absolute neutrophil count, platelet count, Hgb, and Hct.
  - Assess for bruising and bleeding gums.
  - Instruct clients to avoid crowds and contact with infectious individuals.

GI manifestations
- Including nausea, vomiting, and stomatitis
- NURSING CONSIDERATIONS
  - Administer antiemetic such as ondansetron in combination with dexamethasone, granisetron, or metoclopramide before beginning chemotherapy.
  - Provide gentle oral care. Rinse mouth with warmed saline solution.

Severe tissue damage
- Due to extravasations of vesicants
- NURSING CONSIDERATIONS
  - Stop chemotherapeutic medications if extravasation occurs.
  - Use central line for infusion.
  - Only clinically trained personnel should give these medications IV.

Alopecia
NURSING CONSIDERATIONS
- Advise clients that hair loss can occur 7 to 10 days after the beginning of treatment and will last for a maximum of 2 months after the last administration of the chemotherapeutic agent.
- Advise clients who want to do so to select a hairpiece before the occurrence of hair loss.

Doxorubicin

Acute cardiac toxicity, dysrhythmias
NURSING CONSIDERATIONS
- Monitor ECG and echocardiogram.
- The client can be treated with dexrazoxane, but this medication can increase myelosuppression.

Cardiomyopathy, heart failure
- Can have delayed onset
- NURSING CONSIDERATIONS
  - Monitor ECG and echocardiogram.
  - The client can be treated with ACE inhibitors.

Red coloration to urine and sweat
NURSING CONSIDERATIONS: Advise clients that this effect is not harmful.

CONTRAINDICATIONS/PRECAUTIONS

Doxorubicin

- Pregnancy Risk Category D.
- Contraindicated in clients who have severe myelosuppression and clients who have had a lifetime cumulative dose of 550 mg/m². **Qs**

Dactinomycin

- Pregnancy Risk Category D.
- Contraindicated in clients who have acute infections.

INTERACTIONS

Doxorubicin

Calcium channel blockers can increase cardiotoxicity.
NURSING CONSIDERATIONS: Monitor ECG and heart function.

Phenobarbital can decrease metabolism of doxorubicin.
NURSING CONSIDERATIONS: Monitor for toxicities.

Paclitaxel can increase doxorubicin levels by decreasing the clearance.
NURSING CONSIDERATIONS: Monitor for toxicities.

Doxorubicin can increase effect of phenytoin levels.
NURSING CONSIDERATIONS: Monitor phenytoin level.

NURSING ADMINISTRATION

- Reduce dose in liver disease.
- Monitor for bleeding (bruising) or infection (fever, sore throat).
- Monitor CBC and liver enzymes.
- Administer an antiemetic for nausea and vomiting.
- Advise clients to practice good oral hygiene and to avoid mouthwash with alcohol. Stop chemotherapeutic medications if extravasation occurs.
- Advise clients that transient hair loss can occur 7 to 10 days after the beginning of treatment and will last for a maximum duration of 2 months after the last administration of the chemotherapeutic agent.
- Advise clients to select a hairpiece before the occurrence of hair loss.

Doxorubicin

- Monitor ECG and cardiac function.
- Advise clients to continue follow-up care after treatment is completed to monitor for delayed cardiac toxicity.
- Advise clients to notify the provider if they experience chest pain or shortness of breath.

Antimitotics

Vinca alkaloids

SELECT PROTOTYPE MEDICATION: Vincristine (conventional or liposomal; IV)

OTHER MEDICATIONS
- Vinblastine (IV)
- Vinorelbine (IV)

Taxanes

SELECT PROTOTYPE MEDICATION: Paclitaxel (IV)

OTHER MEDICATION: Docetaxel (IV)

PURPOSE

EXPECTED PHARMACOLOGICAL ACTION

Vinca alkaloids

Vincristine
- Useful in combination with other chemotherapy medications
- Stops cell division during mitosis
- Not bone marrow toxic
- M-phase specific

Vinblastine: Structural similar to vincristine

Vinorelbine: Similar structure and actions to vincristine and vinblastine

Taxanes

Paclitaxel
- Stop cell division during mitosis
- Inhibits cell division and produces apoptosis

Docetaxel: Similar structure and action of paclitaxel

THERAPEUTIC USE

Vinca alkaloids

Vincristine: Includes acute lymphocytic leukemia; Wilms' tumor; rhabdomyosarcoma; solid tumors, such as bladder and breast cancers; and Hodgkin's and non-Hodgkin's lymphomas.

Vinblastine
- Kaposi's sarcoma, Hodgkin's and non-Hodgkin's lymphomas
- Carcinoma of the breast and testes

Vinorelbine: Breast cancer, non-small cell lung cancer, ovarian cancer, and Hodgkin's disease

Taxanes

Paclitaxel: Includes ovarian, non-small cell lung tumors, and Kaposi's sarcoma; advanced head and neck cancer; adenocarcinoma of the upper GI tract; leukemias

Docetaxel: Metastatic breast cancer, metastatic non-small cell lung cancer, and prostate cancer

COMPLICATIONS

Vincristine

Peripheral neuropathy effects
- Weakness, paresthesia
- NURSING CONSIDERATIONS
  - Advise clients to report manifestations of decreased reflexes, weakness, paresthesias, and sensory loss.
  - Use caution to prevent injury.

Severe tissue damage
- Due to extravasations of vesicants
- NURSING CONSIDERATIONS
  - Stop chemotherapeutic medications if extravasation occurs.
  - Only clinically trained personnel should administer these medications intravenously.
  - Use a central line for infusion.

Alopecia
NURSING CONSIDERATIONS
- Advise clients that hair loss can occur 7 to 10 days after the beginning of treatment and will last for a maximum of 2 months after the last administration of the chemotherapeutic agent.
- Advise clients to select a hairpiece before the occurrence of hair loss.

Paclitaxel

Bone marrow suppression
- Such as low WBC count or neutropenia; bleeding caused by thrombocytopenia or low platelet count; anemia; or low RBCs
- NURSING CONSIDERATIONS
  - Monitor WBC, absolute neutrophil count, platelet count, Hgb, and Hct.
  - Assess for bruising and bleeding gums.
  - Instruct clients to avoid crowds and contact with infectious individuals.

Bradycardia, heart block, MI
NURSING CONSIDERATIONS
- Monitor for cardiac effects.
- Advise clients to inform the nurse of any chest pain or shortness of breath.

Alopecia
NURSING CONSIDERATIONS
- Advise clients that hair loss can occur 7 to 10 days after the beginning of treatment and will last for a maximum of 2 months after the last administration of the chemotherapeutic agent.
- Advise clients to select a hairpiece before hair loss occurs.

CONTRAINDICATIONS/PRECAUTIONS

Vincristine

- Pregnancy Risk Category D.
- Do not use with radiation therapy
- Use with caution in clients who have liver disease or neuromuscular disease.

Paclitaxel

- Pregnancy Risk Category D.
- Contraindicated in clients who have a neutrophil count less than 1,500/mm³. Use with caution in clients who have myelosuppression.

INTERACTIONS

Vincristine

Vincristine can reduce effects of digoxin.
NURSING CONSIDERATIONS: Monitor digoxin level and ECG.

Mitomycin can increase risk for bronchospasm.
NURSING CONSIDERATIONS: Monitor breath sounds.

Phenytoin can decrease vincristine effect.
NURSING CONSIDERATIONS: Monitor phenytoin level.

Paclitaxel

Cisplatin or doxorubicin can increase myelosuppression.
NURSING CONSIDERATIONS: Use together with caution.

Cardiac medications that decrease heart rate, such as beta-blockers, calcium channel blockers, and digoxin, can increase bradycardia.
NURSING CONSIDERATIONS: Monitor heart rate carefully.

Medications that increase risk for bleeding, such as NSAIDs and anticoagulants, can increase bleeding risk with paclitaxel.
NURSING CONSIDERATIONS: Monitor carefully for bleeding.

NURSING ADMINISTRATION

- Assess for indications of neuropathy, including weakness, numbness, tingling, foot drop, ataxia, and paresthesia. Advise clients to use caution and report manifestations.
- Reduce dose for clients who have liver disease.
- Assess breath sounds for bronchospasm.
- Monitor for bleeding (bruising) or infection (fever, sore throat).
- Monitor CBC and liver enzymes.
- Give an antiemetic for nausea and vomiting.
- Advise clients to use good mouth care.
- Stop chemotherapeutic medications if extravasation occurs.
- Advise clients to use birth control during treatment.

Alkylating agents

Nitrogen mustards

SELECT PROTOTYPE MEDICATION: Cyclophosphamide (oral, IV)

OTHER MEDICATIONS
- Mechlorethamine (IV, intracavitary, intrapleural)
- Bendamustine (IV)
- Chlorambucil (oral)
- Melphalan (oral or IV)

Nitrosoureas

SELECT PROTOTYPE MEDICATION: Carmustine (IV, topical implant to area where a brain tumor was removed)

OTHER MEDICATIONS
- Lomustine (oral)
- Streptozocin (IV)

Platinum compounds

SELECT PROTOTYPE MEDICATION: Cisplatin (IV)

OTHER MEDICATION: Carboplatin (IV)

PURPOSE

EXPECTED PHARMACOLOGICAL ACTION

Nitrogen mustards

Cyclophosphamide, mechlorethamine, bendamustine, chlorambucil
- Kills rapid growing cells by alkylation of DNA and RNA synthesis
- Cell cycle phase nonspecific

Melphalan: Bifunctional agent that has two reactive sites to bind DNA

Nitrosoureas

Carmustine, lomustine
- Kills rapid growing cells by interrupting DNA and RNA synthesis
- Cell cycle phase nonspecific
- Crosses the blood-brain barrier

Streptozocin: Selective uptake by the islet cells of the pancreas

Platinum compounds

Cisplatin
- Kills rapid growing cells by interrupting DNA and RNA synthesis
- Cell cycle phase nonspecific

Carboplatin: Cell kill resulting from cross-linking DNA

THERAPEUTIC USES

Nitrogen mustards

Cyclophosphamide: Includes acute lymphomas; solid tumors, such as head, neck, ovary and breast cancers; Hodgkin's and non-Hodgkin's lymphomas; and multiple myeloma

Mechlorethamine: Bronchogenic carcinoma, Hodgkin's disease, leukemias, and mycosis fungoides

Bendamustine: Chronic lymphocytic leukemia, non-Hodgkin's lymphoma

Chlorambucil: Chronic lymphocytic leukemia, Hodgkin's disease, non-Hodgkin's lymphoma, multiple myeloma

Melphalan: Medication of choice for multiple myeloma, lymphoma, carcinoma of the ovary and breast.

Nitrosoureas

Carmustine: Includes brain tumors; Hodgkin's and non-Hodgkin's lymphomas; multiple myeloma; and adenocarcinoma of the stomach, colon, and rectum

Lomustine: Brain cancer, Hodgkin's disease

Streptozocin: Metastatic islet cell tumors

Platinum compounds

Cisplatin: Includes bladder, testicular, and ovarian cancers

Carboplatin: Small cell cancer of the lung; squamous cell cancer of the head, neck; and endometrial cancer

COMPLICATIONS

Bone marrow suppression
- Such as low WBC count or neutropenia, bleeding caused by thrombocytopenia or low platelet count, and anemia or low RBCs
- NURSING CONSIDERATIONS
  - Monitor WBC, absolute neutrophil count, platelet count, Hgb, and Hct.
  - Assess for bruising and bleeding gums.
  - Instruct clients to avoid crowds and contact with infectious individuals.

GI discomfort, such as nausea and vomiting
NURSING CONSIDERATIONS: Administer an antiemetic such as ondansetron in combination with dexamethasone, granisetron, or metoclopramide before beginning chemotherapy.

Cyclophosphamide

Acute hemorrhagic cystitis
NURSING CONSIDERATIONS
- Increase fluids to 3 L/day.
- Monitor for blood in urine.
- Mesna can be given if needed. Mesna is a uroprotectant agent that detoxifies metabolites to reduce hematuria.

Alopecia
NURSING CONSIDERATIONS
- Advise clients that hair loss can occur 7 to 10 days after the beginning of treatment and will last for a maximum of 2 months after the last administration of the chemotherapeutic agent.
- Advise clients to select a hairpiece before the occurrence of hair loss.

Carmustine

Pulmonary fibrosis
NURSING CONSIDERATIONS: Monitor lung function. The client can be treated with corticosteroids.

Liver and kidney toxicity
NURSING CONSIDERATIONS: Monitor liver and kidney function.

Cisplatin

Renal toxicity
NURSING CONSIDERATIONS: Monitor kidney function. Increase fluids and give a diuretic if indicated.

Hearing loss
NURSING CONSIDERATIONS: Monitor for tinnitus and hearing loss.

CONTRAINDICATIONS/PRECAUTIONS

Cyclophosphamide

- Pregnancy Risk Category D
- Contraindicated in clients who have severe myelosuppression or severe infections **Qs**
- Use with caution in clients who have kidney disorder, prostatic hypertrophy, liver disorders, leukopenia, or thrombocytopenia.

Carmustine

- Pregnancy Risk Category D
- Contraindicated in clients who have severe myelosuppression or impaired pulmonary function.

Cisplatin

- Pregnancy Risk Category D
- Contraindicated in clients who have severe myelosuppression, kidney disorders, or hearing loss.

INTERACTIONS

Cyclophosphamide

Concurrent use of succinylcholine can cause increased neuromuscular blockage.
NURSING CONSIDERATIONS: Do not use together.

Carmustine

Concurrent use of cimetidine can increase bone marrow suppression.
NURSING CONSIDERATIONS: Do not use together.

Cisplatin

Concurrent use of aminoglycosides can increase risk for renal toxicity.
NURSING CONSIDERATIONS: Monitor kidney function.

Concurrent use of furosemide can increase hearing loss.
NURSING CONSIDERATIONS: Do not use together.

NURSING ADMINISTRATION

- Encourage adequate fluid intake of 2 to 3 L/day. Qᴘᴄᴄ
- Monitor for blood in urine. Mesna might be indicated.
- Reduce dose for clients who have liver disease.
- Monitor for bleeding (bruising) or infection (fever, sore throat).
- Monitor CBC, uric acid level, and liver enzymes.
- Give antiemetic for nausea and vomiting.
- Advise clients to use good mouth care.
- Stop chemotherapeutic medications if extravasation occurs.
- Advise clients to use birth control during treatment.
- Assess hearing prior to treatment with cisplatin.

Topoisomerase inhibitors

SELECT PROTOTYPE MEDICATION: Topotecan (IV)

PURPOSE

EXPECTED PHARMACOLOGICAL ACTION

- Kills cancer cells by interrupting DNA synthesis
- Cell cycle phase S-specific

THERAPEUTIC USES

Treats metastatic ovarian cancer, cervical cancer, and small cell lung cancer.

COMPLICATIONS

Bone marrow suppression
- Low WBC count or neutropenia, bleeding caused by thrombocytopenia or low platelet count, and anemia or low RBCs
- Can occur 4 to 6 weeks after infusion
- NURSING CONSIDERATIONS
  - Monitor WBC, absolute neutrophil count, platelet count, Hgb, and Hct.
  - Assess for bruising and bleeding gums.
  - Instruct clients to avoid crowds and contact with infectious individuals. Advise clients to continue precautions after treatment is completed.

GI discomfort (nausea and vomiting)
NURSING CONSIDERATIONS: Administer antiemetic such as ondansetron in combination with dexamethasone, granisetron, or metoclopramide before beginning chemotherapy.

Alopecia
NURSING CONSIDERATIONS
- Advise clients that hair loss can occur 7 to 10 days after the beginning of treatment and will last for a maximum of 2 months after the last administration of the chemotherapeutic agent.
- Advise clients to select a hairpiece before the occurrence of hair loss.

CONTRAINDICATIONS/PRECAUTIONS

- Pregnancy Risk Category D
- Contraindicated in clients who have severe myelosuppression with a neutrophil count less than 1,500/mm³ Qs

INTERACTIONS

Cisplatin can increase myelosuppression.
NURSING CONSIDERATIONS: Use with caution.

NURSING ADMINISTRATION

- Monitor for bleeding (bruising) or infection (fever, sore throat). Qᴘᴄᴄ
- Monitor CBC.
- Give antiemetic for nausea and vomiting.
- Advise clients to perform good oral hygiene and avoid mouthwash with alcohol.
- Advise female clients to use birth control during treatment.

Other antineoplastic agents

- Asparaginase (IV, IM)
- Hydroxyurea (oral)
- Procarbazine (oral)

PURPOSE

EXPECTED PHARMACOLOGICAL ACTION

Asparaginase
- Kills cancer cells by interrupting DNA synthesis in leukemia cells
- Cell cycle phase G_1-specific

Hydroxyurea
- Kills cancer cells by interrupting DNA synthesis
- Cell cycle phase S-specific
- Can cross blood–brain barrier

Procarbazine
- Kills cancer cells by interrupting DNA, RNA, and protein synthesis
- Cell cycle phase nonspecific
- Can cross blood–brain barrier

THERAPEUTIC USES

Asparaginase: Acute lymphocytic leukemia

Hydroxyurea: Includes chronic myelogenous leukemia, ovarian, and squamous cell cancers

Procarbazine: Includes brain tumors, and Hodgkin's and non-Hodgkin's lymphomas

COMPLICATIONS

Asparaginase, hydroxyurea, procarbazine

GI discomfort (nausea and vomiting)
NURSING CONSIDERATIONS: Administer antiemetic such as ondansetron in combination with dexamethasone, granisetron, or metoclopramide before beginning chemotherapy.

Asparaginase

Hypersensitivity reaction
NURSING CONSIDERATIONS: Premedicate if needed. Monitor for wheezing and/or rash. Give test dose. Monitor closely.

CNS effects
• From confusion to coma
• Temporary tremor can occur
• NURSING CONSIDERATIONS: Monitor for CNS effects and evaluate frequently for changes.

Liver and pancreas toxicity
NURSING CONSIDERATIONS
• Monitor liver enzymes.
• Monitor for indications of jaundice.
• Monitor pancreatic enzymes.

Renal toxicity
NURSING CONSIDERATIONS: Monitor kidney function. Increase fluids and administer a diuretic if indicated.

Hydroxyurea and procarbazine

Bone marrow suppression
• Low WBC count or neutropenia, bleeding caused by thrombocytopenia or low platelet count, and anemia or low RBCs
• Can occur 4 to 6 weeks after infusion
• NURSING CONSIDERATIONS
  ○ Monitor WBC, absolute neutrophil count, platelet count, hemoglobin, and hematocrit.
  ○ Assess for bruising and bleeding gums.
  ○ Instruct clients to avoid crowds and contact with infectious individuals.
  ○ Advise clients to continue precautions after treatment is completed.

Procarbazine

Peripheral neuropathy symptoms
• Can include weakness and paresthesia
• NURSING CONSIDERATIONS: Advise clients to report manifestations. Use caution to prevent injury.

CONTRAINDICATIONS/PRECAUTIONS

Asparaginase

• Pregnancy Risk Category C
• Contraindicated in clients who have a history of pancreatitis, exposure to chickenpox, or herpes simplex infection **Qs**
• Use with caution in clients who have liver disease.

Hydroxyurea

• Pregnancy Risk Category D
• Contraindicated in clients who have severe myelosuppression or anemia
• Use with caution in clients who have kidney disease.

Procarbazine

• Pregnancy Risk Category D
• Contraindicated in clients who have severe myelosuppression
• Use with caution in clients who have liver or kidney disease.

INTERACTIONS

Asparaginase

Can decrease effects of methotrexate.
NURSING CONSIDERATIONS: Use with caution. Monitor for medication effect.

Prednisone and vincristine can increase asparaginase toxicity.
NURSING CONSIDERATIONS: Use with caution.

Increased risk for bleeding if used with anticoagulant, antiplatelet medication.
NURSING CONSIDERATIONS: Monitor blood coagulation panel.

Hydroxyurea

Cytotoxic medications can increase hydroxyurea.
NURSING CONSIDERATIONS: Use with caution together.

Procarbazine

Can increase depressant effects of CNS depressants, such as opioids.
NURSING CONSIDERATIONS: Avoid concurrent use.

MAOI or tricyclic antidepressants, foods containing tyramine, and many OTC preparations such as cough medicines can cause hypertensive crisis
NURSING CONSIDERATIONS: Discontinue in advance of procarbazine therapy.

Alcohol can cause a disulfiram-type reaction.
NURSING CONSIDERATIONS: Advise the client to discontinue alcohol in any form before starting treatment.

NURSING ADMINISTRATION

Asparaginase

- Monitor for allergic reaction. Give a test dose. Have resuscitation equipment on hand. Qᴘᴄᴄ
- Give an antiemetic for nausea and vomiting.
- Advise clients to use good mouth care.
- Advise clients to use birth control during treatment.

Hydroxyurea

- Monitor for bleeding (bruising) or infection (fever, sore throat). Withhold medication and notify the provider for a WBC less than 2,500/mm³ or a platelet count less than 100,000/mm³.
- Monitor CBC.
- Give an antiemetic for nausea and vomiting.
- Advise clients to use good mouth care.
- Advise clients to use birth control during treatment.

Procarbazine

- Monitor for neurologic effects, such as confusion or paresthesia.
- Withhold the medication and notify the provider for a WBC less than 4,000/mm³ and a platelet count less than 100,000/mm³.

Noncytotoxic chemotherapy agents

Noncytotoxic chemotherapy medications are nontoxic to cells.

Hormonal agents are effective against tumors that are supported or suppressed by hormones.
- **Hormone agonists** cause an increase in a hormone and can be effective against tumors that require a particular hormone for support. The use of androgenic hormones in a client who has estrogen-dependent cancer can suppress growth of this type of cancer. Conversely, the use of estrogenic hormones for a testosterone-dependent cancer can suppress growth of this type of cancer.
- **Hormone antagonists** block certain hormones and can be effective against tumors that require a particular hormone for support. The use of an antiestrogen hormone in a client who has estrogen-dependent cancer can suppress growth of this type of cancer. The same is true for antitestosterone hormones.

Biological response modulators act as immunostimulants to enhance the immune response and reduce proliferation of cancer cells.

Targeted antineoplastic agents are antibodies or small molecules that attach to specific target sites to stop cancer growth without injuring healthy tissue.

Hormonal agents: Prostate cancer medications

Gonadotropin-releasing hormone agonists

SELECT PROTOTYPE MEDICATION: Leuprolide (subcutaneous, IM)

OTHER MEDICATIONS
- Triptorelin (subcutaneous, IM)
- Goserelin (subcutaneous, IM)
- Histrelin (subcutaneous, IM)

Androgen receptor blockers

SELECT PROTOTYPE MEDICATION: Flutamide (oral)

OTHER MEDICATIONS
- Bicalutamide (oral)
- Nilutamide (oral)

PURPOSE

EXPECTED PHARMACOLOGICAL ACTION

Gonadotropin-releasing hormone agonists
- Testes stop producing testosterone by stopping the release of luteinizing and follicle-stimulating hormones
- Used instead of surgical castration.

Androgen receptor blockers
- Blocks testosterone at receptor site
- Used in conjunction with gonadotropin-releasing hormone agonists to block androgen receptors and suppress the growth of prostate cancer

THERAPEUTIC USES

Gonadotropin-releasing hormone agonists: Palliative treatment for advanced prostate cancer

Androgen receptor blockers: Treatment of prostate cancer

COMPLICATIONS

Leuprolide

Hot flashes, decreased libido, and gynecomastia
NURSING CONSIDERATIONS: Warn clients about adverse effects. Adverse reactions can be transient.

Decreased bone density
NURSING CONSIDERATIONS
- Advise clients to increase calcium and vitamin D intake.
- Advise clients to increase bone mass with weight-bearing exercises.

Dysrhythmias, pulmonary edema
NURSING CONSIDERATIONS: Monitor for dysrhythmias and assess breath sounds.

Disease flare
NURSING CONSIDERATIONS: Manifestations of worsening of the prostate cancer after a dose of the medication.

Flutamide

Hot flashes, decreased libido, and gynecomastia
NURSING CONSIDERATIONS: Warn clients about adverse effects.

Nausea, vomiting, diarrhea
NURSING CONSIDERATIONS: Monitor intake and output.

Hepatitis
NURSING CONSIDERATIONS: Monitor liver enzymes.

CONTRAINDICATIONS/PRECAUTIONS

Leuprolide

- Pregnancy Risk Category X
- Contraindicated in clients who are hypersensitive to gonadotropin-releasing agonists Qs

Flutamide

- Pregnancy Risk Category D
- Contraindicated in clients who have severe liver disease.

INTERACTIONS

Leuprolide

Flutamide and megestrol increase antineoplastic action.

Flutamide

Concurrent use of flutamide and warfarin can increase anticoagulation.
NURSING CONSIDERATIONS: Monitor PT and INR.

NURSING ADMINISTRATION

Leuprolide

- Advise clients to increase calcium and vitamin D intake. Advise clients to minimize bone loss with weight-bearing exercises.
- Perform bone density testing
- Monitor for dysrhythmias and assess breath sounds.
- Warn clients that prostate symptoms can worsen at beginning of treatment (disease flare), which can be prevented by adding flutamide to the client's treatment.
- Monitor prostate-specific antigen (PSA) and testosterone levels, which should both decrease with treatment.

Flutamide

- Administered with a gonadotropin-releasing hormone agonist (e.g., leuprolide) or alone following surgical castration
- Warn clients of side effects of the medication, such as gynecomastia.

Hormonal agents: Breast cancer medications

Estrogen receptor blockers

SELECT PROTOTYPE MEDICATION: Tamoxifen (oral)

OTHER MEDICATIONS
- Raloxifene (oral)
- Fulvestrant (IM)
- Toremifene (oral)

Aromatase inhibitors

SELECT PROTOTYPE MEDICATION: Anastrozole

OTHER MEDICATIONS
- Letrozole
- Exemestane (oral)

Monoclonal antibody

SELECT PROTOTYPE MEDICATION: Trastuzumab (IV)

PURPOSE

EXPECTED PHARMACOLOGICAL ACTION

Estrogen receptor blockers: Stops growth of breast cancer cells, which are estrogen-dependent cancers

Aromatase inhibitors: Stops growth of breast cancer cells by blocking estrogen production

Monoclonal antibody: Targets breast cancer cells, prevents cell growth, and causes cell death

THERAPEUTIC USES

Estrogen receptor blockers: Used to treat or prevent breast cancer

Aromatase inhibitors: Used to treat breast cancer in women who are postmenopausal

Monoclonal antibody
- Used to treat metastatic breast cancer
- Can be used alone or in conjunction with paclitaxel

COMPLICATIONS

Tamoxifen

Endometrial cancer
NURSING CONSIDERATIONS: Monitor for abnormal bleeding. Advise clients to have a yearly gynecological exam and PAP smear.

Hypercalcemia
NURSING CONSIDERATIONS: Monitor calcium level.

Nausea and vomiting
NURSING CONSIDERATIONS
- Monitor fluid status.
- Administer fluids and antiemetics as prescribed.

Pulmonary embolus
NURSING CONSIDERATIONS
- Assess breath sounds.
- Advise clients to report chest pain or shortness of breath.

Hot flashes
NURSING CONSIDERATIONS: Warn clients about adverse effects.

Vaginal discharge or bleeding
NURSING CONSIDERATIONS: Monitor bleeding and discharge.

Anastrozole

Muscle and joint pain, headache
NURSING CONSIDERATIONS: Treat pain with a mild analgesic as prescribed.

Nausea
NURSING CONSIDERATIONS
- Monitor fluid status.
- Administer fluids and antiemetics as prescribed.

Vaginal bleeding
NURSING CONSIDERATIONS: Monitor bleeding and CBC.

Increased risk for osteoporosis
NURSING CONSIDERATIONS: Advise clients to take calcium and vitamin D supplements and perform weight-bearing exercises.

Hot flashes
NURSING CONSIDERATIONS: Warn clients about adverse effects.

Trastuzumab

Cardiac toxicity, tachycardia, heart failure
NURSING CONSIDERATIONS
- Obtain baseline ECG and monitor.
- Monitor for dyspnea and edema. Advise clients to report chest pain or shortness of breath.

Hypersensitivity reaction
NURSING CONSIDERATIONS: Monitor closely during infusion. Have resuscitation equipment nearby.

Nausea and vomiting
NURSING CONSIDERATIONS: Monitor fluid status.

CONTRAINDICATIONS/PRECAUTIONS

Tamoxifen

- Pregnancy Risk Category D
- Contraindicated in clients taking warfarin and in clients who have a history of blood clots or pulmonary embolism Qs

Anastrozole

- Pregnancy Risk Category X
- Contraindicated in women before menopause and in severe liver disease
- Use with caution in clients who have mild to moderate liver disease.

Trastuzumab

- Pregnancy Risk Category D
- Contraindicated in clients hypersensitive to the medication
- Use with caution in clients who have heart disease.

INTERACTIONS

Tamoxifen

Tamoxifen can increase the anticoagulation action of warfarin.
NURSING CONSIDERATIONS
- Monitor PT and INR.
- Warfarin doses might need to be adjusted.

Some SSRI antidepressants (e.g., paroxetine) decrease effectiveness of tamoxifen.
NURSING CONSIDERATIONS: Avoid using together.

Anastrozole

Tamoxifen and estrogen-like medications can reduce anastrozole effects.
NURSING CONSIDERATIONS: Avoid using together.

Concurrent use of anastrozole and anthracyclines can increase the risk for cardiac effects.
NURSING CONSIDERATIONS: Monitor for cardiac effects.

NURSING ADMINISTRATION

- Advise clients to increase calcium and vitamin D intake. Advise clients to reduce bone loss with weight-bearing exercises.
- Monitor for dysrhythmias and assess breath sounds.
- Encourage clients to perform monthly breast self-examination, and schedule annual gynecologic and breast examinations and mammogram with the provider.
- Monitor CBC and calcium levels.
- Monitor fluid status.
- Advise female clients to use birth control during therapy.

Biologic response modifiers

SELECT PROTOTYPE MEDICATION: Interferon alfa-2b (subcutaneous, IM, IV)

OTHER MEDICATIONS
- Aldesleukin (IV infusion)
- Bacillus Calmette-Guerin (BCG) vaccine (intravesical into the bladder)

PURPOSE

EXPECTED PHARMACOLOGICAL ACTION: Increases immune response and decreases production of cancer cells.

THERAPEUTIC USES: Treat or prevent hairy cell leukemia, chronic myelogenous leukemia, malignant melanoma, and AIDS-related Kaposi's sarcoma.

COMPLICATIONS

Flu–like symptoms
- Fever, fatigue, headache, chills, myalgia
- NURSING CONSIDERATIONS: Administer acetaminophen as prescribed.

Bone marrow suppression, alopecia, cardiotoxicity, and neurotoxicity (with prolonged therapy)
NURSING CONSIDERATIONS
- Monitor CBC, fatigue level, and indications of cardiotoxicity (dysrhythmias, palpitations, myocardial infarction, heart failure) and neurotoxicity (confusion, ataxia, inability to concentrate).
- Monitor for manifestations of infection.
- Instruct clients to report dizziness or tingling/numbness of the hands or feet.
- Monitor for bruising; bleeding; and blood in stools, urine, sputum, or emesis.

Depression, anxiety, insomnia, altered mental states
NURSING CONSIDERATIONS: Monitor mood and mental status, and assess for suicidal thoughts.

CONTRAINDICATIONS/PRECAUTIONS

- Pregnancy Risk Category C
- Contraindicated in clients who have hypersensitivity to the medication, suicidal thoughts, colitis, or pancreatitis
- Use caution in clients who have severe liver, kidney, heart, or pulmonary disease; diabetes mellitus; or history of depression. Qs

INTERACTIONS

Concurrent use with theophylline can lead to theophylline toxicity.
NURSING CONSIDERATIONS: Monitor clients for indications of toxicity. Decreased theophylline dosage might be indicated.

Zidovudine can increase the risk of neutropenia or thrombocytopenia.
NURSING CONSIDERATIONS
- Monitor for neutropenia. Instruct clients to avoid crowds and contact with infectious individuals.
- Monitor for bleeding or easy bruising.

Concurrent use with medications that are cardiotoxic or neurotoxic can increase cardiotoxicity or neurotoxicity.
NURSING CONSIDERATIONS: Monitor for cardiotoxicity or neurotoxicity.

Concurrent use with vaccines using a live virus can reduce antibody response.
NURSING CONSIDERATIONS: Avoid use together.

NURSING ADMINISTRATION

- Store the medication in the refrigerator and do not freeze. Administer at room temperature. Do not shake the vial.
- Monitor for flu symptoms. Premedicate with acetaminophen if prescribed.
- Advise clients to practice good oral hygiene.
- Monitor CBC, platelets, and electrolytes.
- Monitor fluid status.

Targeted antineoplastic medications

Epidural growth factor receptor (EGFR)–tyrosine kinase inhibitors

SELECT PROTOTYPE MEDICATION: Cetuximab

OTHER MEDICATION
- Panitumumab (IV)
- Gefitinib (IV)
- Erlotinib (IV)
- Afatinib (IV)

BCR–ABL tyrosine kinase inhibitors

SELECT PROTOTYPE MEDICATION: Imatinib (oral)

CD20–directed antibodies

SELECT PROTOTYPE MEDICATION: Rituximab (IV)

Angiogenesis inhibitors

SELECT PROTOTYPE MEDICATION: Bevacizumab (IV)

PURPOSE

EXPECTED PHARMACOLOGICAL ACTION

EGFR-tyrosine kinase inhibitors: Antibody that stops cancer cell growth and increases apoptosis (cell death)

BCR-ABL tyrosine kinase inhibitors: Stops cancer growth by inhibiting intracellular enzymes

CD20-directed antibodies: Monoclonal antibody that binds to specific antigens on B-lymphocytes and then destroys cancer cells

Angiogenesis inhibitors: Antibody that stops cancer cell growth and increases apoptosis

THERAPEUTIC USES

EGFR-tyrosine kinase inhibitors: Treat EGFR-positive cancers (colorectal and solid tumors of the head and neck)

BCR-ABL tyrosine kinase inhibitors: Treat chronic myeloid leukemia

CD20-directed antibodies: Treat non-Hodgkin's lymphoma, B-cell chronic lymphocytic leukemia

Angiogenesis inhibitors: Treat colorectal and lung cancers

COMPLICATIONS

Cetuximab

Infusion reaction, rash, hypotension, wheezing
NURSING CONSIDERATIONS
- Monitor carefully for indications of a reaction.
- Premedicate if needed with diphenhydramine or corticosteroids.
- Stop treatment and administer antihistamines, epinephrine, glucocorticoids, bronchodilators, and oxygen as prescribed.

Pulmonary emboli
NURSING CONSIDERATIONS: Monitor breath sounds. Monitor SaO_2.

Skin toxicity, rash
NURSING CONSIDERATIONS: Monitor for rash over 2 weeks of treatment. Treat with topical antibiotics if needed.

Imatinib

GI discomfort, such as nausea and vomiting
NURSING CONSIDERATIONS
- Administer antiemetic such as ondansetron in combination with dexamethasone, granisetron, or metoclopramide before beginning chemotherapy.
- Take with food.

Flu-like symptoms
- Fever, fatigue, headache, chills, myalgia
- NURSING CONSIDERATIONS: Administer acetaminophen as prescribed.

Edema
NURSING CONSIDERATIONS: Monitor for edema.

Hypokalemia
NURSING CONSIDERATIONS: Monitor potassium level.

Neutropenia, anemia
NURSING CONSIDERATIONS
- Monitor CBC.
- Assess for bruising and bleeding gums.
- Instruct clients to avoid crowds and contact with infectious individuals.

Rituximab

Infusion reaction, rash, hypotension, wheezing
NURSING CONSIDERATIONS
- Monitor carefully for indications of a reaction.
- Premedicate if needed with diphenhydramine or corticosteroids.
- Stop treatment and administer epinephrine as prescribed.

Flu-like symptoms
- Fever, fatigue, headache, chills, myalgia
- NURSING CONSIDERATIONS: Administer acetaminophen as prescribed.

Tumor lysis syndrome due to rapid cell death
- Can lead to kidney failure, hypocalcemia, and hyperuricemia
- NURSING CONSIDERATIONS
  - Monitor kidney function, and administer dialysis if needed.
  - Monitor fluids and electrolytes.
  - Teach the client to report manifestations, which begin 12 to 24 hr after the first medication infusion.

Bevacizumab

Thromboembolism
- Including cerebrovascular accident, myocardial infarction, transient ischemic attacks (TIA)
- NURSING CONSIDERATIONS: Monitor for thromboembolic disorders.

Alopecia
NURSING CONSIDERATIONS
- Advise clients that hair loss can occur 7 to 10 days after the beginning of treatment and will last for a maximum of 2 months after the last administration of the chemotherapeutic agent.
- Advise clients to select a hairpiece before the occurrence of hair loss.

Hemorrhage
- GI, vaginal, nasal, intracranial, or pulmonary
- NURSING CONSIDERATIONS: Monitor carefully for hemorrhage from any site, including hemoptysis.

Hypertension
NURSING CONSIDERATIONS: Monitor blood pressure.

Gastric perforation
NURSING CONSIDERATIONS: Advise clients to notify the provider if they experience abdominal pain associated with vomiting and constipation.

CONTRAINDICATIONS/PRECAUTIONS

Cetuximab

- Pregnancy Risk Category C
- Contraindicated in clients who have hypersensitivity to the medication **Qs**

Imatinib

- Pregnancy Risk Category D
- Contraindicated in clients who have hypersensitivity to the medication
- Use with caution in clients who have liver disease.

Rituximab

- Pregnancy Risk Category C
- Contraindicated in clients who have hypersensitivity to the medication
- Use with caution in clients who have liver or kidney failure.

Bevacizumab

- Pregnancy Risk Category D
- Contraindicated in clients who have a low WBC, nephrotic syndrome, recent surgery or dental work, or hypertensive crisis.
- Use with caution in clients who have cardiac or renal disease history or hypersensitivity to the medication.

INTERACTIONS

Cetuximab

Sun exposure may increase skin toxicity.
CLIENT EDUCATION: Advise clients to use sunscreen and avoid exposure.

Imatinib

Acetaminophen can increase chance of liver failure.
NURSING CONSIDERATIONS: Monitor liver enzymes.

Concurrent use with warfarin can increase anticoagulant effect.
NURSING CONSIDERATIONS
- Monitor for indications of bleeding.
- Monitor INR and PT, and adjust warfarin dosage accordingly.

Clarithromycin, erythromycin, and ketoconazole can slow imatinib metabolism and cause toxicity.
NURSING CONSIDERATIONS: Monitor for toxicity.

Carbamazepine and phenytoin can increase imatinib metabolism.
NURSING CONSIDERATIONS: Monitor for effectiveness.

Rituximab

Calcium channel blockers and other antihypertensive medications increase chance of hypotension.
NURSING CONSIDERATIONS: Antihypertensives might be withheld up to 12 hr prior to rituximab infusions.

Bevacizumab

Bevacizumab can increase sunitinib level.
NURSING CONSIDERATIONS: Monitor medication levels.

NURSING ADMINISTRATION

- Monitor for infusion reaction and premedicate if prescribed.
- Advise clients to protect skin from the sun and assess for rash. Qpcc
- Advise clients to notify the provider for shortness of breath.
- Advise clients to practice good oral hygiene.
- Monitor CBC, platelets, and electrolytes.
- Monitor fluid status.
- Assess for edema.
- Advise clients to report adverse reactions, such as abdominal pain, skin lesions, headache, and episodes of bleeding.

Application Exercises

1. A nurse is caring for a client who has breast cancer and asks why she is receiving a combination therapy of cyclophosphamide, methotrexate, and fluorouracil. The response by the nurse should include that combination chemotherapy is used to do which of the following? (Select all that apply.)

    A. Decrease medication resistance

    B. Attack cancer cells at different stages of cell growth

    C. Block chemotherapy agent from entering healthy cells

    D. Stimulate immune system

    E. Decrease injury to normal body cells

2. A nurse is preparing to administer cyclophosphamide IV to a client who has Hodgkin's disease. Which of the following medications should the nurse expect to administer concurrently with the chemotherapy to prevent an adverse effect of cyclophosphamide?

    A. Uroprotectant agent, such as mesna

    B. Opioid, such as morphine

    C. Loop diuretic, such as furosemide

    D. H_1 receptor antagonist, such as diphenhydramine

3. A nurse is preparing to administer leucovorin to a client who has cancer and is receiving chemotherapy with methotrexate. Which of the following responses should the nurse use when the client asks why leucovorin is being given?

    A. "Leucovorin reduces the risk of a transfusion reaction from methotrexate."

    B. "Leucovorin increases platelet production and prevents bleeding."

    C. "Leucovorin potentiates the cytotoxic effects of methotrexate."

    D. "Leucovorin protects healthy cells from methotrexate's toxic effect."

4. A nurse is teaching a client who has breast cancer about tamoxifen. Which of the following adverse effects of tamoxifen should the nurse discuss with the client?

    A. Irregular heart beat

    B. Abnormal uterine bleeding

    C. Yellow sclera or dark-colored urine.

    D. Difficulty swallowing

5. A nurse is caring for a client who is being treated with interferon alfa-2b for malignant melanoma. For which of the following adverse effects should the nurse monitor? (Select all that apply.)

    A. Tinnitus

    B. Muscle aches

    C. Peripheral neuropathy

    D. Bone loss

    E. Depression

6. A nurse is caring for a client who receives rituximab to treat non-Hodgkin's leukemia and who asks the nurse how rituximab works. Which of the following should the nurse include?

    A. Blocks hormone receptors

    B. Increases immune response

    C. Binds with specific antigens on tumor cells

    D. Stops DNA replication during cell division

PRACTICE Active Learning Scenario

A nurse in an outpatient facility is teaching a client who has prostate cancer and a new prescription for monthly injections of leuprolide IM. What should the nurse teach this client about leuprolide? Use the ATI Active Learning Template: Medication to complete this item.

THERAPEUTIC USES: Identify for leuprolide.

COMPLICATIONS: Identify two adverse effects.

NURSING INTERVENTIONS: Describe two diagnostic tests to monitor.

CLIENT EDUCATION: Include two teaching points.

Application Exercises Key

1. A. **CORRECT:** Medication resistance is decreased with combination therapy because the chance of developing resistance to several medication is less than to only one medication.

   B. **CORRECT:** Each medication kills cancer cells at a different stage of growth. A combination of medications can kill more cancer cells than only one medication.

   C. Chemotherapy agents are not blocked from entering healthy cells during combination therapy.

   D. Cancer chemotherapy with a combination of cytotoxic agents often causes infection rather than stimulating the immune system.

   E. **CORRECT:** Injury to normal body cells can be decreased by combination therapy because the medications used have different toxicities.

   Ⓝ *NCLEX® Connection: Pharmacological and Parenteral Therapies, Medication Administration*

2. A. **CORRECT:** Mesna is a uroprotectant agent that can help prevent hemorrhagic cystitis when administered IV with a nitrogen mustard chemotherapy medication.

   B. An opioid is not administered concurrently with cyclophosphamide to prevent an adverse effect.

   C. A loop diuretic is not administered concurrently with cyclophosphamide to prevent an adverse effect.

   D. An H_1 receptor antagonist is not administered concurrently with cyclophosphamide to prevent an adverse effect.

   Ⓝ *NCLEX® Connection: Pharmacological and Parenteral Therapies, Parenteral/Intravenous Therapies*

3. A. Leucovorin does not reduce the risk of a transfusion reaction from methotrexate.

   B. Leucovorin does not increase platelet production.

   C. Leucovorin does not potentiate the effects of methotrexate.

   D. **CORRECT:** Leucovorin, a folic acid derivative and an antagonist to methotrexate, is given within 12 hr of high doses of methotrexate to protect healthy cells from the toxic effects of methotrexate.

   Ⓝ *NCLEX® Connection: Pharmacological and Parenteral Therapies, Medication Administration*

4. A. An irregular heart beat is not an adverse effect of tamoxifen.

   B. **CORRECT:** Vaginal discharge and bleeding are adverse effects of tamoxifen. The client who takes tamoxifen is also at increased risk for endometrial cancer, so any abnormal uterine bleeding should be carefully monitored and evaluated.

   C. Liver dysfunction, which can be manifested by yellow sclera or dark urine, is not an adverse effect of taking tamoxifen.

   D. Difficulty swallowing is not an adverse effect of tamoxifen.

   Ⓝ *NCLEX® Connection: Pharmacological and Parenteral Therapies, Adverse Effects/Contraindications/Side Effects/Interactions*

5. A. Tinnitus is not an adverse effect of interferon alfa-2b.

   B. **CORRECT:** Muscle aches and other flu-like manifestations are common adverse effects of interferon alfa-2b. Acetaminophen may be prescribed to relieve these manifestations.

   C. **CORRECT:** Peripheral neuropathy, dizziness, and fatigue are CNS effects that can occur when taking interferon alfa-2b. These should be reported to the provider, and the nurse should teach the client to prevent injury from falls.

   D. Bone loss can occur from treatment with gonadotropin-releasing hormone agonists, such as leuprolide. Bone loss does not occur with interferon alfa-2b treatment.

   E. **CORRECT:** Depression and mental status changes can occur with interferon alfa-2b treatment. The nurse should assess the client for suicidal thoughts.

   Ⓝ *NCLEX® Connection: Pharmacological and Parenteral Therapies, Adverse Effects/Contraindications/Side Effects/Interactions*

6. A. Medications like tamoxifen, an estrogen-receptor modifier, work by blocking hormone receptors. Rituximab does not work in this way.

   B. Interferon alfa-2b is an example of a medication that works by stimulating the client's own immune system. Rituximab does not work in this way.

   C. **CORRECT:** Rituximab is a monoclonal antibody that binds to specific antigens on B-lymphocytes and then destroying cancer cells.

   D. Fluorouracil is an example of a cytotoxic medication that kills cells as they divide. Rituximab does not work in this way.

   Ⓝ *NCLEX® Connection: Pharmacological and Parenteral Therapies, Medication Administration*

PRACTICE Answer

Using the ATI Active Learning Template: Medication

THERAPEUTIC USES: Leuprolide is a gonadotropin-releasing hormone antagonist that prevents testosterone production by stopping the release of luteinizing and follicle-stimulating hormones. It is used instead of surgical castration for clients who have advanced prostate cancer.

COMPLICATIONS
- Hot flashes (or flashes), decreased libido, gynecomastia
- Cardiac manifestations (such as dysrhythmias) and increased edema, which can lead to heart failure
- Decreased bone density, which can lead to fractures
- Disease flare, which means manifestations of the client's prostate cancer can worsen after a dose of the medication

NURSING INTERVENTIONS
- Prostate-specific antigen and testosterone levels, which should both decrease with treatment.
- Bone density testing can be needed for some clients, as well as ECG if cardiac manifestations are present.

CLIENT EDUCATION
- Teach the client about the need for calcium and vitamin D in his diet.
- Encourage the client to increase weight-bearing exercise to minimize bone loss.
- Teach the client to report a flare in prostate manifestations to the provider.
- Advise the client to report adverse effects, such as palpitations, edema, and hot flashes, to the provider.

Ⓝ *NCLEX® Connection: Pharmacological and Parenteral Therapies, Medication Administration*

When reviewing the following chapters, keep in mind the relevant topics and tasks of the NCLEX outline, in particular:

Client Needs: Pharmacological and Parenteral Therapies

ADVERSE EFFECTS/CONTRAINDICATIONS/SIDE EFFECTS/ INTERACTIONS: Identify symptoms/evidence of an allergic reaction.

MEDICATION ADMINISTRATION: Evaluate appropriateness and accuracy of medication order for client.

PARENTERAL/INTRAVENOUS THERAPIES: Evaluate the client's response to intermittent parenteral fluid therapy.

UNIT 12   MEDICATIONS FOR INFECTION

CHAPTER 43 *Principles of Antimicrobial Therapy*

Antimicrobial therapy is the use of medications to treat infections due to bacteria, viruses, or fungi. Antimicrobials (natural or synthetic) must use selective toxicity to kill or otherwise control microbes without destroying host cells.

Changes in the DNA of micro-organisms, called conjugation, which produces resistance to multiple existing medications, mandates the continual creation of new antimicrobials.

Suprainfection is a type of resistance that results when an antibiotic kills normal flora, thus favoring the emergence of a new infection that is difficult to eliminate.

METHODS OF ANTIMICROBIAL ACTIONS

- Destroying the cell wall that is present in bacteria but not in mammals
- Inhibiting the conversion of an enzyme unique for a particular bacterium's survival
- Impairing protein synthesis in the bacteria's ribosomes, which are never identical to mammalian cells

CLASSIFICATION OF ANTIMICROBIAL MEDICATIONS

- Requires defining which microbes are susceptible to each medication
  - **Narrow-spectrum antibiotics,** to which only a few types of bacteria are sensitive
  - **Broad-spectrum antibiotics,** to which a wide variety of bacteria are sensitive
- Requires identifying the mechanism of action of each antibacterial medication
  - **Bactericidal medications** are directly lethal to the micro-organism.
  - **Bacteriostatic medications** slow the growth of the micro-organism, but the immune-system response of phagocytic cells (macrophages, neutrophils) actually destroys the bacteria.
- Multiple factors determine which medication providers prescribe for clinical use (antibacterial, antifungal, or antiviral medication).

SELECTION OF ANTIMICROBIALS

IDENTIFICATION OF CAUSATIVE AGENT

Laboratory testing of body fluids, such as blood, urine, sputum, and wound drainage, identifies the micro-organism causing the infection.

Gram stain

Technicians examine an aspirate of the body fluid under a microscope to identify the micro-organisms directly.

Culture

Technicians apply the aspirate to a culture medium, where colonies of the micro-organism grow over several days. A culture is preferable when a gram stain does not yield a positive identification.
- Nurses should obtain specimens for culture prior to treatment with antimicrobials. QEBP
- Nurses must collect fluid for culture carefully to prevent contamination.

SENSITIVITY OF A MICRO-ORGANISM TO AN ANTIMICROBIAL

For organisms commonly resistant, technicians test the sensitivity of the organism to various antimicrobials.
- **The disk diffusion test** (Kirby-Bauer test) is most common. The size of the bacteria-free zone on the disk determines the degree of medication sensitivity.
- **Serial dilution** is a quantitative method using several test tubes with varying amounts of the antimicrobial that helps determine the amount necessary to treat a specific infection.
  - **Minimum inhibitory concentration (MIC):** The amount of antibiotic that inhibits bacterial growth completely but does not kill the bacteria.
  - **Minimum bactericidal concentration:** The lowest concentration of the antibiotic that kills 99.9% of the bacteria.
  - Providers should adjust the antibiotic dosage to produce the concentration equal to or greater than the MIC.
- **Gradient diffusion** uses a disk and strips with varying concentrations of antibiotic. No further growth of bacteria identifies the essential antibiotic concentration.

HOST FACTORS

Immune system

- In people who have an intact immune system, an antimicrobial works with host defense systems to suppress micro-organisms. Providers prescribe either bactericidal or bacteriostatic antibiotics.
- People with immune-system compromise need strong bactericidal antibiotics, not bacteriostatic medication.

Site of infection

Some sites are difficult for antimicrobials to reach and achieve the MIC.
- Infections in cerebrospinal fluid, where the antimicrobials have to cross the blood-brain barrier (meningitis)
- Bacterial infiltration within the heart (endocarditis)
  - Infectious micro-organisms vegetate on the thrombus that develops on the injured endocardium.
  - New thrombus formation covers and conceals the micro-organisms, making it difficult for defense mechanisms and antibiotics to kill them.
- Purulent abscesses anywhere within the body due to poor blood supply
- Surgical removal of drainage increases the effect of antimicrobials
- Phagocytes that attack foreign objects (pacemaker, joint prosthesis, vascular grafts, heart valves, surgical mesh) and become less able to destroy micro-organisms that colonize around the foreign object

Age

- Infants are at increased risk for antimicrobial toxicity due to undeveloped kidney and liver function, causing slow excretion of the medication.
- Older adult clients easily develop toxicity because of the reduction in medication metabolism and excretion. Ⓖ

Pregnancy

- Antimicrobials can harm a developing fetus by crossing over to the placenta. Ⓠs
  - **Sulfonamides** can produce kernicterus, a severe neurologic disorder, in newborns.
  - **Gentamicin** causes hearing loss in infants.
  - **Tetracyclines** cause discoloration of developing teeth. Toxicity to these antibiotics is more likely during pregnancy.
- Lactation is usually a contraindication for antimicrobials because of possible danger to breastfeeding infants.

Presence of a previous allergic reaction

- Especially with penicillin
- Clients should not receive penicillin after an allergic reaction, narrowing the antibiotic choices for those clients.

Combination therapy

Combining more than one antimicrobial can cause additive, potentiating, or antagonistic effects.
- To treat severe infections
- To treat infections from more than one micro-organism
- Prevents bacterial resistance from causing an infection, such as tuberculosis
- Decreases the risk of toxicity by reducing the dosage of each medication
- Produces more effective treatment than using only one antimicrobial medication

Combining antimicrobials can cause adverse effects.
- Increased resistance to antimicrobials
- Increased cost of therapy
- More adverse or toxic reactions
- Antagonistic effects among the various antimicrobials
- Increased risk for a suprainfection

PROPHYLAXIS

- Indications for prophylactic use include prevention of the following.
  - Infections for clients undergoing gastrointestinal, cardiac, peripheral vascular, orthopedic, or gynecologic surgery
  - Sexually transmitted infections following sexual exposure
- Use antimicrobials for individuals who have the following.
  - Prosthetic heart valves prior to dental or other procedures because of the danger of bacterial endocarditis
  - Recurring urinary tract infections

PREVENTIVE MEASURES

- Perform hand hygiene before and after each client contact to prevent the spread of infection.
- Recognize invasive procedures that increase the risk of infection (indwelling urinary catheter, IV catheter, cardiac catheterization).
- Encourage prevention by having clients maintain an up-to-date immunization status.
- Instruct clients to take the full course of antimicrobials the provider prescribes to prevent medication resistance and recurrence of infection.
- Use infection-control procedures to prevent transmission of resistant micro-organisms. Practice infection-control principles, such as aseptic technique, standard and transmission-based precautions, and careful assignment of rooms within facilities.
- Evaluate the effectiveness of treatment.
  - Check post-treatment cultures to confirm that they are negative for micro-organisms.
  - Monitor clients for clinical improvement (clear breath sounds and resolution of fever).

Application Exercises

1. A nurse is implementing a plan of care for a client who has a wound infection. Which of the following actions should the nurse perform first?

   A. Administer antibiotic medication.

   B. Obtain a wound specimen for culture.

   C. Review WBC laboratory findings.

   D. Apply a dressing to the wound.

2. A nurse is caring for a client who has a urinary tract infection and a history of recurrence of this type of infection. The client asks why the provider has not yet prescribed an antibiotic. The nurse should explain that the provider has to wait for the results of which of the following laboratory tests to identify which antibiotic to prescribe?

   A. Gram stain

   B. Culture

   C. Sensitivity

   D. Specific gravity

3. A nurse is preparing information for the unit's nurses about the effectiveness of antimicrobial therapy for clients who have bacterial infections. Which of the following host factors should the nurse include as conditions that affect antimicrobial effectiveness? (Select all that apply.)

   A. Meningitis

   B. Pacemaker

   C. Endocarditis

   D. Pneumonia

   E. Pyelonephritis

4. A nurse is caring for a group of clients who are receiving antimicrobial therapy. Which of the following clients should the nurse plan to monitor for manifestations of antibiotic toxicity?

   A. An adolescent client who has a sinus infection

   B. An older adult client who has prostatitis

   C. A client who is postpartum and has mastitis

   D. A middle adult client who has a urinary tract infection

5. A charge nurse is teaching a group of nurses about the importance of prophylactic antimicrobial therapy. Which of the following information should the charge nurse include in the teaching? (Select all that apply.)

   A. Administer prophylactic antimicrobial therapy to clients who report exposure to a sexually transmitted infection.

   B. Administer prophylactic antimicrobial therapy to clients who are having orthopedic surgery.

   C. Instruct clients who have a prosthetic heart valve about the need for prophylactic antimicrobial therapy before dental work.

   D. Consult the provider for prophylactic antimicrobial therapy for clients who have recurrent urinary tract infections.

   E. Instruct clients to request prophylactic antimicrobial therapy immediately when they have an upper respiratory infection.

PRACTICE Active Learning Scenario

A staff educator is providing information to a group of nurses about ways to prevent the spread of micro-organisms. What information should the educator include?
Use the ATI Active Learning Template: Basic Concept to complete this item.

RELATED CONTENT: Determine one related concept.

UNDERLYING PRINCIPLES: Describe one related to the concept.

NURSING INTERVENTIONS: Identify five related to the concept.

Application Exercises Key

1. A. The nurse should plan to administer antibiotics, but this is not the priority action.

   B. **CORRECT:** When using the urgent vs. nonurgent approach to care, the nurse's priority action is to obtain a culture of the wound before initiating antibiotic therapy.

   C. The nurse should review the WBC laboratory findings to identify any values outside the expected reference range, but this is not the priority action.

   D. The nurse should apply dressings to the wound to absorb drainage and prevent the spread of infection, but this is not the priority action.

   Ⓝ *NCLEX® Connection: Pharmacological and Parenteral Therapies, Expected Actions/Outcomes*

2. A. A gram stain helps identify the micro-organism that is causing the infection.

   B. A culture determines the type of micro-organism causing the infection.

   C. **CORRECT:** A sensitivity test identifies the most effective antibiotic to prescribe to treat a specific micro-organism.

   D. A specific gravity test determines the dilution of fluid, typically urine, and does not provide information on the type of micro-organism or antibiotic to prescribe to treat the infection.

   Ⓝ *NCLEX® Connection: Pharmacological and Parenteral Therapies, Medication Administration*

3. A. **CORRECT:** Some clients who have meningitis have difficulty responding to antimicrobial therapy because it is difficult for the medication to cross the blood-brain barrier to reaching the infecting micro-organisms.

   B. **CORRECT:** Some clients who have a pacemaker have difficulty responding to antimicrobial therapy due to colonization of micro-organisms around the pacemaker and the inability of phagocytic cells to destroy those micro-organisms.

   C. **CORRECT:** Some clients who have endocarditis have difficulty responding to antimicrobial therapy because the medication cannot penetrate the vegetative thrombus that develops on the injured endocardium.

   D. Clients who have pneumonia should respond effectively to antimicrobial therapy because of the vascularity of pulmonary tissue.

   E. Clients who have pyelonephritis should respond to antimicrobial therapy effectively because of the vascularity of kidney tissue and the filtration system.

   Ⓝ *NCLEX® Connection: Pharmacological and Parenteral Therapies, Medication Administration*

4. A. An adolescent client who has a sinus infection should be able to metabolize and excrete the medication without developing antibiotic toxicity.

   B. **CORRECT:** An older adult client who has prostatitis and is receiving antibiotics is at risk for toxicity due to the age-related reduction in medication metabolism and excretion.

   C. A client who is postpartum and has mastitis should be able to metabolize and excrete the medication without developing antibiotic toxicity.

   D. A middle adult client who has a urinary tract infection should be able to metabolize and excrete the medication without developing antibiotic toxicity.

   Ⓝ *NCLEX® Connection: Pharmacological and Parenteral Therapies, Adverse Effects/Contraindications/Side Effects/Interactions*

5. A. **CORRECT:** Clients who suspect exposure to a sexually transmitted infection require prophylactic antimicrobial therapy to prevent an infection.

   B. **CORRECT:** Clients who are having orthopedic surgery require prophylactic antimicrobial therapy to prevent an infection.

   C. **CORRECT:** Clients who are having dental work and have a prosthetic heart valve should receive prophylactic antimicrobial therapy to prevent an infection.

   D. **CORRECT:** Clients who have recurrent urinary tract infections should receive prophylactic antimicrobial therapy to prevent an infection.

   E. Upper respiratory infections can be viral in origin. Resistance to antimicrobial therapy can occur when clients take antibiotics needlessly.

   Ⓝ *NCLEX® Connection: Pharmacological and Parenteral Therapies, Medication Administration*

PRACTICE Answer

Using ATI Active Learning Template: Basic Concept

RELATED CONTENT: Preventive nursing measures

UNDERLYING PRINCIPLES: Controlling the spread of infection to staff and clients in a health care setting

NURSING INTERVENTIONS
- Perform hand hygiene before and after each client contact to prevent the spread of infection.
- Recognize invasive procedures that increase the risk of infection (indwelling urinary catheter, IV catheter, cardiac catheterization).
- Encourage prevention by having clients maintain an up-to-date immunization status.
- Instruct clients to take the full course of antimicrobials the provider prescribes to prevent medication resistance and recurrence of infection.
- Use infection-control procedures to prevent transmission of resistant micro-organisms.
- Evaluate the effectiveness of treatment.

Ⓝ *NCLEX® Connection: Pharmacological and Parenteral Therapies, Medication Administration*

UNIT 12   MEDICATIONS FOR INFECTION

CHAPTER 44   *Antibiotics Affecting the Bacterial Cell Wall*

Antibiotics that affect the cell wall are bactericidal. This group of antibiotics includes penicillins, cephalosporins, carbapenems, and monobactams.

Penicillins

SELECT PROTOTYPE MEDICATION: Penicillin G potassium, a narrow-spectrum medication for IM or IV use

OTHER MEDICATIONS
- **Narrow-spectrum**
  - Penicillin G benzathine for IM use
  - Penicillin V for PO use
- **Broad-spectrum**
  - Amoxicillin for PO use
  - Amoxicillin-clavulanate for PO use
  - Ampicillin for PO or IV use
- **Antistaphylococcal:** Nafcillin for IM or IV use
- **Antipseudomonal**
  - Ticarcillin-clavulanate for IV use
  - Piperacillin tazobactam for IV use

PURPOSE

EXPECTED PHARMACOLOGICAL ACTION

Penicillins destroy bacteria by weakening the bacterial cell wall.

THERAPEUTIC USES

- Penicillins treat infections due to gram-positive cocci such as *Streptococcus pneumoniae* (pneumonia and meningitis), *Streptococcus viridans* (infectious endocarditis), and *Streptococcus pyogenes* (pharyngitis).
- Penicillins treat meningitis due to gram-negative cocci such as *Neisseria meningitides*.
- Penicillins kill spirochetes, such as *Treponema pallidum*, which causes syphilis.
- Extended-spectrum penicillins (piperacillin, ticarcillin) are effective against organisms such as *Pseudomonas aeruginosa*, *Enterobacter* species, *Proteus*, *Bacteroides fragilis*, and *Klebsiella*. Ticarcillin by itself is no longer available in the U.S., but ticarcillin in combination with clavulanic acid is available.
- Penicillins provide prophylaxis against bacterial endocarditis in at-risk clients prior to dental and other procedures.

COMPLICATIONS

Allergies, anaphylaxis

NURSING CONSIDERATIONS
- Interview clients for prior allergy.
- Advise clients to wear an allergy identification bracelet.
- Observe for allergic reactions for 30 min following parenteral administration of penicillin.

Renal impairment

NURSING CONSIDERATIONS
- Monitor kidney function.
- Monitor I&O.

Hyperkalemia, dysrhythmias, hypernatremia

- **Hyperkalemia, dysrhythmias:** High doses of penicillin G potassium
- **Hypernatremia:** IV ticarcillin-clavulanate
- NURSING CONSIDERATIONS: Monitor cardiac status and electrolyte levels.

CONTRAINDICATIONS/PRECAUTIONS

- A history of severe allergic reactions to penicillin, cephalosporins, or imipenem is a contraindication for penicillins. Qs
- Use cautiously for clients who have or are at risk for kidney dysfunction (clients who are acutely ill, older adults, or young children). Ⓒ
- Clients who are allergic to one penicillin are cross-allergic to other penicillins and are at risk for cross-sensitivity to cephalosporins.

INTERACTIONS

Penicillin in the same IV solution as aminoglycosides inactivates the aminoglycoside.
NURSING CONSIDERATIONS: Do not mix penicillin and aminoglycosides in the same IV solution.

Probenecid delays the excretion of penicillin.
NURSING CONSIDERATIONS: Providers sometimes add probenecid to prolong the action of penicillin therapy.

NURSING ADMINISTRATION

- Instruct clients to take penicillin V, amoxicillin, and amoxicillin-clavulanate with meals. Tell them to take all others with 8 oz of water 1 hr before or 2 hr after meals. QEBP
- Instruct clients to report any signs of an allergic response such as dyspnea, a skin rash, itching, and hives.
- Give IM injections cautiously to avoid injecting into a nerve or an artery.
- Advise clients to complete the entire course of therapy, even if symptoms resolve.
- Advise client to use an additional contraceptive method when taking penicillins.

Cephalosporins

SELECT PROTOTYPE MEDICATION: Cephalexin, first generation

OTHER MEDICATIONS
- **First generation:** Cefazolin for IM or IV use
- **Second generation:** Cefaclor, cefotetan for PO use
- **Third generation:** Ceftriaxone, cefotaxime for IM or IV use
- **Fourth generation:** Cefepime for IM or IV use

PURPOSE

EXPECTED PHARMACOLOGICAL ACTION

- Cephalosporins are beta-lactam antibiotics, similar to penicillins, that destroy bacterial cell walls causing destruction of micro-organisms.
- Cephalosporins comprise four generations. Each subsequent generation is
  - More likely to reach cerebrospinal fluid.
  - Less susceptible to destruction by beta-lactamase.
  - More effective against gram-negative organisms and anaerobes.

THERAPEUTIC USES

Cephalosporins are broad-spectrum bactericidal medications with a high therapeutic index that treat urinary tract infections, postoperative infections, pelvic infections, and meningitis.

COMPLICATIONS

Allergy, hypersensitivity, anaphylaxis, possible cross-sensitivity to penicillin

NURSING CONSIDERATIONS
- If indications of allergy appear (urticaria, rash, hypotension, dyspnea), stop the cephalosporin immediately, and notify the provider.
- Question clients carefully about a history of allergy to a penicillin or another cephalosporin, and notify the provider if present.

Bleeding tendencies from cefotetan and ceftriaxone

NURSING CONSIDERATIONS
- Avoid use for clients who have bleeding disorders and for clients taking anticoagulants.
- Observe clients for bleeding.
- Monitor prothrombin and bleeding times. Delays in clotting can require discontinuation of the medication.
- Administer parenteral vitamin K.

Thrombophlebitis with IV infusion

NURSING CONSIDERATIONS
- Rotate injection sites.
- Administer as a dilute intermittent infusion or slowly over 3 to 5 min and in a dilute solution for bolus dosing.

Renal insufficiency

NURSING CONSIDERATIONS: Give a lower dosage of most cephalosporins to prevent accumulation to toxic levels.

Pain with IM injection

NURSING CONSIDERATIONS: Administer IM injections deep into a large muscle mass such as into the ventrogluteal site.

Antibiotic-associated pseudomembranous colitis

NURSING CONSIDERATIONS
- Observe for diarrhea, and notify the provider if present.
- Stop the medication.

CONTRAINDICATIONS/PRECAUTIONS

NURSING CONSIDERATIONS
- Do not give cephalosporins to clients who have a history of severe allergic reactions to penicillins. Qs
- Use cautiously with clients who have renal impairment or bleeding tendencies.

INTERACTIONS

Disulfiram reaction (intolerance to alcohol) occurs with simultaneous use of alcohol and either cefotetan or cefazolin.
CLIENT EDUCATION: Instruct clients not to consume alcohol while taking these cephalosporins.

Probenecid delays renal excretion.
NURSING CONSIDERATIONS: Monitor I&O.

NURSING ADMINISTRATION

- Instruct clients to complete the entire course of therapy, even if symptoms resolve. QEBP
- Advise clients to take oral cephalosporins with food.
- Instruct clients to store oral cephalosporin suspensions in a refrigerator.

Carbapenems

SELECT PROTOTYPE MEDICATION: Imipenem-cilastatin for IM or IV use

OTHER MEDICATIONS: Meropenem for IV use

PURPOSE

EXPECTED PHARMACOLOGICAL ACTION

Carbapenems are beta-lactam antibiotics that destroy bacterial cell walls, causing destruction of micro-organisms.

THERAPEUTIC USES

- Their broad antimicrobial spectrum is effective for serious infections such as pneumonia, peritonitis, and urinary tract infections due to gram-positive cocci, gram-negative cocci, and anaerobic bacteria.
- Resistance develops from using imipenem alone to treat *Pseudomonas aeruginosa* infections. This pathogen requires a combination of antipseudomonal medications.

COMPLICATIONS

Allergy, hypersensitivity, possible cross-sensitivity to penicillin or cephalosporins

NURSING CONSIDERATIONS
- Monitor for indications of allergic reactions, such as dyspnea, rashes, and pruritus.
- Question clients carefully about their history of allergy to a penicillin or other cephalosporin, and notify the provider if present.

Gastrointestinal upset (nausea, vomiting, diarrhea)

NURSING CONSIDERATIONS
- Observe for manifestations, and notify the provider if they occur.
- Monitor I&O.

Suprainfection

NURSING CONSIDERATIONS: Monitor for indications of colitis (diarrhea), oral thrush, and vaginal yeast infection.

CONTRAINDICATIONS/PRECAUTIONS

- Imipenem-cilastatin is a Pregnancy Risk Category C medication. **Qs**
- Use cautiously in clients who have renal impairment.

INTERACTIONS

Imipenem-cilastatin can reduce blood levels of valproic acid. Breakthrough seizures are possible.
NURSING CONSIDERATIONS: Avoid using together. If concurrent use is unavoidable, monitor for increased seizure activity.

NURSING ADMINISTRATION

Advise clients to complete the entire course of therapy, even if symptoms resolve.

Other inhibitors of cell wall synthesis

SELECT PROTOTYPE MEDICATIONS
- Vancomycin for PO or IV use
- Aztreonam, a monobactam, for IM or IV use
- Fosfomycin for PO use

PURPOSE

EXPECTED PHARMACOLOGICAL ACTION

This group of antibiotics destroys bacterial cell walls, causing destruction of micro-organisms.

THERAPEUTIC USES

- Treat serious infections due to methicillin-resistant *Staphylococcus aureus*, *Staphylococcus epidermidis*, and streptococcal infections.
- Treat antibiotic-associated pseudomembranous colitis due to *Clostridium difficile*.

COMPLICATIONS

Ototoxicity (rare and reversible)

NURSING CONSIDERATIONS
- Assess for indications of hearing loss.
- Instruct clients to notify the provider if changes in hearing acuity develop.
- Monitor vancomycin levels.

Infusion reactions

Red man syndrome: rashes, flushing, tachycardia, and hypotension

NURSING CONSIDERATIONS: Administer vancomycin slowly over 60 min.

IM and IV injection-site pain, thrombophlebitis

NURSING CONSIDERATIONS
- Rotate injection sites.
- Monitor the infusion site for redness, swelling, and inflammation.

Renal toxicity

NURSING CONSIDERATIONS
- Monitor I&O and kidney function tests.
- Monitor vancomycin trough levels.

CONTRAINDICATIONS/PRECAUTIONS

- An allergy to corn or corn products and previous allergy to vancomycin are contraindications. Qs
- Use cautiously for older adults and with clients who have renal impairment or hearing loss. Ⓖ

INTERACTIONS

Increased risk for ototoxicity when taking vancomycin concurrently with another medication that causes ototoxicity (loop diuretics, aminoglycoside antibiotics).
NURSING CONSIDERATIONS: Assess for hearing loss.

NURSING ADMINISTRATION

- Monitor vancomycin trough levels routinely after blood levels have reached a steady state.
- For clients who have renal insufficiency, creatinine clearance levels indicate IV dosage adjustments.

NURSING EVALUATION OF MEDICATION EFFECTIVENESS

Indications of effectiveness include the following.
- Reduction of manifestations such as fever, pain, inflammation, and adventitious breath sounds
- Resolution of infection

Application Exercises

1. A nurse in an outpatient facility is preparing to administer nafcillin IM to an adult client who has an infection. Which of the following actions should the nurse plan to take? (Select all that apply.)

   A. Select a 25-gauge, ½-inch needle for the injection.

   B. Administer the medication deeply into the ventrogluteal muscle.

   C. Ask the client about an allergy to penicillin before administering the medication.

   D. Monitor the client for 30 min following the injection.

   E. Tell the client to expect a temporary rash to develop following the injection.

2. A nurse is preparing to administer cefotaxime IV to a client who has a severe infection and has been receiving cefotaxime for the past week. Which of the following findings indicates a potentially serious adverse reaction to this medication that the nurse should report to the provider?

   A. Diaphoresis

   B. Epistaxis

   C. Diarrhea

   D. Alopecia

3. A nurse is obtaining a medication history from a client who is to receive imipenem-cilastatin IV to treat an infection. Which of the following medications the client also receives puts him at risk for a medication interaction?

   A. Regular insulin

   B. Furosemide

   C. Valproic acid

   D. Ferrous sulfate

4. A nurse is caring for a client who has a cerebrospinal fluid infection with gram-negative bacteria. Which of the following cephalosporin antibiotics should the nurse expect to administer IV to treat this infection?

   A. Cefaclor

   B. Cefazolin

   C. Cefepime

   D. Cephalexin

5. A nurse is preparing to administer penicillin V to a client who has a streptococcal infection. The client tells the nurse that she has difficulty swallowing tablets and doesn't "do well" with liquid or chewable medications because the taste gags her, even when the a nurse mixes the medication with food. The nurse should request a prescription for which of the following medications?

   A. Fosfomycin

   B. Amoxicillin

   C. Nafcillin

   D. Cefaclor

PRACTICE Active Learning Scenario

A nurse in an acute care facility is administering vancomycin IV to a client who has a serious wound infection. What should the nurse teach the client about this medication? Use the ATI Active Learning Template: Medication to complete this item.

THERAPEUTIC USES: Identify for vancomycin for this client.

COMPLICATIONS: Identify two adverse effects the client should watch for.

NURSING INTERVENTIONS: Describe two nursing actions for clients receiving vancomycin.

Application Exercises Key

1. A. A 25-gauge, ½-inch needle is too small and short for an IM injection of nafcillin to an adult client. The nurse should choose the needle size and length that is best for each specific client. A needle for an adult client's IM injection should be 19- to 22-gauge and 1½ inches long.

   B. **CORRECT:** It is important to administer nafcillin IM into a deep muscle mass, such as the ventrogluteal site.

   C. **CORRECT:** It is important to ask the client about an allergy to penicillin or other antibiotics before administering nafcillin. An allergy to another penicillin or to a cephalosporin is a contraindication for administering nafcillin.

   D. **CORRECT:** When administering a penicillin or other antibiotic parenterally, it is important to monitor the client for 30 min for an allergic reaction.

   E. A rash is not an expected reaction after nafcillin administration. A rash can be a manifestation of an allergy to the medication.

   Ⓝ *NCLEX® Connection: Pharmacological and Parenteral Therapies, Medication Administration*

2. A. Diaphoresis is not an adverse effect of cefotaxime. Common adverse effects include rashes, nausea, headache, dizziness, and weakness.

   B. Epistaxis is not an adverse effect of cefotaxime.

   C. **CORRECT:** Diarrhea is an adverse effect of cefotaxime and other cephalosporins that requires reporting to the provider. Severe diarrhea might indicate that the client has developed antibiotic-associated pseudomembranous colitis, which could be life-threatening.

   D. Alopecia is not an adverse effect of cefotaxime.

   Ⓝ *NCLEX® Connection: Pharmacological and Parenteral Therapies, Adverse Effects/Contraindications/Side Effects/Interactions*

3. A. Regular insulin, an antidiabetes medication, does not interact with imipenem-cilastatin. Medications that interact with imipenem-cilastatin include probenecid, aminophylline, theophylline, ganciclovir, and cyclosporine.

   B. Furosemide, a loop diuretic, does not interact with imipenem-cilastatin.

   C. **CORRECT:** Imipenem-cilastatin decreases the blood levels of valproic acid, an antiseizure medication, putting the client at risk for increased seizure activity. If the client must take these two medications concurrently, the nurse should monitor for seizures.

   D. Ferrous sulfate does not interact with imipenem-cilastatin.

   Ⓝ *NCLEX® Connection: Pharmacological and Parenteral Therapies, Adverse Effects/Contraindications/Side Effects/Interactions*

4. A. Cefaclor, a second-generation cephalosporin, is unlikely to be effective against gram-negative bacteria in cerebrospinal fluid.

   B. Cefazolin, a first-generation cephalosporin, is unlikely to be effective against gram-negative bacteria in cerebrospinal fluid.

   C. **CORRECT:** Cefepime, a fourth-generation cephalosporin, is more likely to be effective against this infection than the other medications, which are from the first or second generation. Medications from each progressive generation of cephalosporins are more effective against gram-negative bacteria, more resistant to destruction by beta-lactamase, and more able to reach cerebrospinal fluid.

   D. Cephalexin, a first-generation cephalosporin, is unlikely to be effective against gram-negative bacteria in cerebrospinal fluid.

   Ⓝ *NCLEX® Connection: Pharmacological and Parenteral Therapies, Medication Administration*

5. A. Fosfomycin is available only in a PO formulation. Acceptable alternatives to penicillin V within the penicillin classification include penicillin G, ampicillin, ticarcillin-clavulanate, and piperacillin tazobactam.

   B. Amoxicillin is available only in a PO formulation.

   C. **CORRECT:** Nafcillin is an acceptable alternative within the penicillin classification because it is available for IM or IV use.

   D. Cefaclor is available only in a PO formulation and is not a penicillin.

   Ⓝ *NCLEX® Connection: Pharmacological and Parenteral Therapies,*

PRACTICE Answer

Using the ATI Active Learning Template: Medication

THERAPEUTIC USES: Vancomycin is an antibiotic that kills bacteria by disrupting their cell wall. The IV form treats serious infections due to methicillin-resistant *Staphylococcus aureus*, *Staphylococcus epidermidis*, and streptococci.

COMPLICATIONS
- Infusion reactions (red man syndrome: rashes, flushing, tachycardia, and hypotension)
- Ototoxicity (rare and reversible)
- Renal toxicity
- Thrombophlebitis at the IV site
- IM and IV injection-site pain

NURSING INTERVENTIONS
- Infuse vancomycin over at least 60 min/dose to prevent an infusion reaction.
- Monitor the IV site for redness, pain, or other manifestations of thrombophlebitis.
- Monitor I&O, and notify the provider for oliguria or other signs of acute renal injury.
- Monitor for hearing loss.
- Ask the client about allergy to antibiotics before administering the medication. Watch for allergic manifestations during and after the infusion.

Ⓝ *NCLEX® Connection: Pharmacological and Parenteral Therapies, Medication Administration*

UNIT 12   MEDICATIONS FOR INFECTION

CHAPTER 45 *Antibiotics Affecting Protein Synthesis*

Antibiotics affecting protein synthesis are bacteriostatic, such as tetracyclines and macrolides, or bactericidal, such as aminoglycosides. They treat respiratory, gastrointestinal (GI), urinary, and reproductive tract infections.

Tetracyclines

SELECT PROTOTYPE MEDICATION: Tetracycline

OTHER MEDICATIONS
- Doxycycline
- Minocycline
- Demeclocycline

PURPOSE

EXPECTED PHARMACOLOGICAL ACTION

Tetracyclines are broad-spectrum antibiotics that inhibit micro-organism growth by preventing protein synthesis (bacteriostatic).

THERAPEUTIC USES

Treats the following
- Acne vulgaris (topically and orally)
- Periodontal disease (topically)
- Rickettsial infections, such as typhus fever or Rocky Mountain spotted fever
- Infections of the urethra or cervix due to *Chlamydia trachomatis*
- Brucellosis
- Pneumonia due to *Mycoplasma pneumonia*
- Lyme disease
- Anthrax
- GI infections due to *Helicobacter pylori*

COMPLICATIONS

GI discomfort

Cramping, nausea, vomiting, diarrhea, and esophageal ulceration

NURSING CONSIDERATIONS
- Monitor for nausea, vomiting, and diarrhea.
- Monitor I&O.
- Suggest taking doxycycline and minocycline with meals, although food can reduce absorption.
- Avoid taking at bedtime to reduce the risk of esophageal ulceration.

Yellow or brown tooth discoloration, hypoplasia of tooth enamel

NURSING CONSIDERATIONS: Avoid administration to children younger than 8 years of age and to women who are pregnant.

Hepatotoxicity (lethargy, jaundice)

NURSING CONSIDERATIONS: Avoid administration of high daily doses IV.

Photosensitivity (intense sunburn)

NURSING CONSIDERATIONS: Advise clients to wear protective clothing and use sunscreen while outdoors in sunlight.

Suprainfection

Pseudomembranous colitis (diarrhea), yeast infections of the mouth, pharynx, vagina, bowels

NURSING CONSIDERATIONS: Instruct clients to notify the provider of diarrhea or manifestations of a yeast infection.

Dizziness, lightheadedness (minocycline)

NURSING CONSIDERATIONS: Instruct clients to take care with ambulation and to report these findings if they occur.

CONTRAINDICATIONS/PRECAUTIONS

- Tetracyclines are Pregnancy Risk Category D. Qs
- Taking tetracyclines after the fourth month of pregnancy can stain the deciduous teeth, but they do not affect permanent teeth. They do, however, stain the permanent teeth of children between the ages of 4 months and 8 years who take them.
- Use cautiously with liver and kidney disease. Doxycycline and minocycline are generally safe for clients who have kidney disease, because the liver, not the kidneys, eliminates these two tetracyclines.

INTERACTIONS

Interaction with milk products, calcium and iron supplements, laxatives containing magnesium, and antacids causes formation of nonabsorbable chelates, thus reducing the absorption of tetracyclines.

NURSING CONSIDERATIONS
- Instruct clients to take tetracyclines on an empty stomach with 8 oz water (1 hr before or 2 hr after meals). Clients may take tetracyclines with food if gastric distress occurs, but this will decrease absorption. Minocycline may be taken with food.
- Avoid milk products and antacids, or separate by 2 hr.

Tetracyclines decrease the efficacy of oral contraceptives.
CLIENT EDUCATION: Advise an alternative form of birth control.

Both minocycline and doxycycline increase the risk of digoxin toxicity.
NURSING CONSIDERATIONS: Monitor digoxin level carefully if taking concurrently.

NURSING ADMINISTRATION

- Instruct clients to take tetracyclines (except for minocycline) on an empty stomach with 8 oz water. It may be taken with food if gastric distress occurs. Q EBP
- Tell clients not to take tetracyclines just before lying down because it increases the risk of esophageal ulceration.
- Instruct clients to maintain a 2-hr interval between ingestion of chelating agents and tetracyclines.
- Instruct clients to complete the entire course of therapy, even though manifestations may resolve sooner.
- Advise using additional contraception.

NURSING EVALUATION OF MEDICATION EFFECTIVENESS

Indications of effectiveness include the following.
- A decrease in the manifestations of infection, such as fever, pain, inflammation, and adventitious breath sounds
- Resolution of yeast infections of the mouth, vagina, and bowels
- Resolution of acne vulgaris

Macrolides

SELECT PROTOTYPE MEDICATION: Erythromycin

OTHER MEDICATION: Azithromycin

PURPOSE

EXPECTED PHARMACOLOGICAL ACTION

Erythromycin slows the growth of micro-organisms by inhibiting protein synthesis (bacteriostatic), but it is bactericidal at high doses.

THERAPEUTIC USES

- Treats infections in clients who have a penicillin allergy, such as for prophylaxis against rheumatic fever and bacterial endocarditis
- Treats Legionnaires' disease, pertussis (whooping cough), and acute diphtheria (also eliminating the carrier state of diphtheria)
- Treats chlamydial infections (urethritis, cervicitis), pneumonia due to *Mycoplasma pneumoniae*, and streptococcal infections

COMPLICATIONS

GI discomfort (nausea, vomiting, epigastric pain)

NURSING CONSIDERATIONS
- Administer erythromycin with meals.
- Monitor for and report adverse GI effects.

Prolonged QT intervals

Causing dysrhythmias and possible sudden cardiac death

NURSING CONSIDERATIONS: Avoid use in clients who have prolonged QT intervals.

Ototoxicity with high-dose therapy

NURSING CONSIDERATIONS: Monitor for and report hearing loss, vertigo, and tinnitus.

CONTRAINDICATIONS/PRECAUTIONS

Liver disease and QT prolongation are contraindications. Qs

INTERACTIONS

Erythromycin inhibits the metabolism of antihistamines, theophylline, carbamazepine, warfarin, and digoxin, which can lead to toxicity.
NURSING CONSIDERATIONS: To minimize toxicity, avoid using erythromycin with medications that affect hepatic medication-metabolizing enzymes. If unavoidable, monitor liver function tests carefully for indications of toxicity.

Verapamil, diltiazem, HIV protease inhibitors, antifungal medications, and nefazodone inhibit the metabolism of erythromycin, which can lead to toxicity and cause tachydysrhythmias and possible cardiac arrest.
NURSING CONSIDERATIONS: Avoid concurrent use.

NURSING ADMINISTRATION

- Except for azithromycin, administer oral preparations on an empty stomach (1 hr before meals or 2 hr after) with 8 oz of water, unless GI upset occurs. Ⓠ**EBP**
- Administer erythromycin IV only for severe infections or for clients who cannot take oral doses.
- Instruct clients to complete the entire course of antimicrobial therapy, even if manifestations resolve sooner.
- Carefully monitor the PT or INR of clients who take warfarin concurrently with erythromycin.
- Monitor liver function tests for therapy lasting longer than 2 weeks.

NURSING EVALUATION OF MEDICATION EFFECTIVENESS

Indications of effectiveness include the following.
- A decrease in the manifestations of infection, such as fever, sore throat, cough, inflammation, and adventitious breath sounds
- Resolution of urinary tract manifestations
- Resolution of bacterial endocarditis (negative blood cultures, WBC counts within the expected reference range)

Aminoglycosides

SELECT PROTOTYPE MEDICATION: Gentamicin

OTHER MEDICATIONS
- Tobramycin
- Neomycin
- Streptomycin
- Paromomycin

PURPOSE

EXPECTED PHARMACOLOGICAL ACTION

Aminoglycosides are bactericidal antibiotics that destroy micro-organisms by disrupting protein synthesis.

THERAPEUTIC USES

- Treats aerobic gram-negative bacilli, such as *Escherichia coli*, *Klebsiella pneumoniae*, *Proteus mirabilis*, and *Pseudomonas aeruginosa*.
- Paromomycin (an oral aminoglycoside) treats intestinal amebiasis and tapeworm infections.
- Oral neomycin suppresses the normal flora of the GI tract preoperatively in preparation for colorectal surgery; topically, it treats infections of the eye, ear, and skin.
- Streptomycin can treat tuberculosis in combination with other medications, but newer and safer ones (ethambutol, rifampin, isoniazid) are preferable. Streptomycin also treats severe, uncommon infections (tularemia, plague, and brucellosis).

COMPLICATIONS

Ototoxicity

Cochlear damage (hearing loss), vestibular damage (loss of balance)

NURSING CONSIDERATIONS
- Monitor for tinnitus, headache, hearing loss, nausea, dizziness, and vertigo.
- Do baseline audiometric studies (hearing tests).
- Instruct clients to notify the provider if tinnitus, hearing loss, or headaches occur.
- Stop aminoglycoside if manifestations occur.

Nephrotoxicity

Due to high total cumulative doses resulting in acute tubular necrosis (proteinuria, casts in the urine, dilute urine, elevated BUN, elevated creatinine)

NURSING CONSIDERATIONS
- Monitor I&O, BUN, and creatinine.
- Report hematuria and cloudy urine.

Intense neuromuscular blockade

Resulting in respiratory depression, muscle weakness

NURSING CONSIDERATIONS: Closely monitor use in clients who have myasthenia gravis, clients taking skeletal muscle relaxants, and clients receiving general anesthetics.

Hypersensitivity

Rash, pruritus, paresthesia of hands and feet, urticaria

NURSING CONSIDERATIONS: Monitor for allergic effects.

STREPTOMYCIN

Neurologic disorder

Peripheral neuritis, optic nerve dysfunction, tingling/numbness of the hands and feet

CLIENT EDUCATION: Instruct clients to report any manifestations to the provider promptly.

CONTRAINDICATIONS/PRECAUTIONS

- Use cautiously with clients who have kidney impairment, hearing loss, and myasthenia gravis. Qs
- Use cautiously for clients taking ethacrynic acid (increases the risk for ototoxicity), amphotericin B, cephalosporins, vancomycin (increases the risk for nephrotoxicity), and neuromuscular blocking agents such as tubocurarine.
- Clients who have kidney impairment should receive lower doses of aminoglycosides.

INTERACTIONS

Penicillin inactivates aminoglycosides when in the same IV solution.
NURSING CONSIDERATIONS: Do not mix aminoglycosides and penicillins in the same IV solution.

Concurrent administration with other ototoxic medications, such as loop diuretics, increases the risk for ototoxicity.
NURSING CONSIDERATIONS: Assess frequently for hearing loss with concurrent medication use.

NURSING ADMINISTRATION

- Most aminoglycosides, such as gentamicin and streptomycin (IM only), are parenteral. Neomycin also has oral and topical formulations; tobramycin also has an inhalation formulation.
- Base acquisition of aminoglycoside levels on dosing schedules. Q EBP
  - With ONCE-A-DAY DOSING, it is only necessary to obtain a blood sample for measuring trough levels.
  - DIVIDED DOSES
    - **Peak:** 30 min after administration of aminoglycoside IM or 30 min after completion of an IV infusion
    - **Trough:** Right before the next dose

NURSING EVALUATION OF MEDICATION EFFECTIVENESS

Indications of effectiveness include the following.
- A decrease in the manifestations of infection, such as fever, inflammation, and adventitious breath sounds
- Resolution of urinary tract manifestations
- Wound healing

Application Exercises

1. A nurse is teaching a client about taking tetracycline to treat a GI infection due to *Helicobacter pylori*. Which of the following statements should the nurse identify as an indication that the client understands the instructions?

   A. "I will take this medication with 8 ounces of milk."

   B. "I will let my doctor know if I start having diarrhea."

   C. "I can stop taking this medication when I feel completely well."

   D. "I can take this medication just before bedtime."

2. A nurse is administering gentamicin by IV infusion at 0900. The medication will take 1 hr to infuse. When should the nurse plan to obtain a blood sample for a peak serum level of gentamicin?

   A. 1000

   B. 1030

   C. 1100

   D. 1130

3. A nurse is caring for a client who is starting a course of gentamicin IV for a serious respiratory infection. For which of the following manifestations should the nurse monitor as an adverse effect of this medication? (Select all that apply.)

   A. Pruritus

   B. Hematuria

   C. Muscle weakness

   D. Difficulty swallowing

   E. Vertigo

4. A nurse is caring for a client who has subacute bacterial endocarditis and is receiving several antibiotics, including streptomycin IM. For which of the following manifestations should the nurse monitor as an adverse effect of this medication?

   A. Extremity paresthesias

   B. Urinary retention

   C. Severe constipation

   D. Complex partial seizures

5. A nurse is caring for a client who is undergoing preparation for extensive colorectal surgery. Which of the following oral antibiotics should the nurse expect to administer specifically to suppress normal flora in the GI tract?

   A. Kanamycin

   B. Gentamicin

   C. Neomycin

   D. Tobramycin

PRACTICE Active Learning Scenario

A nurse is teaching a client who has a new prescription for oral erythromycin every 6 hr to treat pneumonia. What should the nurse teach the client about this medication? Use the ATI Active Learning Template: Medication to complete this item.

THERAPEUTIC USES: Describe the therapeutic use for erythromycin in this client.

COMPLICATIONS: Identify two adverse effects the client should monitor for.

NURSING INTERVENTIONS: Describe two diagnostic tests to monitor for clients taking erythromycin.

CLIENT EDUCATION: Include two teaching points for clients taking erythromycin.

Application Exercises Key

1. A. Tetracycline can form a nonabsorbable chelate if clients take it with dairy products. They should take it with water on an empty stomach.

   B. **CORRECT:** Diarrhea can indicate that the client is developing a suprainfection, which can be very serious. The client should notify the provider if diarrhea occurs.

   C. The client should take the full prescription of tetracycline and not stop the medication if he begins to feel well.

   D. Taking tetracycline in the morning helps prevent esophageal ulceration, which can occur if the client takes it just before lying down.

   Ⓝ *NCLEX® Connection: Pharmacological and Parenteral Therapies, Medication Administration*

2. A. The IV infusion should end at 1000, but that is not the time for the nurse to collect a blood specimen for the peak serum level.

   B. **CORRECT:** The nurse should obtain the blood specimen for the peak serum level at 1030, 30 min after the end of the IV infusion. For the trough level, the nurse should collect the blood sample just before starting the infusion.

   C. Collecting the specimen for the peak serum level 1 hr following the end of the IV infusion would yield an inaccurate peak level.

   D. Collecting the specimen for the peak serum level 1.5 hr following the end of the IV infusion would yield an inaccurate peak level.

   Ⓝ *NCLEX® Connection: Pharmacological and Parenteral Therapies, Medication Administration*

3. A. **CORRECT:** Paresthesias of the hands and feet, urticaria, rash, and pruritus are indications of a hypersensitivity reaction that can occur in clients taking gentamicin.

   B. **CORRECT:** Hematuria is an indication of acute kidney toxicity due to gentamicin.

   C. **CORRECT:** Muscle weakness and respiratory depression can occur in clients taking gentamicin as a result of neuromuscular blockade.

   D. Difficulty swallowing is not an adverse effect of gentamicin.

   E. **CORRECT:** Vertigo, ataxia, and hearing loss are indications of ototoxicity that can occur in clients taking gentamicin.

   Ⓝ *NCLEX® Connection: Pharmacological and Parenteral Therapies, Adverse Effects/Contraindications/Side Effects/Interactions*

4. A. **CORRECT:** Paresthesias of the hands and feet are a common adverse effect of streptomycin. This medication treats infections in combination with other antibiotics or to treat severe infections when other antibiotics failed.

   B. Urinary retention is not an adverse effect of streptomycin, but this medication can cause nephrotoxicity.

   C. Severe constipation is not an adverse effect of streptomycin. Common adverse effects include headache, ototoxicity, angioedema, muscle weakness, stomatitis, and optic nerve toxicity.

   D. Complex partial seizures are not an adverse effect of streptomycin.

   Ⓝ *NCLEX® Connection: Pharmacological and Parenteral Therapies, Adverse Effects/Contraindications/Side Effects/Interactions*

5. A. To rid the large intestine of normal flora, the nurse has to administer an antibiotic the client can take orally, so that it passes through the GI tract. Kanamycin, an aminoglycoside, is only available in parenteral formulations.

   B. To rid the large intestine of normal flora, the nurse has to administer an antibiotic the client can take orally, so that it passes through the GI tract. Gentamicin, an aminoglycoside, is only available in parenteral formulations.

   C. **CORRECT:** The nurse should expect to administer neomycin, an aminoglycoside antibiotic, orally prior to GI surgery to rid the large intestine of normal flora.

   D. To rid the large intestine of normal flora, the nurse has to administer an antibiotic the client can take orally, so that it passes through the GI tract. Tobramycin, an aminoglycoside, is only available in parenteral and inhalation formulations.

   Ⓝ *NCLEX® Connection: Pharmacological and Parenteral Therapies, Medication Administration*

PRACTICE Answer

Using the ATI Active Learning Template: Medication

THERAPEUTIC USES: Erythromycin inhibits protein synthesis in the cells of susceptible micro-organisms, usually gram-positive bacteria. Erythromycin can be either bacteriostatic or bactericidal, depending on the organism and on the medication's dosage. It also treats infections for clients who are allergic to penicillin.

COMPLICATIONS
- The most common adverse effects of erythromycin are GI manifestations, including abdominal pain, nausea, vomiting, and diarrhea.
- Hepatotoxicity with abdominal pain, anorexia, fatigue, and possibly jaundice can occur after 1 to 2 weeks of erythromycin therapy.
- Erythromycin can cause a prolonged QT interval on ECG, which can lead to potentially fatal tachydysrhythmias.
- Ototoxicity can occur with high doses, especially after prolonged periods.

NURSING INTERVENTIONS
- Monitor liver function tests for clients who take erythromycin over a period of several weeks.
- If the client is concurrently taking warfarin or digoxin with erythromycin, carefully monitor PT and INR or digoxin levels.
- Monitor WBC counts for effectiveness of erythromycin treatment.

CLIENT EDUCATION
- Advise clients to take erythromycin on an empty stomach, 1 hr before or 2 hr after meals with 8 oz of water.
- Tell clients about adverse effects to watch for, and to call the provider for severe GI distress, manifestations of liver toxicity, and ototoxicity.
- Advise clients to take the entire course of the medication and not to stop when feeling better.

Ⓝ *NCLEX® Connection: Pharmacological and Parenteral Therapies, Medication Administration*

Sulfonamides, trimethoprim, and urinary tract antiseptics are medications that treat urinary tract infections (UTIs). Others include penicillins, aminoglycosides, cephalosporins, fluoroquinolones, and a phosphoric acid derivative. These medications treat active infections and prevent recurrent infections for susceptible individuals. Typical regimens are a single-dose; a short course of 3 days; the traditional course of 7 days; or up to 14 days for severe infections.

Trimethoprim-sulfamethoxazole and nitrofurantoin treat uncomplicated cystitis. Fluoroquinolones treat UTIs resistant to trimethoprim-sulfamethoxazole and nitrofurantoin. Fosfomycin, which requires one dose, is a good alternative for clients who have difficulty with adherence. Qpcc

Sulfonamides and trimethoprim

SELECT PROTOTYPE MEDICATIONS
- Trimethoprim-sulfamethoxazole
- Sulfadiazine
- Trimethoprim

PURPOSE

EXPECTED PHARMACOLOGICAL ACTION

Sulfonamides and trimethoprim inhibit bacterial growth by preventing the synthesis of a folic acid derivative, tetrahydrofolate. Folic acid is essential for the production of DNA, RNA, and proteins.

THERAPEUTIC USES

Trimethoprim-sulfamethoxazole treats the following.
- UTIs, which are most often due to infection with *Escherichia coli*
- Otitis media, chancroid, pertussis, shigellosis, and *Pneumocystis jirovecii* pneumonia

COMPLICATIONS

Hypersensitivity

Including Stevens-Johnson syndrome

NURSING CONSIDERATIONS
- Do not administer trimethoprim-sulfamethoxazole to clients who have allergies to the following.
  - Sulfonamides (sulfa)
  - Thiazide diuretics (hydrochlorothiazide)
  - Sulfonylurea-type oral hypoglycemics (glipizide, glyburide)
  - Loop diuretics (furosemide)
- Stop trimethoprim-sulfamethoxazole at the first indication of hypersensitivity, such as rash.

Blood dyscrasias

Hemolytic anemia, agranulocytosis, leukopenia, thrombocytopenia, aplastic anemia

NURSING CONSIDERATIONS
- Obtain blood samples for baseline and periodic CBC counts to detect hematologic disorders.
- Observe for and instruct clients to report bleeding, sore throat, and pallor.

Crystalluria

Crystalline aggregates in the kidneys, ureters, and bladder, causing irritation and obstruction that causes acute kidney injury

NURSING CONSIDERATIONS
- Encourage adequate oral fluid intake (at least eight 8 oz glasses per day).
- Monitor urine output (should be at least 1,200 mL/day).

Kernicterus

Jaundice, increased bilirubin levels, neurotoxic for newborns

NURSING CONSIDERATIONS: Do not give trimethoprim-sulfamethoxazole to women who are pregnant (during the first trimester or near term) or breastfeeding, or to infants younger than 2 months (due to the risk of kernicterus).

Hyperkalemia

NURSING CONSIDERATIONS: Monitor potassium levels.

CONTRAINDICATIONS/PRECAUTIONS

- Folate deficiency is a contraindication because it increases the risk of megaloblastic anemia.
- Use cautiously in clients who have impaired kidney function (give lower dosages).
- Administer with caution to adults older than 65 years who take ACE inhibitors or angiotensin II receptor blockers because of the risk for hyperkalemia. Ⓖ

INTERACTIONS

Increased effects of warfarin, phenytoin, sulfonylurea oral hypoglycemics

NURSING CONSIDERATIONS

- Give lower dosages during trimethoprim-sulfamethoxazole therapy.
- Monitor laboratory levels (PT, INR, blood glucose, phenytoin levels).

NURSING ADMINISTRATION

- Instruct clients to take trimethoprim-sulfamethoxazole on an empty stomach with 8 oz water.
- Instruct clients to complete the entire course of therapy, even if manifestations resolve sooner.
- Advise clients to use additional contraception. Qs

NURSING EVALUATION OF MEDICATION EFFECTIVENESS

Indications of effectiveness include the following.
- A decrease in the manifestations of UTI, such as frequency, burning, and dysuria
- Negative urine cultures and lower WBC counts

Urinary tract antiseptics

SELECT PROTOTYPE MEDICATION: Nitrofurantoin

OTHER MEDICATIONS: Methenamine

PURPOSE

EXPECTED PHARMACOLOGICAL ACTION

Nitrofurantoin is a broad-spectrum urinary antiseptic with bacteriostatic and bactericidal action. It injures bacteria by damaging DNA.

THERAPEUTIC USES

- Acute UTIs
- Prophylaxis for recurrent lower UTIs

COMPLICATIONS

Gastrointestinal (GI) discomfort

Anorexia, nausea, vomiting, diarrhea

NURSING CONSIDERATIONS
- Administer nitrofurantoin with milk or meals.
- Reduce dosages, and use macrocrystal capsules.

Hypersensitivity reactions

With fever, chills, severe pulmonary manifestations (dyspnea, cough, chest pain, alveolar infiltrations)

CLIENT EDUCATION
- Advise clients to stop taking the medication and to report these reactions.
- Tell clients that pulmonary manifestations should subside within several days after stopping nitrofurantoin.
- Advise clients not to take nitrofurantoin again.

Blood dyscrasias

Agranulocytosis, leukopenia, thrombocytopenia, megaloblastic anemia, hepatotoxicity

NURSING CONSIDERATIONS
- Obtain blood samples for a baseline CBC and periodic blood tests including liver function tests.
- Monitor for and report easy bruising and epistaxis (nose bleeding).

Peripheral neuropathy

Numbness, tingling of the hands and feet, muscle weakness

NURSING CONSIDERATIONS
- Instruct clients to report neuropathy.
- Advise avoiding chronic use of nitrofurantoin.
- Do not administer to clients who have chronic kidney disease (increased risk for peripheral neuropathy).

Headache, drowsiness, dizziness

NURSING CONSIDERATIONS: Instruct clients to report these adverse effects.

CONTRAINDICATIONS/PRECAUTIONS

Impaired kidney function and a creatinine clearance below 40 mL/min are contraindications. Impaired kidney function increases the risk of toxicity because of the inability to excrete nitrofurantoin.

NURSING ADMINISTRATION

- Inform clients that nitrofurantoin turns urine rust-yellow to brown and can stain teeth.
- Encourage clients to take it with food if adverse GI effects occur.
- Instruct clients to complete the entire course of therapy, even if manifestations resolve sooner.
- Recommend that clients avoid crushing, chewing, or opening capsules because of the possibility of tooth staining.
- Instruct clients to avoid nitrofurantoin while pregnant (can cause birth defects).

NURSING EVALUATION OF MEDICATION EFFECTIVENESS

Indications of effectiveness include the following.
- A decrease in the manifestations of UTI, such as frequency, burning, and dysuria
- Negative urine cultures and lower WBC counts
- Resolution of GI disturbances, such as anorexia, diarrhea, nausea, and vomiting

Fluoroquinolones

SELECT PROTOTYPE MEDICATION: Ciprofloxacin

OTHER MEDICATIONS
- Ofloxacin
- Moxifloxacin
- Levofloxacin
- Norfloxacin

PURPOSE

EXPECTED PHARMACOLOGICAL ACTION

Fluoroquinolones are bactericidal due to inhibition of an enzyme necessary for DNA replication.

THERAPEUTIC USES

- Broad-spectrum antimicrobials treat a wide variety of micro-organisms, such as some gram-positive bacteria and gram-negative bacteria such as *Klebsiella*, and *Escherichia coli*.
- Alternative to parenteral antibiotics for clients who have severe infections
- Urinary, respiratory, and GI tract infections; infections of bones, joints, skin, and soft tissues
- Prevention of anthrax for clients who have inhaled anthrax spores

COMPLICATIONS

GI discomfort (nausea, vomiting, diarrhea)

CLIENT EDUCATION: Tell clients to take the medication with milk or meals.

Achilles tendon rupture

CLIENT EDUCATION
- Instruct clients to observe for and report pain, swelling, and redness at the Achilles tendon site.
- Tell clients to stop taking ciprofloxacin and avoid exercise until the inflammation subsides.

Suprainfection (thrush, vaginal yeast infection)

CLIENT EDUCATION: Instruct clients to observe for and report manifestations of yeast infection (cottage-cheese or curd-like lesions on the mouth and genital area).

Phototoxicity (severe sunburn)

From direct and indirect sunlight and sun lamps, even with sunscreen use

NURSING CONSIDERATIONS
- Advise avoiding sun exposure and wearing protective clothing outdoors in sunlight.
- Tell clients to stop taking the medication if phototoxicity occurs.

CONTRAINDICATIONS/PRECAUTIONS

- Do not administer ciprofloxacin to children younger than 18 years of age (due to the risk of Achilles tendon rupture), unless the treatment is for *Escherichia coli* infections of the urinary tract or inhalational anthrax.
- Ciprofloxacin increases the risk for a *Clostridium difficile* infection because it destroys normal intestinal flora.
- Ciprofloxacin and several other fluoroquinolones can affect the CNS (dizziness, headache, restlessness, confusion). Use cautiously with older adults and with clients who have cardiovascular disorders. Ⓖ

INTERACTIONS

Cationic compounds (aluminum-magnesium antacids, iron salts, sucralfate, dairy products) decrease the absorption of ciprofloxacin.
NURSING CONSIDERATIONS: Administer cationic compounds 6 hr before or 2 hr after ciprofloxacin.

Plasma levels of theophylline can increase with concurrent use of ciprofloxacin.
NURSING CONSIDERATIONS: Monitor levels, and adjust dosages.

Plasma levels of warfarin can increase with concurrent use of ciprofloxacin.
NURSING CONSIDERATIONS: Monitor prothrombin time and INR, and adjust dosages.

NURSING ADMINISTRATION

- Ciprofloxacin is available in oral and IV formulations. Discontinue other IV infusions or use another IV site when administering ciprofloxacin IV.
- Give lower dosages to clients who have impaired kidney function.
- Administer ciprofloxacin IV in a dilute solution slowly over 60 min in a large vein. Ⓠᴱᴮᴾ
- For inhalation anthrax infection, give ciprofloxacin every 12 hr for 60 days.
- Instruct clients to complete the entire course of therapy, even if manifestations resolve sooner.

NURSING EVALUATION OF MEDICATION EFFECTIVENESS

Indications of effectiveness include the following.
- A decrease in the manifestations of UTI, such as frequency, burning, and dysuria
- Negative urine cultures and lower WBC counts
- No evidence of suprainfection

Urinary tract analgesic

SELECT PROTOTYPE MEDICATION: Phenazopyridine

PURPOSE

EXPECTED PHARMACOLOGICAL ACTION: The medication is an azo dye that functions as a local anesthetic on the mucosa of the urinary tract.

THERAPEUTIC USES: Relieves manifestations of burning with urination, pain, frequency, and urgency

NURSING ADMINISTRATION

- Acute kidney injury and chronic kidney disease are contraindications.
- It changes urine to an orange-red color.
- Tell clients that the urine can stain clothes.
- Instruct clients to take it with or after meals to minimize GI discomfort.

Application Exercises

1. A nurse reviewing a client's medication history notes an allergy to sulfonamides. This allergy is a contraindication for taking which of the following medications? (Select all that apply.)

   A. Hydrochlorothiazide

   B. Metoprolol

   C. Acetaminophen

   D. Glipizide

   E. Furosemide

2. A nurse is teaching a client who has a new prescription for nitrofurantoin. Which of the following information should the nurse include? (Select all that apply.)

   A. Observe for bruising on the skin.

   B. Take the medication with milk or meals.

   C. Expect brown discoloration of urine.

   D. Crush the medication if it is difficult to swallow.

   E. Expect insomnia when taking it.

3. A nurse is teaching a female client who has a severe UTI about ciprofloxacin. Which of the following information about adverse reactions should the nurse include? (Select all that apply.)

   A. Observe for pain and swelling of the Achilles tendon.

   B. Watch for a vaginal yeast infection.

   C. Expect excessive nighttime perspiration.

   D. Inspect the mouth for cottage cheese-like lesions.

   E. Take the medication with a dairy product.

4. A nurse is planning discharge teaching for a female client who has a new prescription for trimethoprim-sulfamethoxazole. Which of the following information should the nurse include?

   A. Take the medication even if pregnant.

   B. Maintain a fluid restriction while taking it.

   C. Take it on an empty stomach.

   D. Stop taking it when manifestations subside.

5. A nurse is planning to administer ciprofloxacin IV to a client who has cystitis. Which of the following actions should the nurse take?

   A. Administer a concentrated solution.

   B. Infuse the medication over 60 min.

   C. Infuse the solution through the primary IV fluid's tubing.

   D. Choose a small peripheral vein for administration.

PRACTICE Active Learning Scenario

A client who has a UTI has a prescription for phenazopyridine. What information should the nurse review? Use the ATI Active Learning Template: Medication to complete this item.

EXPECTED PHARMACOLOGICAL ACTION

THERAPEUTIC USES: Describe four.

CLIENT EDUCATION: Include three teaching points.

Application Exercises Key

1. A. **CORRECT:** A sulfonamide allergy is a contraindication for taking hydrochlorothiazide. Hypersensitivity, including Stevens-Johnson syndrome, can result from taking hydrochlorothiazide and a sulfonamide concurrently.

   B. A sulfonamide allergy is not a contraindication for taking metoprolol. It is a contraindication for taking chlorpropamide, glimepiride, metolazone, and ethacrynic acid.

   C. A sulfonamide allergy is not a contraindication for taking acetaminophen. It is a contraindication for taking chlorpropamide, glimepiride, metolazone, and ethacrynic acid.

   D. **CORRECT:** A sulfonamide allergy is a contraindication for taking some oral antidiabetes medications, including glipizide and glyburide. Hypersensitivity, including Stevens-Johnson syndrome, can result from taking glipizide and a sulfonamide concurrently.

   E. **CORRECT:** A sulfonamide allergy is a contraindication for taking loop diuretics, such as furosemide. Hypersensitivity, including Stevens-Johnson syndrome, can result from taking furosemide and a sulfonamide concurrently.

   Ⓝ *NCLEX® Connection: Pharmacological and Parenteral Therapies, Adverse Effects/Contraindications/Side Effects/Interactions*

2. A. **CORRECT:** Bruising can indicate a blood dyscrasia, and the client should notify the provider if this occurs.

   B. **CORRECT:** Taking the medication with milk or meals minimizes GI discomfort from nausea, vomiting, anorexia, and diarrhea.

   C. **CORRECT:** A brown discoloration of urine is a common adverse effect of nitrofurantoin.

   D. Crushing the medication can cause staining of the teeth.

   E. Nitrofurantoin is more likely to cause drowsiness than insomnia.

   Ⓝ *NCLEX® Connection: Pharmacological and Parenteral Therapies, Medication Administration*

3. A. **CORRECT:** Pain and swelling of the Achilles tendon indicate an adverse effect of ciprofloxacin to report to the provider.

   B. **CORRECT:** A vaginal yeast infection is an overgrowth of *Candida albicans*, which commonly occurs when taking ciprofloxacin.

   C. An alteration in perspiration is not an adverse effect of this medication. Common adverse effects include headache, tremors, dizziness, and dysphagia.

   D. **CORRECT:** Cottage cheese-like lesions in the mouth indicate an overgrowth of *Candida albicans*, a common adverse effect when taking ciprofloxacin.

   E. Milk and other dairy products contain calcium ions that reduce the effect of ciprofloxacin. The client should take the medication 6 hr before or 2 hr after ingesting dairy products.

   Ⓝ *NCLEX® Connection: Pharmacological and Parenteral Therapies, Adverse Effects/Contraindications/Side Effects/Interactions*

4. A. Trimethoprim-sulfamethoxazole can cause birth defects and fetal kernicterus, especially when taking it during the first trimester or near term

   B. The client should take trimethoprim-sulfamethoxazole with at least eight 8 oz of water each day to prevent crystalluria, which results in kidney damage.

   C. **CORRECT:** The nurse should inform the client that she may take the medication with or without food.

   D. The client should take the entire course of medication the provider prescribed to destroy all the bacteria and prevent a rebound infection.

   Ⓝ *NCLEX® Connection: Pharmacological and Parenteral Therapies, Medication Administration*

5. A. The nurse should administer ciprofloxacin IV in a dilute solution to minimize irritation of the vein.

   B. **CORRECT:** The nurse should administer ciprofloxacin IV over 60 min to minimize irritation of the vein.

   C. The nurse should not infuse ciprofloxacin with any other IV medication or solution. The nurse should use another infusion site.

   D. The nurse should infuse ciprofloxacin into a large vein to minimize the risks of irritation and phlebitis.

   Ⓝ *NCLEX® Connection: Pharmacological and Parenteral Therapies, Medication Administration*

PRACTICE Answer

Using the ATI Active Learning Template: Medication

EXPECTED PHARMACOLOGICAL ACTION: Phenazopyridine is an azo dye, which acts as a local anesthetic on the mucosa of the urinary tract. It is not an antibiotic.

THERAPEUTIC USES: Relieves urinary burning, urgency, pain, and frequency

CLIENT EDUCATION
- Acute kidney injury and chronic kidney disease are contraindications.
- It changes urine to an orange-red color.
- Tell clients that the urine can stain clothes.
- Instruct clients to take it with or after meals to minimize GI discomfort.

Ⓝ *NCLEX® Connection: Pharmacological and Parenteral Therapies, Expected Actions/Outcomes*

CHAPTER 47

Mycobacterial, Fungal, and Parasitic Infections

Mycobacterium tuberculosis is a slow-growing pathogen that necessitates long-term treatment. Long-term treatment increases the risk for toxicity, poor client adherence, and development of medication-resistant strains. Treatment for tuberculosis requires the use of at least two medications to which the pathogen is susceptible. Isoniazid and rifampin are two effective antituberculosis medications.

Metronidazole is the medication of choice for parasitic infections.

Antifungal medications belong to a variety of chemical families and are used to treat systemic and superficial mycoses.

Antimycobacterial (selective antituberculosis)

SELECT PROTOTYPE MEDICATION: Isoniazid

OTHER MEDICATIONS
- Pyrazinamide
- Ethambutol (bacteriostatic only to *M. tuberculosis*)
- Rifapentine

PURPOSE

EXPECTED PHARMACOLOGICAL ACTION

This medication is highly specific for mycobacteria. Isoniazid inhibits growth of mycobacteria by preventing synthesis of mycolic acid in the cell wall.

THERAPEUTIC USES

Indicated for active and latent tuberculosis

Latent: Isoniazid only daily for 9 months, or isoniazid with rifapentine once weekly for 3 months. (Contraindicated in children under age 2, clients who have HIV, pregnant women, and clients resistant to either medication.)

Active: Several antimycobacterial medications are used to treat a client who has active tuberculosis in order to decrease medication resistance. Treatment usually consists of a four-medication regimen often including isoniazid and rifampin.

The initial phase (induction phase) focuses on eliminating the active tubercle bacilli, which will result in noninfectious sputum. **The second phase** (continuation phase) works toward eliminating any other pathogens in the body. Length of treatment varies and can be as short as 6 months for medication-sensitive tuberculosis (2 months for the initial phase and 4 to 7 months for the continuation phase) or as long as 24 months for medication-resistant infections.

COMPLICATIONS

Peripheral neuropathy

Tingling, numbness, burning, and pain resulting from deficiency of pyridoxine, vitamin B_6

NURSING CONSIDERATIONS
- Instruct clients to observe for manifestations and to notify the provider if they occur.
- Administer 50 to 200 mg vitamin B_6 daily.

Hepatotoxicity

Anorexia, malaise, fatigue, nausea, and yellowish discoloration of skin and eyes

NURSING CONSIDERATIONS
- Instruct clients to observe for manifestations and to notify the provider if they occur.
- Monitor liver function tests.
- Instruct clients to avoid consumption of alcohol.
- Elevated liver function test results can result in the need to discontinue the medication.

Hyperglycemia and decreased glucose control

In clients who have diabetes mellitus

NURSING CONSIDERATIONS
- Monitor blood glucose.
- Clients who have diabetes mellitus might require additional antidiabetic medication.

CONTRAINDICATIONS/PRECAUTIONS

Isoniazid is contraindicated for clients who have liver disease.
NURSING CONSIDERATIONS: Use cautiously in older clients, and those who have diabetes mellitus or alcohol use disorder. Qs

INTERACTIONS

Isoniazid inhibits metabolism of phenytoin, leading to buildup of medication and toxicity. Ataxia and incoordination can indicate toxicity.
NURSING CONSIDERATIONS: Monitor levels of phenytoin. Adjust dosage of phenytoin based on phenytoin levels.

Concurrent use of tyramine foods (aged cheeses, cured meats), alcohol, rifampin, and pyrazinamide increases the risk for hepatotoxicity.
NURSING CONSIDERATIONS
- Advise clients to avoid foods with high levels of tyramine.
- Instruct clients to avoid alcohol consumption.
- Monitor liver function.

NURSING ADMINISTRATION

- Usually administered orally. When given IM, warm to room temperature to ensure that the solution is free of crystals, and inject deeply into a large muscle.
- For active tuberculosis, direct observation therapy is done to ensure adherence. Qpcc
- Advise clients to take isoniazid 1 hr before or 2 hr after meals. If gastric discomfort occurs, the client can take isoniazid with meals.
- Instruct clients to complete the prescribed course of antimicrobial therapy, even though manifestations can resolve before the full course is completed.

Broad-spectrum antimycobacterial (antituberculosis)

SELECT PROTOTYPE MEDICATION: Rifampin

PURPOSE

EXPECTED PHARMACOLOGICAL ACTION

Rifampin is bactericidal as a result of inhibition of protein synthesis.

THERAPEUTIC USES

- Rifampin is a broad-spectrum antibiotic effective for gram-positive and gram-negative bacteria.
- Rifampin is given in combination with at least one other antituberculosis medication to help prevent antibiotic resistance. QEBP

COMPLICATIONS

Discoloration of body fluids

CLIENT EDUCATION: Inform clients of expected orange color of urine, saliva, sweat, and tears.

Hepatotoxicity (jaundice, anorexia, and fatigue)

NURSING CONSIDERATIONS
- Monitor liver function.
- Inform clients regarding manifestations of anorexia, fatigue, and malaise, and instruct them to notify the provider if they occur.
- Instruct clients to avoid alcohol.

Mild GI discomfort

Anorexia, nausea, and abdominal discomfort

NURSING CONSIDERATIONS: Abdominal discomfort is mild and usually does not require intervention.

Pseudomembranous colitis

CLIENT EDUCATION: Advise the client to monitor and report fever, diarrhea, abdominal pain, or bloody stool. Discontinue medication if manifestations occur.

CONTRAINDICATIONS/PRECAUTIONS

Use cautiously in clients who have liver dysfunction. Qs

INTERACTIONS

Rifampin accelerates metabolism of warfarin, oral contraceptives, protease inhibitors, and non-nucleoside reverse transcriptase inhibitors (NNRTIs) for HIV, resulting in diminished effectiveness.
NURSING CONSIDERATIONS
- Increased dosages of HIV medications are often necessary.
- Monitor PT and INR.
- Advise clients to use a non-hormonal form of contraception.

Concurrent use with isoniazid and pyrazinamide increases risk of hepatotoxicity.
NURSING CONSIDERATIONS
- Instruct clients to avoid alcohol consumption.
- Monitor liver function.

NURSING ADMINISTRATION

- Administer orally or by IV route.
- Administer oral rifampin 1 hr before or 2 hr after meals. Absorption is decreased if given with food.
- Advise clients to use a non-hormonal form of contraception.

NURSING EVALUATION OF MEDICATION EFFECTIVENESS

Depending on therapeutic intent, effectiveness is evidenced by the following.
- Improvement of tuberculosis manifestations, such as clear breath sounds, no night sweats, increased appetite, and no afternoon rises of temperature
- Three negative sputum cultures for tuberculosis, usually taking 3 to 6 months to achieve

Antiprotozoals

SELECT PROTOTYPE MEDICATION: Metronidazole

PURPOSE

EXPECTED PHARMACOLOGICAL ACTION

Metronidazole is a broad-spectrum antimicrobial with bactericidal activity against anaerobic micro-organisms.

THERAPEUTIC USES

- Treatment of protozoal infections (intestinal amebiasis, giardiasis, trichomoniasis) and obligate anaerobic bacteria (*Bacteroides fragilis*, antibiotic-induced *Clostridium difficile*, *Gardnerella vaginalis*)
- Prophylaxis for clients who will have surgical procedures (vaginal, abdominal, colorectal surgery) and are high-risk for anaerobic infection
- Treatment of *H. pylori* in combination with tetracycline and bismuth subsalicylate in clients who have peptic ulcer disease

COMPLICATIONS

GI discomfort

Nausea, vomiting, dry mouth, and metallic taste

NURSING CONSIDERATIONS: Advise clients to observe for effects and to notify the provider. Clients can take the medication with meals to reduce adverse effects.

Darkening of urine

NURSING CONSIDERATIONS: Advise clients that this is a harmless effect of metronidazole.

Neurotoxicity, CNS effects

Numbness of extremities, ataxia, and seizures

NURSING CONSIDERATIONS
- Advise clients to notify the provider if manifestations occur.
- Stop metronidazole.

Pseudomembranous colitis

NURSING CONSIDERATIONS
- Advise clients to monitor and report fever, diarrhea, abdominal pain, or bloody stool.
- Discontinue medication.

CONTRAINDICATIONS/PRECAUTIONS

- Contraindicated in active CNS disorders, blood dyscrasias, and during lactation.
- Contraindicated in the first trimester of pregnancy ⓠˢ
- Use cautiously in clients who have kidney, cardiac, fungal, or candida infections or seizure disorders.
- Use cautiously in older adults and in clients in second or third trimesters of pregnancy.

INTERACTIONS

Alcohol causes a disulfiram-like reaction (facial flushing, vomiting, dyspnea, tachycardia).
NURSING CONSIDERATIONS: Advise clients to avoid alcohol consumption.

Metronidazole inhibits inactivation of warfarin, phenytoin, and lithium.
NURSING CONSIDERATIONS: Monitor prothrombin time and INR, phenytoin and lithium levels. Adjust dosages accordingly.

NURSING ADMINISTRATION

- Administer by oral or IV route.
- Instruct clients to complete the prescribed course of antimicrobial therapy, even though manifestations can resolve before the full course is completed. ⓠᴾᶜᶜ
- Advise clients to use condoms if using this medication for treatment of trichomoniasis.

NURSING EVALUATION OF MEDICATION EFFECTIVENESS

Depending on therapeutic intent, effectiveness is evidenced by improvement of manifestations.
- Resolution of bloody mucoid diarrhea
- Formed stools
- Negative stool results for amoeba and *Giardia*
- Decrease or absence of watery vaginal/urethral discharge
- Negative blood cultures for anaerobic organisms in the CNS, blood, bones and joints, and soft tissues

Antifungals

SELECT PROTOTYPE MEDICATIONS
- Amphotericin B (a polyene antibiotic for systemic mycoses)
- Ketoconazole (an azole for treating both superficial and systemic mycoses)

OTHER MEDICATIONS
- Flucytosine
- Nystatin
- Miconazole
- Clotrimazole
- Terbinafine
- Fluconazole
- Griseofulvin

PURPOSE

EXPECTED PHARMACOLOGICAL ACTION

Amphotericin B is an antifungal agent that acts on fungal cell membranes to cause cell death. Depending on concentration, these agents can be fungistatic (slows growth on the fungus) or fungicidal (destroys the fungus).

THERAPEUTIC USES

- Antifungals are the treatment of choice for systemic fungal infection (candidiasis, aspergillosis, cryptococcosis, mucormycosis) and nonopportunistic mycoses, (blastomycosis, histoplasmosis, coccidioidomycosis).
- Some antifungals treat superficial fungal infections: dermatophytic infections (tinea pedis [ringworm of the foot] and tinea cruris [ringworm of the groin]); candida infections of the skin and mucous membranes; and fungal infections of the nails (onychomycosis).

COMPLICATIONS

Infusion reactions

Fever, chills, rigors, and headache 1 to 3 hr after initiation

NURSING CONSIDERATIONS
- A test dose of 1 mg amphotericin B, infused slowly IV, can assess client reaction.
- Pretreat with diphenhydramine and acetaminophen. Qs
- Administer meperidine, dantrolene, or hydrocortisone for rigors.

Thrombophlebitis

NURSING CONSIDERATIONS
- Observe infusion sites for of erythema, swelling, and pain.
- Rotate injection sites.
- Administer in a large vein.

Nephrotoxicity

NURSING CONSIDERATIONS
- Obtain baseline kidney function (BUN and creatinine) and do weekly kidney function tests.
- Monitor I&O.
- Infuse 1 L of 0.9% sodium chloride IV on the day of amphotericin B infusion.

Electrolyte imbalance

NURSING CONSIDERATIONS
- Monitor electrolyte levels, especially potassium.
- Administer supplements for deficiencies.

Bone marrow suppression

NURSING CONSIDERATIONS: Obtain baseline CBC and hematocrit, and monitor weekly.

KETOCONAZOLE

Hepatotoxicity

Anorexia, nausea, vomiting, jaundice, dark urine, and clay-colored stools

NURSING CONSIDERATIONS
- Obtain baseline liver function studies, and monitor liver function monthly.
- If manifestations occur, notify the provider and discontinue the medication.

Effects on sex hormones

Male clients: Gynecomastia (enlargement of breast), decreased libido, erectile dysfunction

Female clients: Irregular menstrual flow

NURSING CONSIDERATIONS: Advise clients to observe for these effects and to notify the provider.

CONTRAINDICATIONS/PRECAUTIONS

- Antifungals are contraindicated in clients who have impaired kidney function due to the risk for nephrotoxicity. Qs
- Use antifungals with caution in clients who have anemia, electrolyte imbalance, and bone marrow suppression.
- Fluconazole is Pregnancy Risk Category D in high dose, and contraindicated during lactation.

INTERACTIONS

Aminoglycosides (gentamicin, streptomycin, cyclosporine) have additive nephrotoxic risk when used concurrently with antifungal medications.
NURSING CONSIDERATIONS: Avoid use of these antimicrobials when clients are taking amphotericin B due to additive nephrotoxicity risk.

Antifungal effects of flucytosine are potentiated with concurrent use of amphotericin B.
NURSING CONSIDERATIONS: Potentiated flucytosine effects allow for a reduction in amphotericin B dosages.

Azole antibiotics increase levels of multiple medications, including digoxin, warfarin, and sulfonylurea antidiabetic medications.
NURSING CONSIDERATIONS: If concurrent administration is necessary, carefully monitor for toxicity.

NURSING ADMINISTRATION

- Amphotericin B is highly toxic and should be reserved for severe life-threatening fungal infections.
- Infuse amphotericin B slowly over 2 to 4 hr IV.
- Observe solutions for precipitation and discard if precipitates are present. Use a filter to prevent infusion of undissolved crystals. Kidney injury is lessened with administration of 1 L of 0.9% sodium chloride IV on the day of amphotericin B infusion. QEBP
- Instruct clients to complete the prescribed course of antimicrobial therapy, even though manifestations might resolve before the full course is completed.
- Apply antifungals for topical use to treat superficial vulvovaginal candidiasis as vaginal suppository or cream.

NURSING EVALUATION OF MEDICATION EFFECTIVENESS

Depending on therapeutic intent, effectiveness is evidenced by the following.
- Improvement of findings of systemic fungal infections
- Improvement of findings of superficial infections, such as clear mucus membranes, clear nails, and intact skin

Application Exercises

1. A nurse is caring for a client who has diabetes mellitus, pulmonary tuberculosis, and a new prescription for isoniazid. Which of the following supplements should the nurse expect to administer to prevent an adverse effect of INH?

   A. Ascorbic acid

   B. Pyridoxine

   C. Folic acid

   D. Cyanocobalamin

2. A nurse is infusing IV amphotericin B to a client who has a systemic fungal infection. The nurse should monitor the client for which of the following adverse effects of this medication?

   A. Hypoglycemia

   B. Constipation

   C. Fever

   D. Hyperkalemia

3. A nurse is administering IV amphotericin B to a client who has a systemic fungal infection. The nurse should monitor which of the following laboratory values? (Select all that apply.)

   A. Serum albumin

   B. Serum amylase

   C. Serum potassium

   D. Hematocrit

   E. Serum creatinine

4. A nurse is teaching a client who is beginning a course of metronidazole to treat an infection. For which of the following adverse effects should the nurse instruct the client as a priority to stop taking metronidazole and notify the provider?

   A. Metallic taste

   B. Nausea

   C. Ataxia

   D. Dark-colored urine

5. A nurse is teaching a client who has active tuberculosis about his treatment regimen. The client asks why he must take four different medications. Which of the following responses should the nurse make?

   A. "Four medications decrease the risk for a severe allergic reaction."

   B. "Four medications reduce the chance that the bacteria will become resistant."

   C. "Four medications reduce the risk for adverse reactions"

   D. "Four medications decrease the chance of having a positive tuberculin skin test."

PRACTICE Active Learning Scenario

A nurse in a public health department is teaching a client who has latent tuberculosis (TB) and a new prescription for isoniazid twice weekly for 6 months. What should the nurse teach the client about this medication? Use the ATI Active Learning Template: Medication to complete this item.

THERAPEUTIC USES: Describe the therapeutic use for isoniazid in this client.

COMPLICATIONS: List two adverse effects the client should watch for.

NURSING INTERVENTIONS: Describe one test to monitor for clients taking isoniazid.

CLIENT EDUCATION: Describe two teaching points for clients taking isoniazid.

1. A. Ascorbic acid is given to clients who have a vitamin C deficiency. It is not a supplement administered to prevent an adverse effect of INH.

   B. **CORRECT:** Pyridoxine is frequently prescribed along with INH to prevent peripheral neuropathy for clients who have increased risk factors, such as diabetes mellitus or alcohol use disorder.

   C. Folic acid is administered to clients who have hepatic disease and folic acid deficiency. It is not administered to prevent an adverse effect of INH.

   D. Cyanocobalamin is administered to clients who have malabsorption syndrome. It is not administered to prevent an adverse effect of INH.

   Ⓝ *NCLEX® Connection: Pharmacological and Parenteral Therapies, Expected Actions/Outcomes*

2. A. Amphotericin B can cause hyperglycemia.

   B. Amphotericin B can cause diarrhea.

   C. **CORRECT:** Amphotericin B can cause fever, chills, and nausea during the infusion. Pretreatment with diphenhydramine and acetaminophen can reduce these effects.

   D. Amphotericin B can cause hypokalemia.

   Ⓝ *NCLEX® Connection: Pharmacological and Parenteral Therapies, Adverse Effects/Contraindications/Side Effects/Interactions*

3. A. Amphotericin B does not affect serum albumin levels.

   B. Amphotericin B does not cause pancreatitis.

   C. **CORRECT:** Hypokalemia is a serious adverse effect of amphotericin B. The nurse should monitor serum potassium values for hypokalemia.

   D. **CORRECT:** Amphotericin B can cause bone marrow suppression. The nurse should monitor CBC and platelet count periodically.

   E. **CORRECT:** Amphotericin B can cause nephrotoxicity. The nurse should monitor kidney function (with serum creatinine, BUN, and creatinine clearance).

   Ⓝ *NCLEX® Connection: Pharmacological and Parenteral Therapies, Expected Actions/Outcomes*

4. A. A metallic taste in the mouth is an expected adverse effect of metronidazole and is nonurgent for the client to report to the provider. Another adverse effect is the priority to report.

   B. Nausea is an expected adverse effect of metronidazole and is nonurgent for the client to report to the provider. Another adverse effect is the priority to report.

   C. **CORRECT:** Using the urgent vs. nonurgent approach to client care, the priority adverse effect to report to the provider is ataxia, tremors, paresthesias of the extremities, and seizures, which are manifestations of CNS toxicity.

   D. Dark-colored urine is expected adverse effect of metronidazole and is nonurgent for the client to report to the provider. Another adverse effect is the priority to report.

   Ⓝ *NCLEX® Connection: Pharmacological and Parenteral Therapies, Adverse Effects/Contraindications/Side Effects/Interactions*

5. A. Taking several antituberculosis medications concurrently does not decrease the chance of an allergic reaction to any of the individual medications.

   B. **CORRECT:** If the client took only one medication to treat active tuberculosis, resistance to the medication would occur quickly. Taking three or four medications decreases the possibility of resistance.

   C. Taking several antituberculosis medications concurrently does not minimize the chance of adverse effects to any of the medications. Risk for liver toxicity increases when more than one medication that causes liver toxicity is taken, such as isoniazid, rifampin, and pyrazinamide.

   D. Taking several antituberculosis medications concurrently does not change the fact that the client will have a positive tuberculin skin test indefinitely.

   Ⓝ *NCLEX® Connection: Pharmacological and Parenteral Therapies, Medication Administration*

PRACTICE Answer

Using the ATI Active Learning Template: Medication

THERAPEUTIC USES: A client who has latent tuberculosis has been infected by *Mycobacterium tuberculosis* and is at risk for (but has not yet developed) active tuberculosis. Some clients who have latent tuberculosis, such as those who are immunocompromised or who have recently immigrated to the U.S. from a country where active TB is common, can require treatment with isoniazid, with or without rifapentine, in order to prevent the onset of active TB. The client who has latent TB has a positive tuberculin test but a negative sputum culture and negative chest x-ray for TB. The client cannot infect others with tuberculosis unless the infection becomes active.

COMPLICATIONS

- Paresthesias in the extremities caused by vitamin B_6 deficiency
- Hepatotoxicity
- Hyperglycemia (if client has diabetes mellitus)

NURSING INTERVENTIONS: The client who starts isoniazid should have baseline liver function testing and be tested periodically throughout treatment.

CLIENT EDUCATION

- Teach the client to watch for paresthesias, and to take pyridoxine daily to reverse the effect if they occur.
- Teach the client about indications of hepatitis (anorexia, fatigue, nausea, jaundice) and to notify the provider if these occur.
- Teach the client to take isoniazid as prescribed, and not to stop until the entire course of treatment is completed.
- The client who has latent tuberculosis does not feel ill. The nurse should be sure that the client understands why it is important to continue with treatment.

Ⓝ *NCLEX® Connection: Pharmacological and Parenteral Therapies, Medication Administration*

Viral Infections, HIV, and AIDS

Most antiviral medications act by altering viral reproduction. Antiviral medications are only effective during viral replication. Therefore, they are ineffective when the virus is dormant.

The human immunodeficiency virus (HIV) is a retrovirus. A retrovirus must attach to a host cell in order to replicate. RNA is changed into DNA using the enzyme reverse transcriptase.

Antiretroviral agents are used to treat HIV infections. These medications do not cure HIV infection and do not decrease the risk of passing HIV infection to others. Antiretroviral agents act by preventing the virus from entering the cells (fusion/entry inhibitors and CCR5 antagonists). Others act by inhibiting enzymes needed for HIV replication (nucleoside reverse transcriptase inhibitors [NRTIs], non-nucleoside reverse transcriptase inhibitors [NNRTIs], protease inhibitors [PIs], and an integrase inhibitor [INSTI]). Skipping doses or taking decreased dosages of antiretroviral medications causes medication resistance and possible treatment failure.

Highly active antiretroviral therapy

- Highly active antiretroviral therapy (HAART) involves using three to four HIV medications in combination with other antiretroviral medications to reduce medication resistance, adverse effects, and dosages.
- HAART is an aggressive treatment method using three or more different medications to reduce the amount of virus and increase CD4 counts.
- In addition to HAART, clients who have HIV infection take additional medications to treat adverse effects of antiretrovirals and to treat or prevent secondary infections, such as pneumocystis pneumonia.

Antivirals

SELECT PROTOTYPE MEDICATIONS
- Acyclovir (oral, topical, IV)
- Ganciclovir (oral, IV)

OTHER MEDICATIONS
- Interferon alfa-2b
- Lamivudine
- Oseltamivir
- Ribavirin
- Amantadine
- Boceprevir
- Telaprevir

PURPOSE

EXPECTED PHARMACOLOGICAL ACTION: Acyclovir and ganciclovir prevent the reproduction of viral DNA and thus interrupts cell replication.

THERAPEUTIC USES
- Acyclovir is used to treat herpes simplex and varicella-zoster viruses
- Ganciclovir is used for treatment and prevention of cytomegalovirus (CMV). Prevention therapy using ganciclovir is given for clients who have HIV/AIDS, organ transplants, and other immunocompromised states.
- Interferon alfa-2b and lamivudine are used to treat hepatitis B and C.
- Oseltamivir is used to treat influenza A and B.
- Ribavirin is used to treat respiratory syncytial virus, hepatitis C, and influenza (unlabeled use).
- Boceprevir and telaprevir are protease inhibitors used to treat hepatitis C virus.

COMPLICATIONS

Acyclovir

Phlebitis and inflammation at the site of infusion
NURSING CONSIDERATIONS
- Rotate IV injection sites.
- Monitor IV sites for swelling and redness.

Nephrotoxicity
NURSING CONSIDERATIONS
- Administer acyclovir infusion slowly over 1 hr.
- Ensure adequate hydration during infusion and 2 hr after to minimize nephrotoxicity by administering IV fluids and increasing oral fluid intake as prescribed.
- Use with caution in clients who have renal impairment or are dehydrated.

Mild discomfort associated with oral therapy
- Nausea, headache, diarrhea
- NURSING CONSIDERATIONS: Observe for manifestations and notify the provider.

Gingival hyperplasia
CLIENT EDUCATION: Advise clients to practice good dental hygiene and seek dental care.

Ganciclovir

Suppressed bone marrow
- Including leukocytes and thrombocytes
- NURSING CONSIDERATIONS
  - Obtain baseline CBC and platelet count.
  - Administer granulocyte colony-stimulating factors.
  - Monitor WBC, absolute neutrophil, and platelet counts frequently during treatment.
  - Advise clients to report manifestations of infection and bleeding, and to avoid crowds or individuals who have respiratory infections.

Fever, headache, nausea, diarrhea
NURSING CONSIDERATIONS
- Advise clients to report these findings.
- Administer with food.

CONTRAINDICATIONS/PRECAUTIONS

- Acyclovir should be used cautiously in clients who have renal impairment or dehydration, and clients taking nephrotoxic medications. Q**s**
- Ganciclovir is Pregnancy Risk Category C. It can cause infertility. Advise clients to use barrier contraception during treatment and for 3 months following treatment. It is contraindicated in clients who have a neutrophil count less than 500/mm³ or platelet counts less than 25,000/mm³. Use cautiously in older adults; infants younger than 6 months; and clients who have dehydration, renal insufficiency, or malignant disorders. **G**

INTERACTIONS

Acyclovir

Probenecid can decrease elimination of acyclovir.
NURSING CONSIDERATIONS: Monitor for medication toxicity.

Concurrent use of zidovudine can cause drowsiness.
NURSING CONSIDERATIONS: Use with caution.

Ganciclovir

Cytotoxic medications can cause increased toxicity.
NURSING CONSIDERATIONS: Use together with caution.

NURSING ADMINISTRATION

- Instruct clients to complete the prescribed course of antimicrobial therapy, even though manifestations can resolve before the full course is completed.
- Advise the client to use barrier contraception if using this medication.

Acyclovir

- For topical administration, advise clients to put on rubber gloves to avoid transfer of virus to other areas of the body. Q**EBP**
- Administer IV infusion slowly over 1 hr or longer.
- Inform clients to expect relief of manifestations, but not a cure.
- Instruct clients to wash affected area with soap and water three to four times per day and to keep the lesions dry after washing.
- Advise clients to refrain from sexual contact while lesions are present.
- Clients who have healed herpetic lesions should continue to use condoms to prevent transmission of the virus.

Ganciclovir

- Administer IV infusion slowly, with an infusion pump, over at least 1 hr.
- Administer oral medication with food.
- Encourage extra fluid intake during therapy.
- Administer intraocular for CMV retinitis. Do not use contact lenses with medication.
- Avoid getting ganciclovir solution or powder on skin. Wash well if contact occurs.

NURSING EVALUATION OF MEDICATION EFFECTIVENESS

Depending on therapeutic intent, effectiveness can be evidenced by improvement of findings, such as healed genital lesions, decreased inflammation and pain, and improvement in vision

Antiretrovirals: Fusion/entry inhibitors

SELECT PROTOTYPE MEDICATION:
Enfuvirtide (subcutaneous)

PURPOSE

EXPECTED PHARMACOLOGICAL ACTION: Decreases and limits the spread of HIV by blocking HIV from attaching to and entering CD4 T cell

THERAPEUTIC USES: Treatment of HIV that is unresponsive to other antiretrovirals

COMPLICATIONS

Localized reaction at injection site
NURSING CONSIDERATIONS: Rotate injection sites. Monitor for swelling and redness.

Bacterial pneumonia
NURSING CONSIDERATIONS: Assess breath sounds prior to start of therapy. Monitor for signs of pneumonia, such as fever, cough, or shortness of breath.

Fever, chills, rash, hypotension
NURSING CONSIDERATIONS: Monitor for medication reaction. Discontinue and notify the provider.

CONTRAINDICATIONS/PRECAUTIONS

- Enfuvirtide is contraindicated in clients who have medication hypersensitivity, and for women who are breastfeeding. Qs
- This medication is Pregnancy Risk Category B.

INTERACTIONS

None significant

NURSING ADMINISTRATION

- Enfuvirtide is only administered subcutaneously. Rotate injection sites and avoid previous skin reaction areas. QEBP
- Bring the solution to room temperature before injection.
- Monitor for bacterial pneumonia.
- Monitor for systemic hypersensitivity reaction.
- Teach the client to take exactly as prescribed to minimize development of resistance.
- Advise the client to notify the provider if pregnancy is suspected.

NURSING EVALUATION OF MEDICATION EFFECTIVENESS

Depending on therapeutic intent, effectiveness is evidenced by a reduction of manifestations and the client being free of opportunistic infection.

Antiretrovirals: CCR5 antagonists

SELECT PROTOTYPE MEDICATION: Maraviroc (oral)

PURPOSE

EXPECTED PHARMACOLOGICAL ACTION: Prevents HIV from entering lymphocytes by binding to CCR5 on cell membranes

THERAPEUTIC USE: Treats HIV infection in conjunction with other antiretroviral medications

COMPLICATIONS

Cough and upper respiratory tract infections
NURSING CONSIDERATIONS: Teach client to report respiratory findings.

CNS effects
- Dizziness, paresthesias, orthostatic hypotension
- CLIENT EDUCATION: Advise the client to move carefully from lying or sitting to standing, and prevent injury caused by dizziness.

Hepatotoxicity
- Jaundice, right upper quadrant pain, and nausea, often preceded by allergic reaction (hives, rash)
- CLIENT EDUCATION: Advise the client to stop maraviroc and notify provider for these findings.

Pseudomembranous colitis
NURSING CONSIDERATIONS: Monitor for and report diarrhea and bloody stools.

CONTRAINDICATIONS/PRECAUTIONS

- Contraindicated in clients who have renal impairment. Qs
- Use caution in clients who have existing cardiovascular disorders, renal or liver disease, dehydration, and orthostatic hypotension.
- Use caution in clients who are breastfeeding and in older adults. Ⓒ
- Pregnancy Risk Category B

INTERACTIONS

Most protease inhibitors raise maraviroc levels.
NURSING CONSIDERATIONS: Adjust maraviroc dosage.

Rifampin, efavirenz, phenytoin, some other anticonvulsants, and St. John's wort decrease maraviroc levels.
NURSING CONSIDERATIONS: Adjust maraviroc c dosage.

NURSING ADMINISTRATION

- Administer orally in conjunction with other antiretroviral medications.
- Monitor liver function tests, blood pressure, and CBC at baseline and periodically during treatment.
- Notify provider if pregnancy is suspected.
- Take at regular intervals to maintain therapeutic blood levels.

NURSING EVALUATION OF MEDICATION EFFECTIVENESS

Decrease in manifestations of HIV infection and absent of opportunistic infections

Antiretrovirals: NRTIs

SELECT PROTOTYPE MEDICATION: Zidovudine

OTHER MEDICATIONS
- Didanosine
- Stavudine
- Lamivudine
- Abacavir

COMBINATION MEDICATIONS: Fixed medication dosages in one tablet or capsule
- Abacavir, lamivudine, zidovudine
- Abacavir, lamivudine
- Lamivudine, zidovudine
- Tenofovir/emtricitabine

ROUTE OF ADMINISTRATION: Oral, IV

PURPOSE

EXPECTED PHARMACOLOGICAL ACTION: Reduces HIV symptoms by inhibiting DNA synthesis and thus viral replication

THERAPEUTIC USE: First-line antiretrovirals to treat HIV infection

COMPLICATIONS

Suppressed bone marrow
- Zidovudine can cause suppressed bone marrow, resulting in anemia, agranulocytosis (neutropenia), and thrombocytopenia.
- NURSING CONSIDERATIONS
  - Monitor CBC and platelets.
  - Teach the client to monitor for bleeding, easy bruising, sore throat, and fatigue.

Lactic acidosis
NURSING CONSIDERATIONS
- Monitor for indications of lactic acidosis, such as hyperventilation, nausea, and abdominal pain.
- Pregnancy increases the risk of lactic acidosis.

Nausea, vomiting, diarrhea
NURSING CONSIDERATIONS
- Take medication with food to reduce gastric irritation.
- Monitor fluids and electrolytes.

Hepatomegaly/fatty liver
NURSING CONSIDERATIONS: Monitor liver enzymes.

CONTRAINDICATIONS/PRECAUTIONS

- These medications are Pregnancy Risk Category C. Pregnancy increases risk for lactic acidosis, liver enlargement, and fatty liver. Qs
- These medications are contraindicated in clients who have medication hypersensitivity.
- Use with caution in clients who have liver disease and bone marrow suppression.

INTERACTIONS

Probenecid, valproic acid, and methadone can increase zidovudine.
NURSING CONSIDERATIONS: Reduce dosage. Monitor for medication toxicity.

Ganciclovir or medications that decrease bone marrow production can further suppress bone marrow.
NURSING CONSIDERATIONS: Use together with caution. Monitor blood counts, and report sore throat or fever.

Rifampin and ritonavir can reduce zidovudine levels.
NURSING CONSIDERATIONS: Adjust dosage if needed.

Phenytoin can alter both medication levels.
NURSING CONSIDERATIONS: Monitor medication levels.

NURSING ADMINISTRATION

- Monitor for bone marrow suppression. Obtain baseline CBC and platelets at the start of therapy, and monitor periodically as needed. QEBP
- Treat anemia with epoetin alfa or transfusions.
- Treat neutropenia with colony-stimulating factors.
- Teach client to take exactly as prescribed to minimize development of medication resistance.
- Notify provider if pregnancy is suspected.

NURSING EVALUATION OF MEDICATION EFFECTIVENESS

Depending on therapeutic intent, effectiveness is evidenced by a reduction of manifestations and absent of opportunistic infection.

Antiretrovirals: NNRTIs

SELECT PROTOTYPE MEDICATIONS
- Delavirdine
- Efavirenz

OTHER MEDICATIONS
- Nevirapine
- Etravirine

ROUTE OF ADMINISTRATION: Oral

PURPOSE

EXPECTED PHARMACOLOGICAL ACTION: NNRTIs act directly on reverse transcriptase to stop HIV replication.

THERAPEUTIC USES
- Primary HIV-1 infection
- Often used in combination with other antiretroviral agents to prevent medication resistance

COMPLICATIONS

Rash
- Can become serious and lead to Stevens–Johnson syndrome
- NURSING CONSIDERATIONS
  - Monitor for rash. Treat with diphenhydramine if prescribed.
  - Notify the provider for fever or blistering.

Flu-like symptoms, headache, fatigue
NURSING CONSIDERATIONS
- Monitor for adverse reactions.
- Encourage rest and adequate oral fluid intake.

CNS manifestations
- Dizziness, drowsiness, insomnia, nightmares (especially with efavirenz)
- NURSING CONSIDERATIONS
  - Advise client that these findings should decrease after first few weeks of therapy.
  - Client should not perform activities that require alertness until effects are known.

Nausea, diarrhea
NURSING CONSIDERATIONS: Take at night on an empty stomach.

CONTRAINDICATIONS/PRECAUTIONS

- Efavirenz is Pregnancy Risk Category D, including the first trimester. Delavirdine is Pregnancy Risk Category C. Qs
- These medications are contraindicated in clients who have medication hypersensitivity or severe liver disease.
- Use with caution in clients who have liver or renal disease.

INTERACTIONS

Antacids can decrease absorption of delavirdine.
NURSING CONSIDERATIONS: Allow 1 hr between medications.

NNRTIs can increase effects of benzodiazepines, antihistamines, calcium channel blockers, ergot alkaloids, quinidine, warfarin, and others.
NURSING CONSIDERATIONS: Monitor for medication toxicity.

Rifampin and phenytoin can cause decreased levels of delavirdine.
NURSING CONSIDERATIONS: Do not use together.

Didanosine can reduce absorption of both medications.
NURSING CONSIDERATIONS: Allow 1 hr between medications.

NNRTIs can cause increase in sildenafil level.
NURSING CONSIDERATIONS: Monitor for hypotension and changes in vision. Use together with caution.

Efavirenz and delavirdine can decrease the effects of hormonal contraceptives.
NURSING CONSIDERATIONS: Advise clients to use a barrier form of contraception, such as condoms, in addition to a hormonal contraceptive.

NURSING ADMINISTRATION

- Advise the client to take exactly as prescribed and to not skip doses to minimize development of resistance. Q EBP
- Monitor for rash.
- Efavirenz may be given with a high-fat meal to increase absorption.
- Advise the client to take NNRTIs exactly as prescribed to minimize medication resistance.
- Advise clients to use a barrier form of contraception, such as condoms, in addition to a hormonal contraceptive.

NURSING EVALUATION OF MEDICATION EFFECTIVENESS

Depending on therapeutic intent, effectiveness is evidenced by a reduction of manifestations and absent of opportunistic infection.

Antiretrovirals: Protease inhibitors

SELECT PROTOTYPE MEDICATION: Ritonavir

OTHER MEDICATIONS
- Saquinavir
- Indinavir
- Fosamprenavir
- Nelfinavir
- Lopinavir/ritonavir combination

ROUTE OF ADMINISTRATION: Oral

PURPOSE

EXPECTED PHARMACOLOGICAL ACTION: Protease inhibitors act against HIV-1 and HIV-2 to alter and inactivate the virus by inhibiting enzymes needed for HIV replication.

THERAPEUTIC USES
- Used to treat HIV infections.
- Usually combined with one or two reverse transcriptase inhibitor.
- Ritonavir is usually given with other PIs to increase their effect.

COMPLICATIONS

Bone loss/osteoporosis
NURSING CONSIDERATIONS
- Advise the client to eat a diet high in calcium and vitamin D.
- Severe bone loss is treated with medications such as raloxifene and alendronate.

Diabetes mellitus/hyperglycemia
NURSING CONSIDERATIONS
- Monitor serum glucose. Adjust diet and administer antidiabetic medications as prescribed.
- Advise clients to monitor for increased thirst and urine output.

Hypersensitivity reaction
NURSING CONSIDERATIONS: Monitor for rash. Notify the provider if rash develops.

Nausea and vomiting
CLIENT EDUCATION: Tell the client to take medication with food to reduce GI effects and increase absorption.

Elevated serum lipids
NURSING CONSIDERATIONS: Monitor for hyperlipidemia. Adjust diet.

Altered fat distribution
CLIENT EDUCATION: Warn clients of these effects.

Rhabdomyolysis
NURSING CONSIDERATIONS: Monitor and report muscle pain and weakness.

CONTRAINDICATIONS/PRECAUTIONS

- Protease inhibitors are Pregnancy Risk Category B or C. Qs
- Use with caution in clients who have liver disease, pancreatitis, diabetes mellitus, AV block, and hypercholesterolemia.
- Contraindicated with many other medications. Advise the client to notify the provider before taking any new medications.

INTERACTIONS

All protease inhibitors (especially ritonavir) cause multiple medications (e.g., quinidine) to raise to toxic levels.
NURSING CONSIDERATIONS: Check any new medication with the list of medications that must be avoided in clients taking protease inhibitors.

Ritonavir can increase medication levels of sildenafil, tadalafil, and vardenafil.
NURSING CONSIDERATIONS: Use with caution. Reduce dosages as needed.

Ritonavir decreases levels of ethynyl estradiol in oral contraceptives.
NURSING CONSIDERATIONS: Instruct clients to use an alternative form of birth control.

Phenobarbital, phenytoin, carbamazepine, and St. John's wort all significantly reduce level of protease inhibitors.
NURSING CONSIDERATIONS: Avoid concurrent use, or adjust dosages.

Grapefruit juice can decrease metabolism of PIs.
NURSING CONSIDERATIONS: Advise the client to avoid grapefruit juice.

NURSING ADMINISTRATION

- Instruct clients to report all other medications, including over-the-counter and herbal medications, to the provider.
- Except for indinavir, take protease inhibitors with food to increase absorption.
- Administer with another antiretroviral to reduce the risk of medication resistance.
- Advise clients to use a barrier form of contraception, such as condoms, in addition to a hormonal contraceptive.

NURSING EVALUATION OF MEDICATION EFFECTIVENESS

Depending on therapeutic intent, effectiveness can be evidenced reduction of HIV manifestations and freedom from opportunistic infections.

Antiretrovirals: Integrase inhibitors (INSTIs)

SELECT PROTOTYPE MEDICATION: Raltegravir (oral)

PURPOSE

EXPECTED PHARMACOLOGICAL ACTION: Interferes with the enzyme integrase to prevent HIV replication within the cell

THERAPEUTIC USE: A first-line treatment for HIV when combined with two or three other antiretroviral medications

COMPLICATIONS

Headache and difficulty sleeping
NURSING CONSIDERATIONS: Advise the client to notify the provider if these findings occur.

Skin rash
- Can indicate Stevens-Johnson syndrome or other serious disorder, such as allergy
- NURSING CONSIDERATIONS: Notify the provider if a rash or other skin manifestations occur.

Liver injury
- Anorexia, nausea, right upper quadrant pain, jaundice
- NURSING CONSIDERATIONS
  ○ Monitor liver function tests.
  ○ Notify the provider for signs of liver injury.

Renal failure, hematuria
NURSING CONSIDERATIONS: Monitor for hematuria.

Suicidal ideation
NURSING CONSIDERATIONS: Notify the provider of suicidal thoughts.

CONTRAINDICATIONS/PRECAUTIONS

- Contraindicated during lactation. Qs
- Pregnancy Risk Category C.
- Use cautiously in clients younger than 16 years, older adult clients, or clients who have existing liver disorders.

INTERACTIONS

Raltegravir can be decreased with concurrent use of rifampin or tipranavir/ritonavir.
NURSING CONSIDERATIONS: Increase raltegravir dosage if needed.

NURSING ADMINISTRATION

- Take raltegravir with or without food.
- Monitor baseline and periodic liver function tests and CBC.
- Teach the client to take the medication exactly as prescribed without skipping doses to prevent medication resistance.
- Notify the provider if pregnancy is suspected.

NURSING EVALUATION OF MEDICATION EFFECTIVENESS

Depending on therapeutic intent, effectiveness is evidenced by reduction of HIV manifestations and absence of opportunistic infections.

Application Exercises

1. A nurse is teaching a client who has a new prescription for combination oral NRTIs (abacavir, lamivudine, and zidovudine) for treatment of HIV. Which of the following statements should the nurse include?

   A. "These medications work by blocking HIV entry into cells."

   B. "These medications work by weakening the cell wall of the HIV virus."

   C. "These medications work by inhibiting enzymes to prevent HIV replication."

   D. "These medications work by preventing protein synthesis within the HIV cell."

2. A nurse is caring for a client who takes several antiretroviral medications, including the NRTI zidovudine, to treat HIV infection. The nurse should monitor for which of the following adverse effects of zidovudine? (Select all that apply.)

   A. Fatigue

   B. Blurred vision

   C. Ataxia

   D. Hyperventilation

   E. Vomiting

3. A nurse is caring for a client who is taking ritonavir, a protease inhibitor, to treat HIV infection. The nurse should monitor for which of the following adverse effects of this medication?

   A. Increased TSH level

   B. Decreased ALT level

   C. Hypoglycemia

   D. Hyperlipidemia

4. A nurse is caring for a client who has a new prescription for enfuvirtide to treat HIV infection. The nurse should monitor the client for which of the adverse reactions of this medication? (Select all that apply.)

   A. Bleeding

   B. Pneumonia

   C. Cerebral edema

   D. Localized erythema

   E. Hypotension

5. A nurse is administering IV acyclovir to a client who has varicella. Which of the following actions should the nurse take?

   A. Administer a stool softener.

   B. Decrease fluid intake following infusion.

   C. Infuse acyclovir over 1 hr.

   D. Monitor for a for hypotension

6. A nurse is teaching a client who is beginning highly active antiretroviral therapy (HAART) for HIV infection about ways to prevent medication resistance. Which of the following information should the nurse teach the client about resistance?

   A. Taking low dosages of antiretroviral medication minimizes resistance.

   B. Taking one antiretroviral medication at a time minimizes resistance.

   C. Taking medication at the same times daily without missing doses minimizes resistance.

   D. Changing the medication regimen when adverse effects occur minimizes resistance.

Application Exercises Key

1. A. The fusion/entry inhibitor enfuvirtide and the CCR5 antagonist maraviroc are newer antiretroviral medications that work by blocking HIV entry into cells.

    B. Some bactericidal antibiotics, such as penicillin, work by weakening the cell walls of bacteria.

    C. **CORRECT:** The NRTI antiretroviral medications this client takes work by inhibiting the enzyme reverse transcriptase and preventing HIV replication.

    D. Some antibiotics, such as aminoglycosides, kill bacteria by preventing protein synthesis within the cell.

    Ⓝ NCLEX® Connection: Pharmacological and Parenteral Therapies, Medication Administration

2. A. **CORRECT:** Fatigue is a manifestation of anemia, an adverse effect of zidovudine. Neutropenia can also occur, causing a high risk for infection.

    B. Zidovudine can cause hearing loss and photophobia.

    C. Zidovudine can cause vertigo.

    D. **CORRECT:** Hyperventilation is a finding that can occur if the client develops lactic acidosis, a serious adverse effect of zidovudine.

    E. **CORRECT:** Vomiting and other GI effects are adverse effects of zidovudine.

    Ⓝ NCLEX® Connection: Pharmacological and Parenteral Therapies, Adverse Effects/Contraindications/Side Effects/Interactions

3. A. Increased TSH and T4 levels indicate hyperthyroidism, which is not an adverse effect of ritonavir.

    B. An increase in liver function tests, including AST and ALT levels, can occur as an adverse effect of ritonavir.

    C. Hyperglycemia indicating a possible onset or worsening of diabetes mellitus can occur as an adverse effect of ritonavir.

    D. **CORRECT:** Hyperlipidemia with increased cholesterol and triglyceride levels can occur as an adverse effect of ritonavir.

    Ⓝ NCLEX® Connection: Pharmacological and Parenteral Therapies, Expected Actions/Outcomes

4. A. Bleeding is not an adverse effect of enfuvirtide.

    B. **CORRECT:** Bacterial pneumonia with fever, cough, and difficulty breathing are manifestations of an adverse reaction to enfuvirtide. The nurse should assess breath sounds regularly.

    C. Cerebral edema is not an adverse reaction to enfuvirtide.

    D. **CORRECT:** Enfuvirtide is administered subcutaneously. Injection-site reactions, such as pain, redness, itching, and bruising, are common.

    E. **CORRECT:** A systemic allergic reaction can occur when taking enfuvirtide. Manifestations of hypersensitivity include rash, hypotension, fever, and chills.

    Ⓝ NCLEX® Connection: Pharmacological and Parenteral Therapies, Adverse Effects/Contraindications/Side Effects/Interactions

5. A. Acyclovir can cause diarrhea.

    B. The nurse should increase fluids during and for 2 hr following acyclovir infusion to prevent nephrotoxicity.

    C. **CORRECT:** The nurse should administer IV acyclovir slowly, over at least 1 hr, to prevent nephrotoxicity.

    D. Acyclovir can cause thrombocytopenia in clients who are immunocompromised.

    Ⓝ NCLEX® Connection: Pharmacological and Parenteral Therapies, Medication Administration

6. A. Taking low dosages of the medication can cause medication resistance.

    B. Taking a combination of antiretroviral medications helps prevent resistance to each medication. Resistance occurs quickly if only one medication is taken.

    C. **CORRECT:** The nurse should emphasize the importance of taking each dose of medication exactly as prescribed. Missing even a few doses of antiretroviral medication can promote medication resistance, which can cause treatment failure.

    D. Changing the medication regimen when adverse effects occur can promote medication resistance.

    Ⓝ NCLEX® Connection: Pharmacological and Parenteral Therapies, Medication Administration

PRACTICE Active Learning Scenario

A nurse is caring for a client who is immunocompromised and has a new prescription for ganciclovir IV twice per day to prevent cytomegalovirus. What should the nurse teach the client about this medication? Use the ATI Active Learning Template: Medication to complete this item.

THERAPEUTIC USES: Identify for ganciclovir in this client.

COMPLICATIONS: Identify two adverse effects.

NURSING INTERVENTIONS: Describe two for clients taking ganciclovir, and two tests the nurse should monitor.

PRACTICE Answer

Using the ATI Active Learning Template: Medication

THERAPEUTIC USES: Ganciclovir prevents reproduction of viral DNA and thus prevents viral cell replication. It is used is to prevent or treat cytomegalovirus in clients who are immunocompromised.

COMPLICATIONS

- Minor discomforts, such as fever, headache, and nausea
- Suppresses the bone marrow, causing a decrease in WBCs, especially granulocytes
- Causes thrombocytopenia frequently
- The client should report any discomforts and be sure to report new onset of fatigue, easy bruising, or sore throat.
- Advise the client to report manifestations of infection or bleeding, and to avoid crowds or individuals who have respiratory infections.

NURSING INTERVENTIONS

- Monitor client blood counts, especially WBC, absolute neutrophil count, and thrombocyte count. The nurse should expect ganciclovir therapy to be interrupted for an absolute neutrophil count less than 500/mm³ or a thrombocyte count less than 25,000/mm³.
- Monitor blood counts.
- Prepare to administer granulocyte colony-stimulating factors for a low absolute neutrophil count.
- Monitor I&O, and encourage the client to increase fluid intake.
- Avoid direct contact with the powder from oral ganciclovir or the IV solution, and wash well if contact occurs.
- Advise clients to use a barrier contraception, such as condoms, during treatment and for 3 months following treatment.

Ⓝ NCLEX® Connection: Pharmacological and Parenteral Therapies, Medication Administration

References

Berman, A., Snyder, S., & Frandsen, G. (2016). *Kozier & Erb's fundamentals of nursing: Concepts, process, and practice* (10th ed.). Upper Saddle River, NJ: Prentice-Hall.

Burchum, J. R., & Rosenthal, L. D. (2016). *Lehne's pharmacology for nursing care* (9th ed.). St. Louis: Elsevier.

Dudek, S. G. (2014). *Nutrition essentials for nursing practice* (7th ed.). Philadelphia: Lippincott Williams & Wilkins.

Eliopoulos, C. (2014). *Gerontological nursing* (8th ed.). Philadelphia: Lippincott Williams & Wilkins.

Grodner, M., Escott-Stump, S., & Dorner, S. (2016). *Nutritional foundations and clinical applications of nutrition: A nursing approach* (6th ed.). St. Louis, MO: Mosby.

Halter, M. J. (2014). *Varcarolis' foundations of psychiatric mental health nursing: A clinical approach* (7th ed.). St. Louis, MO: Saunders.

Hinkle, J. L., & Cheever, K. H. (2014). Brunner and *Suddarth's textbook of medical-surgical nursing* (13th ed.). Philadelphia: Lippincott Williams & Wilkins.

Hockenberry, M.J., & Wilson, D. (2015) *Wong's nursing care of infants and children* (10th ed.). St. Louis, MO: Mosby.

Ignatavicius, D. D., & Workman, M. L. (2016). *Medical-surgical nursing* (8th ed.). St. Louis, MO: Elsevier.

Lilley, L. L., Rainforth-Collins, S., & Snyder, J. S. (2014). *Pharmacology and the nursing process* (7th Ed.). St. Louis, MO: Mosby.

Lowdermilk, D. L., Perry, S. E., Cashion, M.C., & Aldean, K.R. (2016). *Maternity & women's health care* (11th ed.). St. Louis, MO: Elsevier.

Pagana, K. D. & Pagana, T. J. (2014). *Mosby's manual of diagnostic and laboratory tests* (5th ed.). St. Louis, MO: Elsevier.

Potter, P. A., Perry, A. G., Stockert, P., & Hall, A. (2013). *Fundamentals of nursing* (8th ed.). St. Louis, MO: Mosby.

Skidmore-Roth, L. (2016). *Mosby's 2016 nursing drug reference* (29th ed.). St. Louis, MO: Elsevier.

Taketomo, C. K., Hodding, J. H., & Kraus D. M. (2014). *Lexi-Comp's pediatric & neonatal dosage handbook: A comprehensive resource for all clinicians treating pediatric and neonatal patients (pediatric dosage handbook)* (21st ed.). Hudson, Ohio: Lexi-Comp.

Touhy, T. A., & Jett, K. F. (2012) *Ebersole & Hess' toward healthy aging: Human needs and nursing response* (8th ed.). St. Lois, MO: Mosby.

Townsend, M. C. (2014). *Essentials of psychiatric mental health nursing: Concepts of care in evidence-based practice* (6th ed.). Philadelphia: F. A. Davis.

STUDENT NAME _____

CONCEPT_____ REVIEW MODULE CHAPTER_____

Related Content

(E.G., DELEGATION, LEVELS OF PREVENTION, ADVANCE DIRECTIVES)

Underlying Principles

Nursing Interventions

WHO? WHEN? WHY? HOW?

STUDENT NAME _____

PROCEDURE NAME _____ REVIEW MODULE CHAPTER_____

Description of Procedure

Indications

Interpretation of Findings

Potential Complications

CONSIDERATIONS

Nursing Interventions (pre, intra, post)

Client Education

Nursing Interventions

STUDENT NAME _____

DEVELOPMENTAL STAGE _____ REVIEW MODULE CHAPTER_____

EXPECTED GROWTH AND DEVELOPMENT

Physical Development	Cognitive Development	Psychosocial Development	Age-Appropriate Activities

Health Promotion

Immunizations	Health Screening	Nutrition	Injury Prevention

Medication

STUDENT NAME _____

MEDICATION _____   REVIEW MODULE CHAPTER_____

CATEGORY CLASS_____

PURPOSE OF MEDICATION

Expected Pharmacological Action

Therapeutic Use

Complications

Medication Administration

Contraindications/Precautions

Nursing Interventions

Interactions

Client Education

Evaluation of Medication Effectiveness

ACTIVE LEARNING TEMPLATE: *Nursing Skill*

STUDENT NAME _____

SKILL NAME_____ REVIEW MODULE CHAPTER_____

Description of Skill

Indications

CONSIDERATIONS

Nursing Interventions (pre, intra, post)

Outcomes/Evaluation

Client Education

Potential Complications

Nursing Interventions

System Disorder

STUDENT NAME _____

DISORDER/DISEASE PROCESS _____ REVIEW MODULE CHAPTER_____

Alterations in Health (Diagnosis)

Pathophysiology Related to Client Problem

Health Promotion and Disease Prevention

ASSESSMENT

Risk Factors

Expected Findings

Laboratory Tests

Diagnostic Procedures

SAFETY CONSIDERATIONS

PATIENT-CENTERED CARE

Nursing Care

Medications

Client Education

Therapeutic Procedures

Interprofessional Care

Complications

STUDENT NAME _____

PROCEDURE NAME _____   REVIEW MODULE CHAPTER_____

Description of Procedure

Indications

Outcomes/Evaluation

Potential Complications

CONSIDERATIONS

Nursing Interventions (pre, intra, post)

Client Education

Nursing Interventions